BIOLOGY
of Women

FIFTH EDITION

BIOLOGY
of Women

FIFTH EDITION

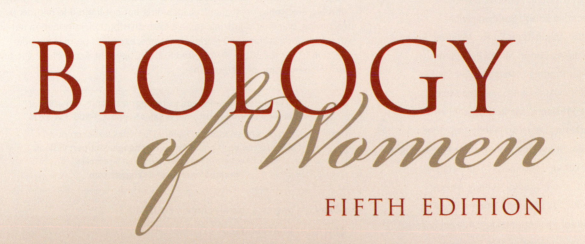

THERESA M. HORNSTEIN

Lake Superior College
Duluth, MN

JERI LYNN SCHWERIN

Lake Superior College
Duluth, MN

Revised from the original text by Ethel Sloane

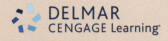

DELMAR
CENGAGE Learning·

Australia • Brazil • Japan • Korea • Mexico • Singapore • Spain • United Kingdom • United States

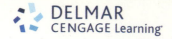

Biology of Women, 5th Edition
Theresa M. Hornstein, Jeri Schwerin

Vice President, Editorial: Dave Garza

Executive Editor: Stephen Helba

Senior Acquisitions Editor: Maureen Rosener

Managing Editor: Marah Bellegarde

Senior Product Manager: Juliet Steiner

Editorial Assistant: Samantha Miller

Vice President, Marketing: Jennifer Baker

Marketing Director: Wendy Mapstone

Senior Marketing Manager: Michele McTighe

Marketing Coordinator: Scott Chrysler

Production Director: Wendy Troeger

Production Manager: Andrew Crouth

Content Project Manager: Allyson Bozeth

Senior Art Director: Jack Pendleton

For product information and technology assistance, contact us at
Cengage Learning Customer & Sales Support, 1-800-354-9706

For permission to use material from this text or product,
submit all requests online at **www.cengage.com/permissions.**
Further permissions questions can be e-mailed to
permissionrequest@cengage.com

Library of Congress Control Number: 2011934073

ISBN-13: 978-1-4354-0033-7

ISBN-10: 1-4354-0033-X

Delmar
5 Maxwell Drive
Clifton Park, NY 12065-2919
USA

Cengage Learning is a leading provider of customized learning solutions with office locations around the globe, including Singapore, the United Kingdom, Australia, Mexico, Brazil, and Japan. Locate your local office at: **international.cengage.com/region**

Cengage Learning products are represented in Canada by Nelson Education, Ltd.

To learn more about Delmar, visit **www.cengage.com/delmar**

Purchase any of our products at your local college store or at our preferred online store **www.cengagebrain.com**

Notice to the Reader
Publisher does not warrant or guarantee any of the products described herein or perform any independent analysis in connection with any of the product information contained herein. Publisher does not assume, and expressly disclaims, any obligation to obtain and include information other than that provided to it by the manufacturer. The reader is expressly warned to consider and adopt all safety precautions that might be indicated by the activities described herein and to avoid all potential hazards. By following the instructions contained herein, the reader willingly assumes all risks in connection with such instructions. The publisher makes no representations or warranties of any kind, including but not limited to, the warranties of fitness for particular purpose or merchantability, nor are any such representations implied with respect to the material set forth herein, and the publisher takes no responsibility with respect to such material. The publisher shall not be liable for any special, consequential, or exemplary damages resulting, in whole or part, from the readers' use of, or reliance upon, this material.

Printed in the United States of America
1 2 3 4 5 6 7 14 13

Dedication

I would like to dedicate this book to my children—Kasha, Nikoli and Elyse—who believed I could do this; my parents, Barb and Hugh; and my sister, Anita. T.H.

I would like to dedicate this book to my family—parents, Frank and Joanne and siblings, Paul, Carolyn, and Jay; my friend, Paul Chang; and my academic advisors, Dr. Francesca J. Cuthbert and Dr. Alan C. Kamil. J.S.

CONTENTS

Chapter 4   THE REPRODUCTIVE CYCLE   77

Chapter 5   MENSTRUAL PROBLEMS: CAUSES AND TREATMENTS · 97

Chapter 6   REPRODUCTIVE TRACT INFECTIONS   118

Chapter 7   BREAST HEALTH   143

PREFACE

Ten years have passed since the publication of the fourth edition of *Biology of Women*. Significant developments in scientific research during that time have changed current understanding of many aspects of women's biology and its implications for women's health. Some highlights include:

- The Women's Health Initiative published surprising findings linking hormone replacement therapy (HRT) to breast cancer, stroke, and heart disease in women.
- A new vaccine has been developed to protect women from the human papilloma virus (HPV); a virus that has been linked to both cervical cancer and genital warts.
- New methods of birth control have become available.

Each chapter of the fifth edition presents updated information that reflects current scientific research. This edition has been significantly expanded and re-organized to make the content more accessible to readers, and new features have been added to address a broader range of cultural and social factors in women's experience.

This book balances the needs of students who are science majors with those of students who do not have a strong scientific background. It is accessible to entry levels students, but offers enough detail and critical thinking opportunities to challenge students who already have some understanding of human anatomy and physiology. In addition, this book can serve as a useful reference for any woman throughout her lifetime.

CONCEPTUAL APPROACH

While anatomy and physiology books cover the body systems, most of the early research that formed the foundation of those texts viewed women simply as a subcategory of men, identical in every way except their reproductive systems. Newer research has found that there are significant differences outside of their reproductive systems between men and women, and that these differences can affect everything from physiological functioning to social interactions. This book explores many of these differences. In addition, social and biological sciences are primarily taught as separate and unrelated disciplines. Many students in the social sciences do not have a strong background in biology, just as many biology students lack an understanding of the interplay between social, cultural, and historical factors and biology. This book brings the biological and social factors together, providing students a foundation for making informed decisions, both in their personal lives and in their chosen fields of study.

ORGANIZATION

The fifth edition is arranged into 18 chapters, most of which are focused on a specific aspect of women's biology or health. Exceptions include

Chapter One and Chapter Two, which present introductory information that provide a foundation for the subsequent chapters. Chapter One introduces students to the scientific method and outlines basic guidelines for evaluating scientific information on the Internet or in the media. Chapter Two gives a general overview of human anatomy and physiology, and serves as an introduction to the body systems.

- Chapter One: Why Biology of Women?
  This chapter provides an introduction to the book as well as an introduction to the scientific method and evaluating scientific research.
- Chapter Two: Anatomy and Physiology
  This chapter gives a general overview of human anatomy and physiology and serves as an introduction to the body systems.
- Chapter Three: Reproductive Anatomy
  The structures and functions of the organs, glands, and tissues of the male and female reproductive systems are examined with an emphasis on the female system.
- Chapter Four: Reproductive Cycle
  The menstrual cycle is examined with an emphasis on the hormones that influence and orchestrate female reproductive function.
- Chapter Five: Menstrual Problems: Causes and Treatments
  Disturbances to the menstrual cycle are explored including discussion about their origins and potential treatments.
- Chapter Six: Reproductive Tract Infections
  This chapter examines the role of the normal flora and their interplay with pathogens of the reproductive tract.
- Chapter Seven: A Woman's Breasts
  This chapter explores the anatomy of breasts, the physiology of lactation, and breast-feeding. Non-cancerous disorders of the breasts, their treatments, and methods of detecting abnormalities are also described.
- Chapter Eight: Cancer and other Diseases of the Reproductive System
  This chapter addresses a range of conditions including endometriosis, fibroids, and cancer.

- Chapter Nine: The Biology of Sex
  This chapter explores the physiology of the female response and discusses sexuality throughout the lifetime. Disorders that affect female sexual function are also addressed.
- Chapter Ten: Genetics and Fetal Development
  The genetic and developmental processes that take place during pregnancy are discussed in this chapter.
- Chapter Eleven: A Woman's Body during Pregnancy, Labor, and Delivery
  This chapter explores the physiology of a typical pregnancy, labor, and delivery.
- Chapter Twelve: Pregnancy Complications
  Conditions and complications that can arise during pregnancy and labor are outlined in this chapter. Methods for monitoring fetal development and potential interventions in case of complications are also discussed.
- Chapter Thirteen: Birth Control
  This chapter outlines birth control methods with regard to their effectiveness, advantages, and disadvantages.
- Chapter Fourteen: Infertility: Causes and Treatments
  Causes of infertility and procedures to overcome infertility are discussed in this chapter.
- Chapter Fifteen: Menopause
  This chapter focuses on menopause as a normal physiological process. Hormone replacement therapy (HRT) and alternatives to HRT are examined.
- Chapter Sixteen: Nutrition: Fuel for a Woman's Body
  This chapter examines the impact of nutrition on maintaining health. This includes the current nutritional guidelines as well as phytonutrients, antioxidants, and fatty acids.
- Chapter Seventeen: Women and Stress
  The chapter examines the physiological effects of stress on women.
- Chapter Eighteen: The Biology of Appearance
  This chapter focuses on the anatomy and physiology of the skin and hair and addresses how and why women alter their appearance.

FEATURES & NEW TO THIS EDITION:

The fifth edition has undergone significant updating, rearrangement, and revision to address the new research from the Women's Health Initiative (WHI) and other research, new options for the prevention and treatment of women's health concerns, and the recognition of other factors that affect women.

The evaluation of scientific information has been added to Chapter 1. A new anatomy and physiology chapter (Chapter 2) provides a system-by-system framework for understanding the body's biological functions and the role of homeostasis in maintaining health. This acts as a foundation for future chapters. The pregnancy chapter from the fourth edition has been divided into three chapters with Chapter 10 addressing genetics, fetal development, and sexual differentiation; Chapter 11 discussing the physiology of a typical pregnancy; and Chapter 12 addressing complications of pregnancy and medical interventions. The fourth edition combined most sexually transmitted infections and reproductive cancers into a single chapter, presented HIV in another, and information on breast cancer in a third. In the fifth edition, sexually transmitted infections, HIV, and normal flora are combined into a single chapter (Chapter 6). Gynecological pathologies and breast cancer are discussed a single chapter (Chapter 8) because of the genetic, hormonal, and treatment similarities. Information from the fourth edition's Health and the Working Woman chapter has been updated and integrated into several of the other chapters. Finally, a chapter which specifically addresses stress and its biological impacts on women has been included. Other significant new features of this edition include:

- Educational research indicates that actively engaging students improves retention and understanding of new information. To that end, critical thinking boxes, case studies, and end-of-chapter questions have been added. To further support active engagement, a separate lab manual is now available with activities that provide hands-on application of information in the text.
- New to this edition, the chapters contain a series of boxes with all new content, many of which were written by sociologists. These include:

  o **Historical Considerations boxes** designed to provide a glimpse into the past and placing the current state of women's biology in context with its historic past.
  o **Social Considerations boxes** that recognize the biological implications of social factors.
  o **Economic Considerations boxes** that address the impact of money on women, especially in regards to health.
  o **Cultural Considerations boxes** seek to broaden the students' view of the world and how culture influences women.
  o **Focus on Exercise boxes** that recognize the influence of exercise on maintaining health and preventing disease.
  o **Focus on Nutrition boxes** that examine the role of nutrition on specific topics related to women's biology.
  o **Evidence Based Practice boxes** focus on new research and current events that are shaping women's biology.
  o **Case Study boxes** provide students with the opportunity to test their understanding of concepts from the chapter by applying them to a scenario.
  o **Critical Thinking boxes** challenge students to think about specific issues related to women's biology and draw informed conclusions.
- Each chapter now concludes with a series of review questions to allow students to check their comprehension.
- The fifth edition contains new, full-color images and graphics designed to support the text.
- The chapters have been reworked and contain new content including:

1. Why Biology of Women?
   o the importance of studying women's biology
   o the importance of taking an active role and responsibility for one's own health
   o how to evaluate information presented in the media
   o an introduction to the scientific method

2. Anatomy & Physiology: An Overview of a Woman's Body
   o an entirely new chapter addressing the basics of anatomy and physiology
   o an introduction to hormone physiology
   o how the body maintains homeostasis

o differences between male and female anatomy other than the reproductive system

3. Reproductive Anatomy
   o updated with new information
   o a revised and updated section on gynecological exams
   o examines both the male and female reproductive systems and the common origins of homologous structures

4. Reproductive Cycle
   o extensively rewritten to focus on the integrated nature of reproductive hormones
   o expanded information on the role of reproductive hormones on other body systems

5. Menstrual Problems: Causes and Treatments
   o focuses on irregularities of the reproductive cycle
   o presents the latest information gleaned from scientific literature

6. Reproductive Tract Infections
   o extensively rewritten and updated
   o new focus on the role of normal flora in maintaining vaginal health
   o updated information on identification of sexually transmitted infections
   o updated information on prevention
   o explanation of expedited partner therapy

7. A Woman's Breasts
   o updated information
   o extensively rewritten and reorganized
   o increased emphasis on the biology of lactation and breast-feeding

8. Cancer and other Diseases of the Reproductive Tract
   o updated information concerning diagnosis and testing
   o focuses on the role of reproductive hormones and genes on cancers of the breasts and the reproductive tract

9. The Biology of Sex
   o updated information concerning the physiology of sex

o expanded information on the biological costs and benefits of sexual activity
o expanded and updated information on sexuality through the lifespan

10. Genetics and Fetal Development
    o explains the process of mitosis and meiosis
    o follows development from fertilization through fetal development
    o expanded information on the influences of teratogens and endocrine disruptors during embryonic development

11. A Woman's Body during Pregnancy, Labor, and Delivery
    o extensively rewritten
    o describes the physiology of normal pregnancy and delivery
    o examines delivery options including midwives and doulas

12. Pregnancy Complications
    o a new chapter which addresses the complications that can arise during pregnancy and delivery
    o examines medical interventions during pregnancy, labor, and delivery

13. Birth Control
    o completely updated
    o includes information on new options including the ring, menstrual suppression, and emergency contraceptives
    o identifies new information on the safety of contraceptives
    o contains updated information on abortion

14. Infertility: Causes and Treatments
    o extensively rewritten
    o examines newly identified causes and treatment options

15. Menopause
    o focuses on menopause as a normal physiological process
    o completely rewritten and updated with new information from WHI studies
    o provides information on alternatives to hormone replacement therapy

16. Nutrition: Fuel for a Woman's Body
    o extensively rewritten
    o new information on phytonutrients, antioxidants, and fatty acids
    o updates the information relating diet to osteoporosis and cardiovascular disease
    o updated with the latest dietary recommendations

17. Women and Stress
    o all new chapter recognizing the role stress plays on women
    o examines the physiological changes that occur with stress
    o examines the differences between the male and female stress response
    o explores methods for coping with stress

18. The Biology of Appearance
    o extensively rewritten
    o examines multiple forms of body art ranging from cosmetics to tattoos and scarring
    o examines the chemical composition of common cosmetics

ANCILLARY PACKAGE

The complete supplements package for *Biology of Women* fifth edition was developed to achieve two goals:

1. To assist the student in learning the information presented in the text.

2. To assist instructors in planning and implementing their courses for the most efficient use of time and other resources.

Student Resources

Laboratory Manual to Accompany Biology of Women

ISBN 10: 1-4354-0035-6
ISBN 13: 978-1-4354-0035-1

A valuable companion to the core book, this student resource provides 17 lab exercises that coordinate with and reinforce the text. Covering topics ranging from lab safety and the scientific method, to skeletal system differences between women and men, and a sexually transmitted infections lab, this resource provides everything needed for a successful lab experience. Objectives and materials are outlined, followed by explanation and activities for students to participate in, and concluding with laboratory report questions including multiple choice, matching, and long answer response questions.

Instructor Resources

Instructor's Resource to Accompany Biology of Women

ISBN 10: 1-4354-0034-8
ISBN 13: 978-1-4354-0034-4

The Instructor's Resource CD-ROM has four robust components to assist the instructor and enhance classroom activities and discussion.

Instructor's Manual

An electronic Instructor's Manual provides excellent tools to help the instructor create a dynamic and engaging learning experience for the student. The Instructor's Manual contains the tools listed here but can be downloaded and modified to meet individual instructional goals.

- Teaching Tips & Strategies: This section provides engaging ideas and tips for the instructor to use in conjunction with the chapter topics.
- Discussion Topics: These excellent and provocative discussion topics can be used to challenge critical thinking and to create an interactive classroom experience.
- Assignments and Activities: These additional ready-to-use activities and assignments provide more opportunities to challenge students and assess their understanding of chapter concepts.
- Additional Resources: With more great resources to help deliver lectures, additional resources include weblinks as well as topic specific additional sources such as journals, books, and organizations.
- Answers to Case Studies and End-of-Chapter Questions: Answers and intended outcomes for chapter case studies and review questions are provided to assist the instructor in grading and evaluation.

- Answers to the *Laboratory Manual to Accompany Biology of Women:* To help instructors make the most of their time, answers and rationales for the student labs are provided.

Computerized Testbank in Exam View™

- Includes a rich bank of over 700 multiple choice, matching, and fill-in-the-blank questions that test students on retention and application of material in the text.
- Answers are provided for all questions, letting instructors focus on teaching, not grading.
- Allows instructors to create custom tests by mixing questions from each of the 18 chapters of questions, modifying existing questions, and even adding additional questions to meet individual instructional needs.

Instructor Slides Created in PowerPoint

- A comprehensive offering of over 500 instructor slides created in PowerPoint outlines concepts from the text to assist the instructor with lectures is included.
- Ideas are presented to stimulate discussion and critical thinking.

Image Library

- Over 160 photos and figures from the text are provided in a searchable database, allowing instructors to incorporate visual support in their lectures, assignments and exams.

AVENUE FOR FEEDBACK

For comments, questions, or suggestions, please feel free to contact:

Theresa Hornstein t.hornstein@lsc.edu
Jeri Schwerin j.schwerin@lsc.edu

ABOUT THE AUTHORS

Theresa Hornstein earned an AS from Muskegon Community College, a BS from Michigan Technological University, and an MS from the University of Wisconsin, Superior. After several years working in labs and field research positions, she moved into teaching both online and in a traditional classroom in the biology department at Lake Superior College in Duluth, MN. Courses she has taught include cell biology, microbiology, general biology, botany, science skills, pathophysiology, anatomy and physiology, student research, and biology of women. In addition, she has taught a number of workshops for GirlTech, a local program designed to get 10-14 year old girls interested in science. She has been awarded four Awards for Excellence grants through the Minnesota State Colleges and Universities, as well as serving on the state wide Task Force for Thinking Assessments and as Center for Teaching and Learning coordinator at Lake Superior College. In 1992, the Minnesota State Board for Community Colleges named her an Outstanding Faculty Member. Her research interests include vermicomposting projects on campus, comparisons of online and on ground student success, applications of the FIRE critical thinking model, edible landscaping, and natural dye projects. She has presented at both regional and national conferences including Fusion2010, I-Teach, the National Science Teachers Association, NISOD, and Women's Lives, Women's Voices, Women's Solutions: Shaping a National Agenda for Women in Higher Education.

Jeri Schwerin earned a B.S. in biology at the University of Minnesota, Duluth; and an M.S. in biology from the University of Massachusetts, Amherst. As a graduate student, she served as a National Science Foundation Teaching Fellow at Hampshire College in Hadley, Massachusetts, and as a program coordinator at the Sigurd Olson Environmental Institute at Northland College in Ashland, Wisconsin. She currently holds a position as a biology instructor at Lake Superior College in Duluth, Minnesota, where she teaches anatomy and physiology, biology and society, and biology of women. In addition to teaching, she serves on the college's Academic Affairs and Standards Council and on the Environmental Council. She has been awarded seven Awards for Excellence by the office of the Chancellor of the Minnesota State Colleges and Universities. In addition to teaching, she currently provides public outreach education with the Lake Superior Research Institute of the University of Wisconsin, Superior onboard their research vessel, the LL Smith Jr.

ACKNOWLEDGEMENTS

We would like to thank all those without whose help and support, this book would not exist:

Our family and friends who have supported us through many long nights and missed holidays. Our students who brought us ideas to expand the book and acted as a sounding board during its writing. Your suggestions have been invaluable. Our colleagues at Lake Superior College who gave us encouragement. Particularly, Marlise Riffel and Mayra Gomez from Lake Superior College, who contributed many of the social, economic, and cultural boxes and provided a sociological perspective to complement our biological ones. Our reviewers who made valuable comments and suggestions that greatly improved our early drafts. Dan Kodatsky who asked the question, "Would you consider writing?" Maureen Rosener who looked at our first proposal and liked it enough to take a chance on us. And, finally, Juliet Steiner, our editor, who played midwife to this project. Your encouragement kept us going. T.H. & J.S.

FOREWORD TO THE FOURTH EDITION OF BIOLOGY OF WOMEN

During the final preparation of the fourth edition of *Biology of Women,* Ethel Sloane died of an illness she had lived with and fought for many years. In the last months of her life, she was working diligently at her computer to update this book. When that no longer was easy for her, a group of extraordinary colleagues from the University of Wisconsin-Milwaukee stepped in to help her, making contributions to several chapters to ensure that the information covered was accurate and up to date. This edition of *Biology of Women* could not have been completed without the expert assistance and great generosity of the following people at the University of Wisconsin-Milwaukee: Rene Gratz, professor, Department of Health Sciences; Donna Van Wynsberghe, professor, Department of Biological Sciences; Ruth E. Williams, assistant vice chancellor; Leslie Schulz, professor, Clinical Laboratory Sciences program; and Reinhold Hutz, professor, Department of Biological Sciences. Later, after Ethel Sloane's death, Rene Gratz, Donna Van Wynsberghe, and Ruth E. Williams put in hours of work to make sure the manuscript was complete and prepared exactly as Ethel would have wished it to be. Cathy Esperti, executive editor at Delmar Cengage Learning, was committed to making sure this edition would be published without a hitch, and marshaled all the resources at her disposal to bring it to print.

After her death, a generation of Ethel Sloane's students wrote or spoke to us, members of her family, to describe the powerful impact this book and the course it was written for had on their development as healthcare professionals or as healthcare consumers. All of them described the feeling of empowerment it gave them, a consequence of learning how to better understand their bodies in sickness and in health, and how to better communicate with healthcare providers. Many of them shared stories of how that knowledge changed their lives or helped them bring about change in the lives of their mothers, sisters, or daughters.

Ethel's friends, family, colleagues, and editor wanted to ensure that the fourth edition of this book would be available to yet another group of students, instructors, and readers. It is a testimony to Ethel that *Biology of Women* continues to enrich people's lives.

The family of Ethel Sloane

HOW TO USE THIS TEXT

This text is designed with you, the reader, in mind. Special elements and boxes appear throughout the text to guide you in reading and to assist you in learning the material. Following are suggestions for how you can use these features to increase your understanding and mastery of the content.

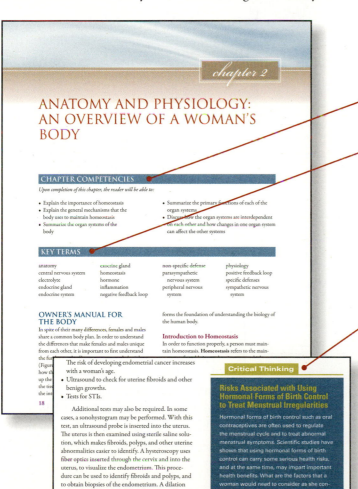

CHAPTER COMPETENCIES AND KEY TERMS

Competencies list the core concepts you should master after reading and studying each chapter. These are a good way to introduce the chapter content and are a great review tool. Key Terms introduce you to the terminology covered in the text, and accompanying definitions can be found in the end of book glossary.

CRITICAL THINKING

Read the information in these boxes and consider the questions. Use your critical thinking skills to answer these complex questions.

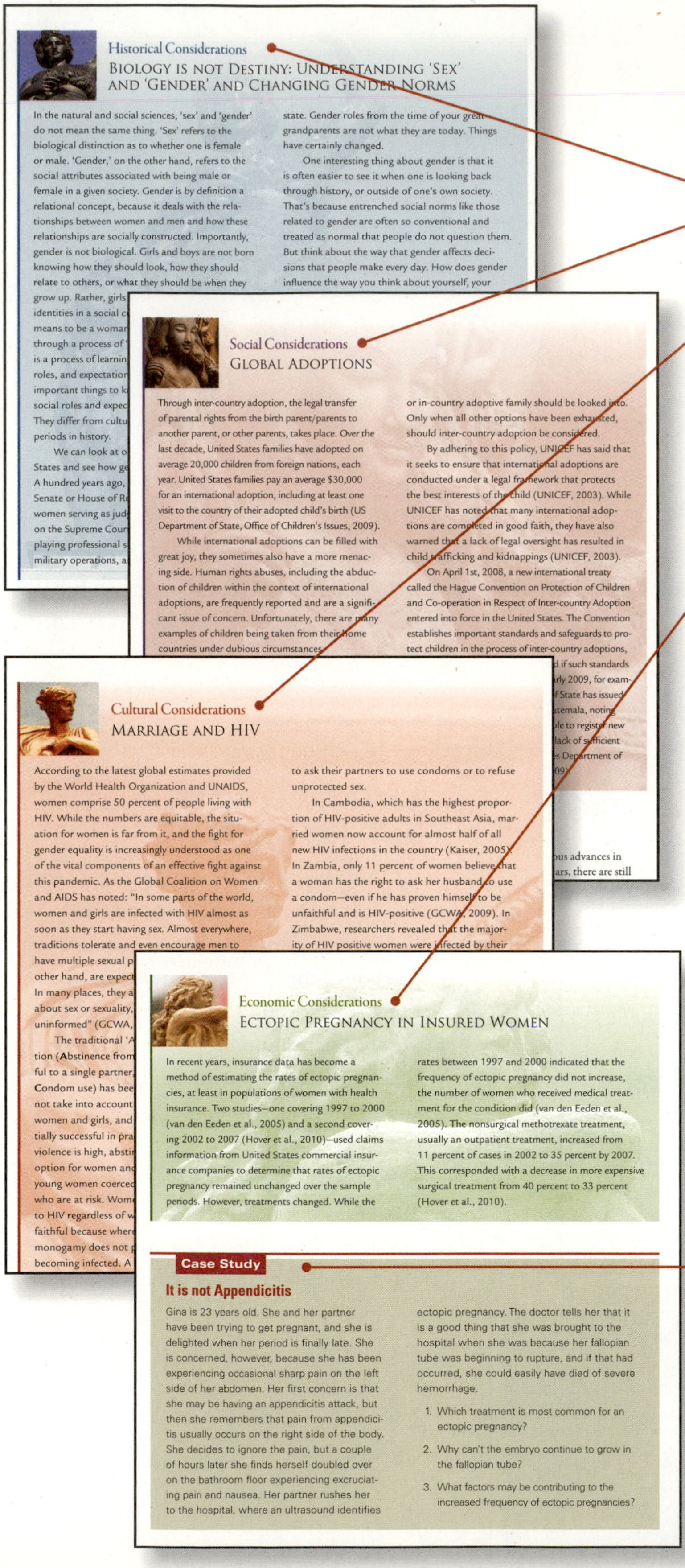

Historical Considerations
BIOLOGY IS NOT DESTINY: UNDERSTANDING 'SEX' AND 'GENDER' AND CHANGING GENDER NORMS

In the natural and social sciences, 'sex' and 'gender' do not mean the same thing. 'Sex' refers to the biological distinction as to whether one is female or male. 'Gender,' on the other hand, refers to the social attributes associated with being male or female in a given society. Gender is by definition a relational concept, because it deals with the relationships between women and men and how these relationships are socially constructed. Importantly, gender is not biological. Girls and boys are not born knowing how they should look, how they should relate to others, or what they should be when they grow up. Rather, girls [text obscured] identities in a social c[text obscured] means to be a woman [text obscured] through a process of [text obscured] is a process of learni[text obscured] roles, and expectatio[text obscured] important things to k[text obscured] social roles and expec[text obscured] They differ from cultu[text obscured] periods in history.

We can look at o[text obscured] States and see how ge[text obscured] A hundred years ago, [text obscured] Senate or House of R[text obscured] women serving as jud[text obscured] on the Supreme Cour[text obscured] playing professional s[text obscured] military operations, a[text obscured]

state. Gender roles from the time of your great grandparents are not what they are today. Things have certainly changed.

One interesting thing about gender is that it is often easier to see it when one is looking back through history, or outside of one's own society. That's because entrenched social norms like those related to gender are often so conventional and treated as normal that people do not question them. But think about the way that gender affects decisions that people make every day. How does gender influence the way you think about yourself, your

Social Considerations
GLOBAL ADOPTIONS

Through inter-country adoption, the legal transfer of parental rights from the birth parent/parents to another parent, or other parents, takes place. Over the last decade, United States families have adopted on average 20,000 children from foreign nations, each year. United States families pay an average $30,000 for an international adoption, including at least one visit to the country of their adopted child's birth (US Department of State, Office of Children's Issues, 2009).

While international adoptions can be filled with great joy, they sometimes also have a more menacing side. Human rights abuses, including the abduction of children within the context of international adoptions, are frequently reported and are a significant issue of concern. Unfortunately, there are many examples of children being taken from their home countries under dubious circumstances[text obscured]

or in-country adoptive family should be looked into. Only when all other options have been exhausted, should inter-country adoption be considered.

By adhering to this policy, UNICEF has said that it seeks to ensure that international adoptions are conducted under a legal framework that protects the best interests of the child (UNICEF, 2003). While UNICEF has noted that many international adoptions are completed in good faith, they have also warned that a lack of legal oversight has resulted in child trafficking and kidnappings (UNICEF, 2003).

On April 1st, 2008, a new international treaty called the Hague Convention on Protection of Children and Co-operation in Respect of Inter-country Adoption entered into force in the United States. The Convention establishes important standards and safeguards to protect children in the process of inter-country adoptions, [text obscured] if such standards [text obscured]rly 2009, for exam-[text obscured]f State has issued [text obscured]temala, noting [text obscured]ple to register new [text obscured]ack of sufficient [text obscured] Department of [text obscured]

Cultural Considerations
MARRIAGE AND HIV

According to the latest global estimates provided by the World Health Organization and UNAIDS, women comprise 50 percent of people living with HIV. While the numbers are equitable, the situation for women is far from it, and the fight for gender equality is increasingly understood as one of the vital components of an effective fight against this pandemic. As the Global Coalition on Women and AIDS has noted: "In some parts of the world, women and girls are infected with HIV almost as soon as they start having sex. Almost everywhere, traditions tolerate and even encourage men to have multiple sexual p[text obscured] other hand, are expect[text obscured] In many places, they a[text obscured] about sex or sexuality, [text obscured] uninformed" (GCWA, [text obscured]

The traditional 'A[text obscured]tion (Abstinence from[text obscured]ful to a single partner[text obscured] Condom use) has bee[text obscured] not take into account[text obscured] women and girls, and [text obscured]tially successful in pra[text obscured] violence is high, abstin[text obscured] option for women and [text obscured] young women coerced[text obscured] who are at risk. Wom[text obscured] to HIV regardless of w[text obscured] faithful because where[text obscured] monogamy does not p[text obscured] becoming infected. A [text obscured]

to ask their partners to use condoms or to refuse unprotected sex.

In Cambodia, which has the highest proportion of HIV-positive adults in Southeast Asia, married women now account for almost half of all new HIV infections in the country (Kaiser, 2005). In Zambia, only 11 percent of women believe that a woman has the right to ask her husband to use a condom—even if he has proven himself to be unfaithful and is HIV-positive (GCWA, 2009). In Zimbabwe, researchers revealed that the majority of HIV positive women were infected by their [text obscured]

[text obscured]us advances in [text obscured]rs, there are still

Economic Considerations
ECTOPIC PREGNANCY IN INSURED WOMEN

In recent years, insurance data has become a method of estimating the rates of ectopic pregnancies, at least in populations of women with health insurance. Two studies—one covering 1997 to 2000 (van den Eeden et al., 2005) and a second covering 2002 to 2007 (Hover et al., 2010)—used claims information from United States commercial insurance companies to determine that rates of ectopic pregnancy remained unchanged over the sample periods. However, treatments changed. While the

rates between 1997 and 2000 indicated that the frequency of ectopic pregnancy did not increase, the number of women who received medical treatment for the condition did (van den Eeden et al., 2005). The nonsurgical methotrexate treatment, usually an outpatient treatment, increased from 11 percent of cases in 2002 to 35 percent by 2007. This corresponded with a decrease in more expensive surgical treatment from 40 percent to 33 percent (Hover et al., 2010).

Case Study
It is not Appendicitis

Gina is 23 years old. She and her partner have been trying to get pregnant, and she is delighted when her period is finally late. She is concerned, however, because she has been experiencing occasional sharp pain on the left side of her abdomen. Her first concern is that she may be having an appendicitis attack, but then she remembers that pain from appendicitis usually occurs on the right side of the body. She decides to ignore the pain, but a couple of hours later she finds herself doubled over on the bathroom floor experiencing excruciating pain and nausea. Her partner rushes her to the hospital, where an ultrasound identifies

ectopic pregnancy. The doctor tells her that it is a good thing that she was brought to the hospital when she was because her fallopian tube was beginning to rupture, and if that had occurred, she could easily have died of severe hemorrhage.

1. Which treatment is most common for an ectopic pregnancy?

2. Why can't the embryo continue to grow in the fallopian tube?

3. What factors may be contributing to the increased frequency of ectopic pregnancies?

CONSIDERATIONS...

Four unique boxes have been provided to connect biological science with the experience of being a woman. Historical Considerations examine woman's experience in a historical context to foster understanding of women's biology today. Social Considerations recognize the biological implications of social factors. Cultural Considerations broaden your understanding of the world and how culture influences women. Economic Considerations explore the impact of money on women, particularly in regards to women's health.

CASE STUDY

Case Study boxes present a fictionalized individual's experience, then ask you to synthesize information read in the chapter to develop your own educated responses to the case study questions.

additional types of accessory structures such as horns, antlers, tusks, and even scales in the case of armadillos. People probably have more awareness of their integument than of any other organ system of the body because it is the most visible. There is a popular misconception that the skin is the largest organ. However, in terms of surface area, the lungs, the circulatory system, and the digestive tract are larger. The skin functions as the primary barrier between the outside environment and the body inside, protecting against thermal, chemical, and physical injury. Relatively waterproof, the skin allows the body to exist in dry air without losing too much water by evaporation and to be immersed in water without appreciably swelling. Because it is abundantly supplied with nerve endings, the skin acts as an enormous sense organ, constantly receiving information from its surface for transmission to the brain. Finally, the skin and the accessory structures serve the important function of creating a person's individual appearance, which makes a person recognizable and distinguishable from others. The integumentary sy[...] Chapter 18[...]

Skeletal S[...]
The skelet[...] attach skele[...] act as pulle[...] act as stora[...] calcium, m[...] row in the[...] marrow, a [...] reserves dr[...] The red bo[...] ing red blo[...] The axial sk[...] sternum, an[...] essential or[...] protecting t[...]

focus on
NUTRITION
Vitamin D, Sun Exposure, and Health

The skin plays a role in the body's ability to make vitamin D. When exposed to UVB rays, the skin converts a form of cholesterol into the precursor of Vitamin D3. The amount of vitamin D a person's body can manufacture depends on season, latitude, sun exposure, and age. It has now been recognized that more than 50 percent of the world's population is vitamin D deficient, fueling a collection of disease conditions affecting nearly every system in the body. Low levels of vitamin D lead to inadequate bone growth, osteoporosis, cardiovascular disease, increased risk of common cancers, and autoimmune conditions (Holick, 2008). There is evidence that vitamin D-fortification of foods is not meeting the nutritional needs of consumers, and it also appears that many people are not manufacturing as much vitamin D as they would be if they were getting more sun exposure. A moderate amount of sun, not enough to produce a sunburn, can have beneficial effects that go far beyond just strong bones and teeth.

lar skeleton includes all of the other bones and it is primarily involved in the movement of the limbs. The major bones of the skeleton are identified in Figure 2-8.

focus on
EXERCISE
Exercise for Bone Health

Aging can bring with it a loss of bone mineral density causing bones to become more fragile. This condition, called osteoporosis, is a major cause of disability in older women, although men can be affected too. Compression fractures in the spine that result from bones becoming too weak to support the body can lead to a stooped posture, and lack of flexibility. Exercise throughout the lifetime, including into old age, is important to maintain and preserve adequate bone density. There are several types of exercise that are beneficial for maintaining bone density. Weight-bearing exercises including aerobic activities such as walking, dancing, gardening, and low impact aerobics put a strain on the bones of the skeleton which stimulates the osteoblasts to deposit more minerals to reinforce the bones. These types of exercises also provide benefits to the cardiovascular system and help to prevent heart disease. Swimming, although it does provide cardiovascular benefits, is not a weight-bearing exercise so it does not benefit the bones directly.

Strength training, which includes using free weight, weight machines, resistance bands, or weight-bearing exercises can stim[...]

density. Osteoblasts respond strongly to estrogen. One reason women are, on average, shorter than men is their difference in estrogen levels. The epiphyseal plates, which are also called growth plates, in a girl's bones grow faster and seal much earlier than those in boys because of the higher concentrations of estrogen in her blood. Consequently, she will complete her growth earlier while her bones are still somewhat shorter. At menopause, decreased estrogen initially slows osteoblast activity for a time period of about five years. After that, the body compensates for the decrease in estrogen, and the rate of bone loss decreases.

Mechanical stress caused by work or exercise is another factor that affects bone growth and maintenance. Increased mechanical stress in the form of weight-bearing exercise increases the activity of the osteoblasts, resulting in increased bone density. Bone density [...] males. [...] body frame [...] weight, [...] in bone [...] r, larger [...] ntage. To [...] women [...] g exercise. [...] s to a level [...] eoporosis. [...] ly debili-[...] d for men, [...] apter 15.

EVIDENCE BASED PRACTICE

Childbirth Fever

Childbirth fever, also known as puerperal fever, is a bacterial infection most often caused by the bacteria *Streptococcus pyogenes*. Throughout history, this disease was a common cause of mortality in women following delivery. In 1795, Alexander Gordon documented an outbreak of the disease in Aberdeen, Scotland. Gordon's data linking transmission of the disease from patient to patient via nurses and physicians was published in *A Treatise on the Epidemic Puerperal Fever in Aberdeen* in which he proposed several methods of controlling the spread of the d[...] were m[...] microbe[...] tial caus[...] before [...] this dis[...]

Oth[...] causes [...] took Go[...] upon it,[...]

sand deliveries and comparing the data from two obstetrical wards in the Allgemeine Krankenhaus, a hospital in Austria. His careful research found that while equal numbers of deliveries were carried out at each ward of the hospital, there were vast differences in the rates of childbirth fever between them. In the ward in which deliveries were attended only by midwives, only 60 deaths from childbirth fever occurred per 3,000 deliveries. Women in the second ward of the hospital who were attended by doctors and medical students suffered over [...] between

control over urination or incontinence. In some cases, childbirth can damage the sphincters causing a condition called stress incontinence in women. Medical procedures such as episiotomy and delivery

Testosterone has effects on muscle development and on the integument. None of the body systems can exist by themselves and all have an important role in maintaining homeostasis.

REVIEW QUESTIONS

1. What is homeostasis, and how does the body maintain homeostasis?

2. Explain the differences between a negative and a positive feedback loop?

3. Which two organ systems exert the most regulating influence over the other systems?

4. How would you differentiate between the central and the peripheral nervous systems?

5. What is the autonomic nervous system, and what does it control?

6. Explain the difference between the sympathetic and parasympathetic nervous systems.

7. What is a hormone, and how do hormones work?

8. Explain how osteoclasts and osteoblasts influence bone growth and bone density.

9. Why are some types of muscle in the body voluntary, while other types are involuntary?

10. Explain the difference between arteries, veins, and capillaries. How are these vessels similar; how are they different?

11. What are some differences between specific immunity and nonspecific immunity?

12. In the digestive system where does the majority of nutrient absorption into the bloodstream occur?

13. List at least two functions of the urinary system.

14. What skeletal differences exist between men and women or are they identical?

15. What is the function of the integumentary system?

CRITICAL THINKING QUESTIONS

1. Why do most organs in the body have both parasympathetic and sympathetic enervation?

2. If a woman had a tumor on her pituitary gland that caused the gland to secrete excess thyroid stimulating hormone, what effect would this have on her thyroid gland's production of thyroid hor-

mone? How would it effect the production of thyroid releasing hormone from the hypothalamus?

3. What might be the long term effects for a woman of taking a medication that inhibits the activities of osteoclasts? Are the long term effects different from the short term effects?

FOCUS ON…

The Focus on Nutrition and Focus on Exercise boxes provide a deeper examination of how specific issues relate to women's biology. They go beyond general information to provide you with a richer understanding of the role of nutrition and exercise in women's issues.

EVIDENCE BASED PRACTICE

This feature box presents current research on a topic covered in the chapter and demonstrates how it has impacted practice or policy surrounding women's issues. These boxes emphasize how continual research can change our understanding of women's health and well-being.

REVIEW QUESTIONS AND CRITICAL THINKING QUESTIONS

Test your understanding of information covered in the chapter with the end of chapter review and critical thinking questions. These questions encourage a synthesis of information and are an excellent way to challenge your comprehension.

chapter 1

WHY BIOLOGY OF WOMEN?

CHAPTER COMPETENCIES

Upon completion of this chapter, the reader will be able to:

- Identify biological differences between women and men
- Describe an overview of the history of women's biology

- Explain the necessity of understanding the language of science as it relates to women's biology
- Discuss guideline for analyzing and evaluating scientific information

KEY TERMS

basic research
cardiovascular disease
Civil Rights Act
clinical investigations
control group
double-blind study

hormone replacement
  therapy
midwifery
myocardial infarction
  (MI)
observational study

peer-reviewed
placebo
primary care
  physician
prognosis
pseudoscience

randomized clinical
  trial
randomized sample
sample size
Title IX
wise woman

Women are biologically unique from men. While all humans carry out similar metabolic functions and have a similar body structure, interactions between hormones and genes in a woman modify the undifferentiated human into an organism with anatomical and physiological characteristics distinct from her male counterpart (Figure 1-1).

Exploring the differences between men and women from a scientific standpoint is not something new. Consider these comments by Albert H. Hayes from his 1869 *Sexual Physiology of Woman and her Diseases.*

"Never, at any period in the history of the world, was Woman such an object of interest and discussion, in speech and in print, as the present time. The press teams with works on woman, - works sociological, physiological, … It is high time that this knowledge were popularized, and placed within the reach of the entire female sex of the United States, so that, in all the junctures and crises of life, they may have the knowledge that will make them equal to the emergency." (pg. 25)

Research presented in *Exploring the Biological Contributions to Human Health: Does Sex Matter?* (Wizemann & Pardue, 2001) identifies a number

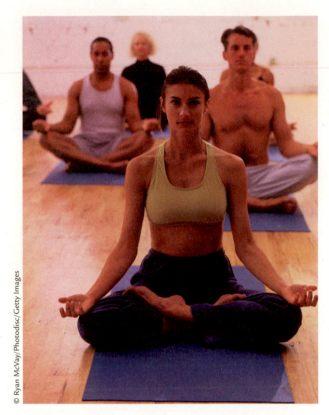

© Ryan McVay/Photodisc/Getty Images

FIGURE 1-1: While structurally and metabolically similar, women are anatomically and physiologically distinct from men.

of biological differences between men and women, differences not limited to the reproductive system. For example, women and men respond differently to pain (Paller et al., 2009). Some brain functions are different between women and men. Women and men recruit different areas of the brain for both motor and memory tasks and to differing degrees (Bell et al., 2006). In addition, blood flow to the brain through the external carotid arteries is greater in women (Yazici, Erdoğmuş, & Tugay, 2005). Women metabolize many medications more quickly than men (Miyazaki & Yamamoto, 2009) indicating that dosages may need to be adjusted for sex. Under physiological stress, women have a more active immune system (Timmons et al., 2006) which should make them better at fighting infections, but may also explain their higher rates of autoimmune conditions, in which the immune system turns against the body. Women build muscle more slowly during strength training, but they are also slower to lose muscle mass when they stop training (Ivey et al., 2000). Research continues to identify other sex-based differences based on biological factors.

Reasons for these differences range from physiological variations due to the genes on the X chromosome to hormonal influences on gene expression. Body cells in a woman have two X chromosomes, one received from her mother, the other from her father. The cells in a man, on the other hand, contain an X from his mother and a Y from his father (Figure 1-2). The X chromosome contains 1100 genes that are not found on the Y chromosome (Migeon, 2007). In a woman's cells, one of the X chromosomes is deactivated, leaving only one X chromosome per cell to express its genes. Deactivation appears to be random, so the maternal X chromosome is deactivated in some cells and the paternal X chromosome is deactivated in others. Because of this, women are a genetic mosaic with some cells expressing the maternal X chromosome, and others expressing the paternal. This provides greater genetic variability and adaptability in women.

Cultural and social structures also play a role in the expression of biological differences and, equally as important, the understanding of those differences. Social customs may lead to sexual differences that are interpreted as being biological in origin. Dietary differences and differences in activities can also produce physiological differences. Is the higher rate of osteoporosis currently seen in women in some cultures due to women doing less weight-bearing exercise (a cultural factor) or to a difference in hormones that influence bone formation (a biological factor)? Is it due to a combination of these factors or something yet unrecognized? How much gender influences biology varies from one cultural to another depending on what is considered encouraged or acceptable behaviors for a woman in that culture.

This leads to a need to clarify some terms. Sex and gender are not the same thing. From a genetic

© Cengage Learning 2013

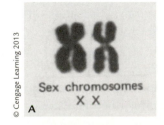

A

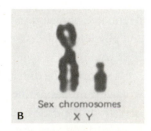

B

FIGURE 1-2: A. Karyotype of a human female B. Karyotype of a human male.

basis, there are two sexes. Those individuals with two X chromosomes are genetically female while those individuals with an X and a Y chromosome are genetically male. However, gender depends on both the genetic sex, biological factors other than chromosomes, and social influences. The American Medical Association (AMA), the World Health Organization (WHO), and Committee on Understanding the Biology of Sex and Gender Differences follow these definitions (Wizemann & Pardue, 2001).

Women have always had a presence in scientific study and, by extension, healing and medicine. The acknowledgement of their contributions, however, has fluctuated over the centuries, primarily due to cultural or religious views of acceptable roles for women. The traditional **wise woman**, the herbalist who treated the illnesses of friends, neighbors, and family, appears in nearly every culture. **Midwifery**, the practice of attending women during childbirth, in particular, became the realm of women in many cultures. Both the Bible and the Torah mention female midwives who were respected medical professionals. However, in early history, a lack of scientific understanding of anatomical structure and the physiology of reproduction spawned myths and misconceptions which still haunt women today.

The rise of the Christian Church in Europe coincided with a decline in rights, position, and education of women. This is not to say women completely vanished from the scientific world. For example, in the 1100s, Abbess Hildegard von Bingen compiled her *Physica* which covered topics ranging from natural history to medicine to metals. She included information on women's health in particular, including detailed information on menstruation, childbirth, and abortion (Throop, 1998). During the Renaissance period, medicine took several important leaps forward, as did the understanding of

focus on

EXERCISE

Recommendations Concerning Exercise and Activity Levels for Women: A Historical Perspective

What is considered to be good exercise for women? Throughout time and place, that has changed. Consider the following recommendation from *The Young Woman's Guide* written in 1846 by William Alcott, a progressive educator in his day and the uncle of Louisa May Alcott. "Two hours of active walking a day are worth a great deal... I must omit, of course, in a work like this, intended for young women, the mention of any motion more rapid than walking. Running, to those who have passed their teens, would be unfashionable... Who could risk the danger of being regarded as a romp?" (p. 212) At the time, light gardening was also considered a questionable activity for young women, although housekeeping, skating, and riding horseback were encouraged. Riding in an open carriage was also considered acceptable exercise.

human anatomy and physiology. Increased interest in dissections of human cadavers led to anatomical works by DaVinci and Vesalius which illustrated the internal anatomy of the human body. Despite these improvements in knowledge, women still faced a relatively high risk of death from infection and complications of pregnancy, and populations as a whole suffered from high death tolls from infectious disease. This period also saw an increasing divide between those with formal medical training and the folk practitioners, many of whom were women. Midwives and wise women continued to be the primary practitioners to help women through childbirth.

The development of the first microscopes and other technologies opened the way for scientific discoveries about how the body works at a cellular level. The new technologies began to uncover the workings within the human body. Improvements in microscopes lead to histological research that identified structures that had never been seen before, and allowed scientists to identify bacteria and other

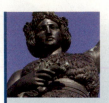

Historical Considerations
Biology is not Destiny: Understanding 'Sex' and 'Gender' and Changing Gender Norms

In the natural and social sciences, 'sex' and 'gender' do not mean the same thing. 'Sex' refers to the biological distinction as to whether one is female or male. 'Gender,' on the other hand, refers to the social attributes associated with being male or female in a given society. Gender is by definition a relational concept, because it deals with the relationships between women and men and how these relationships are socially constructed. Importantly, gender is not biological. Girls and boys are not born knowing how they should look, how they should relate to others, or what they should be when they grow up. Rather, girls and boys develop their gender identities in a social context, and they learn what it means to be a woman, or what it means to be a man through a process of 'socialization'. Socialization is a process of learning one's cultural norms, social roles, and expectations about behavior. One of the important things to know about gender is that these social roles and expectations can and do change. They differ from culture to culture and at different periods in history.

We can look at our own history in the United States and see how gender roles have changed. A hundred years ago, there were no women in the Senate or House of Representatives. There were no women serving as judges, and no women sitting on the Supreme Court. There were no women playing professional sports, no women directing military operations, and no women governing any state. Gender roles from the time of your great-grandparents are not what they are today. Things have certainly changed.

One interesting thing about gender is that it is often easier to see it when one is looking back through history, or outside of one's own society. That's because entrenched social norms like those related to gender are often so conventional and treated as normal that people do not question them. But think about the way that gender affects decisions that people make every day. How does gender influence the way you think about yourself, your life's ambitions, your relationships to others, your interests, and your personal experiences? Is there anything about the way gender operates in our society that you would like to change?

Gender norms and roles are also shaped by historical forces. Take the simple example of women wearing pants. You may enjoy wearing your favorite pair of jeans and think little of it, but in the past, a woman wearing pants was seen as something of a provocation, certainly unfeminine, and not respectable or socially appropriate attire for a woman. Pants did not come into popular use among women until World War II, when women entered the paid workforce in unprecedented numbers. Women entering the factory labor force to support the war effort made wearing pants a practical necessity. Even Rosie the Riveter got into the action and was depicted on posters wearing overalls to work!

---

microscopic organisms. By the 1800s, this research led to the link between microbes and disease.

Dr. Ignác Semmelweis working at the Allegemeine Krankhaus in Vienna, Austria, is credited with instituting a series of procedures designed to minimize contamination during childbirth and publicizing the role of simple hand washing in preventing the spread of the disease. While the recognition of contamination by bacteria during childbirth as the cause of puerperal fever and the need for more sterile conditions to prevent it saved lives, it also ushered in the era of viewing childbirth as an "illness" to be managed by physicians.

The late 1800s brought much more research into women's health. Dr. Albert Hayes published a book titled *Sexual Physiology of Woman and her Diseases* (1869), one of the earliest texts examining health issues specific to women from both a scientific and a social point of view. Some of this research led to curious conclusions about women and their anatomy

EVIDENCE BASED PRACTICE

Childbirth Fever

Childbirth fever, also known as puerperal fever, is a bacterial infection most often caused by the bacteria *Streptococcus pyogenes*. Throughout history, this disease was a common cause of mortality in women following delivery. In 1795, Alexander Gordon documented an outbreak of the disease in Aberdeen, Scotland. Gordon's data linking transmission of the disease from patient to patient via nurses and physicians was published in *A Treatise on the Epidemic Puerperal Fever in Aberdeen* in which he proposed several methods of controlling the spread of the disease. Unfortunately, Gordon's ideas were met with skepticism at a time when microbes had not yet been identified as potential causes of disease. It took another 50 years before the next major breakthrough regarding this disease occurred.

Other researchers continued to explore the causes of childbirth fever. Ignaz Semmelweis took Gordon's information and expanded upon it, conducting studies of several thousand deliveries and comparing the data from two obstetrical wards in the Allgemeine Krankenhaus, a hospital in Austria. His careful research found that while equal numbers of deliveries were carried out at each ward of the hospital, there were vast differences in the rates of childbirth fever between them. In the ward in which deliveries were attended only by midwives, only 60 deaths from childbirth fever occurred per 3,000 deliveries. Women in the second ward of the hospital who were attended by doctors and medical students suffered over 600 deaths from childbirth fever per 3,000 deliveries over the same time period. Semmelweis noted that many of the doctors and medical students worked on cadavers immediately before attending their maternity patients. In 1847, Semmelweis ordered all medical attendants to scrub with chloride of lime, a mild disinfectant, before attending any woman in labor. Within weeks, the death rate dropped to a little over 1 percent, a dramatic decrease (Nuland, 2003).

and physiology. Women's mental health was defined in terms of the social and cultural expectations of the times, and their illnesses were frequently perceived as psychosomatic, a trend that can still be problematic today. During the 1800s, for example, the uterus was blamed as the "starting point for hysteria" in women, with symptoms ranging from paleness and yawning to palpitations and seizures, sadness and sullenness to "immoderate laughter". Socially unacceptable behaviors were treated medically with opium, emetics, and other drugs (Hayes, 1869).

Hayes and others recognized and promoted the use of contraceptives and a woman's right to make her own decisions about her health. However, these ideas were not universally accepted. During 1873, the Act for the Suppression of Trade in, and Circulation of, Obscene Literature and Articles of Immoral Use, more commonly known as the Comstock Law, made it illegal to distribute information relating to conception or to bring contraceptives into the United States (American Law and Legal Information, 2009). Many individuals argued against the Comstock Laws and encouraged increased knowledge of women's biology and health. Perhaps best known is Margaret Sanger who, in 1916, opened a birth control clinic in Brooklyn, New York (Planned Parenthood Federation of America [PPFA], 2009). Sanger and other women who promoted greater access to birth control were jailed for their activities.

Women in Medicine

As medicine became more formalized, most women were pushed further from the ranks of physicians and into the realm of patient. However, women did not vanish entirely from the medical field. In 1849, Dr. Elizabeth Blackwell graduated from the Geneva Medical College, becoming the first recognized female doctor. In 1846, William Alcott, a social reformer and educator, wrote that "Females are better qualified – other things being the same – for attending the sick, than males" (p. 302) and encouraged women to gain a broad education in the sciences. During the mid-1800s, medical schools were opened exclusively for women. The Congressional Medal of Honor was awarded in 1865 to Dr. Mary Walker for her work as a physician during the Civil War. However, the Flexner Report of 1900 resulted in the closing of many medical schools and the narrowing of medical opportunities in the United States for women and minorities. As the Women's Rights Movement of the 19th century gained momentum, control over contraception and reproductive rights became a major point of contention. Against the backdrop of the Comstock Laws, pioneers like Margaret Sanger and Mary Ware Dennett continued to provide contraceptives to women. Their continued efforts and the public outcry against the suppression of contraception knowledge lead to changes in the laws which allowed physicians to prescribe contraceptives to their patients. These changes demonstrated the need for trained female healthcare providers to work with female patients, many of whom would never broach such issues as "female complaints" with a male doctor. In spite of this need, women continued to be underrepresented as physicians and continued to face obstacles to receiving training.

In recent decades, the proportion of women in medical schools has been increasing. In 1972, **Title IX** of the Education Amendments to the **Civil Rights Act** stated that:

> "No person in the United States shall, on the basis of sex, be excluded from participation in, be denied the benefits of, or be subjected to discrimination under any education program or activity receiving Federal financial assistance." (20 U.S.C. §§ 1681–1688)

This legislation initiated a process of leveling the playing field for admission to higher education institutions, including medical schools, that continues today. As a result, change is occurring. In 2005, of the 68,343 students actively enrolled in American medical schools, 49 percent (33,380) were women, up from 31 percent in 1982 (AAMC Fact Sheet, 2008). Currently, 49 percent of pharmacists are women, compared to only 30 percent just twenty years ago (DPE Fact sheet, 2008). Another area of major advancement occurred in dentistry where women in 2003 earned 42 percent of the dental degrees compared to less than one percent in 1960 (U.S. Department of Education National Center for Education Statistics, 2008).

The Last Century

The increased attention to women's health since the 1800s came with some costs. Normal physiological events in a woman's life such as menstruation, pregnancy, and menopause were increasingly treated, at least in the West, as illnesses to be managed through medications and medical procedures. Women have been prescribed hormones for birth control, for menopause, or to prevent miscarriage, and have often not been informed about the potential risks of such treatments. Many healthcare providers have simply treated "problems" without treating the patient as a whole, resulting in women being subjected to unnecessary or excessive surgery without the opportunity to consider alternatives. In addition, recent revelations concerning the risks of **hormone replacement therapy (HRT)**, differing treatment of men and women suffering from heart disease and other conditions, and attempts to control the distribution of information about reproductive options further tarnished the state of women's healthcare.

The increased attention to women's health issues and public frustration with the shortcomings of medicine as it was being practiced has resulted in change. Federal guidelines now protect human subjects from being used without their knowledge or consent in **clinical investigations**, for diseases or conditions, of drugs or medical devices. In response to the demands of pregnant women, birthing centers and certified midwives and doulas are providing alternatives to hospital-based delivery of infants in some cities. Armed with greater knowledge of how their bodies work, many women are becoming active partners in their healthcare, reserving the right to reject advice or to seek a second opinion. There are now more doctors and other healthcare professionals who treat women with greater respect and sensitivity and who explain more to the patient about procedures and therapies (Figure 1-3). For many women, however, underlying health concerns are unchanged. The problems in the areas of reproductive rights, hormonal therapy, unnecessary surgery, prescription drug abuse, pregnancy and childbirth interventions, domestic violence,

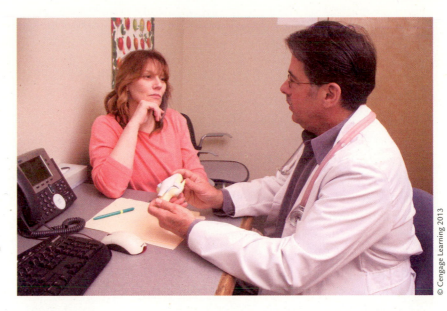

FIGURE 1-3: Lack of knowledge can make a woman feel vulnerable and afraid. Knowing how the body functions in health and disease can give women the self-confidence to participate in the decisions concerning their own healthcare.

© Cengage Learning 2013

and mental health treatment remain unsolved. For example, while the rates of some potentially dangerous childbirth procedures have decreased in recent decades, the rates of others, namely cesarean sections, have increased dramatically in many parts of the world.

In recent years, challenges to what was previously accepted about women's biology, scientific advances in cancer and reproductive biology, and the recognition of the sexual differences in the development, prognosis, and treatment of many diseases have brought a number of women's health issues to national and international attention. Beginning with the success of the original *Our Bodies, Ourselves* by the Boston Women's Health Book Collective in 1970, hundreds of books, articles, and websites have moved the discussion of women's health issues from the halls of medicine to the halls of offices and factories, markets and cafés, and the political arena. Globalization and the Internet have the potential to introduce women to practices and principles different from those they are familiar with.

The increased focus on breast cancer during the 1980s and 1990s illustrated how women could garner public attention and financial support for an important women's health issue. Women's experiences with the life-threatening illness of breast cancer, which in the past had been hidden and certainly not talked about publicly, were nationally spotlighted in the early 1980s when two presidents' wives, Betty Ford and Nancy Reagan, and other celebrities, revealed that they had survived breast cancer.

The Susan G. Komen Breast Cancer Foundation became a leader in breast cancer research funding, education, and legislative advocacy. The activism mustered to fight breast cancer has paved the way for directing public attention to other health issues that disproportionately affect women (Figure 1-4).

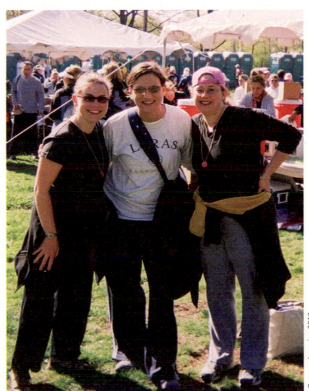

© Cengage Learning 2013

FIGURE 1-4: Activism to fight breast cancer, as in this walk for awareness, has lead to an expanded focus on women's health at a governmental level.

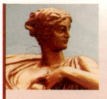

Cultural Considerations
WHICH COUNTRY IS THE BEST FOR WOMEN'S HEALTH?

There are many ways to measure the quality of women's lives in countries around the world. Life expectancy is one measure. A girl born in Swaziland will be unlikely to see her 30th birthday. In Niger, women generally live to be about 45 years old. In Sweden, the average woman will live to be 83 years old and the average Japanese woman will live to be 86.

The World Economic Forum publishes a report each year titled the Gender Gap Report, which examines the lives of women and men in terms of political empowerment, educational attainment, economic participation and opportunity, and health. Each year they rank almost every country in the world according to the gender gap, or differences that they find between the lives of the country's women and men. Iceland was ranked number 1 as the best country for women in 2009. Other Nordic countries, Norway, Finland, and Sweden have ranked next within the top four countries since 2006. The gender gap in the United States has been increasing since 2005 when it ranked 17th in the world. In 2006, the United States dropped to 23rd and then dropped again to 31st by 2009. The country of Yemen ranked last in the Gender Gap Report (Hausmann et al., 2008).

The non-profit organization Save the Children publishes an annual State of the World's Mothers Report, where they compare countries by maternal deaths due to complications of pregnancy and childbirth, infant mortality, and access to healthcare. In their 2007 report, Sweden ranked first as the best country in which to be a mother, with only 1 in 29,800 women dying in childbirth. Children in Sweden have only a 1 in 333 chance of dying within their first year of life. According to the report, nearly one hundred percent of births are attended by a skilled trained midwife in Sweden.

Save the Children's 2007 report ranks Niger as the worst country in which to be a mother, with 1 in 7 women dying as a result of pregnancy or childbirth. Only 16 percent of deliveries are attended to by a skilled healthcare worker, and 15 percent of babies die before their first birthday. In fact, according to the 2007 report, the risks for a woman dying due to complications of pregnancy are:

- 1 in 26 for all of Africa
- 1 in 120 for Asia
- 1 in 290 for Latin America
- 1 in 7,300 for developed countries

The United States ranked 27th out of 42 developed nations in terms of the Mothers Index in 2007, which was a slight drop from ranking 26th in 2006. In terms of infant mortality and children's health, the United States ranked 33rd out of 43 developed nations.

Save the Children also points out another concern, the difference in the amount of money spent on healthcare for girls verses boys in countries that strongly favor boys. In China, girls are 30 percent more likely to die before the age of 5, and in India they are 61 percent more likely to die in the same time frame. In some parts of India, it is estimated that families will spend 2.3 times as much on healthcare for boys than for girls during the first two years of life.

In the United States, public pressure has established women's health offices at the Department of Health and Human Services, the Federal Food and Drug Administration, and the Centers for Disease Control and Prevention, with the goal of expanding the focus on women's health. Women's health issues are being recognized by governments world wide.

The Society for the Advancement of Women's Health Research, a nonprofit organization, was established in 1990 to advocate for increased research of conditions affecting women exclusively, disproportionately, or differently than men (SWHR, 2008). This group continues to inform women, healthcare providers, policy makers, and the media about contemporary women's health issues. The Society was involved in the establishment of the *Journal of Women's Health* and sponsored the first symposium on sex-based biology.

In the United States, increased public attention to the inequities in research on women's health, and additional political pressure from the Congressional Caucus for Women's Issues and the House Subcommittee on Health, motivated the National Institutes of Health (NIH) to take concrete action and began to include women and minorities in clinical studies. Another major change in 1992 was the establishment of the largest community-based clinical intervention and prevention trial ever conducted. Known as the Women's Health Initiative (WHI), it began as a multi-million dollar study that followed 161,808 healthy postmenopausal women over a fifteen year period. This groundbreaking project consisted of three components – a **randomized clinical trial**

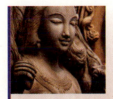

Social Considerations
THE IMPORTANCE OF FOCUSING ON WOMEN'S STUDIES

Women and women's experiences have for too long been seen as somehow outside the 'human standard' which was typically seen as exclusively male. Men's lives, bodies, and experiences were most often the ones romanticized in literature, studied in medicine, and recorded in history. 'Women's studies as an area of scholarship challenged these very notions, emphasizing that women's lives are every bit as important as those of men, and that their contributions to history and to humanity no less significant. Indeed, the development of women's studies as an academic field went hand in hand with the rise of the second wave of feminism in the late 1960s and 1970s, when the women's liberation movement challenged many of the mainstream patriarchal ideas and privileges of the day.

Women's studies developed as a place within the academic community for the flourishing of feminist theory and explored the experiences and achievements of women across history and cultures. It is a discipline which takes the study of gender as a central theme, with the understanding that women's experiences, as well as men's, are profoundly shaped by the social universe in which they find themselves, and the social norms, values, and expectations of their time. Women's studies served as an incubator for feminist thought and debate and helped to uncover what was once minimized by the academic community: women's intellectual, artistic, and historical accomplishments and triumphs.

The Biology of Women textbook draws on many of the proud traditions of women's studies. The book focuses on women's bodies and lives, looking at the intimate connections between women's individual experiences and their social realities, and the concept that a woman's knowledge has the power to change the future, both for herself and for the world she lives in. In many universities and colleges around the country, Biology of Women is taught as a women's studies course. Today, women's studies programs typically take an interdisciplinary approach, drawing on the insights of the social sciences, the natural sciences, the humanities, and the arts. Modern day women's studies programs can be found across the country and today incorporate an analyses of 'intersectionality,' a term which recognizes that people encounter distinct forms of discrimination due to the intersection of gender with such factors as race/ethnicity, age, sexual orientation, nationality, religion, disability, and economic class.

in which participants were assigned to a treatment group randomly to avoid researcher bias, a community prevention study, and an **observational study** in which the researchers observed the outcomes of groups derived from the general public, to gather data on the prevention and treatment of the major causes of death in middle-aged and older women, including cardiovascular disease, cancer, and osteoporosis. Interventions such as smoking cessation programs, low-fat diets, vitamin and calcium supplements, exercise, and hormone therapy were studied to assess their effect on women's health. This project dramatically demonstrated the importance of specifically researching women's health, when mid-study results indicated that not only was hormone replacement therapy (HRT) not as effective as previously believed at preventing heart disease, but in fact increased rates of breast cancer, cardiovascular disease, and pulmonary embolism. These discoveries led to the nearly unprecedented early termination of some of the clinical trials.

Funding for research into specific aspects of women's biology had been, for many years, shortchanged, but this is changing. The 2001 report *Exploring the Biological Contribution to Human Health: Does Sex Matter?* by the Institute of Medicine pointed out the need for understanding how the metabolic differences between men and women influence both their health and healthcare. The National Institutes of Health (NIH) Office of Research on Women's Health (ORWH, 2007) identified health disparities and differences between the sexes as one of the major research priorities for 2008. The need for research on the differences between men and women with regard to common health issues is readily demonstrated by the incidence of cardiovascular disease and its predictable outcome, or **prognosis**. A review of records examining the rate of sudden cardiac death showed that between 1989 and 1998 the rate decreased for men across all age groups. However, in women between the ages of 35 and 44 the rate actually increased (Zheng et al., 2001). According to statistics from the American Heart Association (AHA, 2007), one woman per minute died of cardiovascular disease in

2004. Is there something in women's biology that produces these differences, or could other factors be involved? Two past studies involving tens of thousands of patients showed clear evidence of bias in the treatment of women with heart disease. The studies showed that doctors treated women less aggressively than they treated men, even though the women in the studies generally had more advanced heart disease than the men (Ayanian & Epstein, 1991; Steingart et al., 1991). More recently, the American Medical Association (AMA), in its 2000 report *Women's Health: Sex- and Gender-based Differences in Health and Disease,* reported that women suffered a higher mortality rate from heart attack (**myocardial infarction** or **MI**) than men did, even though women usually suffered their first heart attack 10 years later than men. The report also found that women still received delayed and less aggressive treatment than men. This may account for the higher mortality rate due to MI in women even when the data are adjusted for age. Further research into the hormonal and metabolic differences between men and women may identify other factors that influence women's survival.

While breast cancer and heart disease have caught the public's attention, they are, by no means, the only issues affecting women's health. Stress, eating disorders, sexually transmitted infections (STI's), environmental chemical exposures, AIDS, and domestic violence are just some of the issues that have serious effects on women. Current issues of reproductive health range from human cloning (French et al., 2008), to vaccines that prevent cervical cancer, to the effects of suppressing menstruation. In addition, not all women have access to quality healthcare.

Language of Medicine

This book contains many scientific terms that may be unfamiliar to those who do not have background in science. The question arises, why use all of these technical terms in a book that is used both by science and non-science majors? The language used in this book is the language of science, and more specifically the language of medicine. Researchers and health practitioners in the medical community use terms derived

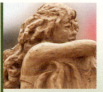

Economic Considerations
WOMEN'S HEALTHCARE COSTS COMPARED TO MEN'S

Healthcare costs are not gender neutral, and mounting evidence seems to show that women are routinely disadvantaged in terms of how much they pay for healthcare services. A *New York Times* article published in October 2008 noted that: "Striking new evidence has emerged of a widespread gap in the cost of health insurance, as women pay much more than men of the same age for individual insurance policies providing identical coverage" (Pear, 2008, p. A23). On selected policies, women paid anywhere from 22-49 percent more than their male counterparts (Pear, 2008).

To make matters worse, according to the National Healthcare Quality and Disparities Reports published by the Agency for Healthcare Research and Policy, the nation's lead federal agency for research on healthcare quality, costs, outcomes, and patient safety, differences in quality of care are also evident for women compared with men (AHRP, 2005). The disparities are particularly stark for women of color (AHRP, 2005). Many times, women in fact get lower quality health services and inferior medical care, despite the fact that they have to pay higher premiums for their insurance coverage (AHRP, 2005).

Some health insurance providers note that the disparities in cost can be due to women's increased use of the medical system, particularly during her childbearing years (Pear, 2008). Nonetheless, the evidence suggests that the disparities in costs exist even when maternal healthcare is not covered. Many times, maternity coverage is offered as a separate option and often as an expensive benefit (Pear, 2008).

The rising costs of healthcare overall have also disproportionately affected women, in part because of their lower average incomes. Individuals in the United States pay more for healthcare than any other industrialized country. Today, women continue to make less money than their male counterparts in the workplace, about 80 cents on every dollar earned by a man (IWPR, 2008). Putting together a woman's lower income on the one hand, and higher insurance premiums on the other, it is not difficult to see why so many women have a difficult time making ends meet when it comes to their healthcare costs. In fact, approximately 17 million women in the United States have no medical insurance whatsoever (USDHHS, 2007), and as many as 52 percent of working-aged women are either uninsured or underinsured (Rustgi et al., 2009). In addition, according to the US Department of Health and Human Services, women are twice as likely as men to be insured as a 'dependent' on a spouse's medical plan (USDHHS, 2007). This means that women are more vulnerable to losing their medical coverage if they get divorced, if they are widowed, or if a spouse loses their job.

---

from Latin and Greek to describe the structures and functions of the human body. New scientific discoveries affect everyone, and it is useful to understand the language of science when evaluating new information that emerges. As women take a more active role and greater responsibility in their own healthcare, familiarity with the language of medicine helps them to communicate better with healthcare providers and to clearly understand the information that they receive. This knowledge also enables women to research healthcare concerns and procedures with more confidence and authority. Health information is presented to the general public in the form of news segments, magazine articles and even pharmaceutical commercials. At the same time, it is not uncommon to hear news reports about deaths

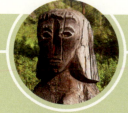

focus on

NUTRITION

Recommendations Concerning Diet and Nutrition for Women: A Historical Perspective

What is considered a healthy diet has changed over time. New information continually becomes available and changes what is accepted practice. Consider this diet for a wet nurse, a woman hired to nurse an infant, published in 1861 by Mrs. Beeton, who was considered an expert in her day. The wet nurse was advised to eat simple foods. She could have boiled meat only once a day, and fish no more than twice a week, because "it is hardly sufficiently nutritious to be often used as a meal" (p.1024). Green vegetables were to be avoided. Between breakfast and dinner, the nurse was to have a half pint of stout with a biscuit. In the early afternoon, she was to have a dinner with a pint of porter. In the evening, another half pint of stout and another biscuit. This was to be followed at 10 pm with a supper of toast with a small bit of cheese and another pint of porter. Hardly what would be recommended today, but, at the time, it was considered the best diet for a nursing woman.

resulting from unforeseen or previously unreported side effects of popular medications. How is a person to filter through and interpret all of this information? Much of the scientific information presented in the popular press is presented without much supporting explanation, and in some cases, with a great deal of misinformation. A familiarity with science – both its language and its limits – can contribute to more informed decisions.

Public access to medical information has increased dramatically in recent years. In the not too distant past, patients looked to their doctors as the ultimate authorities on their healthcare. Now, the Internet allows almost everyone to access medical information on their own, quickly and relatively easily. The difficulty lies in sorting through all of the available information to determine what is reliable and worthy of attention.

Ideally, all research, both basic and applied, would be conducted in a non-biased, scientific

manner, with the ultimate goal of providing accurate information (Figure 1-5). The scientific method calls for an orderly evaluation of the evidence, uninfluenced by preconceived ideas or desired outcomes. Unfortunately, there are times when financial or ideological pressures influence the conclusions that are reached in studies. When these pressures influence the gathering, interpretation, or presentation of information, the result is called bias. Bias can influence scientific studies either through conscious or unconscious means. The scientific community does have safeguards and mechanisms in place to detect and expose bias, but no system is completely infallible.

Rigorous scientific testing is expensive and time consuming. It involves testing large samples of the population using double blind experimental designs to help protect from biased results. A **double blind study** is one in which neither the participants nor the researchers know which subjects in a study are receiving which treatment. A third party assigns participants to a treatment group to avoid bias. For example, when testing the effectiveness of a new medication,

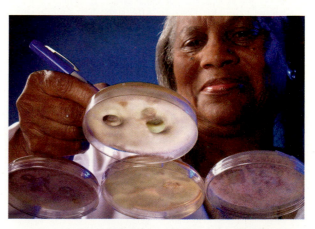

FIGURE 1-5: Ideally, scientific and medical research should be conducted in a non-biased, scientific manner that strives to provide accurate information. *(Courtesy of CDC/Photo by James Gathany, 2006)*

neither the test subjects nor the person administering the experiment should know which participants received the test drug, and which have received a placebo. A **placebo** is an inactive substance or treatment administered as if it were the prescribed, active drug or test treatment. This way, expectations about what "should" happen are less likely to influence the observed results.

Sometimes, marketers of health-related products cloak their advertising in scientific-sounding jargon, implying that the product they want to sell has been scientifically evaluated and "proven" to be effective. These "results" are often presented as "scientific proof" that their product is effective, yet the actual science involved may be scant. This phenomenon of trying to make something sound scientific when it really has not been evaluated scientifically is called **pseudoscience**. The prefix "pseudo" means false.

Guidelines for Evaluating Scientific Information

The following guidelines can be used to evaluate the quality of the health information presented in popular media:

- Consider who is publishing or disseminating the information. Is it a credible source? Some sources are much more reliable than others. News agencies and advertisers have less to lose by publishing inaccurate information than do professional and scientific journals, who must maintain their reputation for accuracy. The most reliable journals are **peer reviewed**, which means that several experts in the field have reviewed the research before it was published. Other reliable sources include established medical websites, such as those associated with large hospitals or non-profit organizations. For example, large organizations such as the American Heart Association or the American Lung Association are more likely to take the necessary steps to avoid losing valuable credibility by publishing fraudulent or inaccurate studies.
- Consider who funded the research, and whether anyone stands to profit either monetarily or ideologically from the public believing the conclusions of the study. This is not always easy to determine, but it can provide important clues about potential bias or "hidden agendas" in the data. A study about the benefits of a given medication released by the company that stands to profit from the sale of that medication may be suspect. Whenever there are those who can profit from a given result, it is a good idea to evaluate the information carefully.
- Consider whether the study has been repeated, and if so, what were the results? Repetition is an important component of good scientific research. The more credible studies that support the results, the more plausible it is that the results are true.
- Consider the **sample size**, or the number of subjects that were studied. Large sample sizes are generally more reliable than small sample sizes because they are likely to better encompass the variation in the population that is being studied. It is also important that the samples were selected randomly for a **randomized sample**, rather than being chosen to lend support to a pre-conceived outcome. The greater the diversity of subjects represented in a study, the more robust and believable the results will be.
- Consider how the study was conducted. Was it a double blind study? Was the sample randomized? Was there a control group that received a placebo instead of the medication or procedure being tested? A **control group** is a group of test subjects who are exposed to the same conditions as everyone else in the experiment, except that they are given a placebo instead of the medication being tested. The control group in an experimental study helps to ensure that the effects that are observed are due to the experimental treatment, and not some other factor.

All of these conditions help to protect the results from bias. Does the study claim to have "proven" something? It is a common misconception that the purpose of scientific studies is to prove a conclusion to be true. In fact, credible science can only eliminate the incorrect conclusions, it can never "prove" something to be true or not. Whenever a claim is made that something has been proven, be aware that this might be an example of pseudoscience. Unfortunately, none of these tips is a guarantee against false information, but taken

Critical Thinking

Science/Pseudoscience: Does Abortion Cause Breast Cancer?

An example of the misuse of scientific information and research bias occurred when abortion opponents began implying that abortions caused breast cancer. Much of the early research was inconclusive. However, a small study with a limited sample size asked women diagnosed with breast cancer if they had had an abortion. This type of study, while appearing scientific, introduces possible bias and lacks both controls and methods of confirming the information. The combination produces results that do not meet rigorous scientific standards. However, abortion opponents seized on the information and began a well-orchestrated campaign of misinformation implying that abortions caused breast cancer.

Larger, more rigorously-designed studies, including the California Teachers Study (Henderson et al., 2008) and a long-term Danish study (Melbye et al.,1997), found no link between abortion and breast cancer. These studies were large, included over a million women, and relied on medical records rather than personal reporting, therefore avoiding bias. The National Cancer Institute (NCI) continues to review the literature as new data becomes available and has concluded that there is no increased risk of breast cancer following an abortion (2008). However, there are those who still choose to ignore the broad pool of research results or choose to misrepresent the data and continue to mislead women seeking abortions by telling them it will cause breast cancer.

together they can help evaluate information with more skill and confidence.

CONCLUSION

No one can be expected to become an expert on everything that might affect a woman's health throughout her lifetime. Even doctors who attend medical school for many years usually specialize in one field of medicine. Still, the more women understand their bodies and their health, the better they can monitor themselves and take steps to intervene if things go awry. Women who can express themselves in detail and explain how their body is varying from what is normal for them can be better partners in their healthcare. To make informed decisions, a woman needs to understand the biology of her own body.

REVIEW QUESTIONS

1. How has the relationship of women and science changed throughout the centuries?

2. In the United States, what legislation made it much easier for women to become equal partners to men in the healthcare professions?

3. How did the findings of the Women's Health Initiative change the medical community's views on prescribing hormone replacement therapy (HRT) to women?

4. What is the language of science, and how is it different from everyday speech?

5. What are the factors that must be considered when evaluating scientific or medical information presented in the popular media?

CRITICAL THINKING QUESTIONS

1. Why is it important to include women and minority populations as subjects in clinical studies? Describe some instances where including women made a difference in the results found.

2. Discuss why it is important to consider the accomplishments of women throughout history when evaluating the state of healthcare for women today?

WEBLINKS

American Heart Association
   www.americanheart.org
American Medical Association (AMA)
   www.ama-assn.org
Center for Disease Control (CDC)
   www.cdc.gov
Department of Health and Human Services
   www.hhs.gov
Federal Food and Drug Administration (FDA)
   www.fda.gov
Human Genome Project **www.ornl.gov/sci/ techresources/Human_Genome/home.shtml**

National Institute of Health (NIH)
   www.nih.gov
Planned Parenthood Federation of America
   www.plannedparenthood.org
Society for the Advancement of Women's Health Research
   www.womenshealthresearch.org
United Nations **www.un.org**
Women's Health Initiative (WHI)
   www.whi.org
World Health Organization (WHO)
   www.who.int

REFERENCES

Agency for Healthcare Research and Quality. (2002). *Focus on research: Mental health.* AHRQ Publication No. 02-M035. Rockville, MD: Agency for Healthcare Research and Quality. Retrieved February 16, 2008 from www.ahrq. gov/research/mentalix.htm.

Agency for Healthcare Research and Quality. (2005). Fact sheet: Women's health.

Alcott, W. (1846). *The young woman's guide to excellence.* Boston, MA: Waite, Pierce and Co.

American Heart Association. (2007). *Heart disease and stroke statistics—2007 update.* Dallas, TX: American Heart Association.

American Law and Legal Information. (2009). Retrieved February 2, 2010 from http://law.jrank. org/pages/5508/Comstock-Law-1873.html.

American Medical Association. (2008). *U.S. medical school applicants and students 1982–83 to 2007–08.* Retrieved February 16, 2008 from http://www. aamc.org/data/facts/charts1982to2007.pdf. (2008, August).

Ayanian, J. Z., & Epstein, A. M. (1991). Differences in the use of procedures between women and men hospitalized for coronary artery disease. *New England Journal of Medicine, 325,* 221–225.

Beeton, I. (1861). *The book of household management.* London: S. O. Beeton.

Bell, E. C., Willson, M. C., Wilman, A. H., Dave, S., & Silverstone, P. H. (2006). Males and females differ in brain activation during cognitive tasks. *Neuroimage, 30*(2), 529–538.

Centers for Disease Control. (2006). Care in the United States - Selected findings from the 2004 National Healthcare Quality and Disparities Reports. Retrieved February 18, 2008 from http://www.cdc.gov/nccdphp/dnpa/bonehealth/

Department of Health and Human Services. OWH Fact Sheet. Retrieved February 18, 2008 from http://www.womenshealth.gov/owh/education. htm.

Department of Professional Employees. (2008). Fact sheet. Retrieved February 20, 2009 from http://dpeaflcio.org/programs-publications/issue-fact-sheets.

French, A. J., Adams, C. A., Anderson, L. S., Kitchen, J. R., Hughes, M. R., & Wood, S. H. (2008). Development of human cloned blastocysts following somatic cell nuclear transfer with adult fibroblasts. *Stem Cells, 26*(2), 485–493.

Hausmann, R., Tyson, L., & Zahidi, S. (2008). *The global gender gap report.* Geneva: World Economic Forum.

Hayes, A. H. (1869). *Sexual physiology of women and her diseases.* Boston, MA: Peabody Medical Institute.

Henderson, K. D., Sullivan-Halley, J., Reynolds, P., Horn-Ross, P.L., et al. (2008). Incomplete pregnancy is not associated with breast cancer risk: the California teachers study. *Contraception, 77,* 391–396.

Institute for Women's Policy Research. (2008). Fact sheet: The gender wage gap - 2007. IWPR No C350. Retrieved December 20, 2010 from http://iwpr.org/pdf/C350.pdf

Ivey, F. M., Tracy, B. L., Lemmer, J. T., NessAiver, M., Metter, E. J., Fozard, J. L., & Hurley, B. F. (2000). Effects of strength training and detraining on muscle quality: Age and gender comparisons. *Journals of Gerontology Series A: Biological Sciences and Medical Sciences, 55*(3), B152–157.

Melbye, M., Wohlfahrt, J., Olsen, J. H., et al. (1997). Induced abortion and the risk of breast cancer. *New England Journal of Medicine, 336,* 81–85.

Migeon, B. R. (2007). Why females are mosaics, X-chromosome inactivation, and sex differences in disease. *Medicine, 4*(2), 97–105.

Miyazaki, R., & Yamamoto, T. (2009). Sex and/or gender differences in pain. *Masui, 58*(1), 34–39.

National Cancer Institute. (2008). Abortion, miscarriage, and breast cancer risk. Retrieved May 15, 2008 from http://www.cancer.gov/cancertopics/factsheet/Risk/abortion-miscarriage.

Nuland, S. B. (2003). *The doctors' plague: Germs, childbed fever, and the strange story of Ignac Semmelweis.* New York, NY: W. W. Norton & Company.

Office of Research on Women's Health. (2009). Health insurance and women. Retrieved March 31, 2009, from http://www.4woman.gov/faq/health-insurance-women.cfm.

Paller, C. J., Campbell, C. M., Edwards, R. R., & Dobs, A. S. (2009). Sex-based differences in pain perception and treatment. *Pain Medicine, 10,* 289–299.

Pear, R. (2008, October 30). Women buying health policies pay a penalty. *New York Times,* p. A23.

Rustgi, S. D., Doty, M. M., & Collins, S. R. (2009, May). Women at risk: Why many women are forgoing needed healthcare. The Commonwealth Fund.

Save the Children. (2007). State of the world's mothers report. Retrieved February 22, 2008 from http://www.savethechildren.org/campaigns/state-of-the-worlds-mothers-report/2007/.

Save the Children. (2009). State of the world's mothers report. Retrieved February 7, 2010 from http://www.savethechildren.org/campaigns/state-of-the-worlds-mothers-report/2009/.

Steingart, R. M., Packer, M., Hamm, P., Coglianese, M. E., Gersh, B., Geltman, E. M., et al. (1991). Sex differences in the management of coronary artery disease. *New England Journal of Medicine, 325,* 226–230.

Timmons, B. W., Tarnopolsky, M. A., Snider, D. P., & Bar-Or, O. (2006). Immunological changes in response to exercise: Influence of age, puberty, and gender. *Medicine & Science in Sports & Exercise, 38,* 293–304.

Throop, P. (1998). *Hildegard von Bingen's Physica: The complete English translation of her classic work on health and healing.* Rochester, VT: Healing Arts Press.

U. S. Department of Education, National Center for Education Statistics. (2005). Postsecondary institutions in the United States: Fall 2003 and degrees and other awards conferred: 2002–2003 (NCES 2005–154).

U. S. Department of Health and Human Services. (2007, July 1). Frequently asked questions.

Wizemann, T. M., & Pardue, M. L. (Eds.) (2001). *Understanding the biology of sex and gender differences, exploring the biological contributions to human health: Does sex matter?* Washington, DC: National Academic Press.

Women's Health Initiative. (2008). Retrieved February 18, 2008 from http://www.nhlbi.nih.gov/whi/whywhi.htm.

Yazici, B., Erdoğmuş, B., & Tugay, A. (2005). Cerebral blood flow measurements of the extracranial carotid and vertebral arteries with Doppler ultrasonography in healthy adults. *Diagnostic and Interventional Radiology, 11*(4), 195–198.

Zheng, Z. J., et al. (2001). Sudden cardiac death in the United States, 1989 to 1998. *Circulation, 104*(18), 2158–2163.

chapter 2

ANATOMY AND PHYSIOLOGY: AN OVERVIEW OF A WOMAN'S BODY

CHAPTER COMPETENCIES

Upon completion of this chapter, the reader will be able to:

- Explain the importance of homeostasis
- Explain the general mechanisms that the body uses to maintain homeostasis
- Summarize the organ systems of the body

- Summarize the primary functions of each of the organ systems
- Discuss how the organ systems are interdependent on each other and how changes in one organ system can affect the other systems

KEY TERMS

anatomy
central nervous system
electrolyte
endocrine gland
endocrine system

exocrine gland
homeostasis
hormone
inflammation
negative feedback loop

non-specific defense
parasympathetic
  nervous system
peripheral nervous
  system

physiology
positive feedback loop
specific defenses
sympathetic nervous
  system

OWNER'S MANUAL FOR THE BODY

In spite of their many differences, females and males share a common body plan. In order to understand the differences that make females and males unique from each other, it is important to first understand the fundamentals of human anatomy and physiology (Figure 2-1). The study of **anatomy** concentrates on how the body is formed and the structures that make up the organ systems. **Physiology** is the study of how the tissues and organ systems work. Understanding the interactions between anatomy and physiology forms the foundation of understanding the biology of the human body.

Introduction to Homeostasis

In order to function properly, a person must maintain homeostasis. **Homeostasis** refers to the maintenance of a stable internal environment, which allows the cells and tissues of the body to function optimally. The body adjusts to the demands placed on it through homeostatic mechanisms. For example, getting caught in traffic and needing to dash across a parking lot to get to an eight o'clock appointment,

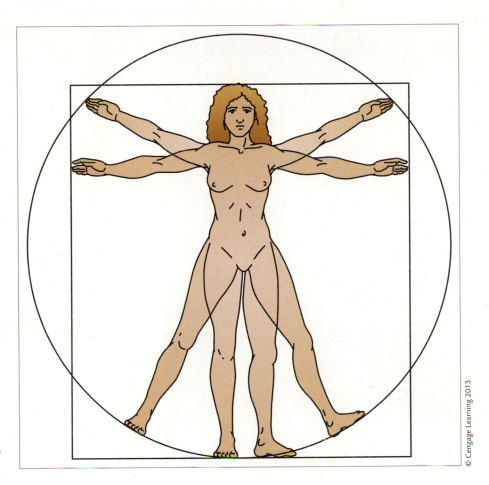

FIGURE 2-1: A female interpretation of the vitruvian man.

will trigger a series of physiological mechanisms that allow the body to adjust to the sudden demands being made upon it. The metabolic rate of the muscles increases as more energy is needed for running. Muscles use oxygen to break down organic molecules to produce energy and carbon dioxide (CO_2) in a process called aerobic respiration. Hemoglobin in the blood carries oxygen through the blood vessels to the muscles. If the muscles are not supplied with enough oxygen to sustain aerobic respiration, they will supplement their energy production with a fermentation reaction. One of the metabolic by-products of muscle fermentation is lactic acid. As lactic acid and CO_2 accumulate in the blood, they cause the pH of the blood to become more acidic, which increases hemoglobin's ability to release oxygen to the muscles. The increased acidity of the blood also stimulates chemoreceptors in the brain, which trigger an increase in the heart and breathing rates, changes which ultimately cause more oxygen to be delivered to the muscles. The increased blood flow and greater oxygen load allow the muscles to return to aerobic

respiration. Upon arriving at the appointment, and beginning to relax, the energy demands on the body decrease (Figure 2-2). Breathing and heart rates slow and buffers in the blood return the pH to normal. This intricate series of events demonstrates the complex and rapid compensations the body can achieve to maintain homeostasis.

What Defines a Healthy Woman

Despite variation between women, there are ranges of physiological measurements that are considered healthy. The average woman, for example, has four and a half to five million red blood cells per cubic millimeter of blood. Her blood pH is usually between 7.35 and 7.45. At rest, the average woman breathes 15 to 20 times per minute, and each breath moves 500 cubic centimeters of air. Her heart beats roughly 70 times per minute. Throughout a typical day, carbohydrates, proteins, and lipids are digested, absorbed and carried through the blood to all parts of the body. As cells break down nutrients to make energy, they generate heat, which combined

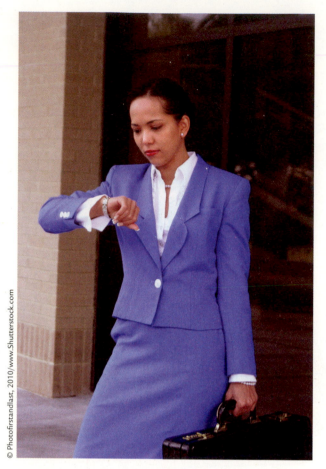

FIGURE 2-2: Homeostasis is the process that allows the body to adjust to environmental demands. It allows the body to meet sudden needs for exertion, and then to relax and return to normal levels when the need for increased energy has passed.

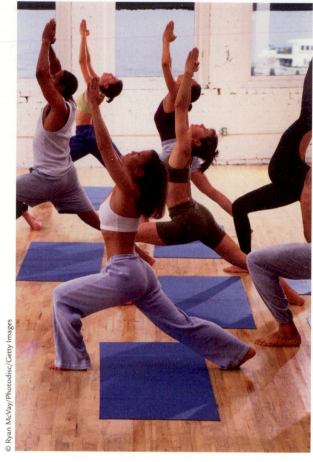

FIGURE 2-3: While there are average parameters for many physiological processes, there is no absolute definition of a "healthy woman." Each individual has values that define normal for her.

with the insulation provided by fat stored under the skin, maintains a body temperature of approximately 37°C.

Few people, if any, fit the normal values perfectly (Figure 2-3). Some women have a body temperature slightly above 37°C (98.6°F) and some are slightly below. Some women breathe more slowly, but each breath is deeper than average. Some women burn 3000 calories a day; others need only 1000 to maintain their body weight. Fluid and electrolyte levels have narrower ranges of variation. **Electrolytes** are the essential chemicals in the blood such as sodium, potassium and calcium ions. Each person has values that define "normal" for them.

In addition to the individual variations that exist, shifts from "normal" occur with changes in activity level, diet, age, and environmental conditions. If it is hot out, body temperature rises. If it is cold, a person

can become hypothermic. If the woman is in good health and the shifts are not too extreme, homeostatic mechanisms work to keep the body within normal ranges. Disease occurs when homeostatic mechanisms fail to return the body back to these normal ranges.

Feedback Loops

Typically, the body maintains homeostasis through systems called feedback loops. A feedback loop is a series of interconnected signals and reactions that coordinate with each other in a predictable pattern. Two patterns predominate: negative feedback loops and positive feedback loops. In the case of **negative feedback loops**, conditions in the body are maintained around a "normal" set point. Negative feedback loops work like the thermostat in a house. Imagine the thermostat set at 65°F. When the temperature in the house drops to 60 °F, the furnace turns on and stays on until the temperature reaches 70 °F. The furnace then shuts off, and when the temperature drops again to 60 °F, the cycle repeats. This on-off pattern keeps the average temperature around 65 °F. Likewise, if a person steps out into a snow-storm without a coat, their body temperature will begin to drop. Temperature sensors in the skin will relay a message to the brain about the temperature drop. The brain will then send a message via the nervous system, causing the muscles to begin shivering, an activity that will bring the body temperature back up to the normal range, at which point the shivering will stop. In this way, negative feedback loops are self-regulating.

With **positive feedback loops**, the effects of the mechanisms that are triggered keep building until some influence outside the feedback loop shuts it off. Positive feedback loops move the body farther away from homeostasis, at least temporarily, and are used less often than negative feedback loops. There are two positive feedback loops that are well documented in the human body. The first is labor and delivery of a baby; the other is the process of ovulation. When labor begins, the hormone oxytocin causes muscle contractions in the uterus. The muscle contracts against the baby, releasing a hormone-like chemical called prostaglandin. Prostaglandin causes both dilation of the cervix and the secretion of more oxytocin by the brain. More oxytocin causes an increase in contractions, which results in the release of more prostaglandin, and, in turn, more oxytocin. The process continues building in intensity until the baby is delivered and there is nothing left for the uterus to contract against. Here the delivery of the baby is the outside event that stops the feedback loop.

OVERVIEW OF THE BODY SYSTEMS

There are eleven organ systems that cooperate to maintain homeostasis. Two systems, the nervous system and the endocrine system are responsible for communication between all of the other organ systems. These two systems also regulate the other systems, and make a good starting point for understanding how the body works.

Nervous System

The nervous system (Figure 2-4) is the body's link to the world, both internal and external. The functional unit in the nervous system is the nerve cell, which is also called a neuron. Each neuron has dendrites that pick up sensations, a body with a nucleus as a control center, and at least one extension called an axon that passes information to the next neuron (Figure 2-5). Between the axon of one neuron and the dendrite of another there is a space called the synapse. Neurons communicate with one another by releasing chemicals

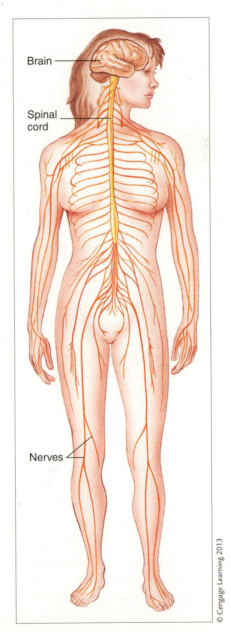

Brain

Spinal cord

Nerves

© Cengage Learning 2013

FIGURE 2-4: The Nervous System (brain, spinal cord, and nerves).

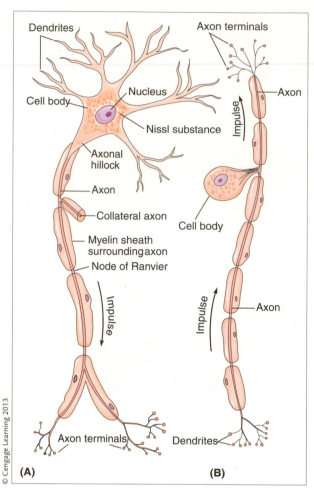

Dendrites

Axon terminals

Cell body

Nucleus

Nissl substance

Axonal hillock

Axon

Collateral axon

Cell body

Myelin sheath surrounding axon

Node of Ranvier

Impulse

Axon

Axon

Impulse

Impulse

Impulse

Axon terminals

Dendrites

(A)   (B)

© Cengage Learning 2013

FIGURE 2-5: Two types of structural neurons: (A) multipolar (B) unipolar.

called neurotransmitters into the synapse between neurons. Neurons can also synapse with muscles, organs, or glands. Axons from many individual neurons are bundled together to form nerves.

The nervous system is divided by structure and by function. Neurons found in the brain and spinal cord make up the **central nervous system** (CNS), and all of the other neurons in the body make up the **peripheral nervous system** (PNS). The function of the CNS is to process information and to issue responses in the form of motor commands. The peripheral nervous system can be divided into the sensory and motor nervous systems. Sensory nerves pick up information from receptors and deliver it to the CNS. Motor nerves carry instructions or motor commands from the CNS out to the responding tissues, including the skeletal muscles. Motor commands to the skeletal muscles are further classified as voluntary because they can be

initiated by conscious thought. Autonomic neurons, in contrast carry motor commands to smooth muscles, organs, and glands, triggering them to increase or decrease their activities. Autonomic motor commands are not under conscious control.

Autonomic nerves can be further subdivided into the **sympathetic nervous system** and the **parasympathetic nervous system**. The sympathetic response is known as a "fight or flight" response. When this response is activated, the body gears up to either fight off or run away from a threatening stimulus and experiences a surge of adrenalin (Figure 2-6). Heart rate, blood pressure, and breathing rates increase. Blood shifts away from the digestive, urinary, and reproductive systems to the brain and skeletal muscles to facilitate fighting or running away. Pain responses decrease, but other sensory responses become more sensitive. In addition, muscles respond more quickly. When the body is under the control of the sympathetic nervous system, there is likely to be a startle response. Parasympathetic responses, in contrast, bring the body back to a calm state. Only necessary nerves fire and the body relaxes. Breathing slows, while heart rate and blood pressure decrease. Systems which were temporarily suppressed during a sympathetic response begin to function fully again. The digestive, urinary, immune, and reproductive systems all work to their full capacity under the influence of the parasympathetic nervous system. A person's mood becomes calm rather than tense. Most organs and tissues in the body receive signals from both sympathetic and parasympathetic nerves. In this way, their functions can be enhanced or diminished by the autonomic nervous system according to circumstances.

Endocrine System

The **endocrine system** is a collection of glands that function to regulate the body through hormones. Two master glands, the hypothalamus and the pituitary gland, regulate the production of many of the hormones by the other glands. There are two kinds of glands, endocrine and exocrine. **Exocrine glands** have ducts through which their products are secreted to the outside of the body. For example, the mammary glands and sweat glands are considered exocrine because they have ducts that lead to the outside of

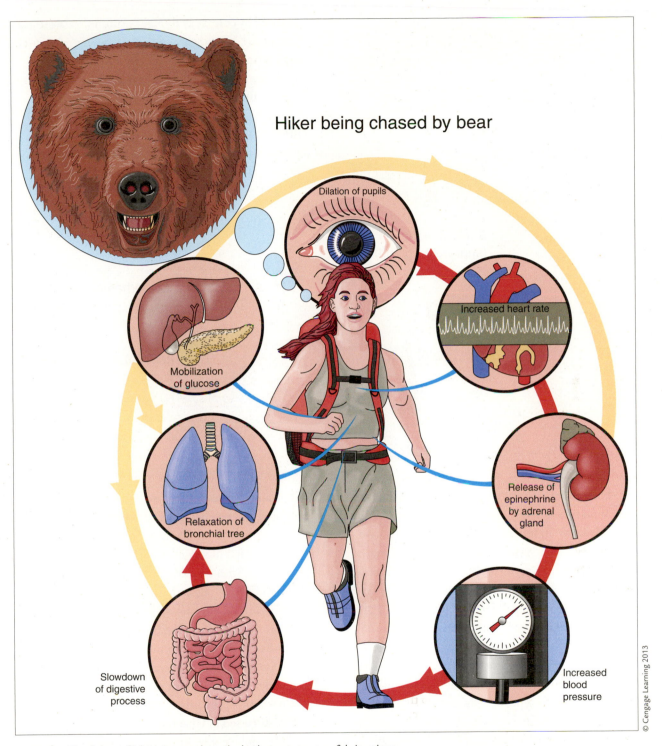

FIGURE 2-6: The fight or flight response: how the body reacts to stressful situations.

the body. **Endocrine glands** produce hormones and secrete them into the surrounding tissues and into the bloodstream to be delivered to distant tissues (Figure 2-7). To complicate matters further, some glands have both exocrine and endocrine functions. The pancreas is a good example. The exocrine cells of the pancreas secrete digestive enzymes into the lumen of the small intestine, which in anatomical terms is considered the outside of the body. The endocrine cells in the pancreas secrete the hormones insulin and glucagon into the bloodstream. These hormones work together to regulate blood sugar levels.

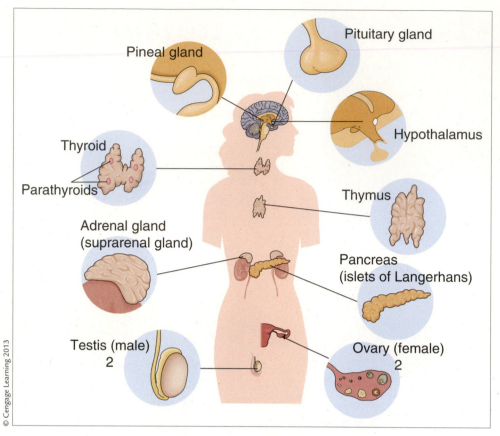

Pineal gland

Pituitary gland

Thyroid

Parathyroids

Hypothalamus

Thymus

Adrenal gland
(suprarenal gland)

Pancreas
(islets of Langerhans)

Testis (male)
2

Ovary (female)
2

© Cengage Learning 2013

FIGURE 2-7: Structures of the Endocrine System.

Hormones travel through the bloodstream until they bind to target cells that can respond to that specific hormone. In some cases these target cells have receptors on their surface which act as a docking station for the hormone. In other cases, hormones diffuse directly in the cells to trigger a response. Some hormones target many different kinds of cells. For example, human growth hormone can bind to and stimulate growth in every cell in the body. Thyroid hormones also influence metabolism in almost all of the cells throughout the body. Other hormones bind to only a few types of cells. Thyroid stimulating hormone (TSH), for example, only binds to specialized cells in the thyroid gland, where it stimulates the production and release of thyroid hormone.

Specific Hormones and their Roles

Commonly, when people think about hormones, they think about the fluctuating hormones experienced by adolescents going through puberty. Specifically, they think about the effects of the sex hormones estrogen and testosterone. However, the body uses a wide range

of hormones to accomplish diverse functions, many unrelated to reproduction. For example, a non-reproductive hormone familiar to most people is insulin, which regulates blood glucose levels. Many people are also familiar with thyroid hormones, which play an important role in regulating metabolic rate. Table 2-1 describes several hormones, their source and target, and their primary effects on the body. This is by no means an exhaustive list of the hormones produced by the body. Scientists continue to discover new hormones and find new functions for previously identified ones. The hormones primarily associated with reproduction will be discussed in Chapter 4.

Hormone concentrations in the blood depend on several factors and represent a balance between hormone production and hormone deactivation and excretion. On one side of the equation is the production and release of the hormones. Hormone precursors can be manufactured by the body or taken in via the diet. The production and secretion of many hormones can be stimulated by messages from the nervous system, or by the presence of releasing,

Table 2-1 A sample of hormones.

Hormone	Source	Target	Action
parathyroid hormone (PTH)	parathyroid glands	osteoclasts (bone dissolving cells)	disassemble bone / increase blood calcium levels
calcitonin	thyroid	osteoblasts (bone building cells)	increase bone formation / decreases blood calcium levels
growth hormone	anterior pituitary	all cells	increased cell growth
adrenalin	adrenal medulla	sympathetic nervous system	fight or flight response/ increased respiration, heart rate and blood pressure
aldosterone	adrenal cortex	nephron	fluid and electrolyte balance
antidiuretic hormone (ADH)	pituitary	nephron	water retention, increase blood pressure
insulin	pancreas	all cells	move glucose and amino acids into cells; decrease blood sugar
glucagon	pancreas	liver & skeletal muscle	break down glycogen stores to increase blood glucose
cortisol	adrenal cortex	all cells	stress response/ raises blood sugar; alters lipid metabolism/ depresses immune function

© Cengage Learning 2013

stimulating, or inhibiting hormones from the hypothalamus or pituitary gland. On the other side of the equation, some hormones are inactivated by the target tissue. Others are excreted by the kidneys or removed by the liver. Most hormones are regulated by negative feedback loops that involve the hypothalamus, pituitary, and other endocrine glands. A change in homeostasis causes the release of hormones that stimulate a metabolic change to correct the imbalance. When homeostasis is restored, hormone levels drop until homeostasis is disturbed again.

Hormone Interactions

Hormones usually work in conjunction with other hormones as part of a negative feedback loop to maintain homeostasis. These feedback loops can be relatively simple or they can be quite complex, depending on the number of hormones involved. The interactions between hormones usually occur within three major patterns: permissive, synergistic, and antagonistic. A good example of the permissive effect is demonstrated by the interactions between thyroid

releasing hormone (TRH), thyroid stimulating hormone (TSH), and the thyroid hormones. When the level of TRH secreted by the hypothalamus increases, it triggers the increased release of TSH from the pituitary gland. This increase in TSH secretion then stimulates the thyroid gland to increase its secretion of thyroid hormone.

Several hormones act simultaneously to produce a synergistic effect. For example, glandular tissues in the breast must be stimulated by the coordinated activity of the hormones prolactin, estrogen, progesterone, insulin, thyroid hormone, and growth hormone to begin to produce milk. Lactation occurs only when all of these hormones are present in the correct concentrations in the bloodstream.

Two hormones with opposing effects are referred to as antagonistic. Antagonistic hormones work in opposition to each other to maintain overall homeostasis. Often antagonistic hormones work together to keep nutrient, fluid, or electrolyte levels in the blood within target ranges. The hormones insulin and glucagon work antagonistically with each other to maintain blood glucose levels. Insulin lowers blood glucose levels by moving glucose out of the bloodstream and into the cells. Glucagon raises blood glucose levels by breaking down glycogen, a stored carbohydrate in the body, and releasing the resulting glucose back into the blood. One hormone raises and the other lowers blood glucose levels, and together they keep the blood glucose within healthy levels.

Hormone Imbalances

To maintain healthy function, hormones must be present within proper concentration ranges in the bloodstream. Either excessive or inadequate levels of hormones can result in disease. Because hormones work together in permissive, synergistic, and antagonistic patterns, it can sometimes be difficult to pinpoint what the source of a hormonal imbalance might be. In general, disturbances in hormone function fall into two categories: hypofunction or hyperfunction.

Hypofunction   Hypofunction is a decrease in hormone function and can range from a minor hormone deficit to a complete lack of hormone activity. Inadequate hormone levels can result from hyposecretion or from hormone resistance. In the case of hyposecretion, the amount of hormone secreted by the endocrine gland falls below the usual level. Often hyposecretion of one hormone is accompanied by sharp rises in the levels of stimulating or releasing hormones that would normally trigger the production and release of the hormone in question. Hyposecretion can occur when the diet is lacking the precursors needed to make hormones. For example, hyposecretion of thyroid hormone can be caused by a diet deficient in iodine, since iodine is an important component of thyroid hormone. Hyposecretion can also occur when a gland fails to develop. Without the gland, there is no hormone production or secretion. Atrophy of the endocrine gland may also cause hyposecretion. For example, one of the side effects of taking testosterone-based anabolic steroids is testicular atrophy. The anabolic steroid participates in the feedback loop, causing a drop in three hormones: GnRH (gonadotropin releasing factor), LH (luteinizing hormone), and FSH (follicle stimulating hormone). Without FSH and LH, the testes atrophy, and the body stops making its own testosterone. Tumors,

inflammation, autoimmune conditions and infection may also cause hyposecretion by physically disrupting the action of the gland responsible for manufacturing and secreting a specific hormone.

Hypothyroidism is a good example of a disease caused by hyposecretion of hormones; in this case, the undersecretion of thyroid hormone. Women exhibit higher rates of hypothyroidism. In the case of hypothyroidism, the metabolic rate is decreased; producing weight gain, decreased healing, slowed reflexes, excessively dry skin and fatigue. Another familiar example of endocrine hypofunction is Type 1 diabetes. This form of diabetes results from the undersecretion of insulin by the pancreas.

Hormone resistance is another cause of hormone hypofunction. In this case, receptors on the target tissue may not be able to bind with the hormone in question, preventing the hormone from having an effect. A classic example of hormone resistance is Type 2 diabetes. When a prolonged diet of simple sugars keeps insulin levels elevated for long periods of time, the receptors on target cells display fatigue and fail to respond to the insulin. This creates a situation in which blood glucose levels remain elevated, even in the presence of normal levels of insulin in the blood.

Hyperfunction   Hyperfunction usually occurs when endocrine glands secrete too much hormone and the high circulating levels of hormone produce an exaggerated response. In some cases, chemicals in the body mimic releasing hormones, binding to the receptor sites in the endocrine glands and causing them to release excess hormone. Hyperfunction can be caused by endocrine tumors or a failure of the negative feedback mechanism that regulates hormone secretion. A good example is the oversecretion of thyroid hormones, which can lead to Grave's disease, a form of hyperthyroidism. The excess thyroid hormones increase metabolism throughout the body causing elevated heart rate, anxiety, insomnia, excessive weight loss, exaggerated reflexes, and heat intolerance. Women are more likely than men to develop Grave's disease.

Integumentary System

In humans, the integumentary system is made up of the skin and the accessory structures such as the hair and finger nails. Other species of mammals have additional types of accessory structures such as horns, antlers, tusks, and even scales in the case of armadillos. People probably have more awareness of their integument than of any other organ system of the body because it is the most visible. There is a popular misconception that the skin is the largest organ. However, in terms of surface area, the lungs, the circulatory system, and the digestive tract are larger. The skin functions as the primary barrier between the outside environment and the body inside, protecting against thermal, chemical, and physical injury. Relatively waterproof, the skin allows the body to exist in dry air without losing too much water by evaporation and to be immersed in water without appreciably swelling. Because it is abundantly supplied with nerve endings, the skin acts as an enormous sense organ, constantly receiving information from its surface for transmission to the brain. Finally, the skin and the accessory structures serve the important function of creating a person's individual appearance, which makes a person recognizable and distinguishable from others. The integumentary system will be discussed in more detail in Chapter 18.

Skeletal System

The skeleton provides support for the body. Tendons attach skeletal muscles to the bones and the muscles act as pulleys to produce movement. The bones also act as storage sites for important minerals such as calcium, magnesium, and phosphorus. The marrow in the long bones of an adult contains yellow marrow, a form of stored fat that is one of the last reserves drawn upon under starvation conditions. The red bone marrow produces blood cells, including red blood cells, white blood cells, and platelets. The axial skeleton consists of the skull, vertebrae, sternum, and ribs. The axial skeleton shelters the essential organs such as the brain, heart and lungs, protecting them from potential injury. The appendicu-

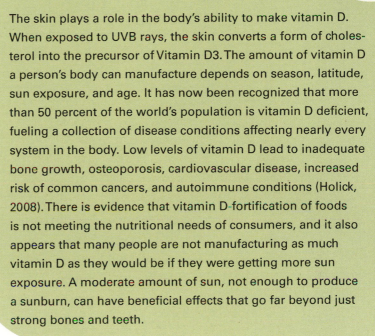

focus on

NUTRITION

Vitamin D, Sun Exposure, and Health

The skin plays a role in the body's ability to make vitamin D. When exposed to UVB rays, the skin converts a form of cholesterol into the precursor of Vitamin D3. The amount of vitamin D a person's body can manufacture depends on season, latitude, sun exposure, and age. It has now been recognized that more than 50 percent of the world's population is vitamin D deficient, fueling a collection of disease conditions affecting nearly every system in the body. Low levels of vitamin D lead to inadequate bone growth, osteoporosis, cardiovascular disease, increased risk of common cancers, and autoimmune conditions (Holick, 2008). There is evidence that vitamin D-fortification of foods is not meeting the nutritional needs of consumers, and it also appears that many people are not manufacturing as much vitamin D as they would be if they were getting more sun exposure. A moderate amount of sun, not enough to produce a sunburn, can have beneficial effects that go far beyond just strong bones and teeth.

lar skeleton includes all of the other bones and it is primarily involved in the movement of the limbs. The major bones of the skeleton are identified in Figure 2-8.

Bone Growth, Repair, and Maintenance

Bone tissue is a composite matrix of collagen protein and hydroxyapatite minerals with living cells dispersed throughout. The collagen protein gives bones some flexibility and prevents them from shattering under pressure, while the mineral calcium apatite makes the bones rigid so that they do not bow under the weight of the body. Three types of bone cells, the osteoblasts, the osteoclasts, and the osteocytes, contribute to the growth, repair, and maintenance of the bone tissues (Figure 2-9). Osteoblasts are cells that build new bone tissue by laying down new collagen fibers and then coating them with the mineral hydroxyapatite. Osteoclasts are cells that destroy old, damaged, or brittle bone tissues, so that osteoblasts can replace them with new bone tissue. Osteocytes maintain mature bone.

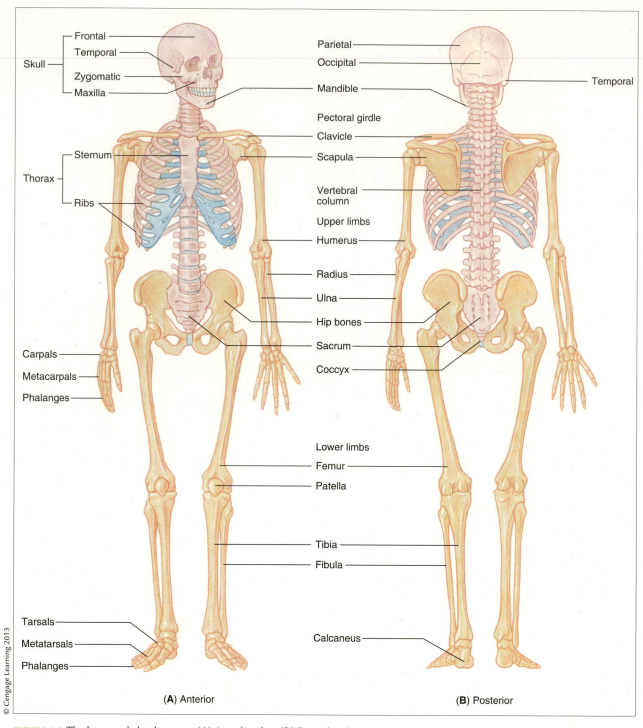

Skull
- Frontal
- Temporal
- Zygomatic
- Maxilla

Thorax
- Sternum
- Ribs

Carpals
Metacarpals
Phalanges

Tarsals
Metatarsals
Phalanges

Parietal
Occipital
Mandible
Pectoral girdle
Clavicle
Scapula
Vertebral column
Upper limbs
Humerus
Radius
Ulna
Hip bones
Sacrum
Coccyx
Lower limbs
Femur
Patella
Tibia
Fibula
Calcaneus

Temporal

(A) Anterior

(B) Posterior

© Cengage Learning 2013

FIGURE 2-8: The human skeletal system: (A) Anterior view (B) Posterior view.

The bone matrix is arranged in layers called lamellae, around a central canal which contains blood vessels and nerves. If the lamellae are tightly packed, the bone is referred to as compact bone (Figure 2-10). Spongy bone contains pockets between the irregularly spaced lamellae, giving it a spongy appearance. These pockets contain bone marrow.

The growth of bone depends on a number of factors, including diet, exercise and the actions of a variety of hormones. Calcium, magnesium, phosphorus, proteins, and vitamins C and D must be present in the diet in adequate amounts for bones to grow properly. Vitamin C is important for depositing collagen, the major protein component of bones. Vitamin D is

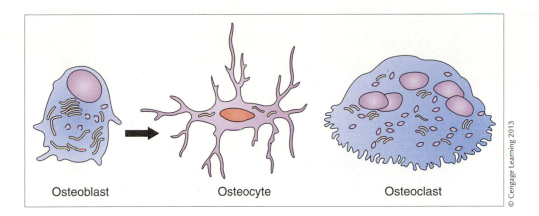

FIGURE 2-9: The different types of bone cells.

Osteoblast   Osteocyte   Osteoclast

© Cengage Learning 2013

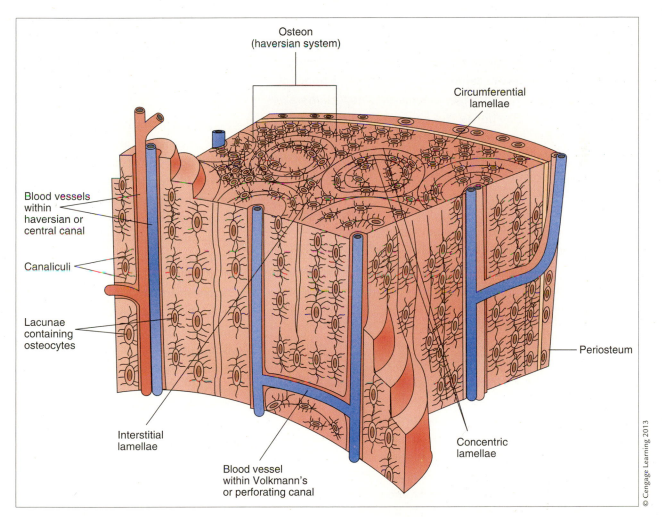

Osteon
(haversian system)

Circumferential
lamellae

Blood vessels
within
haversian or
central canal

Canaliculi

Lacunae
containing
osteocytes

Periosteum

Interstitial
lamellae

Concentric
lamellae

Blood vessel
within Volkmann's
or perforating canal

© Cengage Learning 2013

FIGURE 2-10: The microscopic structure of bone.

necessary for calcium absorption from the intestines. An imbalance in any of the bone components can weaken the bones.

Several hormones play a role in bone formation. Calcitonin, one of the hormones secreted by the thyroid gland, is responsible for stimulat-ing the osteoblasts. Parathyroid hormone, from the parathyroid glands, moves calcium out of the bone and into the blood for other functions such as muscle contraction, blood clotting, and nerve function. The antagonistic interactions between the two hormones maintain blood calcium levels

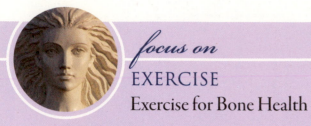

focus on

EXERCISE
Exercise for Bone Health

Aging can bring with it a loss of bone mineral density causing bones to become more fragile. This condition, called osteoporosis, is a major cause of disability in older women, although men can be affected too. Compression fractures in the spine that result from bones becoming too weak to support the body can lead to a stooped posture, and lack of flexibility. Exercise throughout the lifetime, including into old age, is important to maintain and preserve adequate bone density. There are several types of exercise that are beneficial for maintaining bone density. Weight-bearing exercises including aerobic activities such as walking, dancing, gardening, and low impact aerobics put a strain on the bones of the skeleton which stimulates the osteoblasts to deposit more minerals to reinforce the bones. These types of exercises also provide benefits to the cardiovascular system and help to prevent heart disease. Swimming, although it does provide cardiovascular benefits, is not a weight-bearing exercise so it does not benefit the bones directly.

Strength training, which includes using free weight, weight machines, resistance bands, or weight-bearing exercises can stimulate the osteoblasts and help bones maintain their density. These exercises can also strengthen the muscles that maintain posture, thus preventing some of the strain that can lead to compression fractures in the spine. Flexibility exercises such as stretches can also contribute to better posture, and less strain on the bones. These exercises also help to maintain range of motion, which makes other activities easier and more enjoyable.

New research indicates that weight-bearing exercise combined with consuming soy isoflavone is more effective for building bone density than either of these alone. Soy products, chick peas, and alfalfa are common sources of isoflavone. Research also indicates that a combination of walking 45 minutes per day, three days per week, and consuming soy isoflavone can improve cardiovascular health as well (Aubertin-Leheudre et al., 2007). It is important to maintain the exercise routine however, as the benefits from exercise disappear within five years after exercise ceases (Evans et al., 2007).

density. Osteoblasts respond strongly to estrogen. One reason women are, on average, shorter than men is their difference in estrogen levels. The epiphyseal plates, which are also called growth plates, in a girl's bones grow faster and seal much earlier than those in boys because of the higher concentrations of estrogen in her blood. Consequently, she will complete her growth earlier while her bones are still somewhat shorter. At menopause, decreased estrogen initially slows osteoblast activity for a time period of about five years. After that, the body compensates for the decrease in estrogen, and the rate of bone loss decreases.

Mechanical stress caused by work or exercise is another factor that affects bone growth and maintenance. Increased mechanical stress in the form of weight-bearing exercise increases the activity of the osteoblasts, resulting in increased bone density. Bone density overall is typically greater in males. Men typically have a larger body frame than women and carry more weight, which helps them to maintain bone density as they age. However, larger women also share this advantage. To maintain their bone density, women can engage in weight-bearing exercise. When bone density declines to a level that endangers the integrity of the bone, the result is called osteoporosis. Osteoporosis can be a seriously debilitating disease for women and for men, and will be addressed in Chapter 15.

Skeletal Differences Between Men and Women

There are several differences between the male and female skeleton, and these differences are related to adaptations for childbearing. For example, differences can be observed in

within normal ranges. Human growth hormone, estrogen, and testosterone all stimulate the lengthening of bones, and contribute to maintaining bone the shape of the pelvis, the femur, and the knee joint. The female pelvis is generally wider than the male pelvis and tipped forward slightly. This configuration allows for the maximum opening at the pelvic outlet, which is important for the delivery of infants through the birth canal. In addition, the subpubic angle – the angle under the pubic symphysis – is usually greater than 90° degrees in a woman and less than 90° in a male. Figure 2-11 shows the differences between a female and a male pelvis.

The wider pelvis in a woman moves the position of her femur laterally. If a woman's femur formed a 90° angle to the pelvis, her knees would be several centimeters apart, and she would walk with a waddle. To compensate for the wider pelvis, the female femur angles inward, allowing the knees to be situated closer to the midline of the body. In addition to the pelvic and femoral differences, there are variations in bone density and ridge formation. Typically, the brow ridges, jaw, and bony protuberances for muscle attachment are more prominent in males.

The Muscular System

Most people are familiar with skeletal muscles that attach to the bones and are responsible for the movement of the head, trunk, and limbs. However, the human body has three distinct types of muscles – skeletal muscle, smooth muscle, and cardiac muscle. Each muscle type has unique characteristics with regard to both structure and contractility. The three types of muscle also differ in the degree to which they are controlled by conscious thought or by the autonomic nervous system.

Skeletal Muscle   Skeletal muscles connect to bones, and when they contract, they shorten and exert a pulling force on the bones, causing movement (Figure 2-12). These muscles will not contract without a signal from the brain or spinal cord. Skeletal muscles are also called voluntary muscles because their contraction can be initiated by conscious thought. In addition to causing movement, skeletal muscles also generate heat and play a major role in the maintenance of body temperature.

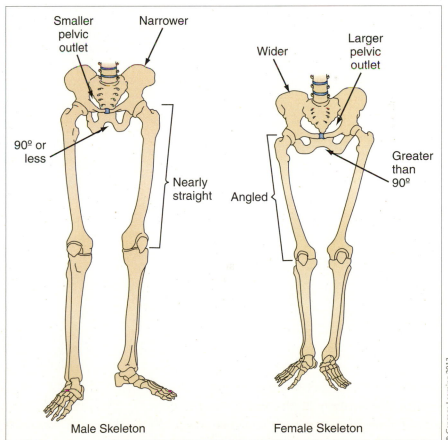

FIGURE 2-11: The primary differences between the male and female skeleton can be seen in the pelvic bones and femur.

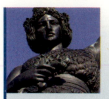

Historical Considerations
THE HISTORY OF DOMESTIC VIOLENCE

In medieval times, husbands were expected to physically chastise their wives, and this was not considered out of the ordinary. In fact, the phrase 'rule of thumb' came about through the English common law tradition, summarized by William Blackstone in 1767 as the ancient right that permits a husband to chastise his wife with a whip or [stick] no bigger than his thumb (Van Hasselt, 1988). Social institutions, including government and religious institutions, more often than not condoned and supported domestic violence, seeing a husband's 'discipline' of his wife as a necessary duty. Rape of one's wife was not considered to be rape at all, as husbands were seen as being immune from such culpability. The traditional definition of rape was 'sexual intercourse with a female not his wife without her consent' (Bovarnick, 2006). In 1867, a North Carolina Court ruled in one case where a man beat his wife that: "If no permanent injury has been inflicted, nor malice nor dangerous violence shown by the husband, it is better to draw the curtain, shut out the public gaze, and leave the parties to forget and forgive" (NiCarthy, 2004).

Domestic violence in the United States was, and continues to be a phenomenon which is fuelled by unequal power relationships between women and men, and which indicated women's lower status within society. In the United States, it was not until 1871 that domestic violence was first outlawed – and then only in two States, Alabama and Massachusetts (Renzetti & Edleson, 2008). It was not until almost a hundred years later, during the women's movement of the late 1960s and 1970s, that advocates were able to begin to truly change public consciousness about the pervasive problem of domestic violence. At the time, domestic violence was largely seen as a family problem, and not as a crime. Feminists have long understood that domestic violence is overwhelmingly (although not exclusively) committed by men against women, and

that domestic violence cannot be understood properly without a sociological understanding of gender inequality and oppression. In 1974, the first shelter for battered women was established, and today there exist hundreds of battered women's shelters throughout the United States (Renzetti & Edleson, 2008).

Today, legal, medical, and community responses to domestic violence have improved, and so too has our knowledge of the fundamental dynamics of abusive relationships. We know that domestic violence is about much more than physical abuse, but that it includes controlling and belittling behavior, including coercion and threats, intimidation, emotional abuse, isolation, minimizing, denying and blaming, economic abuse, using children, and using male privilege for advantage (NiCarthy, 2004). It can take a long time for a woman to leave a violent relationship. In fact, a woman often leaves her abusive partner seven or eight times before she is finally able to leave for good (NiCarthy, 2004).

Anti-domestic activists around the country work hard to raise awareness about domestic violence in their communities, all the while changing attitudes that condone it, and reaching out to women caught in its cycle. While domestic violence has a long history, the battle against domestic violence is sadly not a thing of the past. Today, worldwide, violence against women at the hands of intimate partners continues to be a leading cause of ill-health (and death) of women. In the United States, domestic violence affects two to four million women every year, and an average of 2,000 women every year die at the hands of their abusive partners. There is a lot that can be done to stop domestic violence. If you or someone you know is in a violent relationship, you can get help. Seek advice from a local battered women's shelter or call the National Domestic Violence hotline at 1-800-799-SAFE.

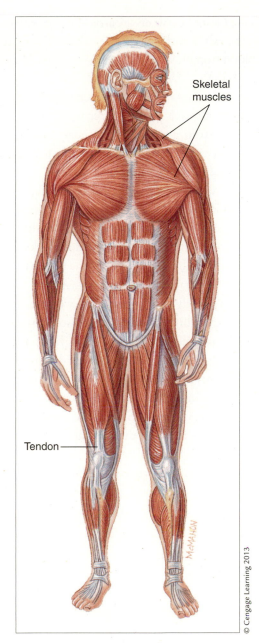

FIGURE 2-12: The muscles and tendons of the skeletal system.

Smooth Muscle   Smooth muscle is found in the walls of the blood vessels, and is also a component of the walls of many of the organs in the body. This type of muscle is under the control of the autonomic nervous system and is not under conscious control. In addition, smooth muscle can contract in response to stretching, without input from the nervous system. The uterus is an example of an organ that is composed primarily of smooth muscle. It has a tremendous capacity to stretch to accommodate a growing fetus. It also has the capacity for the strong contractions that are required to deliver a baby. Menstrual cramps represent less powerful contractions of the smooth muscles that make up the uterine walls.

Cardiac Muscle   Cardiac muscle is only found in the heart. Cardiac muscle is unique because individual cardiac muscle cells can communicate with each other and coordinate their contractions in the absence of nervous stimulation. In addition, heart muscle cell that is removed from the body will continue contracting spontaneously for a short period of time, in the absence of any nerves or hormones. However, unlike other muscles in the body, cardiac muscle requires a constant and uninterrupted supply of oxygen or the cells will die. Any decreases in the supply of oxygen to the heart muscle creates problems ranging from angina, which is pain and cramping of the heart muscle, to cardiac cell death, known as a heart attack or myocardial infarction.

Cardiovascular System

The cardiovascular system consists of the heart, the blood vessels, and the blood that flows through them (Figure 2-13). The cardiovascular system is also referred to as the circulatory system. This system acts as a supply network, delivering oxygen, nutrients, hormones, and other building materials to all of the cells in the body, while simultaneously transporting waste products of cell metabolism to the liver, kidneys, or lungs for removal from the body. This system is so essential to maintaining homeostasis that it is one of the first organ systems to begin functioning during fetal development delivering nutrients to and removing wastes from the developing fetus. At the other end of the lifespan, cardiovascular disease is a major cause of mortality for women over 50, especially in cultures where a sedentary lifestyle is common. The estrogen that a woman produces from puberty until menopause protects her from many of the factors that contribute to heart disease, which explains why heart attacks are rare in premenopausal women, and more common in postmenopausal women. Lacking high levels of estrogen, men are more likely to develop cardiovascular disease at a younger age.

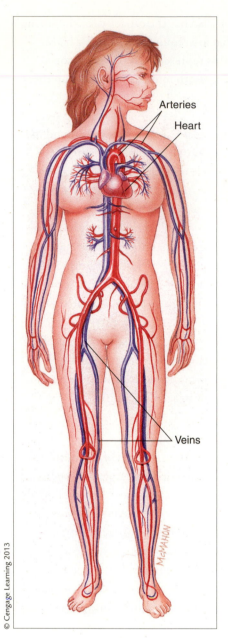

Arteries

Heart

Veins

© Cengage Learning 2013

FIGURE 2-13: The heart and blood vessels of the circulatory system. The vessels carrying oxygen-rich blood are shown in red. Those with oxygen-poor blood are in blue.

The Heart

The heart is a hollow, muscular organ that consists of four chambers, including two smaller chambers called atria and two larger chambers called ventricles. Blood enters the heart through the atria, and leaves the heart from the ventricles. The ventricles are made up of thick walls of cardiac muscle, and when they contract they create enough pressure to push the blood out of the heart to the farthest reaches of the body. Flexible

valves are located between the atria and the ventricles and at the exit points from the ventricles. These prevent blood from flowing backwards through the heart (Figure 2-14).

The heart does not derive its sustenance from the blood that travels through its chambers with each heartbeat. Instead, a network of coronary vessels covers the surface of the heart and brings needed oxygen and nutrients to the cardiac muscles. The coronary vessels also remove metabolic wastes generated by the heart. Coronary vessels can become blocked, either through a buildup of cholesterol deposits inside the vessels or because a blood clot blocks the flow of blood. If this occurs the cardiac tissues that are supplied by that vessel will become starved for oxygen and quickly die. Cardiac muscle does not regenerate after this kind of cell death, so damage that is done to the heart is permanent. This type of tissue death is called an infarct, and the disruption to normal heart function that this damage causes is called a myocardial infarction, or a heart attack. High levels of circulating estrogen hormones in women have a protective effect on the coronary vessels, and they also help to keep cholesterol levels lower, making women less prone to heart attacks prior to menopause. At menopause, however, estrogen levels begin to diminish, and women's rates of heart disease begin to match that of men.

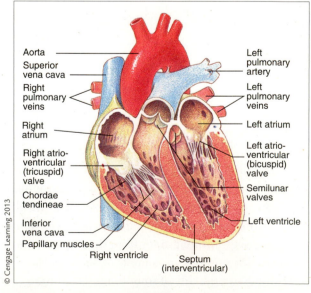

Aorta

Superior vena cava

Right pulmonary veins

Right atrium

Right atrio-ventricular (tricuspid) valve

Chordae tendineae

Inferior vena cava

Papillary muscles

Right ventricle

Septum (interventricular)

Left pulmonary artery

Left pulmonary veins

Left atrium

Left atrio-ventricular (bicuspid) valve

Semilunar valves

Left ventricle

© Cengage Learning 2013

FIGURE 2-14: The structure of the human heart.

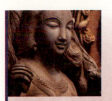

Social Considerations

HORMONE REPLACEMENT THERAPY AND CARDIOVASCULAR DISEASE IN WOMEN

Women are naturally protected from heart disease by their high circulating levels of estrogen. By the time women reach menopause in their forties or fifties, they become as vulnerable as men to suffering a fatal heart attack. For decades it was believed that hormone replacement therapy (HRT), prescribed to women to relieve menopause symptoms, would also protect postmenopausal women from heart disease. In 1991, the National Heart, Lung and Blood Institute (NHLBI) began the Women's Health Initiative, one of the largest studies of its kind to carefully examine the effects of ERT and HRT on women's risks for breast cancer, strokes, heart attack, blood clots, colorectal cancer, and bone fractures due to osteoporosis. Although the trials were meant to follow women's health from 1991 to 2005, the trials were stopped early because overwhelming evidence indicated the risks associated with using HRT outweighed the benefits.

While HRT was shown to reduce the risk of developing colorectal cancer or fractures due to osteoporosis, the risk of suffering a heart attack while using HRT increased by 29 percent, the risk of blood clots doubled, and the risk of stroke increased by 41 percent. Breast cancer risk was also increased with HRT. ERT protected women from bone fractures, but increased their risk of stroke by 39 percent and blood clots by 47 percent. Recommendations for prescribing ERT and HRT were changed as a result of these findings, and now doctors recommend ERT or HRT only at the lowest levels for the shortest amount of time, if at all, to relieve discomfort brought on by menopause.

The Blood Vessels

The blood vessels form a closed loop that transports blood throughout the body. In general, arteries carry highly oxygenated blood away from the heart, and veins carry oxygen depleted blood toward the heart. Between the arteries and the veins are capillaries, which deliver oxygen and nutrients to the cells in the body. Exchanges into and out of the bloodstream occur only at the level of the capillaries; other vessels have walls that are too thick for the materials to diffuse across. Arteries must withstand the pressure that is generated each time the ventricles of the heart contracts and this wave of pressure is measured as blood pressure. This pressure can also be felt as the pulse. Pressure from the heartbeat is dissipated by the time the blood travels through the capillaries, so blood returning toward the heart has to be moved by other means. Skeletal muscle contractions around the veins help to push blood toward the heart, and valves found in the veins prevent the backward flow of blood. In some cases, blood can pool around the valves and cause local swelling and distension of the vessels, resulting in varicose veins. In addition to the pressure created by the contraction of skeletal muscles, the act of breathing causes pressure changes in the chest cavity that help to draw the blood in the veins back toward the heart. This is called the respiratory pump.

Blood Flow

The heart is a double pump that moves blood through two circuits in the body, the pulmonary circuit and the systemic circuit (Figure 2-15). With each heart beat, the heart pumps blood through the pulmonary circuit, which brings blood to the lungs and back; and also through the systemic circuit, which brings blood to all of the rest of the cells of the body and back. As blood travels through the lungs on the pulmonary circuit, it picks up oxygen to be distributed by the systemic circuit. As blood travels through the systemic circuit, it slowly releases oxygen to the cells and tissues that need it. By the time the blood in the systemic system returns to the heart it is depleted of oxygen and ready to be pumped through the pulmonary circuit again, where it can become re-oxygenated.

Blood returns to the heart through the largest vein, the vena cava. Blood enters the heart through the right atria, which contracts to push the blood into the right ventricle. The right ventricle then contracts to push the blood out of the heart through the

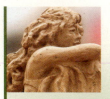

Economic Considerations
WOMEN OF COLOR AND HEART DISEASE

Heart disease is the number one killer of women in the United States. For women with heart disease, arteries become increasingly narrow, constricting blood flow to the heart. According to the United States National Institutes of Health, heart disease is more prevalent among African-American and Latinas, and these women are also more likely to experience factors that increase the risk of developing heart disease, including high blood pressure, lack of physical activity, obesity, and diabetes (USNIH, 2009). According to the National Heart, Lung and Blood Institute, more than 80 percent of midlife African-American women are overweight or obese, 52 percent have hypertension, and 14 percent have been diagnosed with diabetes (NHLBI, 2009). For Latina women, some 83 percent of midlife women are overweight or obese, and more than 10 percent have been diagnosed with diabetes. Latinas also exhibit symptoms of heart disease at an earlier age than their Caucasian counterparts (NHLBI, 2009).

Women of color and poor women also have less access to information about heart disease and preventative medical care, and frequently do not know their risks. They are often less able to seek preventative healthcare due to lack of health insurance. While not all risk factors, such as family history, can be controlled, there are things all women can do to cut their risk of heart disease. Women are encouraged to take the following preventative steps to minimize their risk of heart disease:

- know your blood pressure
- don't smoke
- get tested for diabetes
- eat a healthful diet
- be physically active and maintain a healthy weight
- have regular cholesterol screenings
- find healthy ways to cope with stress
- limit your alcohol intake to no more than one drink per day
- always consult your physician for more information (USDHHS, 2008)

---

pulmonary artery to the lungs. After picking up oxygen in the lungs, blood returns to the heart through the pulmonary veins. Blood in the pulmonary veins enters the left atrium, where it stays until it is pushed into the left ventricle. When the left ventricle contracts it forces the blood out through the body's largest artery, the aorta, and out toward the body. The blood flow through the heart follows this pathway:

vena cava → right atrium→ tricuspid valve→ right ventricle → pulmonary arteries → lungs to pick up oxygen → pulmonary veins → left atrium → mitral valve → left ventricle → aorta → arteries → capillaries (oxygen to tissues) → veins → vena cava

Blood

Blood is made up of a fluid component and cellular components called formed elements. The fluid component of the blood is the plasma, which is colorless. Plasma consists of a mixture of electrolytes, plasma proteins, nutrients, and wastes suspended in water. Suspended in the plasma are the cellular components of the blood, including the red blood cells, white blood cells, and platelets. The red blood cells contain an iron based molecule called hemoglobin, which gives blood its color. Hemoglobin has the unique ability to attach to oxygen molecules when oxygen is abundant, for example, in the lungs. It releases oxygen when it encounters regions in the body where oxygen levels are low, for example, in the capillaries surrounding the cells and tissues of the body.

Under the microscope, red blood cells have a biconcave shape and lack a nucleus when mature. The hormone testosterone encourages red blood cell formation, and consequently men have higher circulating levels of red blood cells than women.

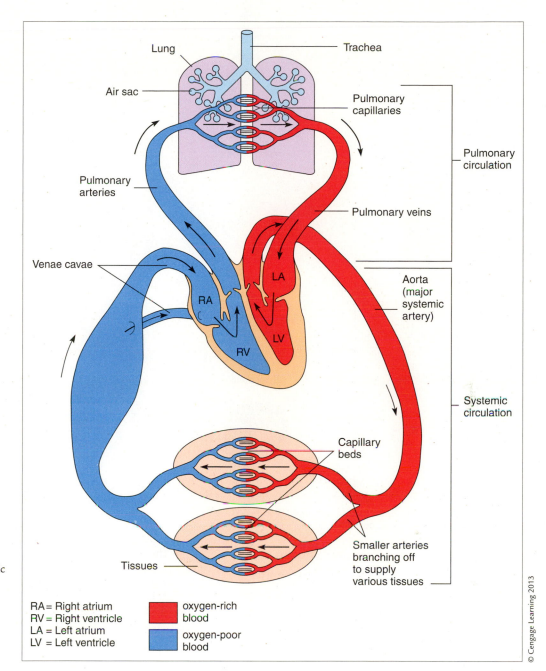

Lung

Trachea

Air sac

Pulmonary
capillaries

Pulmonary
circulation

Pulmonary
arteries

Pulmonary veins

Venae cavae

LA

Aorta
(major
systemic
artery)

RA

LV

RV

Systemic
circulation

Capillary
beds

Smaller arteries
branching off
to supply
various tissues

Tissues

RA = Right atrium
RV = Right ventricle
LA = Left atrium
LV = Left ventricle

oxygen-rich
blood

oxygen-poor
blood

FIGURE 2-15: Schematic drawing of the blood flow and oxygenation pattern of blood through the pulmonary and systemic circulation.

© Cengage Learning 2013

Women also lose small amounts of blood during each menses, a circumstance that can predispose them to anemia, a low red blood cell count.

There are five types of white blood cells, each with specific functions, and almost all related to immune function (Figure 2-16). Neutrophils are the most numerous in the bloodstream. Leukocytes patrol the blood, lymph, and tissues, engulfing and digesting invaders that they encounter. This process of engulfing and digesting is called phagocytosis. Lymphocytes are specialized white blood cells that identify and destroy disease causing microbes and abnormal or damaged cells such as cancer cells. Lymphocytes produce antibodies which are proteins that can target and destroy specific disease causing invaders. Basophils release a chemical called histamine and other immunoactive chemicals as part of the body's immune defense. Eosinophils fight allergies and parasitic worm infections by phagocytizing the invaders. Macrophages are the largest phagocytic cells. These aid in the defense against invaders and serve to activate the lymphocytes.

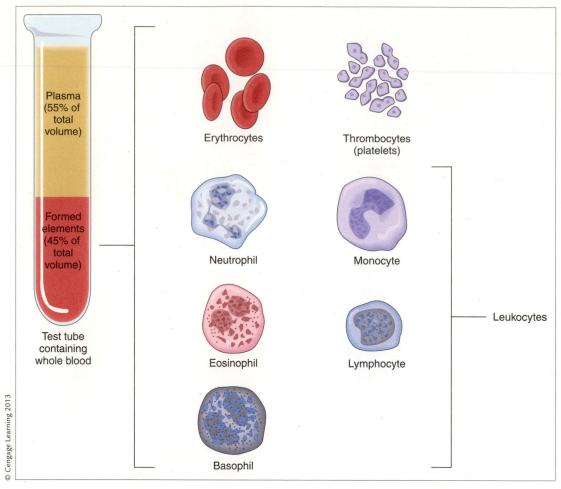

© Cengage Learning 2013

FIGURE 2-16: The composition of human blood.

Lymphatic System / Immune System

Lymphatic vessels run roughly parallel to the arteries, veins, and capillaries of the cardiovascular system and carry a colorless fluid called lymph throughout the body. Lymph is similar to blood plasma and is, in fact, fluid that has moved from the capillaries into the spaces surrounding the tissues and is then absorbed into the lymph vessels to become lymph (Figure 2-17). The lymphatic vessels eventually return this fluid to the bloodstream. As lymph travels through the lymph vessels, it encounters lymph nodes, which are small nodules that contain lymphocytes. The lymphatic system and the immune system are often considered together because many of the pathogen fighting cells of the immune system are found in the vessels and the nodes of the lymphatic system (Figure 2-18). Many components of the immune system are found outside of the lymphatic system however, including white blood cells that travel through the blood or tissues.

The immune system consists of both nonspecific defenses and specific defenses. **Nonspecific defenses** guard against a wide range of potential pathogens. Microbes or other agents that cause disease are called pathogens. For example, physical and chemical barriers act to prevent microbes from entering the body. The skin consists of many layers of dead cells through which a microbe must pass before reaching the bloodstream. Mucus membranes that line the respiratory system contain sticky mucus that traps pathogens, and cilia that sweep them away. In addition, mucus contains antimicrobial chemicals that can kill bacteria. Chemical defenses such as histamine, digestive secretions, and enzymes provide a second line of defense, attacking organisms which have gained access to the body. Fever increases the body's temperature making an inhospitable environment for most microbes. When tissues are injured either by pathogens or physical injury, **inflammation** occurs. The process leading to inflammation

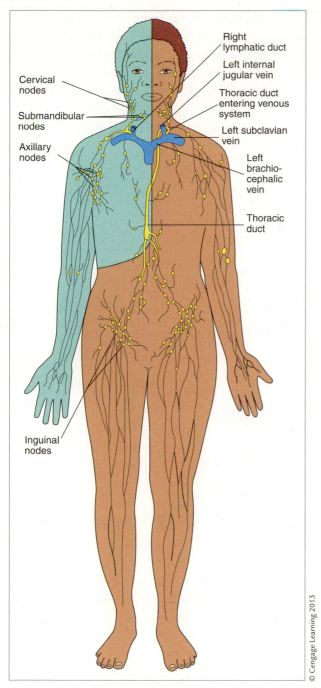

Cervical nodes

Submandibular nodes

Axillary nodes

Right lymphatic duct

Left internal jugular vein

Thoracic duct entering venous system

Left subclavian vein

Left brachio-cephalic vein

Thoracic duct

Inguinal nodes

© Cengage Learning 2013

FIGURE 2-17: Lymphatic drainage in the human body.

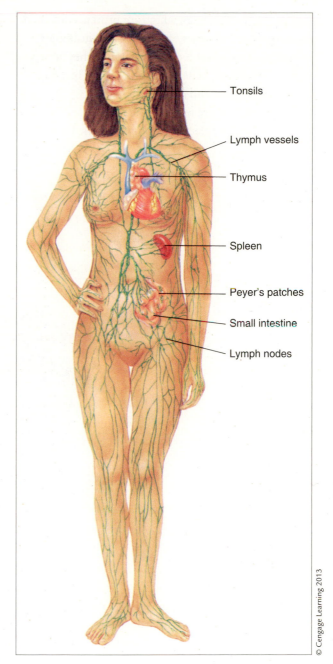

Tonsils

Lymph vessels

Thymus

Spleen

Peyer's patches

Small intestine

Lymph nodes

© Cengage Learning 2013

FIGURE 2-18: The structure of the lymphatic system showing the vessels, nodes, and organs.

involves a series of steps. Damaged tissues release chemicals which cause blood vessels to dilate, increasing blood flow to the area and creating a localized increase in temperature. The dilated vessels allow plasma to leak out into the surrounding tissues and this causes swelling. Inflammation attracts white blood cells that can engulf and destroy the foreign microbes. If a large number of white blood cells accumulate and eventually die, they and the dead bacteria in the inflamed area form pus.

If nonspecific defenses are unable to prevent or eradicate an infection, the specific defenses are activated to destroy the pathogen. **Specific defenses** target individual types of pathogens and can store immunological memory of pathogens to protect the body from subsequent infections. There are two major types of specific defenses, the antibody response and the cell-mediate response. In the case of the antibody response, lymphocytes called B cells manufacture antibodies, which are proteins designed to destroy specific types of pathogens. Antibodies are released into the bloodstream where they attach to surface markers, called antigens, on the invading pathogen's surface and destroy them.

The cell-mediate response can occur rapidly or may be delayed by weeks or even years. Viruses and other pathogens leave the bloodstream and enter body cells to reproduce and to avoid destruction by circulating antibodies. Specialized lymphocytes called cytotoxic T cells patrol the tissues and destroy virus infected body cells, thus preventing the virus from reproducing (Figure 2-19). In the case of specific defenses, specialized memory cells are created

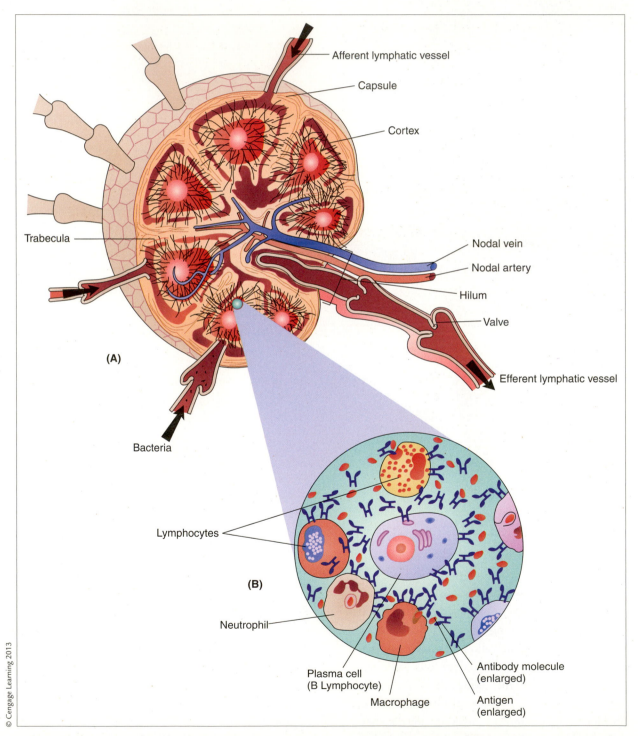

FIGURE 2-19: The structure of a lymph node: (A) Section through a lymph node showing the flow of lymph (B) Microscopic detail of bacteria being destroyed within the lymph node.

that store information about the pathogen and the antibodies used to combat it, for a quick response in case of future infection. Usually this will prevent an individual from becoming ill with the same disease a second time. Unfortunately, some invaders like the flu virus and the organisms that cause the common cold mutate frequently, so even if the immune system develops memory cells to this year's cold or flu, that information will probably not be able to protect against infection when next year's version of the flu comes around.

It is important to remember that the many components of the nonspecific and specific immune systems are at work simultaneously and these components usually reinforce the others. For example, if the skin barrier is broken, the phagocytic white blood cells will be attracted to the area and engulf and digest invading bacteria that may have entered at the wound site. If the phagocytes are overwhelmed, the more specialized lymphocytes will produce antibodies, which seek out and destroy the invaders. At the same time, fever and inflammation help the other components of the immune system to work more effectively, making the body less hospitable to the pathogens that are trying to reproduce. The components of the immune system work together to provide protection against a wide range of infections, and when these defenses fail or are overrun, homeostasis fails and illness results.

The immune system is complex, and it is vulnerable to malfunctions that can cause disruptions to homeostasis. In the case of allergies, for example, the immune system treats relatively harmless substances such as dust or pollen grains as if they were pathogens that must be destroyed. As the immune system mounts an attack on the perceived "invader", unpleasant symptoms such as excess mucus production, sneezing, and watering eyes can result. In addition, the immune system mistakes one of the body tissues as foreign invaders and attacks them, causing an autoimmune disorder. For example, women of northern European descent are more prone to the disease multiple sclerosis, in which immune cells attack and destroy myelin, the fatty coating around nerve cells. Destroying the myelin reduces the efficiency of nerve transmission and can result in a loss of sensation or mobility. In contrast, immune deficiency diseases occur when some component of the overall immune system is absent or not functioning properly.

BOX 2-1

Immune Terminology

Antigen - foreign molecule which elicits an immune response and combines with the antibodies produced

Antigenic determinants - surface markers on cells which are used to identify self and non-self cells

Antibody - globular proteins produced by B-cells in response to an antigenic challenge; also called immunoglobins (Ig's)

Specific defense - immune response aimed at a single target identified by antigenic determinants

Nonspecific defense - protective mechanisms that defend against all potential invaders

Respiratory System

One function of the respiratory system is to move air into and out of the lungs so that oxygen can be absorbed into the bloodstream (Figure 2-20). The respiratory system, however, is involved in additional functions. For example, communication through verbal speech is accomplished by forcing air through the vocal cords, which are part of the respiratory tract. The sense of smell relies on the respiratory system since nerve endings called olfactory receptors are embedded in the mucus membranes of the nose. As air is drawn over the receptors, molecules in the air trigger the olfactory receptors.

The upper respiratory system is made up of the nasal cavity and the pharynx, and the lower respiratory system is made up of the larynx, trachea, bronchi, and the lungs (Figure 2-21). In the lungs, the bronchi form progressively smaller branches called bronchioles, and these end in small sacs called alveoli (Figure 2-22). The alveoli have very thin walls, only one cell layer, and each alveoli is surrounded by capillaries. At the same time carbon dioxide (CO_2),

An Unpredictable Disease

Joanne, a 31-year-old mother of three, has just returned from a trip to Finland to visit her relatives. She is tired from travelling and feeling stressed because of missing an airline connection on her way home. As she is leaving the airport, she stumbles and falls down. Bystanders help her to her feet but she can't seem to stand unassisted. Even with help, she discovers that she can't walk and is taken to the hospital.

A medical history reveals nothing unusual, although she has noticed tingling first in her right leg, then in her left over the past month. When asked about her family health history, she reveals her sister has noticed blurred vision lately. While she's waiting in the emergency room, the numbness fades and she regains the ability to walk. Although she wants to go home, the doctor convinces her to stay for further testing. The doctor orders an MRI which reveals scleric plaques, scar tissue within the myelin sheaths of her neurons. The plaques interfere with transmission of nerve impulses, producing paralysis and numbness. She is diagnosed with multiple sclerosis. The doctor explains that her immune system has mistakenly begun to attack and destroy her myelin as if it were an invading bacteria or virus.

1. How does her history – the stress of travel, family of northern European descent, sister also showing neurological symptom – play into the diagnosis?

2. What is the prognosis? How might the disease progress?

3. What lifestyle decisions can she make to positively influence the outcome of this disease?

which is a metabolic waste product of cell metabolism, diffuses from the blood into the alveoli to be exhaled.

The inner surface of the alveoli is coated with a slippery fluid called surfactant, which is secreted by the cells that make up the wall of the alveoli. Surfactant reduces the surface tension within the alveoli and prevents the alveolar walls from collapsing and sticking together during exhalation. Premature babies often lack sufficient surfactant in their lungs, as the production of surfactant does not occur until the end of gestation.

To function efficiently, the lungs must have both a large surface area for gas exchange, and they must be open to the external environment. These characteristics make the respiratory system particularly vulnerable to invasion by pathogens such as bacteria and viruses. Several lines of defense protect this system from potential infections. The larynx, trachea, and bronchi are lined with cells that have fine hair-like cilia on them. These cells also secrete mucus, which acts like a sticky trap for dust, and microbes that might find their way to this portion of our respiratory tract. The cilia beat in a coordinated fashion to move the mucus up out of the lungs where it is swallowed and dissolved by the strong acids in the stomach. Smoking destroys the cilia's ability to move mucus and trapped microbes and debris away, leaving smokers much more vulnerable to infections of the lower respiratory system. Traveling through and between the alveoli are alveolar macrophages, which are immune cells that patrol the lung tissues for pathogens, damaged cells, or debris. For reasons that are not well understood, women are more prone than men to the development and survival of cancer cells in the lungs.

Lung capacity is largely determined by the size of the chest cavity, producing the characteristic differences between women and men. During puberty, the shoulders broaden and the chest cavity expands more in boys, on average, than it does in girls. This change at puberty translates into an average vital capacity, which is the maximum amount of air that can be inhaled and exhaled from the lungs, of 4.8 L for men and 3.1 L for women. However, for reasons that are not thoroughly understood, men are more likely than

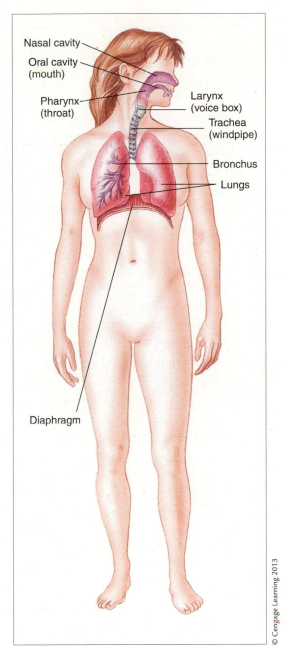

Nasal cavity
Oral cavity (mouth)
Pharynx (throat)
Larynx (voice box)
Trachea (windpipe)
Bronchus
Lungs
Diaphragm

© Cengage Learning 2013

FIGURE 2-20: The respiratory system consists of the nasal cavity, oral cavity, sinuses, larynx, trachea, bronchi, and lungs.

women to develop conditions that diminish lung capacity such as emphysema and chronic obstructive pulmonary disease (COPD).

Digestive System

The overall function of the digestive system is to convert food into forms that can be absorbed by the body and to remove the remaining indigestible wastes. The digestive system consists of the digestive tract, which is a passageway that extends through the body from the mouth to the anus, and the accessory organs (Figure 2-23). Food passes through the digestive tract as it is processed, and water and nutrients are absorbed into the bloodstream. The accessory organs contribute digestive enzymes and other substances required for digestion to the digestive tract and regulate metabolism.

The Digestive Tract

The digestive tract begins at the mouth. Here, teeth grind food into smaller pieces, which makes the food easier to swallow and increases the surface area. Increasing the surface area makes it easier for the enzymes further along the system to chemically break down the food. Saliva, which contains enzymes, bicarbonate buffer, and water, moistens the food and begins the digestion of starches into simple sugars.

The esophagus is the tube which connects the mouth to the stomach. During swallowing, the smooth muscle of the esophagus uses rhythmic peristaltic contractions to push food toward the stomach. In order to enter the stomach, the food must pass the esophageal sphincter, a ring of smooth muscle which controls movement into the stomach. In babies, this muscle is not yet well developed. When the baby's stomach begins churning to digest the milk, some of the stomach contents may get pushed past the sphincter, causing the baby to spit up. In adults, the sphincter may not close tightly, allowing stomach acid and food to enter and irritate the esophagus. This sensation is experienced as heartburn.

The stomach is a hollow organ made primarily of smooth muscle and lined with a mucus membrane. The gastric secretions include several substances that aid in the digestion of food. Hydrochloric acid breaks down proteins and kills microbes that may have entered the stomach with food. Pepsin is an enzyme that chemically digests proteins. Additional stomach secretions include hormones and a chemical called intrinsic factor which helps with the absorption of vitamin B_{12}. The mixture of these secretions and the swallowed food is called chyme. The muscular contractions of the stomach mechanically break down and homogenize the chyme. Although mixing of food and some preliminary digestion of proteins does occur in

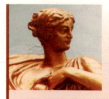

Cultural Considerations

The Hazards of Feeding the Family: Chronic Obstructive Pulmonary Disease in Women

Chronic obstructive pulmonary disease is a condition that makes it increasingly difficult to breathe, and can cause coughing, shortness of breath, and wheezing. It can take the form of chronic bronchitis or emphysema, or both. In the United States, cigarette smoking is the leading cause of chronic obstructive pulmonary disease, but in the developing world, poor women also develop this condition as a result of cooking for their families. Indeed, a woman's health profile can be influenced significantly by her gender role and her social status.

Throughout the world, women are often in charge of feeding the family, and spend a significant amount of their day cooking and preparing meals. However, when women don't have access to modern conveniences like a stove or cook top, they often cook over open fires or with traditional stoves, using solid fuels such as wood and coal. In particular, women living in rural communities may cook and heat their homes with fuels such as wood, agricultural crop residues, animal dung, or charcoal. When they do, they also breathe in a mix of literally hundreds of pollutants every single day.

For their lungs, this exposure to indoor smoke can have similar health effects to cigarette smoking, even if a woman has never so much as held a cigarette. In fact, research has shown that women exposed to domestic wood smoke while cooking for many years develop chronic obstructive pulmonary disease with very similar symptoms to those of cigarette smokers (WHO, 2008).

For women, this indoor smoke is responsible for half a million deaths each year, and millions more suffer due to impaired breathing and other respiratory problems. Improving the ventilation of home stoves or providing cleaner burning fuel sources, so that inhabitants no longer breathe the resulting indoor air pollutants, are important strategies in the fight against this disease in developing countries. One study in Xuanwei, China, where rates of lung cancer and chronic obstructive pulmonary disease are strongly associated with household use of smoky coal, researchers showed that simple measures, such as installing a chimney, could dramatically reduce the incidence of chronic obstructive pulmonary disease among women (Chapman et al., 2005).

the stomach, it is not the primary site for the chemical digestion of food. Most of the chemical breakdown of food takes place in the small intestine. In addition, very little is absorbed from the stomach into the bloodstream. Substances that are absorbed from the stomach include water, sugar, alcohol, aspirin, and some medications.

From the stomach, measured amounts of chyme pass through the pyloric sphincter that separates the stomach from the small intestine. In the first few centimeters of the small intestine, the acidic pH of the chyme is adjusted to neutral with the addition of bicarbonate ions. Pancreatic juice, which is a mixture of bicarbonate ions, and enzymes, is secreted into the small intestine by the pancreas.

Pancreatic enzymes continue the chemical digestion of the chyme. One enzyme, amylase, breaks down starches and carbohydrates. Another enzyme, trypsin, continues the digestion of proteins. Bile, which is secreted from the gall bladder, acts as a detergent, and breaks apart fat droplets so that the enzyme lipase can digest them. As chyme passes through the small intestines, nutrients are absorbed into the bloodstream.

After passing through the small intestine, the chyme moves into the large intestine where water is removed and the remaining waste is compacted into feces. The large intestine is home to cooperative bacteria, the normal flora, that thrive on food wastes. Intestinal normal flora also manufactures vitamin K

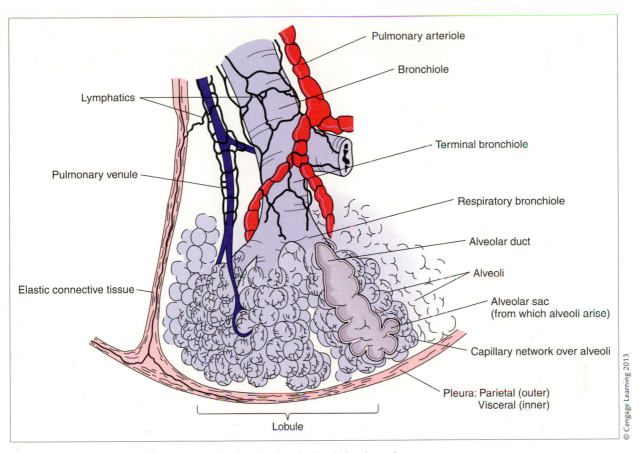

FIGURE 2-21: The anatomy of the lungs showing the alveoli and related blood vessels.

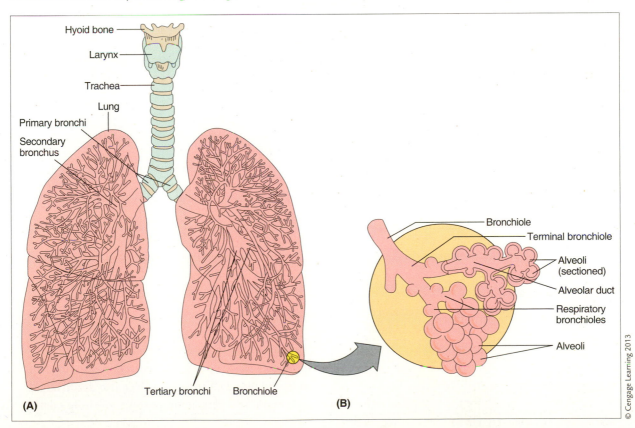

FIGURE 2-22: The lower respiratory tract.

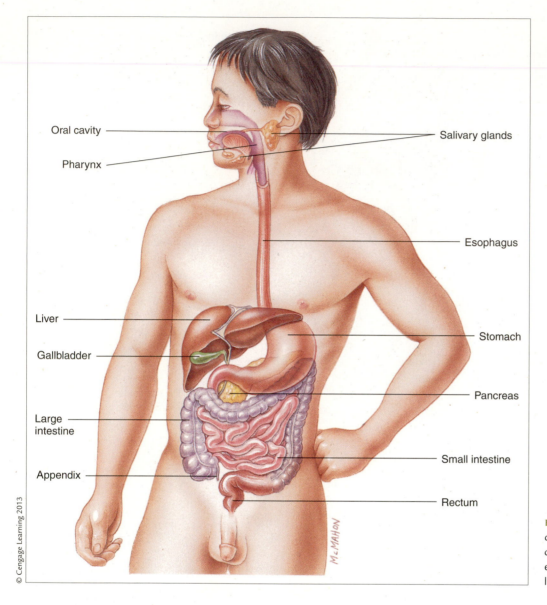

Oral cavity

Pharynx

Salivary glands

Esophagus

Liver

Stomach

Gallbladder

Pancreas

Large intestine

Small intestine

Appendix

Rectum

McMAHON

FIGURE 2-23: The digestive system consists of the mouth, esophagus, intestines, liver, and pancreas.

and limits the activity of pathogenic microbes that could cause disease.

The Accessory Organs of the Digestive System

Two of the accessory organs, the pancreas and the gall bladder contribute enzymes, bile, or other materials to the digestive tract to facilitate the digestion of the chyme. The largest accessory organ, the liver, also contributes substances to the digestive tract, in addition to serving many other functions in the body. Bile is manufactured by the liver and stored in the gall bladder before it is secreted into the small intestine. The liver acts as a detoxification center for the blood and is the site where old or damaged red blood cells are recycled

(Figure 2-24). The blood returning from the small and large intestines is filtered through the liver before it re-enters the general circulation. This allows the liver to detoxify harmful substances that have been absorbed into the bloodstream from the digestive tract. The liver also processes many of the nutrients that are absorbed from the small intestines. For example, excess glucose is converted into glycogen molecules which can be stored for future use. Lipids are also stored in the liver. In addition, the liver produces plasma proteins involved in immune function and blood clotting. The liver also deactivates hormones and plays an important role in regulating hormone levels.

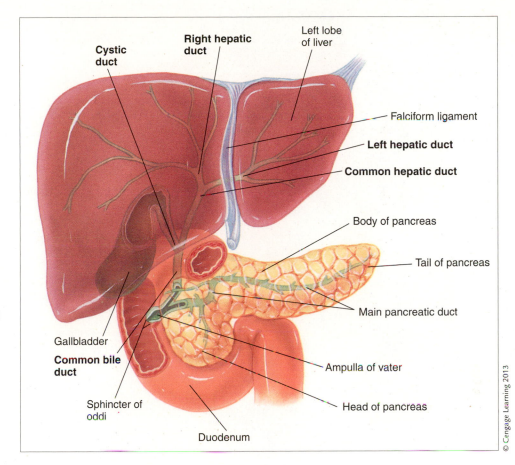

FIGURE 2-24: Bile produced by the liver drains through the hepatic ducts to the gall bladder where it is stored. When needed to emulsify fats, the gall bladder releases bile which passes through the common bile duct and into the small intestine.

Labels in figure:
Cystic duct · **Right hepatic duct** · Left lobe of liver · Falciform ligament · **Left hepatic duct** · **Common hepatic duct** · Body of pancreas · Tail of pancreas · Main pancreatic duct · Gallbladder · **Common bile duct** · Ampulla of vater · Sphincter of oddi · Head of pancreas · Duodenum

Although the liver does have some capacity to regenerate itself, that capacity is not unlimited. Because it has so many important roles to play in the body, long term damage can have serious health consequences. The liver can be damaged by overexposure to alcohol, toxins, or by viral attacks. Infection by various strains of the hepatitis virus can have devastating effects. Hepatitis B and C can be transmitted sexually and are a major cause of liver failure.

Urinary System

The urinary system removes water-soluble wastes from the blood and eliminates them from the body as urine (Figure 2-25). In coordination with the respiratory system, the kidneys are responsible for adjusting the pH balance in the blood. In addition, the kidneys are responsible for regulating the fluid and electrolyte balance of the plasma and other body fluids.

The kidneys filter between 80–120 liters of blood per day and typically produce one to two liters of urine, depending on the level of fluid consumption. From the kidneys, urine travels through the ureters to the urinary bladder. The urinary bladder is a hollow organ whose walls are primarily smooth muscle. The bladder serves as a temporary storage place for urine, and a full bladder can hold about one liter of urine. Urine passes from the urinary bladder to the outside of the body through the urethra. In females, the urine exits the body from the urethral opening which is located in the vestibule of the vulva. In males, the urethra extends through the penis and the urethral opening is found in the glans of the penis. The urethra is, on average, shorter in women than it is in men, which may contribute to women's increased susceptibility to urinary tract infections. Bacteria from the skin surface have a shorter distance to travel to the bladder in women than in men. Urinary tract infections will be addressed in more detail in Chapter 6.

The process of urination is coordinated by a reflex called the micturition reflex. As the bladder

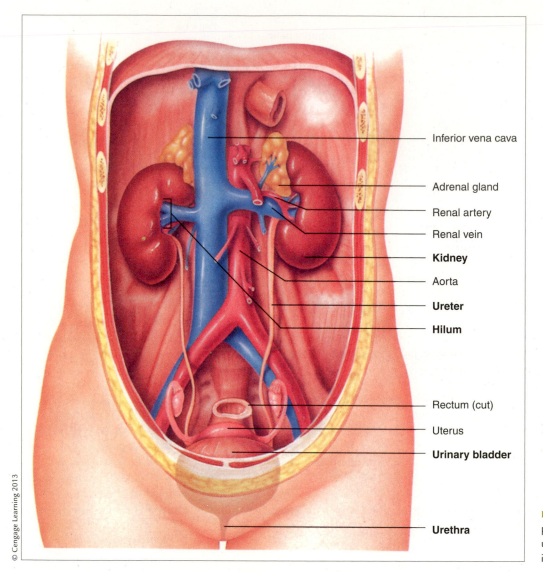

Inferior vena cava

Adrenal gland

Renal artery

Renal vein

Kidney

Aorta

Ureter

Hilum

Rectum (cut)

Uterus

Urinary bladder

Urethra

© Cengage Learning 2013

FIGURE 2-25: The position of the urinary system organs in a woman.

fills with urine, stretch receptors in the bladder notify the brain about the need to urinate. There are two sphincters that control the exit of urine from the bladder (Figure 2-26). The internal urethral sphincter is not under voluntary control, but the external urethral sphincter is. Normally, when the external sphincter is voluntarily relaxed, the internal sphincter will relax automatically and urine is released. However, if there is enough urine in the bladder (over 500 mL), the resulting pressure can force open the internal urethral sphincter, and then the external sphincter will open as well, in spite of voluntary efforts to stop it. Children do not develop the necessary pathways in their nervous systems to voluntarily control urination until they are about two years old. Damage to either of the sphincters or damage to the nervous system can cause loss of

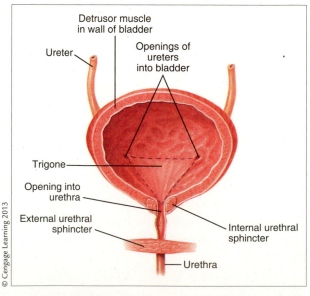

Detrusor muscle in wall of bladder

Ureter

Openings of ureters into bladder

Trigone

Opening into urethra

External urethral sphincter

Internal urethral sphincter

Urethra

© Cengage Learning 2013

FIGURE 2-26: The structure of the urinary bladder.

Lifestyle Choices

How would lifestyle choices such as smoking, drinking to excess, over eating or under-eating affect homeostasis? What specific effects could be predicted? What overall effects might emerge?

control over urination or incontinence. In some cases, childbirth can damage the sphincters causing a condition called stress incontinence in women. Medical procedures such as episiotomy and delivery by forceps or vacuum extraction increase the likelihood of this kind of damage.

CONCLUSION

An additional body system, the reproductive system, will be addressed in detail in Chapter 3. Although the primary function of the reproductive system is the creation of offspring, many of the hormones that are involved in reproduction also play important roles in other body systems. Estrogen, for example, is important for bone development and cardiovascular health. Testosterone has effects on muscle development and on the integument. None of the body systems can exist by themselves and all have an important role in maintaining homeostasis.

REVIEW QUESTIONS

1. What is homeostasis, and how does the body maintain homeostasis?

2. Explain the differences between a negative and a positive feedback loop?

3. Which two organ systems exert the most regulating influence over the other systems?

4. How would you differentiate between the central and the peripheral nervous systems?

5. What is the autonomic nervous system, and what does it control?

6. Explain the difference between the sympathetic and parasympathetic nervous systems.

7. What is a hormone, and how do hormones work?

8. Explain how osteoclasts and osteoblasts influence bone growth and bone density.

9. Why are some types of muscle in the body voluntary, while other types are involuntary?

10. Explain the difference between arteries, veins, and capillaries. How are these vessels similar; how are they different?

11. What are some differences between specific immunity and nonspecific immunity?

12. In the digestive system, where does the majority of nutrient absorption into the bloodstream occur?

13. List at least two functions of the urinary system.

14. What skeletal differences exist between men and women or are they identical?

15. What is the function of the integumentary system?

CRITICAL THINKING QUESTIONS

1. Why do most organs in the body have both parasympathetic and sympathetic enervation?

2. If a woman had a tumor on her pituitary gland that caused the gland to secrete excess thyroid stimulating hormone, what effect would this have on her thyroid gland's production of thyroid hormone? How would it effect the production of thyroid releasing hormone from the hypothalamus?

3. What might be the long term effects for a woman of taking a medication that inhibits the activities of osteoclasts? Are the long term effects different from the short term effects?

WEBLINKS

American heart Association
www.womenshealth.gov/index.htm
American Diabetes Association
www.diabetes.org

National Women's Health Information Center
www.womenshealth.gov/index.htm
Women's Health Initiative
www.nhlbi.nih.gov/whi

REFERENCES

Aubertin-Leheudre, M., Lord, C., Khalil, A., & Dionne, I. J. (2007). Effect of 6 months of exercise and isoflavone supplementation on clinical cardiovascular risk factors in obese postmenopausal women: A randomized, double-blind study. *Menopause, 14*(4), 624–629.

Bovarnick, S. (2007). Universal human rights and non-Western normative systems: A comparative analysis of violence against women in Mexico and Pakistan. *Review of International Studies, 33*, 59–74.

Chapman, R. S., He, X., Blair, A. E., & Lan, Q. (2005). Improvement in household stoves and risk of chronic obstructive pulmonary disease in Xuanwei, China: Retrospective cohort study. *British Medical Journal, 331*, 1050–1052.

Evans EM, Racette SB, Van Pelt RE, Peterson LR, Villareal DT. (2007). Effects of soy protein isolate and moderate exercise on turnover and bone density mineral density in postmenopausal women. *Menopause, 14*(3 Pt1), 481–488.

Holick, M. F. (2008). Sunlight, UV-radiation, vitamin D and skin cancer: How much sunlight do we need? *Advances in Experimental Medicine and Biology, 624*, 1–15.

National Heart, Lung and Blood Institute. (2009). Lower heart disease risk. Retrieved March 31, 2009 from http://www.nhlbi.nih.gov/educational/hearttruth/lower-risk/.

National Institutes of Health. (2009). The heart truth: Women of color partners. Retrieved March 31, 2009 from http://www.nhlbi.nih.gov/educa-tional/hearttruth/partners/women-of-color-partners.htm.

NiCarthy, G. (2004). *Getting Free: You Can End Abuse and Take Back Your Life.* Berkeley, CA: Seal Press.

Renzetti, C. M., & Edleson, J. L. (2008). *Encyclopedia of interpersonal violence.* Thousand Oaks, CA: SAGE Publishers.

U. S. Department of Health and Human Services. (2008). Frequently asked questions: Heart disease. Retrieved March 31, 2009, from http://www.4women.gov/FAQ/heart-disease.cfm.

Van Hasselt, V. B. (1988). *Handbook of family violence.* Basel: Birkhäuser Publishing.

World Health Organization (2008). Fact sheet: Chronic obstructive pulmonary disease (COPD), No. 315.

chapter 3

REPRODUCTIVE ANATOMY

CHAPTER COMPETENCIES

Upon completion of this chapter the reader will be able to:

- Identify and understand the functions of the organs and glands of the female reproductive system
- Explain the relationship between the reproductive and urinary systems in terms of their anatomy

- Explain the role of the pelvic bones, ligaments and membranes in supporting the reproductive system and other organs and glands
- Identify and understand the functions of the organs and glands of the male reproductive system

KEY TERMS

cervix	labia majora	penis	vagina
clitoris	labia minora	prostate	vas deferens
ejaculation	ovary	seminal vesicles	vestibule
epididymis	oviduct	testes	vulva
fallopian tube	ovum	urethra	
hymen	pelvic floor	uterus	

INTRODUCTION

The female reproductive system is frequently portrayed as difficult to understand and "mysterious" because its structures are internal, in contrast with many of the structures of the male reproductive system. While it is true that two components of the male reproductive system, the scrotum and the penis, are external, it should be noted that most of the male reproductive structures are internal, just as they are in the female system. In fact, when compared, the number of external verses internal structures in the female and the male reproductive systems are very similar. In addition, most other body systems, with the exception of the integument, are primarily internal, so the argument that having the majority of its organs within the body cavity makes the system harder to understand does not hold up under scrutiny. It is more likely that misconceptions about the female reproductive anatomy were, and still are, a product of cultural and societal expectations about women, rather than the result of an inability to understand the organs and glands because they were not visible outside the body.

Renaissance anatomist Andreas Vesalius was one of the first Europeans to publish accurate writings and illustrations of female internal anatomy. Vesalius's unprecedented visualization of anatomy, *De Humani Corporis Fabrica*, was not only an accurate representation of the structure of males but included illustrations from the dissections of at least nine female cadavers. These formed the foundation for modern anatomical knowledge of both men and women. In the 450 years since Vesalius, numerous misconceptions and misunderstandings have shaped research into female anatomy. These misconceptions have influenced a wide range of social policies and attitudes including those concerning women's abilities to hold jobs, the types of activities that women could engage in, and even the sources of mental illness in women. As scientific knowledge about the female reproductive system expanded in recent years, a better understanding of female reproductive anatomy has emerged. For example, work by Australian urologist Dr. Helen O'Connell et al. (1998) added surprising new insights to the understanding of female reproductive anatomy. Dr. O'Connell was concerned that modern textbooks did not provide sufficient information about the locations of nerves serving the clitoris to allow surgeons to design nerve sparing pelvic surgeries. She dissected 10 female cadavers ranging in age from 22 to 88. Her detailed dissections revealed the internal portions of the clitoris to be much larger than was previously described. Despite modern imaging techniques such as MRIs and advances in histological research, misleading and inaccurate information about female anatomy is still common.

This chapter provides the anatomical basis to distinguish some of the myths from the realities. If female reproductive anatomy is to be understood in a biological framework, it is important to consider that the organs and other structures of the female and the male reproductive tracts originate from the same groups of cells in the developing fetus. In fact, the body plan of the human embryo remains essentially both female and male, unless the SRY gene on a Y chromosome triggers a series of events that result in the production of large amounts of the hormone testosterone, around the seventh week of gestation. It is only then that the reproductive structures of a male fetus will develop into the anatomical characteristics that are associated with being male. If no Y chromosome, and hence no SRY gene, is present to trigger the production of testosterone, the reproductive system and body plan will develop as female. When different structures originate from the same embryonic tissues, they are referred to as homologous. In some cases, homologous structures have similar functions, and in other cases, they do not. Table 3-1 outlines homologous structures in the female and the male reproductive systems.

Table 3-1 Homologous Structures of the Reproductive System.	
Structure Found in the Female Reproductive System	**Structure Found in the Male Reproductive System**
Ovary	Testicle
Uterus	Prostatic Utricle
Skene's Gland or Female Prostate	Prostate
Bartholin's Gland	Bulbourethral Gland or Cowper's Gland
Labia Majora	Scrotum
Labia Minora	Spongy Urethra
Clitoris	Penis
Glans of the Clitoris	Glans of the Penis
Clitoral Hood	Foreskin of the Penis

OVARIES

The **ovaries** are the female gonads, which means that they are the organs producing both gametes and hormones (Figure 3-1). The testicles fulfill a homologous role in males. In females, the gamete is called **ovum**, although they are commonly referred to as eggs. Male gametes are called sperm (Figure 3-2). The ovaries are the size and shape of almonds in the

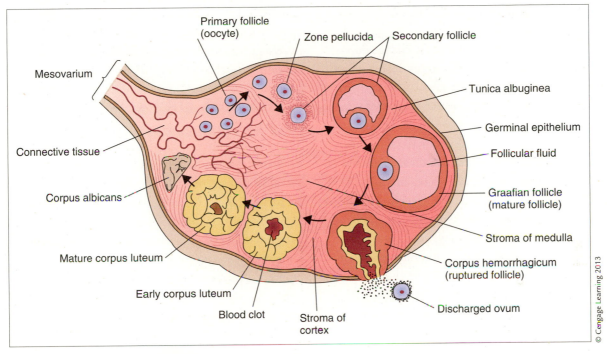

FIGURE 3-1: An individual ovary diagramming the stages of follicular development.

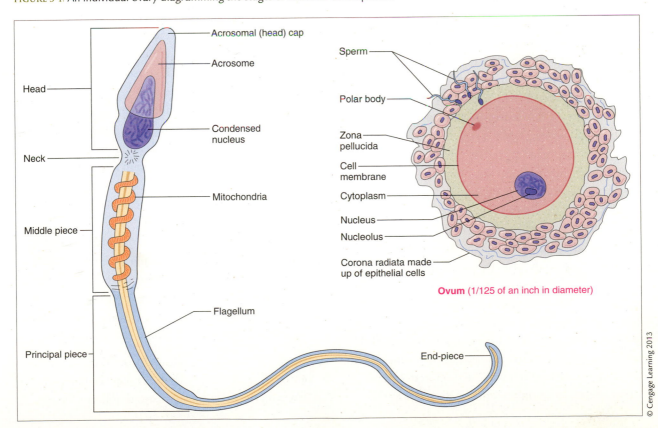

FIGURE 3-2: Human sperm and ovum.

shell, approximately 3 cm long by 1-1/2 cm wide by 1 cm thick. They are suspended in the pelvic cavity three ways: attached to the peritoneal covering over the back of the uterus by connective tissue called the mesovarium; attached to the uterus by the ovarian ligament; and attached to the lateral body wall by the suspensory ligament of the ovary. Over a woman's lifetime, the position of the ovaries may change due to displacement by the expanding uterus during pregnancy and by stretching of the ligaments.

The internal surface of the ovaries is covered with the germinal epithelium, a flattened layer of protective cells. This layer was originally misnamed because it was thought that it gave rise to ova throughout life. Deep to the germinal epithelium is a region called the cortex, the area in which the ova develop. Inside the cortex is the region called the medulla, with many large blood vessels, lymphatic vessels, and nerves. A framework of fibrous cells forms the connective tissue called the stroma, which gives the ovaries their shape.

When a girl is born, her ovaries contain groups of cells called primordial follicles, and the ova she is destined to produce throughout her reproductive life will develop from these follicles. The primordial follicles arose before she was born from special cells called primordial germ cells, which were segregated from the rest of the body cells as early as 10 days after fertilization. After migrating to the wall of the primitive ovary, the germ cells, now called oogonia, become surrounded with a layer of follicle cells to form the primordial follicle. The primordial follicles in the fetal ovary divide at a prodigious rate, and by 20 weeks, there are more than seven million of them. After that, further cell division to form new follicles is very rare, and for the next 50 years or so, the majority of ova undergo a process of regression and degeneration called atresia. The remaining ova are released from the ovary during the process of ovulation discussed in Chapter 4.

Investigators differ in their estimates of the number of follicles remaining by the time that a baby girl is born. Some propose that 150,000 exist, others maintain that about one million are present to form the stock from which all future eggs to be ovulated will be selected. At birth, the primordial follicles each contain an ovum arrested in the stage of development known as a primary oocyte. By puberty, the number of follicles has dropped to 50,000 or fewer by the process of atresia. Usually only one egg is ovulated each month, with a total of approximately 400 ova ovulated during a woman's reproductive years, between puberty and menopause. It has been commonly believed that a woman is born with all the eggs she will ever have. However, recent research with mice suggests that it may be possible for new ova to develop throughout a woman's lifetime.

OVIDUCTS OR FALLOPIAN TUBES

The **fallopian tubes** are also known as the **oviducts** or the uterine tubes. The fallopian tubes and the ovaries are sometimes referred to as the adnexa because they are adjacent, or next to, the uterus (Figure 3-3 and Figure 3-4). The fallopian tubes are named after the sixteenth century anatomist Gabrielle Fallopius, who thought they resembled tubas or curved trumpets and proposed they released noxious fumes from the uterus. The prefix salpinx, which in Greek means "tube", is used when describing conditions of the oviducts. The fallopian tube is anatomically divided into four sections:

1. The interstitial or uterine portion is the shortest portion and narrow compared to the rest of the oviduct. The uterine portion lies completely within the muscle of the uterus.
2. The isthmus is the straight section with a thick muscular wall and a narrow lumen. This section is the usual site of a tubal ligation, a surgical procedure that prevents the sperm from meeting the ovum by cutting or ligating the oviduct. This procedure will be discussed in Chapter 13.
3. The ampulla occupies about one-half the entire length of the tube. This portion is thin-walled with a highly folded lining.
4. The infundibulum, nearest the ovary, is a trumpet-shaped expansion with finger-like projections called fimbriae that wave back and forth to attract the ovum into the opening, or ostium of the fallopian tube. One fimbria is longer, closer to the ovary, and is called the ovarian fimbria.

When an ovum is released from the ovary, it is not in direct contact with the end of the fallopian tube, and the exact mechanisms that keeps the egg

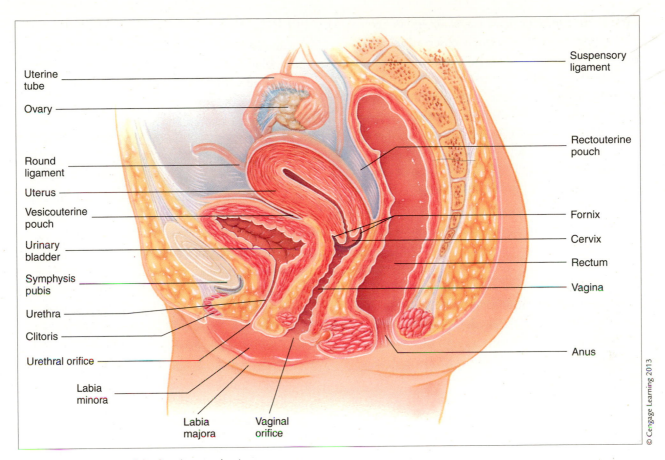

FIGURE 3-3: The organs of the female reproductive system.

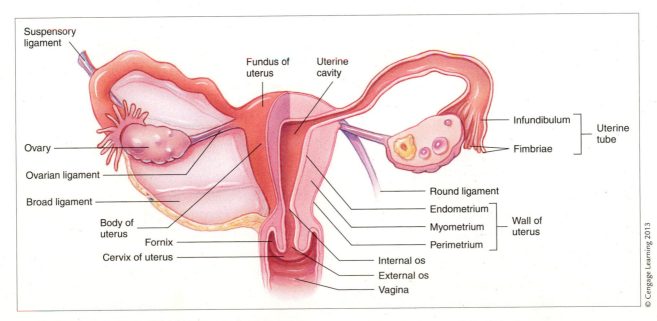

FIGURE 3-4: Internal organs of the female reproductive system.

from drifting into the pelvic cavity are still not completely understood. Laproscopic observations at the time of ovulation have revealed that the fimbrae are brought closer to the ovary to curve around it by contraction of muscle fibers in the connective tissue which covers and suspends the fallopian tubes from the abdominal wall. It has also been suggested that muscular contractions in the walls of the fimbriae, coupled with wave-like action of the ciliated cells lining the tube, pull the ovum into the tube by a gentle suction.

The walls of the tubes contain longitudinal and circular smooth muscle fibers and a rich supply of blood vessels. The tube is lined with ciliated epithelial tissue that secretes a fluid to provide an environment necessary for the movement, fertilization, and survival of the ovum. The rhythmic contractions of the smooth muscles in the walls of the oviducts, combined with the motion of the cilia help the egg to move toward the uterus. This muscular activity is influenced by hormones and is greatest at the time of ovulation.

Once in the infundibulum, the egg rapidly travels through the ampulla until it reaches the ampullary-isthmus junction, where its transit is delayed for about 30 hours. This pause is referred to as the "tube-locking" mechanism, or the "isthmic block," and if sperm are present, fertilization occurs here. If the egg is not fertilized within 24 hours after ovulation, it deteriorates. If fertilization occurs, the newly fertilized egg divides and passes rapidly through the isthmus and interstitial portion into the uterine cavity. It takes 45–80 hours between ovulation and the fertilized egg's entry into the uterus. Two to three additional days pass before the embryo implants in the uterine lining, a process called implantation.

Structural abnormalities or scarring of the tubes that result from surgery or infection can block movement of the egg, sperm or embryo through the fallopian tubes. Occasionally, an egg is fertilized and implants in the fallopian tube, rather than in the uterus. This is referred to as an ectopic or tubal pregnancy. It is not possible for a fetus to develop to term in the fallopian tube, and if left untreated, the inevitable rupture of the fallopian tube can lead to the death of both the mother and the embryo. Additional information about ectopic pregnancies can be found in Chapter 12.

UTERUS

The **uterus** is a hollow muscular organ that houses the developing fetus during gestation. The uterus is constructed of three distinct layers. The outer layer of the uterus, the perimetrium, consists of epithelial and connective tissues. The middle layer, the myometrium, is the thickest of the three layers. It consists primarily of involuntary smooth muscle, and it is responsible for the powerful contractions of labor. The inner lining of the uterus, the endometrium, can be further divided into the rapidly dividing basal layer and the thick functional layer. The layers of the uterus wall are illustrated in Figure 3-3. During the reproductive years, the endometrium, under the influence of hormones, thickens and then sheds causing menstruation. If a pregnancy occurs, the embryo implants in the functional layer of the endometrium and is maintained until delivery.

The uterus has an upper expanded portion called the body, or fundus, and a lower constricted portion called the neck, or **cervix**. The cervix projects into the vagina and has an opening, the external os. As with the other organs of the reproductive system, there is considerable variation in the size of the non-pregnant uterus, but on average it is 76 mm long, 51 mm wide at the fundus, 25 mm thick at its thickest part, and the walls of the uterus are about 13 mm thick. The uterus has the ability to grow from a non-pregnant weight of about 57 grams when non-pregnant, to 907 grams immediately after delivery. It can then shrink back to its original size within six weeks after delivery.

Position of the Uterus

The position of the uterus between the rectum and the bladder varies, depending on a woman's posture, how full her bladder or the rectum is, and how many pregnancies she has had (Figure 3-5). Figure 3-6 shows the body of the uterus in a typical position, which is inclined forward. When the urinary bladder is distended, the backward movement of the uterus is called retroversion; when the rectum is distended, the forward movement of the body of the uterus is called anteversion. Further and marked anteversion with relation to the cervix is called acute flexion; marked retroversion is called retroflexion. The uterus is

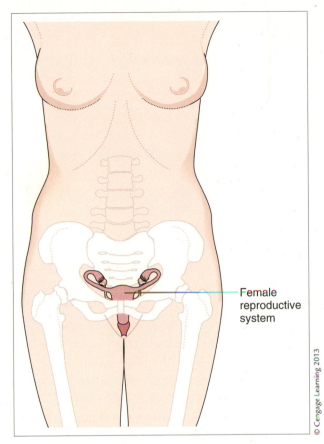

FIGURE 3-5: Position of the female reproductive organs in the pelvis.

© Cengage Learning 2013

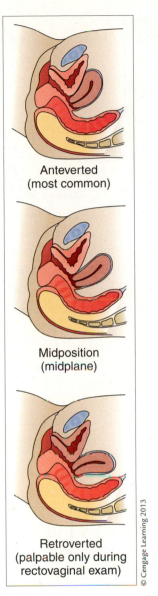

Anteverted
(most common)

Midposition
(midplane)

Retroverted
(palpable only during
rectovaginal exam)

© Cengage Learning 2013

FIGURE 3-6: The position of the uterus can vary in position: Uterus is anteverted (most common); Uterus in midposition; Uterus is retroverted.

normally anteverted and anteflexed. When a woman's uterus tends to remain in a retroflexed position, it is sometimes called a "tipped" uterus. In the past, having a tipped uterus was considered a contributing factor to such physical symptoms as backache, constipation, and menstrual cramps. During the nineteenth century, gynecologists used vaginal pessaries to correct retroflexions of the uterus. During the early part of the twentieth century, many unnecessary surgeries were performed to "correct" the position of the uterus and to relieve the symptoms blamed on its atypical position. It is now accepted that a tipped uterus does not contribute to the negative symptoms ascribed to it in the past.

Some historical medical records and scholarly writings described the uterus in fanciful and errone-ous terms. Early accounts even described the uterus as an independent animal moving within a woman's body and capable of independent activity. A physician in the fourteenth century a.d. wrote:

In the middle of the flanks of women lies the womb, a female viscus, closely resembling an animal, for it is moved of itself hither and thither in the flanks . . . and in a word, is altogether erratic. It delights also in fragrant smells and advances toward them, and it has an aversion to fetid smells and flees from them; and on the whole the womb is like an animal within an animal (Speert, 1973).

Centuries earlier, Hippocrates wrote that the uterus went wild unless it was often fed with male semen. Hippocrates then went on to describe hysteria as a condition of female madness that he believed resulted

Female reproductive system

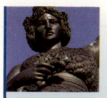

from dysfunction of the uterus. The idea of linking mental illness with problems related to the uterus was reiterated by Freud in the 1890s. Freud's influence on the perceptions of women and their mental health was strong through much of the twentieth century.

CERVIX

The lower part of the uterus, the cervix, projects into the vagina and is circumferentially attached to it, dividing the uterus into an upper, or supravaginal part, and a lower or vaginal portion. The vaginal part of the cervix is called the portio vaginalis. In an adult woman who has not delivered any children, the cervix comprises approximately one-half the length of the uterus; in a woman who has given birth to at least one child, it may be only one-third the length of the uterus. In its typical position in most women, the cervix is directed downward and backward. This position is supported and maintained by ligaments, which attach it to the body wall.

The cervix is predominantly composed of fibrous connective tissue with many smooth muscle fibers.

It is firm to the touch except after approximately the sixth weeks of pregnancy, when it softens, owing to an increased blood supply to the uterus and cervix. The texture of the non-pregnant cervix has been compared to the texture of the tip of the nose, or to the glans of the erect penis.

The opening of the cervix into the vagina is called the external os. The opening into the uterine cavity is called the internal os. The canal between the external and the internal os is the endocervical canal, lined with the endocervical epithelium. It contains many mucus-secreting glands and is approximately 2.5 cm long. Dilation of the cervix means an enlargement of the os, and this small opening has the capacity to enlarge enough to accommodate the delivery of a baby. Before childbirth, the external os appears as a small, round dimple, approximately 3 mm in diameter. After childbirth, it appears as a transverse slit with irregular margins. Enlarging the cervical opening with dilators to perform an abortion or a dilation and curettage has the same effect.

The epithelium on the surface of the vaginal aspect of the cervix is pale pink, whereas the epithelium of the endocervical canal that leads into the uterus from the external os is redder in color. Because of this color difference, inflammations, benign polyps, or cysts are highly visible on the surface of the portio vaginalis, even though these conditions originate inside the endocervical canal. The glands that line the endocervical canal are highly branched and extend deeply into the recesses and folds of the cervical walls. If microorganisms invade the glands, they can lead to a chronic infection.

Cervical Mucus

The endocervical glands secrete cervical mucus. During the reproductive cycle, the physical properties of the cervical mucus change as a result of fluctuations of the levels of two hormones: estrogen and progesterone. During most of the cycle, the mucus is thick in texture and not hospitable to sperm that might try to pass through it on their way toward the uterus and the fallopian tubes (Figure 3-7A). Near the time of ovulation, however, the mucus becomes thinner and less viscous and is easier for the sperm to pass through (Figure 3-7B). When this "fertile mucus" is spread out on a glass microscope slide it will undergo "ferning"

or "arborization" forming distinct patterns as it dries that resemble ferns or tree branches. After ovulation, the mucus becomes much thicker again, and no longer demonstrates ferning. These changes can be used both to test hormonal activity and to determination of the time of ovulation.

VAGINA

The **vagina** is a muscular tube that passes upward to the uterus at an approximate 45° angle from the vulva. The shape of the vagina is so variable and so capable of distension that it is difficult to measure its dimensions. This great distensibility enables the vagina to withstand vigorous stresses during intercourse or childbirth. When the vagina is empty, its walls collapse against each other, and the vagina becomes a potential space, rather than an open cavity. In a woman who has never had a child, there are many folds in the vaginal walls and the vaginal walls are firm. After giving birth, the walls become more or less smoothed out, but usually retain their firmness, especially near the opening of the vagina. This is not always true for women who have had many children.

The cervix projects into the upper vagina. The circular indentation formed all around the cervix is anatomically divided into the anterior, posterior,

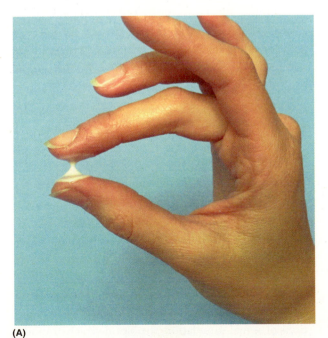

(A)

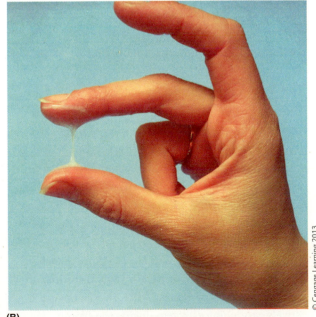

(B)

FIGURE 3-7: Cervical mucus consistency changes throughout the reproductive cycle: (A) Before ovulation the mucus is thick, and blocks the passage of sperm (B) At ovulation the cervical mucus becomes thinner and elastic, allowing sperm to move through it.

and lateral fornices. The walls of the fornices are thin because they consist only of the vaginal wall, with the pelvic cavity on the other side. During an internal pelvic examination, the position and relations of the various pelvic organs and ligaments can be palpated and outlined through the fornices. Normally, the posterior fornix is empty, and the body of the uterus can be felt through the anterior fornix; the fallopian tubes and the ovaries, through the lateral fornices.

The posterior fornix extends deeper into the pelvis and is larger and longer than the anterior fornix. This anatomical arrangement can favor the passage of sperm into the cervix after intercourse because a pool of ejaculated semen collects in the posterior fornix and, if a woman is lying on her back, the opening of the cervix is directly exposed to the ejaculate.

Only a thin partition of vaginal wall separates the posterior fornix from the peritoneum, which dips down to form the rectouterine pouch, also called the pouch of Douglas. For this reason, the posterior fornix can be used as an entry point into the abdomen for several kinds of diagnostic and surgical procedures. In culdocentesis, for example, a needle is inserted through the pouch of Douglas to determine the nature of any fluid that might be present, such as blood or pus. Colpotomy is a surgical incision through the posterior fornix into the peritoneum of the pelvic cavity. Through this opening, the pelvic viscera can be visually explored by means of an endoscope, which is a tube equipped with optical devices and light—a sort of internal microscope.

The Vaginal Lining

The lining of the vagina is called the vaginal epithelium. This mucus membrane consists of many layers of protective epithelial cells resting on connective tissue, which contain blood vessels and nerves. The deeper layers of the epithelial cells are constantly dividing and pushing up to replace the superficial layers, creating a very tough, resistant, and protective lining. Estrogen stimulates the growth of the epithelial cells. Before puberty and after menopause when there is less estrogen present, the vaginal epithelium is thinner and less resilient. When the ovaries are actively producing estrogen during the reproductive years, a smear of cellular material taken from the thick vaginal epithelium will show large numbers of shed cells, and it is possible to recognize phases of the menstrual cycle by the shape and staining qualities of these cells. An index of estrogenic activity can be determined by the type of cells present in a stained smear of the vaginal lining.

Vaginal Discharge

The contents of the vagina after puberty and before menopause are normally quite acidic, with a pH of approximately 4.5. As shed cells from the vaginal epithelium accumulate, vaginal bacteria break down the stored sugars in the cells and form lactic acid. The presence of the lactic acid is responsible for the lowered pH of the vagina. Multiple species of bacteria ordinarily inhabit the vagina and are called the normal flora. Information about the important role that these microorganisms play in maintaining vaginal health will be discussed in Chapter 6.

Normally, the vaginal discharge is clear and consists of fluid arising from the capillaries in the vaginal walls, with lesser amounts contributed from the cervical glands, the uterine cavity, and the fallopian tubes. Mucus, superficial shed cells, normal flora, and other microorganisms can also be found in the discharge. The acidic pH of the discharge combined with the tough epithelial lining protects the vagina from infection by harmful bacteria throughout most of a woman's life. However, before puberty and after menopause, the pH of the vagina tends to be less acidic, and the vagina is somewhat more vulnerable to infection. Throughout a woman's lifetime, disruptions of the normal flora by chemical contraceptives, antibiotics, or excess douching can increase the likelihood of vaginal infections.

Vaginal Lubrication

There is always some lubrication of the vagina from vaginal discharge, but sexual stimulation produces considerably more. Before the observations of sex researchers William Masters and Virginia Johnson in the 1960s, it was incorrectly assumed that Bartholin's glands and cervical mucus from the cervical glands increased the vaginal lubrication. However, Masters and Johnson (1966) observed that, under the conditions of sexual stimulation, the blood vessels around the vagina become engorged with blood. The increasing pressure forces a mucoid liquid, or transudate, to pass from the vessels through the vaginal epithelium into the vagina. This liquid at first forms individual droplets and then, as the droplets coalesce, forms a coating for the entire vagina. Because this appeared to be similar to drops of perspiration beading on a forehead, Masters and Johnson called this the "sweating phenomenon" of the vagina. This occurs very early in the female sexual response and usually provides sufficient lubrication for intercourse. The vaginal response tends to be prevented when certain kinds of vaginal infections are present, and some women using hormonal forms of birth control may also find that vaginal lubrication is diminished. Without lubrication, sexual intercourse can be uncomfortable.

Nerves of the Vagina

At least two types of nerves found in the vagina play a role in female sexual function. Sensory neurons facilitate the perception of sensations in the vagina, and autonomic neurons regulate blood flow to the vaginal walls and to the tissues surrounding the vagina. Sensations of pressure within the vagina are also detected by nerve receptors in the rectum or urinary bladder. Anatomical studies (Pauls et al., 2006) have revealed that nerves are distributed evenly throughout the vagina, and that the concentration of nerves does not appear to correlate with a woman's age, previous births, or sexual function. However, this study only sampled twenty-one women, and it did not distinguish between sensory and autonomic nerves, so additional research is needed. The upper two-thirds of the vagina is supplied almost entirely by autonomic neurons which control the rich supply of blood vessels surrounding the vagina. In addition to contributing to vaginal lubrication during sexual arousal, these blood vessels fill the erectile tissues that surround the vagina and are associated with the clitoris. Neurons controlling these vessels are important to female sexual function. In fact, when Pieterse et al. (2008) tested the level of vaginal blood flow in women who had nerve sparing hysterectomies rather than conventional hysterectomies, they found that the women with intact nerves had better vaginal blood flow, and, presumably, better sexual function. Additional research has found that autonomic nerves descend between the vagina and the urethra and also play an important role in urinary continence (Yoshida et al., 2007).

FEMALE PROSTATE

Surrounding the urethra and homologous to the male prostate, there are a collection of glands and ducts that manufacture secretions that are expelled by the urethra and which contribute to the lubrication of the vulva. These glands comprise the female prostate, a name that was officially accepted by the Federative International Committee on Anatomical Terminology in 2002 (*Terminologica Histologica*, 2002). The female prostate does not appear to be as distinct an organ as the male prostate, but it is derived from homologous embryological tissues. These glands are also referred to as the paraurethral glands, or the Skene's glands. When Alexander Skene announced his discovery of the glands in the nineteenth century, they had already been described by Dutch physiologist Reijnier de Graaf 200 years earlier as the producers of "female semen," the lubricating fluid discharged during sexual stimulation. In 1982, Ladas, Whipple, and Perry described this secretion in their book, *The G-Spot & Other Recent Discoveries about Human Sexuality*. They dubbed the secretion the female ejaculate and sparked many years of controversy about the phenomenon of female ejaculation. There has been some speculation that the fluid that is expelled is urine and that women who experience this phenomenon might simply be experiencing coital incontinence. In a study based on the responses of twelve women, six of whom experienced ejaculation and six who did not, Cartwright et al. (2007) found that these emissions were not consistent with coital incontinence. Recent research by Wimpissinger et al. (2007) found that when analyzed, the ejaculated substance was chemically more similar to prostate plasma than it was to urine. The sample size for this study was small, only two women were sampled, but it points to the need for more research. It is important to note that much of the glandular tissue of the female prostate lies in close proximity to the anterior wall of the vagina. This proximity may play an important role in understanding the Graafenburg or G-Spot.

THE G-SPOT

In 1950, Ernst Graafenberg, a German gynecologist, described a "zone of erogenous feeling located along the anterior vaginal wall." His work did not receive much attention at the time, but the publication of Ladas, Whipple, and Perry's book revived inquiry about the phenomenon during the early 1980s. Since that time, there has been considerable controversy in scientific circles about the existence or non-existence of the G-spot (Rabinerson & Horowitz, 2007, Hines, 2001, Alzante & Hoch, 1986, Belzer, 1984). New studies describing the more extensive size of the clitoris and its proximity of the urethra and vagina, along with the functions of the female prostate, may increase understanding about the anatomical and physiological origins of this structure. In a recent study, Gravina et al. (2008) used ultrasound to examine this area of the vagina and discovered variations in the thickness of what they termed the clitoris-urethrovaginal complex. They correlated the differences in thickness with a woman's tendency to experience vaginal orgasms. In their study, women who exhibited a thickened mucosa in the region of the G-spot were more likely to experience vaginal orgasms than women who did not.

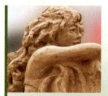

Economic Considerations
THE G-SPOT SHOT

Advertisements for the G-Spot shot have been appearing on the Internet in recent years. Claims that the majority of women surveyed after receiving G-Spot augmentation reported enhanced sexual arousal/gratification abound on these sites. The G-Spot shot is a procedure that is accomplished by injecting a cosmetic dermal filler such as collagen into the wall of the vagina to enlarge the G-Spot, enabling some women to have a higher level of sexual arousal and stronger and more frequent orgasms. The cost of this "cosmetic" procedure is not covered by insurance, putting the procedure beyond the means of most women. The effect of the shot can last four-six months, requiring repeated, costly injections to maintain the effect.

THE VULVA

The female external genitals are called the **vulva**. The name vulva means "covering" in Latin, and refers to the area bounded by the mons pubis anteriorly, the perineum posteriorly, and the labia minora and majora laterally. The clitoris and the vestibule are also considered to be part of the vulva. The vulva protects the urethral and vaginal openings. Older references also use the term pudendum. The vulva has a rich supply of sensory nerve fibers from the pudendal nerve and is highly sensitive to touch. If the internal wall of the vagina is inflamed or infected, although the site of the irritation is inside, the itching or pain is often referred to the outside on the vulva because of the nerve distribution.

Clitoris

The **clitoris** originates from the same embryological tissues as the penis does in males. Like the penis, it is made up of erectile tissue that can fill with blood and swell during sexual excitement. Some texts describe the clitoris as a vestigial homologue of the penis, implying that it is an incompletely developed or useless structure. However, the clitoris is rich in both blood supply and nerve endings, and serves an important role in female sexuality. It has, for its size, a generous blood and nerve supply relatively greater than that of the penis. There are more sensory receptors located in the clitoris than in any other part of the body, and it is, unsurprisingly, often the most erotically sensitive part of a woman's body (Figure 3-8).

The glans is the portion of the clitoris that is external and visible. The clitoris consists of two crura, which are also called roots; a shaft, which is also called the body of the clitoris; and a glans. The two crura join to form the shaft of the clitoris. Within the shaft are the two corpora cavernosa that consist of erectile tissue. When the corpora cavernosa become engorged with blood it causes the clitoris to double in size and become erect. At the end of the shaft is the rounded glans which is extremely sensitive to the touch. The ischiocavernosus muscles and the bulbocavernosus muscles contribute to clitoral erection not by flexing and moving the clitoris directly, but by contracting and trapping blood in the free spaces of the corpus cavernosa. During sexual excitement, these muscles contract and compress the dorsal vein of the clitoris, which is the only vein that drains the blood

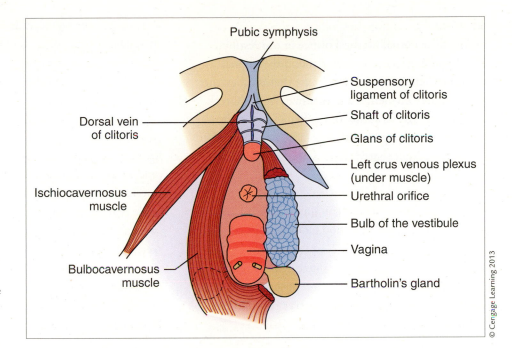

Pubic symphysis

Suspensory
ligament of clitoris

Shaft of clitoris

Glans of clitoris

Left crus venous plexus
(under muscle)

Urethral orifice

Bulb of the vestibule

Vagina

Bartholin's gland

Dorsal vein
of clitoris

Ischiocavernosus
muscle

Bulbocavernosus
muscle

© Cengage Learning 2013

FIGURE 3-8: Mechanism of clitoral erection. Stimulation of the clitoris results in an increased blood flow to the erectile tissues (corpora cavernosa) in the shaft of the clitoris. The contraction of the two clitoral muscles compresses the only vein that drains the corpus carvernosa. The trapped blood causes the engorgement of the erectile tissues, and the enlargement and erection of the clitoris.

from the spaces in the corpora cavernosa. The arterial blood continues to pour in filling the venous spaces until they become engorged with blood. This mechanism causes the erection of the clitoris in a process analogous to the process that causes the erection of a penis during sexual excitement.

Recent anatomical studies on female cadavers by Australian urologist Helen O'Connell et al. (1998), have shown the clitoris is much larger than was previously thought. Her studies revealed that most of the clitoris extends back into the body, and wraps around both the vagina and the urethra. In addition, O'Connell and her colleagues found that there is more erectile tissue associated with the clitoris than was previously described in most anatomical texts. When they compared the arrangement and amount of erectile tissue in the urethra and genitalia of the cadavers with current anatomical descriptions, they found variations based on the age of the woman, and that there was more erectile tissue associated with the clitoris in younger women than is described in modern anatomical texts and diagrams. The researchers concluded, although the sample size was small, that the dissections upon which anatomical descriptions of female human urethral and genital anatomy relied were inaccurate because they were likely to have been performed on elderly women in which the erectile tissue had shrunk. The investigators also recommended

that because the erectile tissues of what were formerly called the vestibular bulbs were more closely related to the clitoris and urethra, the bulbs of the vestibule should be renamed the bulbs of the clitoris. In addition to calling attention to the inaccuracy of anatomical textbooks, an important implication of this research is the potential to prevent damage to the erectile tissues important to sexual function for women having surgery for bladder problems, hysterectomy, or other surgeries in the vicinity of the urethra.

Vestibule

The **vestibule** is the area enclosed by the labia minora. Opening into the vestibule are the urethra from the urinary bladder, the vagina, and the two ducts of the Bartholin's glands, which are also called the greater vestibular glands. Bartholin's glands produce a few drops of mucus during sexual excitement that moisten the vestibule in preparation for intercourse. Occasionally, the duct of a Bartholin's gland can become obstructed, and the gland continues to secrete behind the duct. The result is a Bartholin's cyst, which usually produces no symptoms, but which may form an abscess and need to be removed. A gonorrhea infection may sometimes cause a Bartholin's cyst. Approximately 2.5 cm below the clitoris, there is a small elevation like a dimple. In its center is the opening of the urethra called the external urethral orifice.

Hymen

Below the external urethral orifice in the vestibule is the opening to the vagina. Around the vaginal opening there is a small membrane that is called the **hymen**, after Hymen, the god of marriage in Greek mythology. The structure of the hymen is highly variable. It will appear different in each individual woman, without regard to her sexual history. The hymen can be:

- Thin as a spider web, or thick and fleshy
- Quite vascular, with a good blood supply, or relatively avascular
- Extremely variable in how much of the vaginal opening is covered
- So pliable and flexible that it never ruptures but instead stretches, even after childbirth

It is commonly believed that the hymen tears at the first coitus, producing copious and visible bleeding. If no bleeding occurs, this is sometimes taken as evidence that a woman is not a virgin. Many also believe that the hymen makes it impossible for a virgin to wear tampons during her menstrual period, or that if the attempt is made, this sign of virginity will disappear. In fact, an intact hymen is not proof of virginity, and a ruptured hymen is not indicative that sexual intercourse has occurred. Although it is usually possible to determine with accuracy whether or not a woman has had a child by examining the shape of her cervical os, it is generally impossible to say whether or not she is a virgin by just looking at the vaginal opening and the condition of the hymen.

In rare cases, the hymen can completely cover the opening to the vagina. This is called an imperforate

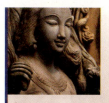

Social Considerations
VAGINAL COSMETIC SURGERIES

Vaginal surgeries, also known as vaginoplasties, are not new. They have been available for decades to treat urinary incontinence, uterine prolapse, and damage to the vagina caused by childbirth or trauma. However, the availability of vaginal surgeries for elective and cosmetic purposes is a relatively new phenomenon. The American Society of Plastic Surgery reported 793 elective vaginal rejuvenation surgeries in the United States in 2005. That number jumped to 1,030 in 2006. Although the numbers represent only a fraction of total cosmetic surgeries undergone, the rate of increase of these surgeries is significant, with some estimating a rate of increase by 30% per year at present. These surgeries fall into two broad categories. Labioplasty involves altering the appearance of the labia majora or the labia minora, while vaginal rejuvenation alters the size or shape of the vagina. Reducing the width, or "tightening" the vagina is frequently purported to increase a woman's sexual pleasure during intercourse, although anecdotal reports about the results of the surgery have been mixed. Some women report

increased satisfaction, while others report pain due to scar tissue resulting from the surgery. Scientific studies on the results of vaginal surgeries have yielded mixed conclusions as well (Adamo & Corvi, 2009; Tunuguntia & Gousse, 2006; Pardo et al., 2006; Crouch et al., 2004; Weber et al., 2000). In addition to resulting in pain during intercourse, the development of scar tissue can also interfere with vaginal lubrication. Another concern is the potential damage to nerves in the vagina, some of which are responsible for relaying sensations to the brain (Crouch et al., 2004). Other nerves in the vagina influence blood flow to the clitoris and to the tissues surrounding the vaginal walls themselves, and thus play important roles in arousal and sexual function. In 2007, the American College of Obstetricians and Gynecologists issued the following statement advising against cosmetic vaginal procedures: "So-called vaginal rejuvenation, designer vaginoplasty, revirgination, and G-spot amplification procedures are not medically indicated, nor is there documentation of their safety and effectiveness" (ACOG, 2007).

hymen and is usually discovered during adolescence. A girl with an imperforate hymen will menstruate into the vagina month after month, and the discharge will accumulate in the vagina, a condition called hematocolpos. If it is not recognized, menstrual blood may fill the uterus and the fallopian tubes as well. Cutting of the hymen alleviates the problem. Another variation that can occur is a septate hymen. In this case, a band of extra tissue in the hymen stretches across the vaginal opening, making it appear that there are two vaginal openings instead of one. If the septum is not too thick and is flexible enough, intercourse is not hampered. There is usually no problem with insertion of tampons, although there may be some difficulty encountered while removing them. The treatment for a septate hymen is minor surgery to remove the extra band of tissue. After childbirth, the hymen usually loses its continuous rim and remains as isolated fragments, with gaps in between. These fragments of the hymen are referred to as carunculae hymenales.

The hymen is present throughout a woman's life, although the wide variability in structure between individuals makes it hard to assign it a clear function. In some cases the hymen does have psychological, sociological, or cultural significance depending on the traditions of a woman's family or community. In recent years there has been a rise in the availability of hymen restoration surgeries. During this surgery the hymen is constructed or reconstructed using membranes or other tissues (O'Connor, 2008).

Mons Pubis

Another name for the mons pubis is the mons veneris, which translates as "the mountain of Venus," named for Venus, the goddess of love. The mons pubis is the cushion of fatty tissue and skin that lies over the pubic symphysis and, after puberty, is covered with pubic hair (Figure 3-9). In many women, the upper border of pubic hair is straight across, forming a triangle, and this is the so-called female escutcheon. In most males and about 25% of females, the upper border of the pubic hair extends upward toward the navel. When a woman has this abdominal growth of hair, it is very rarely a sign of an overabundance of male sex hormones.

Labia Majora

Extending down from the mons pubis are two longitudinal folds of skin, narrowing to enclose the vulvar cleft, and meeting posteriorly in the perineum. These folds are called the **labia majora**, and they protect the

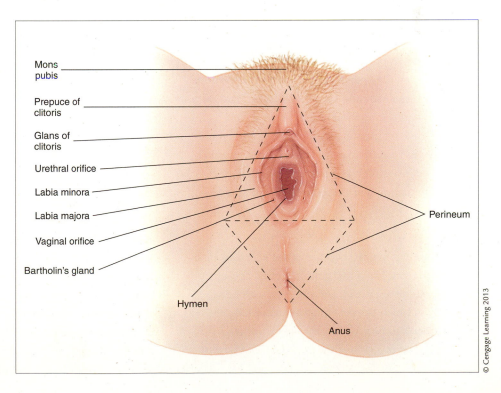

FIGURE 3-9: External structures of the female genitalia or vulva.

Mons pubis
Prepuce of clitoris
Glans of clitoris
Urethral orifice
Labia minora
Labia majora
Vaginal orifice
Bartholin's gland
Hymen
Perineum
Anus

© Cengage Learning 2013

inner parts of the vulva. The outer surface of the labia is covered with pubic hair. The inner surface is not, but it has many sebaceous glands and sweat glands. The tissue inside the labia majora is loose connective tissue with pads of subcutaneous fat. This fat, like the fat on the hips and in the breasts, is particularly sensitive to estrogen, which is why the labia and the rest of the vulva become enlarged at puberty and can shrink after menopause. Underneath the subcutaneous fat and deep within the labial tissue are masses of erectile tissue, which have recently been found to be part of the clitoris. Under the skin of the labia majora, there are temperature sensitive, subcutaneous muscle fibers, similar to the dartos muscle of the male scrotum.

Labia Minora

The **labia minora** are the delicate inner folds of skin that enclose the urethral opening and the vagina. These folds are sometimes called the nymphae. The labia minora extend down from the anterior inner part of the labia majora on each side. Each fold joins above and below the clitoris. The joining of the folds above

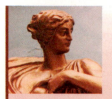

Cultural Considerations
HARMFUL TRADITIONAL PRACTICES: FEMALE GENITAL MUTILATION

According to the World Health Organization, female genital mutilation (FGM) is a procedure which involves the removal or alteration of external female genitalia for non-medical reasons. It is sometimes referred to as genital cutting, or female circumcision, and FGM is categorized by the World Health Organization into four major types:

1. Clitoridectomy, which involves partial or total removal of the clitoris

2. Excision, which involves partial or total removal of the clitoris and the inner labia

3. Infibulation, which involves the narrowing of the vaginal opening by cutting and repositioning the inner, and sometimes outer, labia, with or without removal of the clitoris

4. Other, which includes all other harmful procedures to the female genitalia for non-medical purposes, such as stretching, piercing, pricking, scraping or cauterizing the genital area (WHO, 2008)

FGM has been classified as a 'harmful traditional practice', because of the pain and injury it causes to women and girls. It is often carried out in the name of custom and tradition within the societies which perform it, and occasionally it is defended on the grounds of religion, although no religious texts condone the practice. FGM is most common in East and West Africa, as well as in some countries in Asia and the Middle East. Immigrant communities from these regions sometimes carry the practice with them when they relocate to North America and Europe. Typically, FGM is performed on girls, often before the age of puberty, by a traditional midwife or community elder experienced in the practice. The surgical tools are frequently rudimentary and unsterilized, and no anesthesia or antibiotics are used (WHO, 2008).

FGM is said to increase male pleasure during sexual intercourse, while at the same time making a woman more 'clean' and 'beautiful'. FGM is also said to ensure a girl's virginity until marriage, and to mark the transition into womanhood. Some 100 to 140 million girls and women worldwide are currently living with the consequences of FGM, and in Africa where the practice is prevalent, about three million girls are at risk for FGM annually (WHO, 2008).

FGM creates many health complications for women and is internationally recognized as a violation of the human rights of girls and women. Typical complications can include severe pain, shock, bleeding, tetanus, and infection (WHO, 2008). In the long term, women can suffer from recurrent bladder and urinary tract infections, painful intercourse, and an increased risk of complications during childbirth (WHO, 2008).

the clitoris forms the prepuce; the junction below the clitoris forms the frenulum. Each labium minora then extends downward to surround the vagina and join again at the posterior end of the vagina, where it blends into the skin of the labia majora. At this junction, there is a slightly raised ridge of skin, the fourchette. After the birth of a baby, the fourchette flattens out. There are no pubic hairs on the labia minora, but there are many sebaceous glands that may feel like tiny grains of sand when pressed between the thumb and forefinger.

The large numbers of sebaceous glands on the vulvar skin produce sebum, a mixture of oils, waxes, triglycerides, cholesterol, and cellular debris. Sebum lubricates the skin, and in combination with the secretions from the sweat glands and the vagina forms a waterproofing protective layer that enables the vulvar skin to repel urine, menstrual blood, and bacterial infections. Because of the many sebaceous glands, however, the labia minora, particularly in the area of the clitoris, are frequently the site of sebaceous cysts: painful nodules about the size of a pea in the skin. A vulvar sebaceous cyst usually drains spontaneously and disappears within a few days. However, it may become infected and require treatment or removal.

There are wide variations in the size and shape of the labia minora, and one side is generally larger than the other. Sometimes they are completely hidden by the labia majora, or they may be enlarged so that they project forward. Enclosed within the skin of the labia minora are venous sinuses or blood spaces that become engorged with blood during sexual excitement, causing a color change and an increase in the thickness of the labia, sometimes as much as two to three times their diameter.

PELVIC FLOOR: SUPPORT OF THE PELVIC ORGANS

The uterus, fallopian tubes, ovaries, the urinary bladder, and rectum are connected to each other and to the walls of the pelvic cavity by a number of ligaments and folds of the peritoneum (Figure 3-10). The peritoneum is the membrane that lines the body wall and covers most of the organs of the abdomen and pelvis. If these structures are repeatedly strained during childbirth, or if they become lacerated or atrophied, they can progressively weaken resulting in a variety of conditions. For example, the uterus,

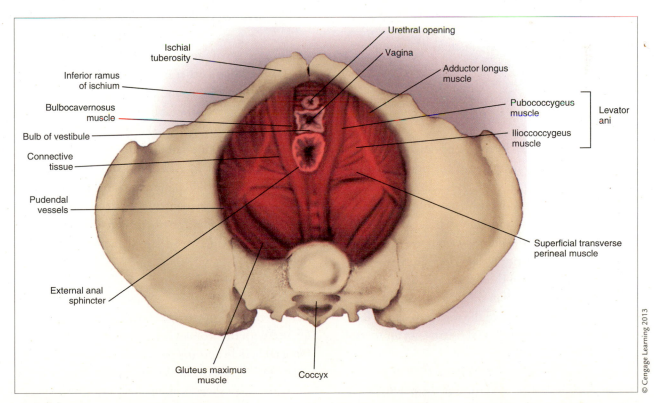

FIGURE 3-10: Muscles of the pelvic floor, from below.

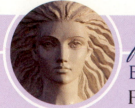

focus on

EXERCISE

Focus on Exercise: Kegel Exercises

Stress incontinence is the involuntary loss of urine that can occur during exercise or as a result of coughing, laughing or sneezing. Most surgical treatment for stress incontinence is aimed at restoring the integrity of the pubococcygeus muscle and the urethrovesical angle. Voluntary contractions of the pubococcygeus muscle, commonly called Kegel exercises, can alleviate many cases of mild to moderate stress incontinence and are certainly worth trying before resorting to surgery. The exercises, as described by Arnold Kegel, the physician who advocated them, are meant to strengthen the pelvic diaphragm. Fifty to 100 times a day, the pubococcygeus should be contracted for at least 3 seconds, and the anus and vagina drawn up into the pelvis. No one can observe these exercises being performed and they can be done in any position—standing, sitting, and lying down. An easy regimen to follow would be to perform the contractions for 15 repetitions, six times a day (i.e., first thing in the morning, mid-morning, lunchtime, mid-afternoon, dinnertime, and bedtime). Also, whenever voiding, the flow of urine should be stopped and started several times. For many women, Kegel exercises strengthen the pubococcygeus muscle enough to pull up the neck of the bladder and increase the urethrovesical angle, thereby preventing leakage of urine. Reductions of incontinent episodes by 50%–60% as a result of such pelvic floor exercises have been reported (Burns et al., 1990; Bo, Talseth, & Holme, 1999).

can become damaged or strained. Another problem that can result from pelvic floor weakening or pelvic floor damage is urinary incontinence. Fecal incontinence can also occur. There are steps that a woman can take throughout her lifetime to protect her pelvic floor. Some medical practices during childbirth such as episiotomy and assisted delivery by forceps or vacuum extraction contribute to a woman's chance of developing damage to her pelvic floor. Avoiding these procedures, except in the rare cases where they are necessary, is an important precaution. In addition, the skeletal muscles of the pelvic floor can be exercised, just like any other skeletal muscles, to maintain their strength and effectiveness.

Gynecological Exams

Gynecological exams usually consist of both a physical exam looking for infections, abnormal changes in the reproductive system, and a Pap smear to screen for cervical cancer. An internal exam can identify uterine fibroids and other irregularities. Cervical, ovarian, and endometrial cancers have few noticeable symptoms during the early, more curable stages. A thorough exam provides one of the best methods to identify these conditions. Sexually transmitted infections (STIs) may also be asymptomatic, requiring lab tests to identify the infectious agent. Gynecological exams also provide an opportunity to discuss reproductive questions and birth control options.

External Examination

In most cases a gynecological examination is performed with the woman lying down on the examining table in lithotomy position; that is, her feet are up in stirrups, her buttocks close to the end of the table, and a sheet is draped like a tent over the knees and the upper part of her body. This position

bladder, or rectum can be displaced downward and begin to protrude or drop out of position. This dropping down or falling of an organ is called prolapse. When the urinary bladder prolapses into the anterior wall of the vagina and causes a bulge, it is called a cystocele. When the anterior wall of the rectum bulges into the posterior wall of the vagina, it is called a rectocele. Even though the uterus has more supporting structures than the other organs, it is the most likely to prolapse into the vagina. Chapter 8 will address the symptoms and treatments for uterine prolapse.

The muscles that form the lower wall of the pelvis are collectively referred to as the **pelvic floor**. Like the ligaments of the reproductive system, they straightens the curvature in the lumbar region of the spine and relaxes the abdominal muscles. The procedure usually includes palpation of the abdomen, inspection of the external genitals, and a speculum examination of the vagina and cervix, including cell smears for lab tests.

The healthcare provider will look for any enlargement or tenderness in the abdomen. The vulva and the perineum are examined, and the labia majora and minora are spread apart to see the entrance to the vagina, the hymen, and the urethra, to look for inflammation, scarring, sores, or growths such as warts, cysts, or tumors.

Pushing up the urethral opening against the pubic bone with the tip of the forefinger is called stripping or milking the urethra. In acute urethritis or in gonorrhea, a few drops of pus could be squeezed out from the paraurethral glands. The thumb and forefinger are used on either side of the labia majora to palpate for Bartholin's glands, which normally cannot be felt but which may be enlarged and tender if infected.

Internal Examination

To examine the cervix and the inside of the vagina, an instrument called the speculum is used to separate and hold apart the vaginal walls (Figure 3-11). The bivalve or duck-bill speculum may be made out of steel or plastic. It has two blades, and the posterior, or bottom one, is slightly longer than the anterior blade.

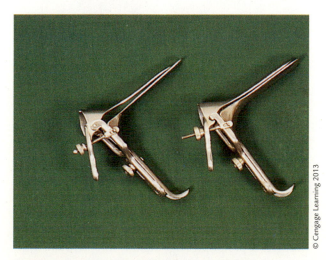

© Cengage Learning 2013

FIGURE 3-11: Vaginal speculum. Specula are available in different sizes.

It is designed so that it opens after insertion and can be fastened to remain open. The speculum cannot be lubricated with jelly because this would interfere with any analysis of vaginal secretions or cells. Usually, enough natural lubrication is present at the vaginal opening to ease the speculum into place. If not, water can be used.

The closed speculum is inserted, posterior blade first, into the vagina at about a 45° angle downward. In lithotomy position, the angle of the vagina is down toward the sacrum. When the speculum is in up to the hilt, it is rotated and opened. If the speculum is painful its position should be changed. The entire circumference of the cervix can then be viewed. At this point, a sample of cervical and vaginal cells (Pap smear) or discharge may be taken to screen for cervical cancer, vaginal infections, gonorrhea, and chlamydia (Figure 3-12).

The speculum is then slowly withdrawn as the vaginal walls are inspected again to make certain that any redness, cyst, or other damage has not been missed because it was hidden by the blades (Figure 3-13). A digital examination is then performed with the insertion of the middle and index finger into the vagina. As the examiner's fingers reach the full length of the vagina, the fornices are explored and palpated for masses or tenderness, and the cervix is palpated for size, shape, and consistency. The woman may be asked to hold her breath and "bear down." This increase in intra-abdominal pressure will reveal any weakness in the muscular supports of the bladder, rectum, or uterus.

The size, shape, position, mobility, and sensitivity of the uterus, ovaries, and fallopian tubes are ascertained by the bimanual, or two-handed, examination (Figure 3-14). The fingers of one hand inside the vagina are placed against the cervix to elevate it while the other hand presses downward on the lower abdomen. In this way, the body of the uterus can be outlined between the two hands. Then, the healthcare provider will try to identify the ovaries. The normal fallopian tube cannot usually be felt as a distinct structure, and the woman may feel a twinge of discomfort as the ovaries are pressed between the external and the internal hands to determine size, shape, and mobility.

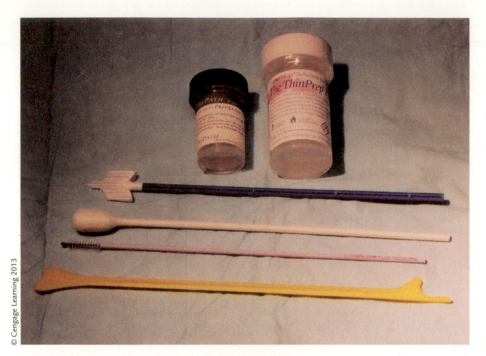

FIGURE 3-12: Pap smear.

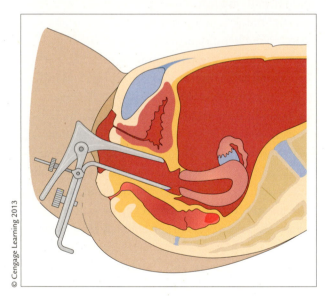

FIGURE 3-13: Lateral view of the speculum in position.

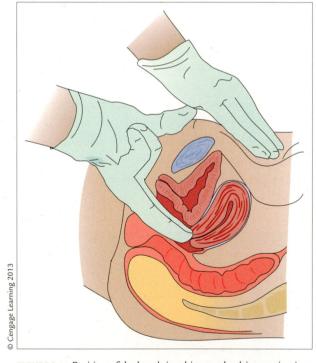

FIGURE 3-14: Position of the hands in a bimanual pelvic examination.

The pelvic examination should be concluded with the rectal or rectovaginal examination (Figure 3-15). There are some pelvic structures such as the posterior surface of the uterus, the broad ligaments, the uterosacral ligaments that can be felt accurately only through the rectum. At the same time, any abnormal growth that may be present in the rectum could also be located by this examination.

THE MALE REPRODUCTIVE TRACT

The reproductive tract of the male is adapted for the purposes of producing large numbers of sperm and then transporting the sperm into the female's reproductive tract so that the sperm can fertilize the egg. What follows

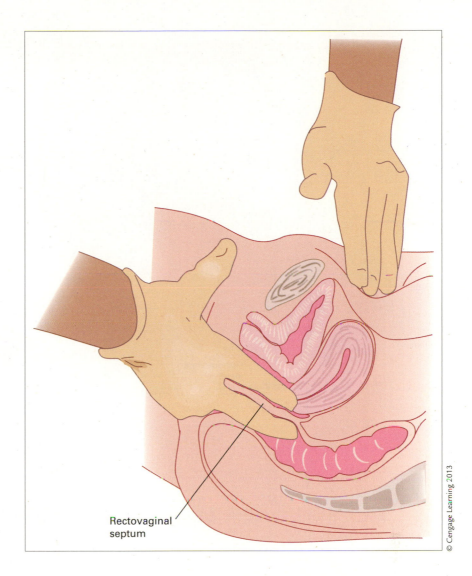

Rectovaginal
septum

FIGURE 3-15: Position of the hands in a
rectovaginal examination.

is a brief description of the male reproductive structure and function along with some comparisons of the
homologies of female and male anatomy (Figure 3-16).

Testes

The **testes** are the male gonads, responsible for producing both gametes and hormones, namely testosterone (Figure 3-17). The testes are also referred to as
testicles and one testicle is referred to as a testis. The
testes are smooth, oval organs about 4–5 cm long and
2.5 cm in diameter. The testes are suspended in the
scrotum, a loose pouch of skin divided by a septum
into a right and left half, each containing a testis. The
right and left scrotal sacs are homologous to the right
and left labia majora. As in the labia, a sheet of dartos
muscle lying just under the skin causes skin wrinkling
and contraction in response to cold temperature.
Another muscle, the cremaster muscle, contracts or

relaxes to change the proximity of the testes to the
body in order to regulate their temperature.

Although the testes are carried in the scrotum,
they originated during fetal life as primordial germ cells
in the abdominal cavity, just as in the female. Shortly
before birth, however, the testes descend along with
their ducts, nerves and blood vessels through the inguinal canal, out of the abdominal cavity, and into the
relatively cooler scrotal sacs. This is necessary because
growth and development of viable sperm require temperatures lower than normal body temperature. To
help maintain the lower temperature, the scrotum lacks
insulating fat and has many sweat glands.

In two to five percent of male babies, one or
both testes do not descend into the scrotum and
remain in the body cavity. This condition is known
as cryptorchidism, which translated from the Greek
means "hidden testis." Cryptorchidism sometimes

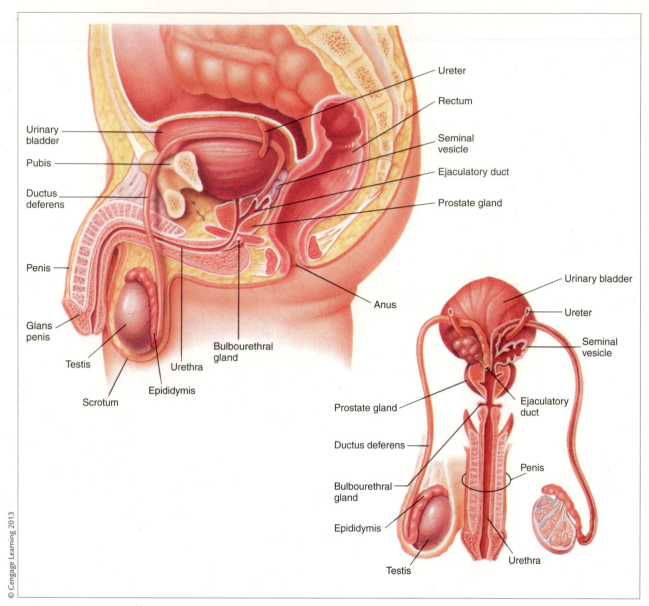

FIGURE 3-16: The male reproductive system.

corrects itself during childhood. If not, surgery can be performed to correct the problem. If uncorrected by the time of puberty, irreversible infertility can result.

Spermatogenesis, which is the production of sperm, occurs within the long, highly coiled seminiferous tubules inside the testes. The differentiation process, from the progenitor germ cells called spermatogonium, to a mature spermatozoon, takes about 74 days. Spermatogenesis begins at puberty, and continues throughout life. Every day a healthy male makes hundreds of millions of sperm. Specialized Sertoli cells in the testis mechanically

support and nurture the maturing sperm. Between the seminiferous tubules are clumps of interstitial cells, which produce male sex hormones, including testosterone.

Male Accessory Genital Ducts

The accessory duct system transports the sperm from the testes to the penis and then to the outside of the body. The duct system includes the epididymis, vas deferens, and urethra. As the sperm mature in the seminiferous tubules of each testis, they move to a structure called the **epididymis**. The epididymis is a 20-foot-long coiled tube that runs alongside the

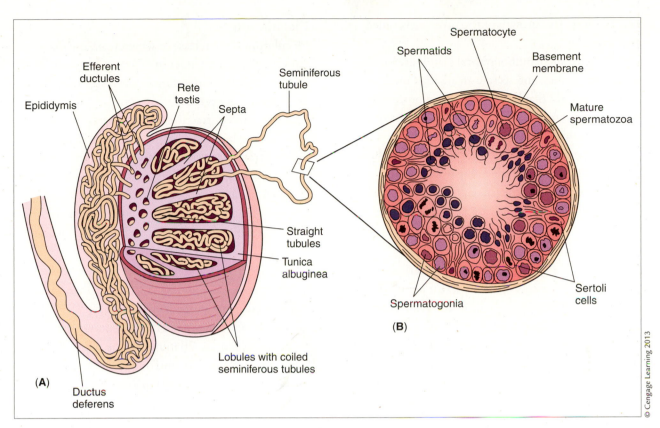

FIGURE 3-17: Anatomy of the testis.

testis within the scrotum and serves as a storage site for sperm. Sperm may be retained in the epididymis for up to six weeks before being ejaculated. If the sperm are not ejaculated, they die and are disposed of through phagocytosis, the normal scavenger activity of white blood cells. If ejaculation does take place, the sperm leave the scrotum through the vas deferens and ascend upward through the inguinal canal into the body cavity. The **vas deferens** are also called the ductus deferens. The end of each vas deferens expands and joins with a duct from a gland called a seminal vesicle to form a short ejaculatory duct. The two ejaculatory ducts penetrate the prostate gland to join the **urethra** as it exits from the urinary bladder. The urethra extends from the bladder to the end of the penis.

Male Accessory Glands

The accessory glands contribute fluids to the accessory duct system to combine with the sperm and form semen. Semen contains substances to nourish and protect the sperm and facilitate their movement. Only about five percent of the volume of semen is made up of sperm; the rest of the ejaculate is a mixed secretion of several accessory glands. In addition to the sperm, semen contains many of the substances ordinarily found in blood plasma with the addition of chemicals such as prostaglandins, enzymes, enzyme inhibitors, and hormones that play a role in sperm vitality, motility, migration, and fertilizing capacity.

The **seminal vesicles**, located at the base of the bladder, produce a viscous, alkaline fluid rich in fructose that provides a direct source of energy for the sperm. More than half of the bulk of semen is contributed by the seminal vesicles. The **prostate** is a single gland that surrounds the urethra as it leaves the bladder. The prostate secretes a milky, alkaline fluid to neutralize the acidity of the vagina during intercourse and enhance sperm motility, which is best at a pH of 6.0–6.5. The prostate is the homologue of the paraurethral, or Skene's, glands in the female. Although small in childhood, it begins to grow at puberty and reaches adult size by age 20. Around age 50, the prostate may slowly begin to grow larger and may eventually cause urinary obstruction. This growth of the prostate is called hypertrophy.

The two small bulbourethral glands are located along the urethra, and secrete an alkaline mucus-containing fluid that is lubricating and protective. These glands are also called Cowper's glands, and their equivalent in females are the Bartholin's glands. In some species the secretions of the bulbourethral gland form an impenetrable plug over the cervix, preventing sperm from other males from impregnating the female. This is not the case in humans.

Penis

The penis and the scrotum form the external genitalia in the male. The **penis** is the organ for copulation and also serves as the outlet for urine. It has an attached root, a body or shaft, and a glans, similar to its female homologue, the clitoris. The skin of the penis is thin with no hairs except near the root of the organ. The prepuce, which is also called the foreskin, is a circular fold of skin that extends over the glans. In some cultures, the foreskin is removed by a process called circumcision.

The body of the penis contains three cylindrical masses of erectile tissue that extend throughout its length. Two corpora cavernosa and one corpus spongiosum that surrounds the urethra are capable of filling with blood to create an erection. The bulbocavernosus muscles in the female and the bulbospongiosus muscles in the male are counterparts, and serve a similar function during intercourse. The corpora cavernosa in the male and the ischocavernosus muscles are mainly responsible for erection and behave identically to the erectile tissues and muscles responsible for erection of the clitoris.

Ejaculation

Ejaculation is the release of semen from the male reproductive tract. Under involuntary nervous control, muscle contractions in the testes and the reproductive ducts move the sperm into the urethra. Simultaneous contractions in the seminal vesicles, prostate, and bulbourethral glands expel seminal fluid into the tract along with the sperm. The volume of ejaculate averages 3 mL, but can normally range from 1–10 mL. The number of sperm in a single ejaculation is subject to individual variation and may be anywhere from 100 million sperm to half a billion sperm, but the normal average is 300–400 million. The first fraction of ejaculate contains most of the sperm, which have better motility and survival ability than those in the later portions. Immediately after ejaculation, the fluid semen coagulates and then spontaneously liquefies again within 15–20 minutes. The sperm do not reach their full motility until liquefaction occurs, so the rate of coagulation and liquefaction can be significant in the clinical evaluation of male fertility.

CONCLUSION

The study of human anatomy is one of the oldest scientific fields of research, and interest in understanding the anatomy of the female reproductive tract has waxed and waned over the centuries. New discoveries about the female anatomy have emerged in recent decades and will continue to emerge as scientists seek to build on existing knowledge. The understanding of anatomy is fundamental to the understanding of the physiology of the female reproductive system, both in health and in illness. Chapter 4 introduces the underlying physiology of the female reproductive cycle.

REVIEW QUESTIONS

1. Which structures are a part of the external genitalia in women? Which structures are internal structures? Are there any organs that have both external and internal components?

2. What are the functions of the ovaries? You should be able to describe at least two functions.

3. What is the purpose of the cilia in the Fallopian tubes?

4. Name and describe the three layers of the uterus.

5. Why is it difficult to accurately measure vagina size?

6. New information has recently become available about the anatomy of the clitoris. How are the new descriptions of the clitoris different from previous diagrams and descriptions available in anatomy textbooks?

7. What factors contribute to a woman's risk of developing urinary incontinence as they age?

8. What is uterine prolapse?

CRITICAL THINKING QUESTIONS

1. Operation protocols for sparing nerve and blood supply in pelvic operations for men have been available for many years. What factors have contributed to the delay in developing sexual function sparing pelvic operations for women?

2. If a spinal injury were to damage the neurons that supply a woman's lower pelvis, what physiological effects would result?

WEBLINKS

World Health Organization:
www.who.int

REFERENCES

ACOG Committee Opinion #378, "Vaginal Rejuvenation and Cosmetic Vaginal Procedures." Obstetrics & Gynecology, September (2007).

Adamo, C., & Corvi, M. (2009). Cosmetic mucosal vaginal tightening (lateral colporrhaphy): improving sensitivity in women with a sensation of wide vagina. *Plastic Reconstructive Surgery, 123*(6), 212–213.

Alzante, H., & Hoch, Z. (1986). The "G-spot" and "female ejaculation": A current appraisal. *Journal of Sex and Marital Therapy, 12*(3), 211–220.

American College of Obstetricians and Gynecol-ogists. (2007, September). Committee opinion no. 378. Vaginal rejuvenation and cosmetic vaginal procedures. *Obstetrics & Gynecology, 110*(3), 737–738.

Androgen insensitivity syndrome. (2008). Retrieved April 1, 2009 from http://ghr.nlm.nih.gov/condition/androgen-insensitivity-syndrome.

Banks, E., Merik, O., Farley, T., Akande, O., Bathiji, H., & Ali, M. (2006). Female genital mutilation and obstetric outcome: WHO collaborative prospective study in six African countries. *Lancet, 367*(9525), 1835–1841.

Belzer, E. G., Jr. (1984). A review of female ejaculation and the Grafenberg spot. *Women's Health, 9*(1), 5–16.

Bo, K., Talseth, T., & Holme, I. (1999). Single blind, randomized controlled trial of pelvic floor exercises, electrical stimulation, vaginal cones, and no treatment in management of genuine stress incontinence in women. *British Medical Journal, 318*(7182), 487–493.

Burns, P. A., Pranikoff, K., Nochajski, T., et al. (1990). Treatment of stress incontinence with pelvic floor exercises and biofeedback. *Journal of the American Geriatric Society, 38,* 341–344.

Caldwell, W. E., & Moloy, H. C. (1933). Anatomical variations in the female pelvic and their effect on labor with a suggested classification. *American Journal of Obstetrics and Gynecology, 26,* 479–482.

Cartwright, R., Elvy, S., & Cardozo, L. (2007). Do women with female ejaculation have detrusor overactivity? *Journal of Sexual Medicine, 4*(6), 1655–1658.

Crouch, N. S., Minto, C. L., Laio, L. M., Woodhouse, C. R., & Creighton, S. M. (2004). Genital sensation after feminizing genitoplasty for congenital adrenal hyperplasia: A pilot study. *British Journal of Urology, 93*(1),135–138.

Federative International Committee on Anatomical Terminology. (2002). *Terminologica histologica: International terms for human cytology and histology.* Philadelphia, PA: Lippincott, Williams & Wilkins.

Gravina, G. L., Brandetti, F., Martini, P., Carosa, E., Di Stasi, S. M., Morano, S., Lenzi, A., & Jannini, E. A. (2008). Measurement of the thickness of the urethrovaginal space in women with or without vaginal orgasm. *Journal of Sexual Medicine, 5*(3), 610–618.

Hines, T. M. (2001). The G-spot: A modern gynecological myth. *American Journal of Obstetrics and Gynecology, 185*(2), 359–362.

Ladas, A., Whipple, B., & Perry, J. (1982). *The G spot: And other recent discoveries about human sexuality.* New York, NY: Holt, Rinehart and Winston.

Maines, R. P. (1998). *The technology of orgasm: "Hysteria," the vibrator, and women's sexual satisfaction.* Baltimore, MD: Johns Hopkins University Press.

Masters, W. H., & Johnson, V. E. (1981). *Human sexual response.* New York, NY: Bantam Books.

O'Connell, H. E., Hutson, J. M., Anderson, C. R., & Plenter, R. J. (1998). Anatomical relationship between urethra and clitoris. *Journal of Urology, 159*(6), 1892–1897.

O'Connor, M. (2008). Reconstructing the hymen: Mutilation or restoration? *Journal of Law, Medicine & Ethics, 16*(1), 161–175.

Pardo, J. S., Sola, V. D., Ricci, P. A., Guiloff, E. F., & Freundlich, O. K. (2006). Colpoperineoplasty in women with sensation of a wide vagina. *Acta Obstetricia et Gynecologica Scandinavica, 85*(9), 1125–1127.

Pauls, R., Mutema, G., Segal, J., Silva, W. A., Kleeman, S., Dryfhout, M. A., & Karram, M. (2006). A prospective study examining the anatomic distribution of nerve density in the human vagina. *Journal of Sexual Medicine, 3*(6), 979–987.

Pieterse, Q. D., Ter Kuile, M. M., Deruiter, M. C., Trimbos, J. B., Kenter, G. G., & Maas, C. P. (2008). Vaginal blood flow after radical hysterectomy with and without nerve sparing. A preliminary report. *International Journal of Gynecological Cancer, 18*(3), 576–583.

Rabinerson, D., & Horowitz, E. (2007). G-spot and female ejaculation: Fiction or reality? *Harefuah 46*(2), 145–147.

Speert, H. (1973). *A pictorial history of gynecology and obstetrics.* Philadelphia, PA: F. A. Davis Co.

Tunuguntia, H. S., & Grousse, A. E. (2006). Female sexual dysfunction following vaginal surgery: A review. *Journal of Urology, 175*(2), 439–446.

Weber, A. M., Walters, M D., & Piedmonte, M. R. (2000). Sexual function and vaginal anatomy in women before and after surgery for pelvic organ prolapse and urinary incontinence. *American Journal of Obstetrics and Gynecology, 182*(6), 1610–1615.

Williamson, S., & Nowak, R. (1998, August 1). The truth about women. *New Scientist.*

Wimpissinger, F., Stifter, K., Grin, W., & Stacki, W. (2007). The female prostate revisited: Perineal ultrasound and biochemical studies of female ejaculate. *Journal of Sexual Medicine, 4*(5), 1388–1393.

World Health Organization. (2008, May). Fact sheet: Female genital mutilation (FGM). No. 241. Retrieved April 4, 2009 from http://www.who.int/mediacentre/factsheets/fs241/en/.

Yoshida, S., Koyama, M., Kimura, T., Murakami, G., Niikura, H., Takenaka, A., & Murata, Y. (2007). A clinicoanatomical study of novel nerve fibers linked to stress urinary incontinence: The first morphological description of a nerve descending properly along the anterior vaginal wall. *Clinical Anatomy, 20*(3), 300–306.

chapter 4

THE REPRODUCTIVE CYCLE

CHAPTER COMPETENCIES

Upon completion of this chapter, the reader will be able to:

- Identify the function of each hormone in the reproductive cycle
- Explain the feedback loops controlling reproduction
- Describe the ovarian and uterine changes that occur over the course of the reproductive cycle

- Explain how the female reproductive cycle differs from the male
- Discuss the process of puberty

KEY TERMS

androgen

basal body
    temperature

cholesterol

corpus luteum

endometrium

estradiol

estriol

estrogen

estrone

follicles

follicle-stimulating
    hormone (FSH)

gonadotropin-
    releasing hormone
    (GnRH)

gonadotropins

graafian follicle

granulosa cells

inhibin

luteal phase

luteinizing hormone
    (LH)

menarche

menses

menstrual synchrony

ovulation

oxytocin

progesterone

progestins

prostaglandins
    (PGs)

puberty

testosterone

theca externa

thelarche

INTRODUCTION

Menstruation is a phenomenon unique among primates. In humans, roughly once a month during her reproductive years, a woman sheds the endometrial lining which then flows through the cervix and vagina and out of the body, a phenomena called **menses**. People throughout history recognized that blood was essential to life; to bleed and not to die, indeed, to lose blood regularly and still

remain healthy, must have seemed supernatural. Magical powers were attributed to menstruation and menstrual blood, and superstitions and taboos surrounding the natural physiological function of menstruation endured for centuries. Menstruating women were blamed for crop failures, spoiled milk, natural disasters, and disease outbreaks. They were often considered irrational, unstable, weak, and unhealthy. These menstrual myths have been used to limit women's activities and opportunities in some cultures.

Some menstrual myths had a grain of fact behind them. For example, *Lactobacillus*, a common bacterial species living on humans, produces organic acids as products of its metabolism. This is the same group of microbes responsible for fermenting milk to yogurt or sour cream. In times before microbes were identified and hand washing was not a common practice, it is not hard to imagine a menstruating woman unknowingly transferring a few *Lactobacillus* to the milk as she milked the cow. As the bacteria grew, the acids it produced would sour the milk. The truth is anyone who had the bacteria on their hands and introduced those microbes to the milk would have caused it to sour, not just menstruating women, yet in some cultures a woman was not allowed near the cows during menstruation.

Most of the menstrual myths are just that – tall tales lacking a basis in fact. Menstruating women are not ill or weak. For many years, menstruating girls were excused or even prohibited from sports and gym classes at school. However, in a study of healthy female athletes, menstruation had no effect on performance during competitions or training (Figure 4-1) (Kishali et al., 2006). Menstruating women do not "contaminate" those around them, including their sexual partners. Yet many people still believe menstruating women should not have sexual intercourse.

Individual women's attitudes toward menstruation are influenced by their experiences. Menstrual discomfort and menstrual migraines do affect some women. Women who are undernourished or anemic may feel weaker during menses. Others only experience menstrual bleeding. While many regard menstruation as a normal biological function, others continue to reinforce the negative mythology around it. Some cultures still segregate menstruating women or require ritual purifications after menstruation. Despite increased candor about sexuality in the media, discussion of menstruation is, for the most part, still focused on the stereotypic negative events or on premenstrual syndrome (PMS). Advertising often promotes the idea of debilitating cramps, disfiguring bloating, or menstrual odors to sell products. Like other body functions, menstruation is not considered a topic of polite conversation and many women find menstruation difficult to talk about. This leaves many women either uninformed or misinformed about a normal reproductive cycle. A 1990 study of 80 college women found most had an incomplete knowledge of menstruation and had a distinctly negative bias towards it (Koff, Rierdan, & Stubbs, 1990). However, the situation is changing. A more recent study found that women with higher levels of education and who participated in higher levels of exercise viewed menstruation more positively (Figure 4-2) (Morrison et al., 2010). An understanding of the hormones involved in the reproductive cycle, how the hormones interact, and how the body responds facilitates the separation of reproductive facts from fiction.

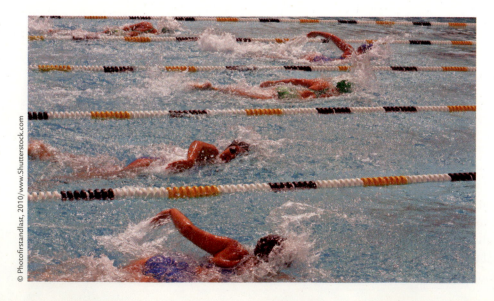

FIGURE 4-1: Despite a once-held belief that menstruating girls shouldn't participate in sports, studies show that menstruation has no effect on performance or endurance of healthy female athletes.

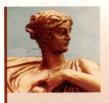

Cultural Considerations
CULTURAL ATTITUDES TOWARD MENARCHE

Menarche is a girl's first menstrual period. How women view menstruation and menarche varies culture to culture. A study of junior high school students in Hong Kong found that 85 percent viewed menstruation negatively (Tang, Yeung, & Lee, 2003). Among Latina teens, most girls viewed menarche negatively, something to keep hidden from men (Marván et al., 2007). One study also found that a negative view was also typical of low income African American girls, who felt uninformed about menstruation and menstrual issues (Chenoa Cooper & Barthalow, 2007). The idea that menstruation should be kept secret may explain why many girls don't know what to expect at menarche.

Other cultures view menstruation in a more positive light. Among some Native American groups, menarche is celebrated. Menstruating women are considered to possess great power and pose a potential risk to men if they were not responsible with their power (Hornstein, interview with a Native American student, February 2000). In the Anand district of India, menarche is celebrated although a large scale study of 900 girls there found that only a little over 60 percent of the girls received any information about menarche before it occurred (Tiwari, Oza, & Tiwari, 2006). A study which collected menarche stories from women found that Lithuanian girls felt more valued and more mature. Sudanese girls felt menstruating made them more beautiful. Malaysians felt that menstruation gained them both more respect and wisdom (Christler & Zittel, 1998). A unifying concept among women who viewed menarche and menstruation positively is that menstruation moves them from the realm of child to that of adult with all its rights and responsibilities.

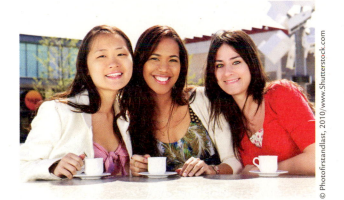

FIGURE 4-2: Women with higher levels of education who are more physically active have a more positive view about menstruation.

REPRODUCTIVE HORMONES

The female reproductive cycle, also called the menstrual cycle, refers to the cyclic changes that occur in the ovaries and uterus under the influence of the reproductive hormones. Recognition of the complex relationship between the organs of reproduction and the endocrine system did not develop until the early 1920s. This was rapidly followed by the identification of the major sex hormones and some of their functions as well as the role of the hypothalamus and pituitary in controlling hormone secretion. The ephemeral nature of hormones has made their identification difficult. Newer micro assay techniques continually identify new hormones involved in reproduction and identify new, non-reproductive functions for hormones already associated with reproduction. The hormones involved in reproduction fall into two major categories – the sex steroids and the protein-based regulatory hormones (gonadotropins).

Sex Steroids

The basic building block for the synthesis of steroids is **cholesterol**. Cholesterol has negative associations for most people as a contributing factor to cardiovascular disease. However, cholesterol is necessary for the formation of steroid hormones. All the

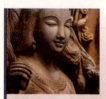

Social Considerations
RECLAIMING MENSTRUATION

Menstruation, nicknamed "the curse," has been treated like a nuisance and an irritation for about as long as we can remember. Everything about it is viewed as dirty, messy, painful, polluting, embarrassing, crazy-making, or at best inconvenient (Delaney, Lupton & Toth, 1988). But that's not our legacy. If we dig back far enough in the records of human culture, we see that humans have viewed women's menstruation with wonder, awe, respect, deference, and sometimes fear. Imagine yourself as a woman at the dawn of time. You and your sisters and all of the women in your community bleed at the same time each 28 days, at the new moon. You are a living calendar in a time before calendars. And when your blood stops flowing, you come to realize that new life has begun. Menstruation rituals and ceremonies from around the world tell us that menstrual blood has been treated as sacred, powerful, transformative, healing, and taboo—forbidden. The rituals and practices surrounding menstrual blood are many and varied, but they share the characteristic of being very clear: in each culture, women know what menstruation means and what to do around their menstruation (Uskal, 2004). Judy Grahn, in her book, *Blood, Bread, and Roses: How Menstruation Created the World*, embarked on an exploration of menstrual practices and lore with the assumption that women established the practices, not men as had often been assumed. Grahn concluded that we can trace the evolution of human culture back to the dawn of time when menstruation linked women with the cosmos— as their bodies mirrored the cycle of the moon and the oceans, of light and water (Grahn, 1993).

In the first decade of the new millennium, we have finally begun to address the stigma of menstruation and to ask ourselves what menstruation teaches us. We are transforming "the curse" back into a cosmic connection. And we're taking our daughters with us. "Period parties" celebrate menarche. You can even purchase a "Red Goddess Celebration Box" to help a girl celebrate menarche and her entrance into womanhood.

endocrine tissues that produce sex steroids assemble them through biosynthetic pathways that start with cholesterol. The primary sex steroids are estrogen, progesterone, and testosterone. Both females and males secrete all three hormones, though in differing ratios.

Estrogen

Estrogen is a general term encompassing a variety of "female hormones", including the three most common estrogens in humans: estradiol, estrone, and estriol. **Estradiol**, produced by the ovary, fat cells, and the adrenal glands, is considered the strongest estrogen, having the most pronounced effects. **Estriol** is produced by the placenta during pregnancy and is considered the weakest form of estrogen. **Estrone** is produced by the ovary, the adrenal glands, and the placenta, and is considered to produce a moderate level of activity in its target cells. There are other types of estrogens that are administered as medications, such as the conjugated equine estrogens (derived from the urine of pregnant mares) and synthetic estrogens like diethylstilbestrol (DES), tamoxifen, and raloxifene, which do not have a steroid structure but still have an estrogenic effect. Plants produce phytoestrogens which are considered to be weak estrogens.

Estrogens produce a wide range of physiological effects depending on the target tissue. They stimulate cell division in the uterine lining resulting in a thickening of the endometrium. They also reduce the viscosity of cervical mucus and change the amount of sugar released by vaginal cells. In breast tissue, estrogen increases the growth of mammary duct cells and increases the deposition of fat. Fat deposition in other parts of the body is also affected by estrogens resulting in thicker fat deposits under the skin, in the hips, and in the back of the arms in women. These fat cells can then secrete more estrogen in the form of estradiol.

Estrogen causes an increase in bone formation by stimulating the osteoblasts. In girls, the rapid growth associated with puberty is enhanced by estrogen. However, estrogen also causes the epiphyseal cartilages in the long bones to seal sooner resulting in an earlier cessation of growth. This earlier sealing of the bones is one reason that women, on average, are shorter than men.

The strength of capillary walls is increased by estrogen, and when estrogen levels are low before and during menstruation, there may be a greater tendency to bruise. Estrogen causes a reduction in blood cholesterol levels, specifically the low-density lipoproteins (LDL's) or "bad cholesterol". Liver cells are stimulated by estrogen to produce a greater concentration of some blood proteins, particularly those involved in blood clotting, red blood cell formation, and transportation of hormones. Estrogen also reduces the liver's ability to metabolize alcohol, some drugs, and dietary cholesterol. Estradiol inhibits immune function by lowering the levels of the chemical interferon and inhibiting both T-helper and macrophage activity. As research continues, additional functions for estrogen may be identified.

Progesterone

Progestin is a general term referring to a variety of chemicals, both natural and synthetic, that produce characteristic secretory and glandular changes in the endometrium. In vertebrates, the naturally-occurring progestin is **progesterone** produced by the ovary after ovulation has occurred and by the adrenal glands. The terms "progesterone" and "progestin" are often used synonymously, even though they may refer to different chemicals.

focus on
NUTRITION
Gall Stones, Estrogen, and Phytoestrogens

The greatest risk factor for developing gall stones is gender. Higher levels of estrogen make women two to three times more likely to develop gall stones. Rather than depositing cholesterol as plaques in blood vessels, estrogen encourages the delivery of cholesterol to the liver. The liver processes the cholesterol as part of the bile and secretes it into the gall bladder. Higher levels of cholesterol in bile can create a supersaturated condition in which the cholesterol precipitates out to form stones (Novacek, 2006). HRT (hormone replacement therapy) and high dose oral contraceptives dramatically increase the risk of estrogen-induced gall stones (Dunn & McNair, 2007). Altering the diet to include more phytoestrogens and soluble fiber can decrease total serum cholesterol levels resulting in less cholesterol available to be deposited in the gall bladder and a decrease in the formation of gall stones (Segasothy & Phillips, 1999).

Progesterone prepares the uterus for the implantation of a fertilized egg by increasing the formation of secretory glands, the storage of glycogen (a complex form of sugar), and the formation of spiral arteries in the endometrium. These changes improve the chances of implantation and survival of an embryo. Elevated progesterone levels inhibit the shedding of the endometrial lining. Under the influence of progesterone, the uterus develops increased numbers of oxytocin and prostaglandin receptors. These receptors play a role in contractions during labor (Chapter 11). Progesterone also causes an increase in the thickness of cervical mucus resulting in a temporary plugging of the cervical os.

In addition, progesterone causes a proliferation of the milk glands of the breasts (Chapter 7) and is associated with the breast tenderness some women feel during their menstrual cycle. It causes an increase in the excretion of water and sodium from the kidneys. Progesterone also alters blood glucose levels by increasing the cellular sensitivity to insulin (Trout et al., 2007). Finally, it causes a slight rise in basal body temperature and a slight increase in respiratory rates. As research continues, additional functions may be identified.

Androgens

Androgen is a term used synonymously with male sex steroid, but functionally it means any compound that has masculinizing effects. The androgen produced by the interstitial cells of the male testes is **testosterone**, but the adrenal glands produce other androgens including DHEA, dihydrotestosterone, and andostenedione. In the same way that estrogens are responsible for those physical and physiological features identified as "female", androgens are responsible for many of the characteristics identified as "male". The testosterone secreted by the fetal testes during prenatal development causes male differentiation of the embryonic reproductive tract.

For males at puberty, androgens cause the increased growth of facial and body hair, but can also reduce the growth of scalp hair. Testosterone causes enlargement of the larynx and an increase in the length and thickness of the vocal cords, producing the deeper voice found in most males. With increased testosterone the thickness and coarseness of the skin is increased, skin tone darkens, and sebaceous gland secretion increases. Testosterone causes an increase in muscle mass and an increase in the size and strength of the skeleton due to an increase in protein metabolism. Other physiological effects include an increased metabolic rate and increased production of red blood cells. This increase results in a greater oxygen carrying capacity in males and a decreased likelihood of developing iron-deficiency anemia.

Both the ovaries and the adrenal glands in females produce small amounts of androgens. When the levels of androgens in women approach the levels found in men, there are masculinizing effects. These can include excessive development and distribution of hair, voice and skin changes, and changes in fat distribution. Increased androgen levels can result from diseases of the ovary or adrenal glands or abuse of anabolic steroids.

In a study of female athletes, a reduction in the number of periods was associated with increased testosterone levels.

Prostaglandins

Prostaglandins (PGs) are closely related to steroid hormones and belong to a group of biologically active compounds called eicosanoids. Originally identified as a component of semen, research shows that prostaglandins are formed from fatty acids found in most cells. Although they have regulatory effects and are sometimes classified as hormones, prostaglandins are not technically hormones because they are produced by all tissues rather than by specific endocrine glands.

Research has identified a broad range of effects that prostaglandins have on the body. They are involved in maintaining blood pressure, controlling blood clot formation, regulating inflammation, and altering transmission of nerve impulses. In the lungs, they are associated with asthma. High levels of PGs have been shown to be associated with pain and fever. In the reproductive system, prostaglandin $F2\alpha$ is linked to menstrual cramps. Prostaglandins also play a major role in labor and delivery.

Endocrine Disruptors

Endocrine disruptors are chemicals that resemble steroid hormones and can bind to the same receptors on target cells. They are not produced in the body and do not respond to the normal homeostatic mechanisms. Pesticides, plastics, and many other common chemicals act as endocrine disruptors and affect both men and women. A study by Roeleveld and Bretveld (2008) found that pesticide exposure was associated with decreased semen quality and reduced fertility in men. In women, endocrine-disrupting pesticides caused menstrual irregularities and miscarriages (Bretveld et al., 2006). Bisphenol A, an endocrine disruptor commonly found in plastics, binds to the same receptors as estrogen in the pancreas and alters blood sugar levels (Alonso-Magdalena et al., 2008). Considering the range of influence steroid hormones have in the human body, endocrine disruptors can pose a serious threat to maintaining homeostasis.

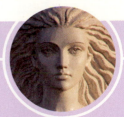

Gonadotropic Hormones

The secretion of estrogen, progesterone and testosterone do not occur in isolation. Their release is part of a complex pattern of hormone interactions that include **gonadotropins**, protein-based hormones that regulate reproduction. The primary gonadotropins are **follicle-stimulating hormone** (FSH), **luteinizing hormone** (LH), **oxytocin,** and **gonadotropin – releasing hormone** (GnRH). In the complex web of control mechanisms, additional hormones also play a role in controlling secretion of the reproductive hormones.

GnRH, also known as luteinizing hormone releasing factor (LHRH), is released from the hypothalamus. It controls the release of FSH and LH from the pituitary gland. Secretion of GnRH is controlled by a feedback loop involving estrogen and progesterone in woman and testosterone in men. Both phytoestrogens (Jefferson, 2010) and endocrine disruptors (Mahoney & Padmanabhan, 2010) can impact the release of GnRH.

LH is secreted from the pituitary gland in response to GnRH levels. LH targets the ovarian follicles in women, leading to the release of estrogen and the maturation of the follicle. In men, LH targets Leydig, or interstitial cells, and is responsible for the release of testosterone. Leptin, insulin, and endorphins also have a role in controlling both GnRH and LH secretion (Crown, Clifton, & Steiner, 2007). FSH, like LH, is secreted by the pituitary gland in response to GnRH levels. FSH targets gonadal cells. In men, it leads to spermatogenesis and the production of sperm. In women, FSH targets the ovarian follicles and is responsible for triggering the primordial follicles to develop into mature **graafian follicles.** Oxytocin is another pituitary hormone.

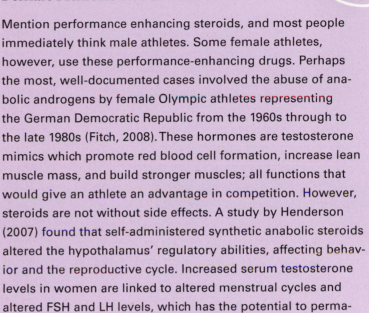

focus on

EXERCISE
Female Athletes and Steroid Use

Mention performance enhancing steroids, and most people immediately think male athletes. Some female athletes, however, use these performance-enhancing drugs. Perhaps the most, well-documented cases involved the abuse of anabolic androgens by female Olympic athletes representing the German Democratic Republic from the 1960s through to the late 1980s (Fitch, 2008). These hormones are testosterone mimics which promote red blood cell formation, increase lean muscle mass, and build stronger muscles; all functions that would give an athlete an advantage in competition. However, steroids are not without side effects. A study by Henderson (2007) found that self-administered synthetic anabolic steroids altered the hypothalamus' regulatory abilities, affecting behavior and the reproductive cycle. Increased serum testosterone levels in women are linked to altered menstrual cycles and altered FSH and LH levels, which has the potential to permanently alter women's reproductive cycles (Rickenlund, 2004). The effects of steroids are not solely limited to hormonal disruptions. Anabolic steroids are hepatotoxic, altering liver metabolism, damaging liver enzyme production, and killing liver cells (Pagonis et al., 2008). Athletes who abuse steroids for short-term competitive gains risk producing long-term damage.

Best known for causing smooth muscle contraction during labor and delivery and in the milk let down reflex, oxytocin has also been identified as having a role in improved mood, bonding behaviors, and as an anti-stress hormone.

THE FEMALE REPRODUCTIVE CYCLE

The reproductive cycle involves a monthly fluctuation of reproductive hormones and the physiological changes that they produce, particularly in the ovaries and the uterus. The length of a typical reproductive cycle varies from 21 days to 45 days. Within a typical cycle, menses may last from two

EVIDENCE BASED PRACTICE

Menstrual Migraines

Migraines are a severe headache characterized by throbbing pain usually localized to one side of the head, visual disruptions, and nausea. In women who suffer from migraines, 20-30 percent are classified as menstrual migraines, migraines which occurs just prior to or during menstruation (Russell, 2010). Pringsheim, Davenport, and Dodick (2008) found that menstrual migraines are usually more severe, last longer, and respond more poorly to pain medications than migraines not associated with menstruation. Menstrual migraines are more likely to reoccur more within a day of medication treatment, something not usually seen with non-menstrual migraines (Pinkerman & Holroyd, 2010). The cause of menstrual migraines

remains unidentified. Estrogen, prostaglandins, and serotonin levels are thought to contribute. Treatment of migraines usually uses a two-pronged approach. First, attempts can be made to prevent migraines. Identifying and avoiding migraine triggers, increasing phytoestrogens in the diet, and maintaining blood sugar levels can be effective. Second, if a migraine does occur, medication can be used. Drug therapies include nonsteroidal anti-inflammatories (NSAID), and other prescription medications (Pringsheim, Davenport, & Dodick, 2008; Silberstein et al., 2004; Newman et al., 2001). A woman should consult with her health provider to determine which treatment works best to control her menstrual migraines.

to seven days. **Ovulation**, the release of an egg from the ovary, usually occurs on the 14th day before menstruation. Illness, diet, exercise, stress, and a variety of other factors can alter hormone levels and change the length of a woman's cycle. A 28-day reproductive cycle is considered average and is used as the standard in most textbooks. During an average cycle, shown in Figure 4-3, menses begins day 1 of the cycle and ends day 5, and ovulation usually occurs on day 14.

The reproductive cycle can be divided into three distinct but interconnected sets of events that occur simultaneously: the ovarian cycle, the endometrial cycle, and the hormonal cycle. In a series of feedback loops, changes in hormone levels cause cyclical changes in the ovary and in the endometrium of the uterus. Cyclical changes in the ovary then produce additional changes in the hormone feedback loops.

Hormonal Cycle

The monthly changes that constitute the ovarian and endometrial cycles are dependent on the changing concentrations of the steroid hormones estrogen and

progesterone. Estrogen and progesterone are secreted in response to the release of the gonadotropins GnRH, FSH and LH from the hypothalamus and the pituitary gland in the brain. GnRH is secreted in short pulses, one pulse-every 60–90 minutes throughout most of the cycle, that decrease in frequency as menstruation approaches. Sex steroids and neurotransmitters control the secretion of GnRH from the hypothalamus. Variations in the release of FSH and LH are the result of feedback interactions with estrogen and progesterone. In response to each GnRH pulse, a pulse of FSH and LH is discharged by the pituitary gland into the bloodstream and transported to the ovaries where these hormones stimulate the ovarian follicles to develop and produce estrogen. Variations in the pulse rate outside the normal range can disrupt follicle development and hormone production.

As estrogen increases in the circulation, it reaches the pituitary gland, and stimulates the release of additional FSH and LH. However, when estrogen levels peak around day 12 of the cycle, it triggers a positive feedback effect with the pituitary gland, which causes a surge of LH and FSH

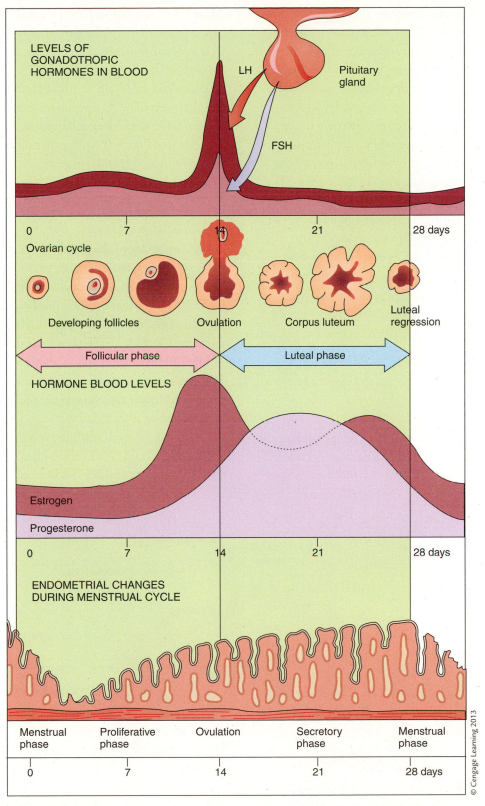

FIGURE 4-3: Hormone levels and changes in the ovary and uterus over a 28 day reproductive cycle.

secretion into the bloodstream. This surge of LH and FSH triggers ovulation, and a mature follicle leaves the ovary. Under the influence of LH, the ruptured follicle that remains becomes the **corpus luteum** which secretes both progesterone and estrogen. Progesterone levels peak around day 21 into the cycle, and act on the uterus to prepare the endometrium for a possible pregnancy. The increased progesterone levels in the bloodstream reduce the frequency of the hypothalamic GnRH pulses. This reduction in GnRH, in turn, reduces the secretion of FSH and LH from the pituitary gland as part of a negative feedback loop. If a pregnancy occurs, the corpus luteum continues to secrete progesterone in order to maintain the endometrium. In the absence of a pregnancy, the corpus luteum degenerates, progesterone levels decline, and a portion of the endometrium sheds, causing menses to occur. The GnRH pulses then return to their original frequency and a new cycle begins.

Ovarian Cycle

The ovary undergoes distinctive changes during the ovarian cycle (Figure 4-4). The ovarian cycle is usually divided into three stages: the follicular phase (days 1-13), ovulation (day 14), and the luteal phase (days 15-28). The germinal epithelium of the ovary contains primordial follicles. Each **follicle** consists of an oocyte surrounded by an inner layer of **granulosa cells** and an outer layer of cells called the **theca externa**. As a woman's ovaries mature, primordial follicles begin to mature into primary follicles (see Figure 4-5). Further development of the follicles depends on stimulation by FSH and LH.

Follicular Phase (Days 1-13)

At the beginning of the ovarian cycle, several follicles respond to the increasing presence of FSH, but usually the growth of one follicle will outpace the others. The dominant follicle produces more estrogen than the other developing follicles. Estrogen in combination with FSH induces the development of more LH receptors on the granulosa cells. These LH-binding sites are critical for ovulation and for the subsequent conversion of the follicle into the corpus luteum.

As estrogen levels continue to increase, the primary follicle develops a fluid-filled pocket called an antrum, and becomes a secondary follicle

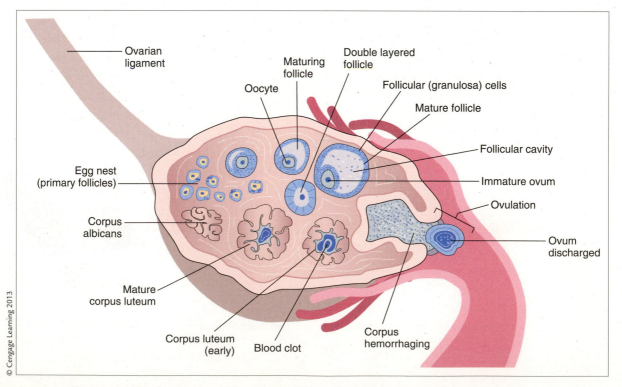

© Cengage Learning 2013

FIGURE 4-4: An ovary showing the changes which occur over the course of a reproductive cycle.

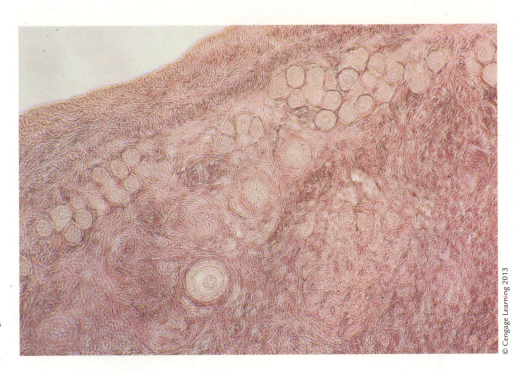

© Cengage Learning 2013

FIGURE 4-5: The tiny primordial follicles respond to increased levels of FSH to become slightly larger primary follicles.

(Figure 4-6). At this stage, the granulosa and theca cells secrete a peptide hormone called **inhibin**, which suppresses FSH secretion from the pituitary gland. Activin, another peptide hormone, enhances FSH secretion, but the follicular fluid contains more inhibin than activin. One hypothesis proposes that this increase in inhibin and the subsequent decrease in FSH usually insures that only one follicle per month matures, and decreases the chances of a multiple pregnancy. The secondary follicle continues to grow into a mature, or graafian, follicle as it prepares for ovulation.

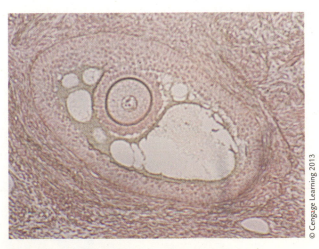

© Cengage Learning 2013

FIGURE 4-6: A secondary follicle with its fluid-filled antrum.

Ovulation (Day 14)

The accelerated production of estrogen from the dominant follicle in the ovary produces a positive feedback loop that increases LH secretion. At midcycle, an estrogen surge triggers an LH surge, which in turn, triggers a series of events in the ovary that leads to ovulation. The LH surge normally occurs 12 hours before the discharge of an egg, or **ovulation**. Over the counter ovulation test kits use LH levels to predict when ovulation will occur. Increased LH levels also result in metabolic changes in the granulosa cells, and they begin to produce and secrete progesterone. This increase in progesterone enhances the positive feedback effect of estrogen on the LH surge. Progesterone also encourages the activity of proteolytic enzymes in the follicular fluid that can digest the follicle wall, and allow the ovum to escape during ovulation. In addition, the high levels of LH stimulate the synthesis of prostaglandins, which reach their peak concentration in the follicular fluid at ovulation and are essential for follicle rupture. As ovulation approaches, the follicle wall becomes stretched, proteolytic enzymes in the follicular fluid are activated, prostaglandins exert their influence, and the oocyte with its surrounding protective cells ruptures from the surface of the ovary and into the body cavity. The oocyte is then swept by the ciliated fimbriae into the fallopian tube.

The Luteal Phase (Days 15 – 28)

After ovulation, the granulosa cells left behind in the ruptured follicle enlarge, undergo metabolic changes, and become the corpus luteum. The corpus luteum produces both progesterone and estrogen, and reaches its peak of activity around day 21of the cycle, approximately seven days after ovulation. If fertilization does not occur and there are no hormones from the developing embryo to maintain the corpus luteum, it regresses to form a corpus albicans. During the **luteal phase**, FSH and LH in the bloodstream drop to their lowest levels, while estrogen and progesterone levels are at their highest. Although FSH and LH levels are in decline, there is a continuous presence of small amounts of these hormones throughout the cycle. There is some evidence that the estrogen produced by the corpus luteum and local concentrations of prostaglandin influence the timing

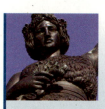

Historical Considerations
VARIATION IN THE REPRODUCTIVE CYCLE

The events which occur during the reproductive cycle, as well as variations in the normal cycle have been an area of active research for years. One of the most thorough books about this topic written for the average woman is the 1935 *The Modern Method of Birth Control* by Welton. This book includes frank and practical descriptions of the reproductive system, the hormone cycles, and the physiological effects of the hormonal changes. One chapter discusses whether menstruation is necessary. The last half of the book consists of a series of charts that diagram menstrual cycles, ranging from a 21 day cycle to a 35 day cycle. It further identifies for each cycle variation when ovulation occurs and describes how the hormonal levels change over the course of the cycle. Finally, this book encouraged women to chart their own cycle and identify when they were most likely to be fertile to either avoid or achieve pregnancy.

of the corpus luteum's transformation into the corpus albicans. With the decline of the corpus luteum, the levels of estrogen and progesterone decrease rapidly. As their negative feedback effect is diminished, FSH and LH can again increase to initiate a new cycle.

Endometrial Cycle

During the endometrial cycle, the uterus is prepared for a potential pregnancy. Like the ovarian cycle, it is divided into three stages: menses, the proliferative stage, and the secretory phase. Physiological changes that take place during the endometrial cycle are influenced by the hormonal and ovarian cycles.

Menses

The first phase of the endometrial cycle is **menses**, commonly referred to as the menstrual period. The **endometrium** consists of two layers: a superficial stratum functionalis and a stratum basale. The stratum functionalis contains secretory glands and occupies two-thirds of the endometrium, while the thin stratum basale is in contact with the muscle layers of the uterus. From day 1 to day 4, the endometrium undergoes menses as the stratum functionalis is shed, forming the menstrual flow. Over the course of three to four days, approximately 50 mL (3 ½ tablespoons) of blood, glandular secretions, and tissue fragments flow from the uterine cavity through the cervical os and out the vagina. Menstrual blood does not usually clot because clotting factors ordinarily found in blood are deactivated by enzymes in the uterus. The clots that may appear with a heavier menstrual flow are a combination of red blood cells, mucus, glycogen, and glycoproteins that form in the vagina rather than in the uterus.

Proliferative Phase

The proliferative phase occurs between menses and ovulation. Even while menstruation is occurring, estrogen from the developing follicles in the ovaries triggers cell division in the endometrium that repairs the denuded areas of the lining. Regeneration of the superficial layer of the endometrium occurs rapidly, and the stratum functionalis thickens as the estrogen levels increase. Within a few days after menstruation, the entire uterine cavity is covered with new epithelial cells. These cells continue to grow, the layer continues to thicken. Secretory glands form in the endometrium, but do not yet become functional.

Secretory Phase

The secretory phase of the endometrial cycle lasts from ovulation until the first day of menses. The glands of the endometrium respond to progesterone and become dilated. Spiral arteries form within the lining, bringing blood and increased nutrients to the stratum functionalis (Figure 4-7). During this phase, the endometrium becomes twice as thick as it was during the proliferative phase, forming a hospitable site for implantation of a fertilized ovum.

If pregnancy has not occurred, the endometrium begins to regress at the end of the secretory phase. The breakdown of the stratum functionalis is caused by falling levels of estrogen and progesterone as the corpus luteum becomes the corpus albicans. As the endometrium regresses, the spiral arteries deteriorate. Some of the arteries intermittently constrict, cutting off the blood flow to the areas that they formerly supplied, and the tissue dies from lack of blood. Prostaglandins, especially F2α, may play a role in inducing this arterial constriction. When the arteries dilate again, the blood escapes from the top where the tissue has already disintegrated. The pools

of blood rupture through the endometrial surface into the uterine cavity. As more of the superficial layer disintegrates, small pieces of endometrium become detached, and glandular secretions and blood slowly ooze into the uterine cavity, and then out the vagina. Menses begins, signaling day 1 of the next cycle.

BASAL BODY TEMPERATURE (BBT) CURVE

Increased levels of progesterone have the effect of raising the basal body temperature above what it would be in the absence of this hormone. **Basal body temperature** (BBT) is the body temperature upon waking, before significant physical activity can raise the temperature further. If a woman takes her BBT each morning of her menstrual cycle and plots the temperature on a graph she will create a BBT curve. For women who are experiencing menstrual cycles, the BBT pattern will show a definite elevation in temperature that occurs within one to three days of ovulation. This elevation of temperature remains until approximately three days prior to the onset of the next menses, when the curve again deflects back to the postmenstrual level. The morning temperature usually varies from about 36.2°C before ovulation to about 37°C–37.1°C after ovulation. Women before menarche or after menopause, and women who are not ovulating, do not show this biphasic basal body temperature curve.

While the actual time of ovulation cannot be accurately predicted by using BBT alone, it can certainly be approximated after a BBT chart has been kept through several cycles. With this information, intercourse can be timed to either increase or decrease the chances of pregnancy. Waiting for the increase in temperature before trying to conceive is a mistake, however. The release of the ovum from the ovary probably occurs 24–38 hours before the temperature elevation. The most favorable schedule for conception would be intercourse every other day for the three to four days before the rise, including the two days after it. After the basal body temperature has been elevated for two days, conception is unlikely. BBT charts can, therefore, be useful for both infertility treatment and fertility control.

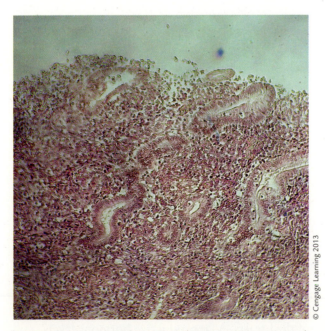

© Cengage Learning 2013

FIGURE 4-7: Late cycle endometrium showing spiral arteries and secretory cells.

Critical Thinking

Are Periods Necessary?

The development of oral contraceptives has given women unprecedented control over their reproductive cycles. The first oral contraceptive pills consisted of three weeks of pills containing hormones followed by a week of placebo pills lacking hormones. The placebo week, mimicked the drop in sex steroids of a natural cycle and triggered menstruation. However, many women quietly informed other women that by skipping the placebo week and beginning the next cycle of pills, they could suppress their menstrual cycle. A 2003 study of undergraduate women reported that 12 percent were using oral contraceptives for menstrual suppression without medical supervision (Johnston-Robledo et al., 2003).

Newer contraceptives (Chapter 13) are specifically designed to suppress menstruation for months at a time. Hormonal methods of menstrual suppression are now commonly used by female members of the military due to the difficulties of menstrual hygiene under deployment conditions (Christopher & Miller, 2007; Trego & Jordan, 2010). As menstrual suppression has become more common, concerns have been raised about its long term consequences and the medicalization of menstruation (Trego, 2007; Andrist et al., 2004).

Is menstruation necessary? What happens if women don't menstruate? Is menstrual suppression safe? To date, the data are limited and much of it is based on anecdotes. During times of famine, many women stop menstruating with no apparent negative effects. A four-year study found no health differences between women using cyclic oral contraceptive for menstrual suppression and those using the placebo week for menstruation (Davis et al., 2010). Debate continues on whether menstruation is biologically necessary and if there are either benefits or risks associated with the practice of menstrual suppression (Benagiano et al., 2009).

MALE REPRODUCTIVE CYCLES

While women have a complex reproductive cycle involving both positive and negative feedback mechanisms, men's reproductive cycles are simpler. As GnRH levels increase, it causes an increase in the secretion of FSH and LH. FSH travels to the semeniferous tubules of the testes to promote the production of sperm, while LH travels to interstitial or Leydig cells, which are clusters of tissue between the tubules. These cells produce and secrete both testosterone and inhibin. Once testosterone levels reach a maximum set point, negative feedback causes a decrease in GnRH levels. This, in turn, decreases LH and FSH, leading to a decrease in testosterone secretion. As testosterone levels reach a minimum set point, negative feedback again triggers an increase in GnRH. This negative feedback loop maintains testosterone levels within a fairly narrow range.

PUBERTY

Puberty is the transition from childhood to adulthood, when physical and psychological changes that allow reproduction take place. For most girls, puberty occurs between ages eight and 13. Delayed puberty is classified as the lack of the development of secondary sexual characteristics after age 14. Precocious puberty is the development of secondary sexual characteristics before age seven and a half (Park, Goldsmith, & Weiss, 2002). **Menarche** is the term for the onset of the menstrual periods, but monthly ovulation may not take place for a year or more afterward. The physical changes associated with puberty begin slowly. Usually the first sign in girls is **thelarche**, the development of the breasts. As reproductive hormone levels change, pubic hair develops, fat deposition shifts, and menarche usually occurs. The time frame from the initiation of breast development to menarche averages 2.3 years (Park, Goldsmith, & Weiss, 2002).

The endocrine events that control the onset of puberty are an area of active research, and there are several hypotheses that attempt to explain this process. Much attention is focused on the role of the hypothalamus, but the onset of puberty is also influenced by genetic factors, and social and economic factors related to nutrition and general health. Historically, the distribution of body fat was considered a result of puberty. However, newer research indicates that the amount of body fat can influence the onset of puberty as well (Kaplowitz, 2008). A study of children approaching puberty found that leptin, a hormone produced by adipose cells, influences GnRH pulse frequencies (Maqsood et al., 2007). More adipose cells produced more leptin, which increases the GnRH pulse frequency. Individuals who lacked the ability to make leptin did not enter puberty. However, after treatment with leptin, puberty proceeded (Kaplowitz, 2008). The hormone leptin is associated with good nutritional status. The hormone gherlin, which is associated with poor nutritional status, inhibits LH secretion and delays puberty (Tena-Sempere, 2008; Fernandez – Fernandez et al., 2005). These data help to explain how nutritional status influences the onset of puberty (Figure 4-8).

Behavioral and environmental cues can influence hormone cycles, and can play a role in the onset of puberty (Euling et al., 2008). For example, a study of both delayed puberty and precocious puberty found that sleep influences hormone cycles. LH pulses increase during REM sleep (Park, Goldsmith, & Weiss, 2002), potentially facilitating the onset of puberty. In another study, the sense of smell played a role in hormone secretion. The neurons that trigger the production of GnRH extend into the nasal cavity next to the olfactory nerves that detect odors. Studies in both humans (Cariboni, Maggi, & Parnavelas, 2007) and mice (Yoon, Enquist, & Dulac, 2005) found that damage to these neurons, or failure of the neurons to reach the nasal cavity decreased GnRH secretion and delayed or prevented puberty.

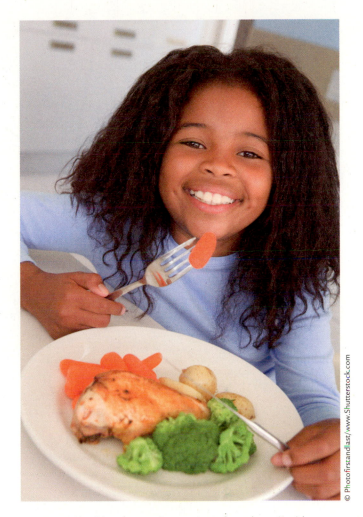

FIGURE 4-8: Nutritional status is one trigger for puberty in girls.

MENSTRUAL HYGIENE
Menstrual pads, tampons, and menstrual caps are commercial products used to contain menstrual flow. Prior to the development of commercial products, natural sponges, rags or highly absorbent materials such as lichen or moss were used to catch the menstrual flow. Alternatives to commercial products are still available today. A woman's choice for dealing with her menstrual period depends on her preferences.

MENSTRUAL SYNCHRONY
Martha McClintock (1971) reported that women living in close proximity tended to develop **menstrual synchrony** and menstruated at approximately the same time. Her study of the timing of the onset of menses involved 135 young women 17–22 years of age who were living together in a dormitory,

Case Study

A Cluster of Precocious Puberty Cases

Almira's mother is concerned. Her six-year-old is developing breasts and some very adult curves. Her neighbors have noticed the same thing among their young daughters - Paloma, age seven, and Tadea, age six. The doctor says all three girls are undergoing central precocious puberty (CPP). They are experiencing early development of secondary sexual characteristics. Each of the girls shows thelarche, early breast development. Something has caused their bodies to begin puberty much earlier than normal. In hopes of delaying further development until a more appropriate age, the girls are put on leuprolide, a GnRH antagonist that will lower the levels of estrogen they are producing (Kunz, Sherman, & Klein, 2007). Blood tests show the girls have high levels of zearalone, an estrogenic fungal toxin (Massart et al., 2008). Fungal contamination has been associated with the higher level of CPP in Puerto Rico. The doctor suspects the girls have picked up the toxin from contaminated poultry (Pérez-Comas et al., 1991).

1. What is the normal pattern of the development of secondary sexual characteristics at puberty?

2. Why would a GnRH antagonist lower estrogen levels?

and she found their menstrual cycles were synchronized. Other researchers subsequently confirmed that menstrual synchronization occurred among women who spent considerable time together (Graham & McGrew, 1980), although other research into this phenomenon have found no effect.

Quadagno, Subeita, Deck, and Francoeur (1981) reported that menstrual synchrony occurred among three and four women living together as well as between pairs. Investigators speculated that menstrual synchronization may be influenced by the sense of smell, and most likely involves pheromones, which are hormone-like chemicals secreted outside the body. Newer studies have focused on the pheromone 3α- androstenol found in axillary sweat glands (Preti et al., 2003). Not all people can detect this pheromone. Morofushi et al. (2000) found that 38 percent of women living in a college dorm synchronized their cycles within three months. Those who synchronized were those who could detect t3α- androstenol. Another study found that 3α- androstenol decreased LH pulse frequency during the follicular phase of the reproductive cycle (Shinohara et al., 2000). Janafar et al. (2007) found that in a group of 88 women,

nearly 60 percent synchronized their cycles. It is interesting to note that in the Janafar study poorer personal hygiene correlated with greater synchrony. Since the pheromone is found in perspiration, washing would remove it, resulting in less synchrony.

Pheromones other than those found in perspiration have been identified. One study found that breast milk contains pheromones that also altered LH levels. Researchers were able to document a change in the timing of the LH surge at ovulation in women who spent considerable time with a woman who was breastfeeding (Jacob et al., 2004).

CONCLUSION

The reproductive cycle in women is comprised of complex interactions between hormone cycles and physiological changes to the uterus and the ovaries. Hormonal changes facilitate the maturation and release of eggs from the ovaries, and to the development and subsequent shedding of the endometrial lining. A familiarity with these changes forms the framework for understanding alternations of the cycle that can occur throughout a woman's lifetime.

REVIEW QUESTIONS

1. Relate the body changes that occur during puberty to the hormone level changes. Which hormones are responsible?

2. What hormonal signals trigger menstruation?

3. What is the function of FSH?

4. Why are there only minimal levels of progesterone until after ovulation?

5. What chemical is the base for all steroid hormones?

CRITICAL THINKING QUESTIONS

1. Relate the ovarian changes that occur during the menstrual cycle to the hormonal changes that occur.

2. How does the uterus change in response to the hormones?

WEBLINKS

Metaformia: A Journal of Menstruation and Culture
www.metaformia.com
Online Museum of Menstruation
www.mum.org

U.S. National Library of Medicine National Institutes of Health
www.pubmed.gov

REFERENCES

Alonso-Magdalena, P., Ropero, A. B., Carrera, M. P., Cederroth, C. R., Baquié, M., Gauthier, B. R., Nef, S., Stefani, E., & Nadal, A. (2008). Pancreatic insulin content regulation by the estrogen receptor ER alpha. *PLoS ONE, 3*(4), e2069.

Andrist, L. C., Hoyt, A., Weinstein, D., & McGibbon, C. (2004). The need to bleed: Women's attitudes and beliefs about menstrual suppression. *Journal of the American Academy of Nurse Practitioners, 16*(1), 31–37.

Benagiano, G., Carrara, S., & Filippi, V. (2009). Safety, efficacy and patient satisfaction with continuous daily administration of levonorgestrel/ethinylestradiol oral contraceptives. *Journal of Patient Preference and Adherence, 3,* 131–143.

Bretveld, R. W., Thomas, C. M., Scheepers, P. T., Zielhuis, G. A., & Roeleveld, N. (2006). Pesticide exposure: the hormonal function of the female reproductive system disrupted? *Reproductive Biology and Endocrinology, 4,* 30.

Cariboni, A., Maggi, R., & Parnavelas, J. G. (2007). From nose to fertility: The long migratory journey of gonadotropin-releasing hormone neurons. *Trends in Neurosciences, 30*(12), 638–644.

Cooper, S., & Barthalow Koch, P. (2007). "Nobody told me nothin": Communication about menstruation among low-income African-American women. *Women Health, 46*(1), 57–78. Retrieved January 21, 2010 from http://www.ncbi.nlm.nih.gov/pubmed/18032175.

Chrisler, J. C., & Zittel, C. B. (1998). Menarche stories: Reminiscences of college students from Lithuania, Malaysia, Sudan, and the United States. *Health Care for Women International, 19*(4), 303–312. doi:10.1080/073993398246287

Christopher, L. A., & Miller, L. (2007). Women in war: Operational issues of menstruation and unintended pregnancy. *Military Medicine, 172*(1), 9–16.

Crown, A., Clifton, D. K., & Steiner, R. A. (2007). Neuropeptide signaling in the integration of metabolism and reproduction. *Neuroendocrinology, 86*(3), 175–182.

Cumming, D. C., & Wheeler, G. D. (1987). Opioids in exercise physiology. *Seminars in Reproductive Endocrinology, 5,* 171–176.

Cutler, W. B., Freidmann, E., & McCoy, N. L. (1998). Pheromonal influences on sociosexual behavior in men. *Archives of Sexual Behavior, 27*(1), 1–13.

Cutler, W. B., Garcia, C. R., Huggins, G. R., & Preti, G. (1986). Sexual behavior and steroid levels among gynecologically mature premenopausal women. *Fertility and Sterility, 45*(4), 496–502.

Cutler, W. B., Garcia, C. R., & Krieger, A. M. (1979). Sexual behavior frequency and menstrual cycle length in mature premenopausal women. *Psychoneuroendocrinology, 4,* 297–309.

Cutler, W. B., Preti, G., Krieger, A., Huggins, G. R., Garcia, C. R., & Lawley, H. J. (1986). Human axillary secretions influence women's menstrual cycles: The role of donor extract from men. *Hormones and Behavior, 20*(4), 463–473.

Davis, M. G., Reape, K. Z., & Hait, H. (2010). A look at the long-term safety of an extended-regimen OC. *Journal of Family Practice, 59*(5), E3.

Delaney, J., Lupton, M. J., & Toth, E. (1988). *The curse: A cultural history of menstruation.* Urbana, IL: University of Illinois Press.

Dunn, J. M., & McNair, A. (2007). Prolonged cholestasis following successful removal of common bile duct stones: Beware patients on estrogen therapy. *World Journal of Gastroenterology, 13*(46), 6277–6280.

Euling, S. Y., Selevan, S. G., Pescovitz, O. H., & Skakkebaek, N. E. (2008). Role of environmental factors in the timing of puberty. *Pediatrics, 121,* Suppl 3, S167–171.

Fernández-Fernández, R., Tena-Sempere, M., Navarro, V. M., Barreiro, M. L., Castellano, J. M., Aguilar, E., & Pinilla, L. (2005). Effects of ghrelin upon gonadotropin-releasing hormone and gonadotropin secretion in adult female rats: In vivo and in vitro studies. *Neuroendocrinology, 82*(5-6), 245–255.

Fitch, K. D. (2008). Androgenic-anabolic steroids and the Olympic Games. *Asian Journal of Andrology, 10*(3), 384–390.

Graham, C. A., & McGrew, W. C. (1980). Menstrual synchrony in female undergraduates living on a coeducational campus. *Psychoneuroendocrinology, 5,* 245–252.

Grahn, J. (1993). *Blood, bread, and roses: How menstruation created the world.* Boston, MA: Beacon Press.

Henderson, L. P. (2007). Steroid modulation of GABAA receptor-mediated transmission in the hypothalamus: Effects on reproductive function. *Neuropharmacology, 52*(7), 1439–1453.

Jacob, S., Spencer, N. A., Bullivant, S. B., Sellergren, S. A., Mennella, J. A., & McClintock, M. K. (2004). Effects of breastfeeding chemosignals on the human menstrual cycle. *Human Reproduction, 19*(2), 422–429.

Jahanfar, S., Awang, C. H., Rahman, R. A., Samsuddin, R. D., & See, C. P. (2007). Is 3alpha-androstenol pheromone related to menstrual synchrony? *Journal of Family Planning and Reproductive Health Care, 33*(2), 116–118.

Jefferson, W. N. (2010). Adult ovarian function can be affected by high levels of soy. *Journal of Nutrition, 140* (12), 23225–23255. doi: 10.3945/jn.110.123802 .

Johnston-Robledo, I., Ball, M., Lauta, K., & Zekoll, A. (2003). To bleed or not to bleed: Young women's attitudes toward menstrual suppression. *Women and Health, 38*(3), 59–75.

Kaplowitz, P. B. (2008). Link between body fat and the timing of puberty. *Pediatrics, 121 Suppl 3,* S208–217.

Kishali, N. F., Imamoglu, O., Katkat, D., Atan, T., & Akyol, P. (2006). Effects of menstrual cycle on sports performance. *International Journal of Neuroscience, 116*(12), 1549–1563.

Koff, E., Rierdan, J., & Stubbs, M. I. (1990). Conceptions and misconceptions of the menstrual cycle. *Women and Health, 16*(3–4), 119–136.

Kunz, G. J., Sherman, T. I., & Klein, K. O. (2007). Luteinizing hormone (LH) and estradiol suppression and growth in girls with central precocious puberty: Is more suppression better? Are pre-injection LH levels useful in monitoring treatment? *Journal of Pediatric Endocrinology & Metabolism, 20*(11), 1189–1198.

Lebrun, C. M. (1994). The effect of the phase of the menstrual cycle and the birth control pill on athletic performance. *Clinical Sports Medicine, 13*(2), 419–441.

Mahoney, M. M., & Padmanabhan, V. (2010). Developmental programming: Impact of fetal exposure to endocrine-disrupting chemicals on gonadotropin-releasing hormone and estrogen receptor mRNA in sheep hypothalamus. *Toxicology and Applied Pharmacology, 247*(2), 98–104.

Maqsood, A. R., Trueman, J. A., Whatmore, A. J., Westwood, M., Price, D. A., Hall, C. M., & Clayton, P. E. (2007). The relationship between nocturnal urinary leptin and gonadotrophins as children progress towards puberty. *Hormone Research, 68*(5), 225–230.

Marván, M. L., Vacio, A., García-Yañez, G., & Espinosa-Hernández, G. (2007). Attitudes toward menarche among Mexican preadolescents. *Women & Health, 46*(1), 7–23.

Massart, F., Meucci, V., Saggese, G., & Soldani, G. (2008). High growth rate of girls with precocious puberty exposed to estrogenic mycotoxins. *Journal of Pediatrics,152*(5), 690–695, 695.e1.

McClintock, M. K. (1971). Menstrual synchrony and suppression. *Nature, 229,* 244–245.

Miller, E. (1998). Menstrual synchrony: A methodological comment. *Mankind Quarterly, 38*(4), 363–481.

Morofushi, M., Shinohara, K., Funabashi, T., & Kimura, F. (2000). Positive relationship between menstrual synchrony and ability to smell 5alpha-androst-16-en-3alpha-ol. *Chemical Senses, 25*(4), 407–411.

Morrison, L. A., Sievert, L. L., Brown, D. E., Rahberg, N., & Reza, A. (2010). Relationships between menstrual and menopausal attitudes and associated demographic and health characteristics: The Hilo Women's Health Study. *Women & Health, 50*(5), 397–413.

Newman, L., Mannix, L. K., Landy, S., Silberstein, S., Lipton, R. B., Putnam, D. G., Watson, C., Jöbsis, M., Batenhorst, A., & O'Quinn, S. (2001). Naratriptan as short-term prophylaxis of menstrually associated migraine: A randomized, double-blind, placebo-controlled study. *Headache, 41*(3), 248–256.

Novacek, G. (2006). Gender and gallstone disease. *Wiener medizinische Wochenschrift, 156*(19–20), 527–533.

Pagonis, T. A., Koukoulis, G. N., Hadjichristodoulou, C. S., Toli, P. N., & Angelopoulos, N. V. (2008). Multivitamins and phospholipids complex protects the hepatic cells from androgenic-anabolic-steroids-induced toxicity. *Clinical Toxicology (Philadelphia, PA), 46*(1), 57–66.

Park, S., Goldsmith, L., & Weiss, G. (2002). Age-related changes in the regulation of luteinizing hormone secretion by estrogen in women. *Experimental Biology and Medicine, 227,* 455–464.

Pérez-Comas, A., Saénz de Rodríguez, C. A., & Sánchez, L. F. (1991). Abnormalities of sexual development in Puerto Rico: Status report. *Boletín de la Asociación Médica de Puerto Rico, 83*(7), 306–309.

Pinkerman, B., & Holroyd, K. (2010). Menstrual and nonmenstrual migraines differ in women with menstrually-related migraine. *Cephalalgia, 30*(10), 1187–1194.

Preti, G., Cutler, W. B., Garcia, C. R., Huggins, G. R., & Lawley, H. J. (1986). Human axillary secretions influence women's menstrual cycles: The role of donor extract of females. *Hormones and Behavior, 20*(4), 474–482.

Preti, G., Wysocki, C. J., Barnhart, K. T., Sondheimer, S. J., & Leyden, J. J. (2003). Male axillary extracts contain pheromones that affect pulsatile secretion of luteinizing hormone and mood in women recipients. *Biology of Reproduction, 68*(6), 2107–2113.

Pringsheim, T., Davenport, W. J., & Dodick, D. (2008). Acute treatment and prevention of menstrually related migraine headache: Evidence-based review. *Neurology, 70*(17), 1555–1563.

Quadagno, D. M., Subeita, H. E., Deck, J., & Francoeur, D. (1981). Influence of male social contacts, exercise, and all female living conditions on the menstrual cycle. *Psychoneuroendocrinology, 6,* 239–244.

Rickenlund, A., Thorén, M., Carlström, K., von Schoultz, B., & Hirschberg, A. L. (2004). Diurnal profiles of testosterone and pituitary hormones suggest different mechanisms for menstrual disturbances in endurance athletes. *Journal of Clinical Endocrinology & Metabolism, 89*(2), 702–707.

Roeleveld, N., & Bretveld, R. (2008). The impact of pesticides on male fertility. *Current Opinion in Obstetrics and Gynecology, 20*(3), 229–233.

Russell, M. B. (2010). Genetics of menstrual migraine: The epidemiological evidence. *Current Pain and Headache Reports, 14*(5), 385–388.

Segasothy, M., & Phillips, P. A. (1999). Vegetarian diet: Panacea for modern lifestyle diseases? *Quarterly Journal of Medicine, 92*(9), 531–544.

Shinohara, K., Morofushi, M., Funabashi, T., Mitsushima, D., & Kimura, F. (2000). Effects of 5alpha-androst-16-en-3alpha-ol on the pulsatile secretion of luteinizing hormone in human females. *Chemical Senses, 25*(4), 465–467.

Silberstein, S. D., Elkind, A. H., Schreiber, C., & Keywood, C. (2004). A randomized trial of frovatriptan for the intermittent prevention of menstrual migraine. *Neurology, 63*(2), 261–269.

Speroff, L., Glass, R. H., & Kase, N. G. (1994). *Clinical gynecologic endocrinology and infertility* (5th ed.). Baltimore, MD: Williams & Wilkins.

Stern, K., & McClintock, M. K. (1998). Regulation of ovulation human pheromones. *Nature, 392*(6672), 177–179.

Tang, C. S., Yeung, D. Y., & Lee, A. M. (2003). Psychosocial correlates of emotional responses to menarche among Chinese adolescent girls. *Journal of Adolescent Health, 33*(3), 193–201.

Tena-Sempere, M. (2008). Ghrelin and reproduction: ghrelin as novel regulator of the gonadotropic axis. *Vitamins & Hormones, 77,* 285–300.

Tiwari, H., Oza, U. N., & Tiwari, R. (2006). Knowledge, attitudes and beliefs about menarche of adolescent girls in Anand district, Gujarat. *Eastern Mediterranean Health Journal, 12*(3–4), 428–433.

Trego, L. L. (2007). Military women's menstrual experiences and interest in menstrual suppression during deployment. *Journal of Obstetric, Gynecologic, & Neonatal Nursing, 36*(4), 342–347.

Trego, L. L., & Jordan, P. J. (2010). Military women's attitudes toward menstruation and menstrual suppression in relation to the deployed environment: Development and testing of the MWATMS-9 (short form). *Women's Health Issues, 20*(4), 287–293.

Trout, K. K., Rickels, M. R., Schutta, M. H., Petrova, M., Freeman, E. W., Tkacs, N. C., & Teff, K. L. (2007). Menstrual cycle effects on insulin sensitivity in women with type 1 diabetes: A pilot study. *Diabetes Technology & Therapeutics, 9*(2), 176–182.

Uskul, A. K. (2004). Women's menarche stories from a multicultural sample. *Social Science & Medicine, 59*(4), 667–679.

Weller, A., & Weller, L. (1997). Menstrual synchrony under optimal conditions: Bedouin families. *Journal of Comparative Psychology, 111*(2), 143–151.

Welton, T. (1935). *The modern method of birth control.* New York, NY: Walter J. Black.

Wilson, H. C. (1992). A critical review of menstrual synchrony research. *Psychoneuroendocrinology, 17*(6), 565–591.

Yoon, H., Enquist, L. W., & Dulac, C. (2005). Olfactory inputs to hypothalamic neurons controlling reproduction and fertility. *Cell, 123*(4), 669–682.

chapter 5

MENSTRUAL PROBLEMS: CAUSES AND TREATMENTS

CHAPTER COMPETENCIES

Upon completion of this chapter the reader will be able to:

- Describe the characteristics that differentiate normal menstruation from menstrual problems
- Define the medical terms that describe irregularities in menstruation and understand the potential ambiguities associated with some of the terms

- Describe advantages and disadvantages of current treatment options for menstrual problems

KEY TERMS

abnormal uterine bleeding
amenorrhea
dysfunctional uterine bleeding (DUB)

dysmenorrhea
female athlete triad
hysterectomy

premenstrual dysphoric disorder (PMDD)

premenstrual syndrome (PMS)

WHAT CONSTITUTES A MENSTRUAL PROBLEM?

There is tremendous variability between women in their menstrual cycles in terms of length of the cycle, number of days that bleeding occurs and amount of bleeding. Menstrual cycles are frequently described as being 28 days long, but the mean length of a menstrual cycle is between 25–30 days. In fact, only 10–15 percent of menstrual cycles are exactly 28 days, and anywhere from 20–40 days is still considered within a normal range. Currently, there is an international push to standardize the terminology describing menstruation because confusion over definitions has created difficulties when comparing the effectiveness of treatments for menstrual disorders (Woolcock et al., 2008; Fraser et al., 2007). It has been suggested that much of the older terminology describing menstrual cycles be abandoned in favor of simpler, more descriptive terms (Woolcock et al., 2008; Fraser et al., 2007). However, the older terminology persists. Box 5-1 provides definitions for terms used to describe menstruation.

Menstrual Cycle Alterations

- Hypermenorrhea or menorrhagia: Excessive menstrual bleeding, either in duration or amount, during regularly occurring menstrual cycles.
- Hypomenorrhea: Decreased menstrual bleeding, either in duration or amount, occurring at regular intervals.
- Intermenstrual bleeding: Irregular vaginal bleeding, usually not caused by menses and not excessive in amounts, occurring between regular menstrual cycles.
- Menometrorrhagia: A combination of menorrhagia and metrorrhagia. Irregular, frequent, possibly excessive, or prolonged vaginal bleeding, which may or may not be menstrual.
- Metrorrhagia or intermenstrual bleeding: Bleeding of normal amount but occurring at irregular intervals.
- Oligomenorrhea: Light menstrual bleeding or infrequent menses, which occur in cycles at least 35 days apart.
- Polymenorrhea: Frequent menses that occur in cycles no more than 21 days apart.

Used with permission from Littleton, L.Y, and Engebretson, J.C. (2005). *Maternity Nursing Care*. Clifton Park, NY: Delmar/Cengage Learning.

Cycles that are less than 21 days are considered short cycles. Cycles that are greater than 40 days are identified as long cycles. Two-thirds of all cycles vary in length from one to six days. The average duration of menstrual flow is four to six days. However, menses lasting as few as two days or as many as eight days is not considered abnormal. The amount of menstrual blood that is lost at each period ranges from as little as 20 mL to as much as 80 mL. The average flow is 50 mL. Some women experience regular and consistent menstrual flow, while others experience considerable variation. Individual women may experience variability in their menstrual cycles over their lifetime, sometimes due to external life events, but often for unknown reasons. Women usually experience more regularity in the menstrual cycles between the ages of

20 and 40. It is the preovulatory phase in a cycle that is more variable; the postovulatory phase is usually between 13 to 15 days. This variability in cycle length affects when a woman will ovulate. In a 28 day cycle, ovulation should occur on day 14. However, for a woman with a 21 day cycle ovulation should occur on day 7 and not halfway through her cycle. A woman experiencing a 35 day cycle should ovulate on day 21.

The reasons for variations in the menstrual cycle length vary from minor fluctuations in hormone secretion to serious medical conditions. If a woman is experiencing a persistent change in her menstrual cycles, it is important that the cause be identified, rather than just masked. The difficulty arises in determining which changes in the menstrual cycle warrant investigation.

MENSTRUAL DISORDERS

Many women experience deviations from the average in their menstrual cycles during their reproductive years. Because there is so much variation in frequency of cycles, amount of flow, and duration of flow, it can be difficult for a woman to know when it is necessary to seek medical attention. Generally, persistent changes from a woman's normal pattern that continue for several months indicate that there may be a problem. An easy way to track changes to the menstrual cycle is to keep a record of periods, either on a calendar or in some other systematic format (Figure 5-1).

Additionally, if a woman is charting her basal body temperature (BBT), she can identify if and when she is ovulating. Variations in the menstrual cycle are summarized in Table 5-1.

Amenorrhea

Amenorrhea is the lack of menstruation during a woman's reproductive years and normally occurs only while a woman is pregnant or breastfeeding. Amenorrhea itself is a symptom, not a disease. There are many possible causes for a lack of menstruation, some of which may require treatment. Another concern is that over a long period of time, amenorrhea and the lack of menstrual cycles can result in lowered estrogen levels, which can set the stage for reduced bone density and osteoporosis. There are two types of amenorrhea, primary and secondary.

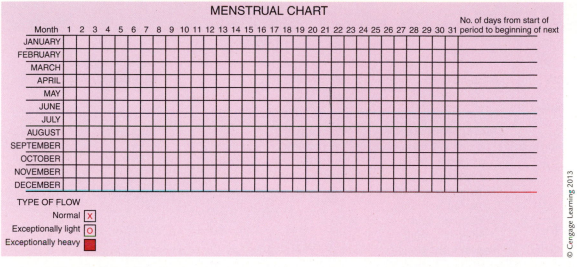

FIGURE 5-1: Menstrual record chart.

Table 5-1   Menstrual Cycle Conditions.

| CONDITION | DATA | | |
	SUBJECTIVE	OBJECTIVE	LABORATORY OR PROCEDURE
Amenorrhea			
Primary amenorrhea	No menarche	Secondary sex characteristics Reproductive tract anomalies	Thyroid function tests Blood glucose level Karyotype (Turner syndrome) Laparoscopy (ovarian pathology)
Secondary amenorrhea	3 or more missed menstrual periods Menstrual pattern	Previous gynecologic procedures or problems Weight gain or loss Major life events Exercise level Thyroid size Exophthalmia Hirsutism Delayed deep tendon reflexes Breast atrophy Thinning hair Temporal baldness	Decreased thyroid function tests Increased blood glucose level Increased serum prolactin level Laparoscopy to detect polycystic ovary syndrome Ultrasound to detect ovarian cysts
Abnormal or Dysfunctional Uterine Bleeding			
Bleeding between menstrual periods	Possible uterine abnormality Irregular bleeding Heavy bleeding Prolonged bleeding Light bleeding Short or long cycles	Anemia Pregnancy test CBC (complete blood count) for anemia or infection Ultrasound Endometrial biopsy to rule out endometrial cancer	Low thyroid function, pituitary function (FSH or LH) hCG studies (for anovulation) Increased prolactin level

(continued)

Table 5-1 (*continued*)

CONDITION	SUBJECTIVE	OBJECTIVE	LABORATORY OR PROCEDURE
		DATA	
Dysmenorrhea			
Primary dysmenorrhea	Mild to severe cramping, lasting 2–4 days before menses to third day of menses GI symptoms: bloating, nausea, vomiting Back, thigh, and headache pain Family history	Nulliparity Age (adolescence to early 20s) Normal results on physical examination	Ultrasound
Secondary dysmenorrhea	Increasingly painful menses Dyspareunia Painful defecation Rectal pressure Heavy or irregular bleeding	Third or fourth decade of life Endometriosis PID, STD Increased uterine size Endometritis Salpingitis Leiomyomata	Elevated WBC count if STD or PID is present Cultures for gonorrhea and chlamydia Ultrasound Laparoscopy (endometriosis)
Endometriosis			
Dysmenorrhea	Infertility Cyclic dyspareunia Dyschezia GI symptoms Pelvic heaviness Chronic pelvic pain (may radiate to thighs) Abnormal bleeding	Uterus may be fixed Possible adenexal mass(es) Pelvic tenderness	Ultrasound monitoring of implants Laparoscopy
Premenstrual syndrome			
Cluster of symptoms at luteal phase	Depressed mood Mood swings Irritability Difficulty in concentration or coping Fatigue Edema Breast tenderness Headache (premenstrual) Sleep disturbances Abdominal bloating Increased appetite Weight gain Food cravings Acne Heart palpitations Anxiety Hostility	Signs of stress Emotional lability	None

Used with permission from Littleton, L.Y, and Engebretson, J.C. (2005). *Maternity Nursing Care*. Clifton Park, NY: Cengage Learning.

Primary Amenorrhea

The timing of menarche is variable, and the onset of menstruation can be linked to family history and genetics. Primary amenorrhea occurs when menarche does not take place by age 16 (MayoClinic.com, 2010; Zegeye, 2009; Master-Hunter & Heiman, 2006). When a girl has not started to menstruate when most of her peers have reached puberty, the reason for the lack of menstruation needs to be investigated. This form of amenorrhea can be related to chromosomal abnormalities, a malformation of the reproductive tract, or both. Less frequently, primary amenorrhea is caused by disorders of the thyroid, adrenal cortex, or more rarely, diseases of the pituitary gland. Primary amenorrhea can also result from extreme malnutrition and eating disorders such as anorexia nervosa which lead to a severe reduction in body fat (Andersen, & Ryan, 2009; Frisch, 1996; Frisch, 1997).

Cryptomenorrhea (Greek: kryptos, hidden) is a term for "silent" menstruation, and this condition can contribute to primary amenorrhea. Normal hormone cycles, ovulation, and menstrual bleeding occur, but the menstrual flow is blocked from exiting the cervix or vagina. The most common reason for the condition is an imperforate hymen, but an infection that causes subsequent scar tissue formation in the vagina or cervix may result in cryptomenorrhea. It can rarely result from an absence of the vagina, caused by a genetic disorder or a malformation of the reproductive tract during development. Cryptomenorrhea is usually diagnosed several years after other signs of puberty such as breast development and other secondary sexual characteristics appear. It is treated surgically.

Secondary Amenorrhea

Secondary amenorrhea is a term applied to the cessation of menstrual periods any time between menarche and menopause when the cause is not pregnancy or breastfeeding. Some of the reasons for secondary amenorrhea are listed in Table 5-2. Like primary amenorrhea, it can be caused by thyroid, adrenal, or pituitary gland disorders. Secondary amenorrhea can also result from an over secretion of the hormone prolactin from the anterior pituitary gland. This condition is called hyperprolactinemia. Polycystic ovary disease and the associated ovarian hormone irregularities can also contribute to secondary amenorrhea.

Table 5-2 Some Causes of Secondary Amenorrhea.

Physiologic (Normal)	Anatomic	Central Nervous System (Hypothalamic)
Pregnancy	Chromosome disorders	Psychogenic
Lactation	Hysterectomy	Environmental
Menopause	Cryptomenorrhea	Nutritional
	Destruction of endometrium Trauma (overly enthusiastic curettage) Disease (e.g., TB) Irradiation	Sudden weight loss Anorexia nervosa Obesity iatrogenic (medically-induced)
	Ovarian Disease (cysts, tumors, etc.) Ovarian failure, premature menopause Destruction, through surgery, infection, Irradiation	Oral contraceptives ("post- pill amenorrhea") Psychotropic drugs Thyroid dysfunction Adrenocortical dysfunction
	Pituitary Tumors, disease Pituitary insufficiency	Chronic systemic disease Hyperprolactinemia

Secondary amenorrhea has often been traced to psychogenic factors such as stress, fear, anxiety, or trauma. A great fear of pregnancy or a tremendous desire for pregnancy can contribute to it; so can a major change in environment such as moving or travel, or emotional events such as a death in the family. It is important to note that this type of amenorrhea usually resolves itself within a few months. Secondary amenorrhea can result from extreme malnutrition, extreme exercise, or eating disorders such as anorexia nervosa. Limited secondary amenorrhea can also result from a rapid and extreme weight loss, especially when coupled with physical or psychological stress. Under these conditions, the hypothalamus stops releasing gonadotropin-releasing hormone and FSH and LH release from the pituitary is disrupted (Andersen & Ryan, 2009; Reame et al., 1985; Reid & Van Vugt, 1987; Warren et al., 1999). This condition is termed functional hypothalamic amenorrhea (Nattiv et al., 2007; Warren et al., 1999). In general, 17 percent body fat is the minimum for the initiation of cycles at menarche, and 22 percent body fat is necessary to sustain regular menstrual cycles. While there are exceptions in which women with lower body fat do menstruate and maintain their fertility, the average woman requires this minimum of body fat to maintain menstruation for three reasons:

- Androgens produced by the ovaries are chemically converted to estrogen by adipose tissue. Thus, body fat becomes an additional source of estrogen for later release.
- Body fat influences the way estrogen is metabolized; lean women make more of a less potent form of estrogen.
- Adipose tissue can store steroid hormones such as estrogens for later release.

Because a decrease in body fat can result in amenorrhea, the occurrence of irregular cycles with obesity becomes harder to explain. One theory suggests that adipose tissue can synthesize too much additional estrogen, and the excess production interferes with the hormonal regulation of menstruation. Chronic obesity may influence how the body cells respond to estrogen and other hormones that are important for regulating menstruation.

Intense exercise can also contribute to secondary amenorrhea. Women who dramatically reduce body fat through exercise are more prone to irregular or absent menstrual periods. This is often termed athletic amenorrhea (De Souza et al., 2010; Stokic et al., 2005). Weight loss itself, although common with intensive training, is apparently not the determining factor because not all athletes have irregular periods. Those who do are often no different in height and weight than those who menstruate normally, but may have greatly decreased subcutaneous fat and greatly increased lean muscle mass. Female athletes have generally been found to have body fat ranging between five percent and six percent of their body weight compared with an average range in women of 24–34 percent. Several studies (Warren, 1985; Abraham, Beumont, Fraser, & Llewellyn-Jones, 1982) of ballet dancers found that cessation of exercise (usually due to injury) resulted in a return of normal cycles. Recent evidence suggests that both an energy deficit brought on by intense exercise and the psychological stress of training may contribute to secondary amenorrhea in athletes (Pauli & Berga, 2010).

Female Athlete Triad   Athletes who participate in sports, especially endurance sports, which emphasize appearance and weight, are particularly vulnerable to what is termed the **female athlete triad** by sports medicine physicians (Nattiv et al., 2007; Furia, 1999). The first component of the triad is an abnormal eating pattern that results in the athlete not taking in enough calories to meet the calories expended through exercise. Lack of adequate nutrition can lead to functional hypothalamic amenorrhea, which is the second component of the triad. Women who experience amenorrhea do not experience a monthly estrogen surge and, since estrogen is an important hormone for maintaining bone density, they may become vulnerable to decreased bone mineral densities in their skeletons (Lambrinoudaki & Papadimitriou, 2010). This reduction in bone density can lead to osteoporosis, which is the third component of the triad. Long recognized as a problem for some postmenopausal women, osteoporosis currently is seen as a concern for amenorrheic women athletes who have low bone mineral density. This may increase their risk for fractures during their competitive years. If this reduction in bone density is prolonged, it can reduce a woman's peak bone density, which is usually attained in the early thirties. This reduction in peak bone density can increase the risk of post-menopausal osteoporosis. A sedentary lifestyle that does not include weight bearing exercise can contribute to reduced bone mineral density in young women (Hoch et al., 2009). The American Academy of Sports Medicine has recommended that women athletes with exercise-induced amenorrhea should be screened for the other elements of the triad – inadequate nutrition and osteoporosis (Nattiv et al., 2007; Drinkwater et al., 1997). Resolving the nutritional deficiency has been shown to play a key role in reversing amenorrhea and improving bone mineral density in female athletes (Fenichel & Warren, 2007).

It should also be pointed out that female athlete triad is associated with the intensive physical training that accompanies competitive sports, marathon running, or professional dancing. It does not occur as a result of moderate activities, such as walking, jogging, aerobics, or other kind of recreational sports. Moderate exercise maximizes health and decreases the risk of developing heart disease, osteoporosis, and other diseases. Research comparing former college athletes with nonathletic women has found that strenuous exercise early in life is linked to a lower incidence of diabetes and cancer.

Dysmenorrhea

The medical term for pelvic pain or cramps that occur during menstruation is **dysmenorrhea**. Many women experience moderate to severe discomfort just before the menstrual period starts or on the first days of menstruation. The pain generally lasts for 24 hours, but in some cases continues for several days (Singh et al., 2008; Proctor & Faquhar, 2007). Dysmenorrhea can be felt in the lower pelvic area together with pain in the thighs and a backache. The intensity of the pain ranges from minor discomfort to incapacitating, although individual response to discomfort can be a factor in how seriously the pain is perceived. If a woman has experienced painful menstrual periods since menarche, the condition is called primary dysmenorrhea. Secondary dysmenorrhea occurs when the condition first arises years after

menarche. Severe dysmenorrhea, accompanied by headache, nausea, and vomiting may not indicate a disease; but if these symptoms are new, or if they seriously disrupt a woman's life, she should have them investigated by a healthcare provider. A physical examination and complete medical history can help determine the cause.

What Causes Dysmenorrhea?

Several medical conditions can cause dysmenorrhea, including pelvic inflammatory disease, endometriosis, and uterine fibroids. Adenomyosis and uterine fibroids, both benign growths in the uterus, can cause severe cramping during the menses. In some cases, the presence of an intrauterine device, or IUD, can cause dysmenorrhea. Dysmenorrhea can also be a symptom of vertebral disorders (Grgic, 2009). In the absence of these conditions, the causes of dysmenorrhea are not definitively known, although a number of theories have been proposed. Psychological, anatomical, and hormonal causes are all possibilities, but none of these provide an adequate explanation for all cases. Shifts in the concentrations and ratios of estrogen and progesterone during the menstrual cycle may also play a role in menstrual cramps. It is likely that dysmenorrhea is caused by a variety of factors.

The smooth muscle of the myometrium undergoes continuous contractions and the intensity of these contractions increases during menstruation to facilitate the shedding of the stratum functionalis of the endometrium. These contractions are triggered by chemical messengers called prostaglandins. Some women with severe dysmenorrhea experience exaggerated uterine contractions and have significantly higher prostaglandin levels in their menstrual blood than those without menstrual pain (Majoribanks et al., 2010). Prostaglandins can also cause a reduction in the normal blood flow to the uterus, a condition called uterine ischemia. This ischemia can contribute to menstrual cramping (Grjic, 2009). However, some severely dysmenorrheic women do not show increased levels of prostaglandins or intensified contractions during menstruation, indicating that other factors are responsible.

For some women, an occluded or partially blocked cervical opening contributes to menstrual

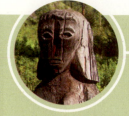

focus on

NUTRITION

Effects of Dietary Fiber and Fat Intake on the Menstrual Cycle

Preliminary studies have revealed some interesting connections between dietary fat and fiber intake and the menstrual cycle. In one study, 341 Japanese women between the ages of 18 and 29 years old recorded their estimated food intake and menstrual cycles, and the mean lengths of the women's menstrual cycles were compared. It was found that the women who consumed the most dietary fat had the shortest menstrual cycles and hence more frequent periods. These results were statistically significant (Nagata et al., 2006). The study also suggested that diets high in fiber were associated with longer menstrual cycles and less frequent periods. Another study did find, however, that women who consume more fiber are less likely to suffer from dysmenorrhea. Further studies have indicated that dietary fat intake tends to increase estrogen levels in the bloodstream and fiber intake reduces estrogen levels, presumably by aiding in the breakdown and elimination of estrogen from the body. By changing estrogen levels in her bloodstream, the length of the woman's menstrual cycle was altered and symptoms of dysmenorrhea influenced (Nagata et al., 2005; Nagata et al., 2004). These findings have significance beyond their effect on the menstrual cycle since high levels of circulating estrogens are also associated with breast, endometrial, and ovarian cancers.

However, methods that work for one woman may not work for another. Heat, in the form of a hot water bottle, a heating pad, or a soak in a hot bath tub, can be effective for many because heat promotes an increase in blood flow and decreases muscle spasms. A hot beverage can be soothing and relaxing, and may help to break the positive feedback loop between pain and tension. Dysmenorrhea can produce tension and anxiety, so relaxation techniques to relieve anxiety can be helpful. Meditation is a method of altering one's mental activities and autonomic functions, and it can be used to reduce both physical and emotional tension. In meditation, energy and concentration are directed inward to achieve relaxation (Figure 5-2).

Having an orgasm can also relieve dysmenorrhea. During an orgasm, the uterus undergoes spontaneous contractions beginning at the fundus and terminating at the cervix. Immediately after an orgasmic response, the external os of the cervix dilates slightly, remaining opened for five to ten minutes. This may be a physiological basis for the reports that orgasm is helpful in alleviating menstrual cramps.

pain. When this is the case, delivery of their first baby usually decreases or eliminates dysmenorrhea, presumably because of changes to the cervix that occur during childbirth. During pregnancy, new blood vessels grow to supply the uterus and these vessels remain after delivery. It may be that the greatly increased blood supply to the uterus during and after pregnancy also plays a role in decreasing symptoms.

Treatments for Dysmenorrhea

For centuries, women have been sharing remedies for menstrual pain with each other. Because there are many factors that can cause dysmenorrhea, it should not be surprising that there are many ways that it can be treated, often without using drugs or hormones.

For many women with primary dysmenorrhea, aspirin and other nonsteroidal anti-inflammatory drugs (NSAIDs) can be used to treat menstrual cramps (Majoribanks et al., 2010). Aspirin has a weaker prostaglandin-inhibiting effect than the other compounds but can be effective for mild dysmenorrhea, although it may cause heavier menstrual bleeding in some women. All of the NSAIDs have possible side effects, which may include gastrointestinal distress, blurred vision, headaches, or dizziness. Increased levels of progesterone after ovulation may contribute to dysmenorrhea. Suppressing ovulation with hormonal contraceptives can reduce dysmenorrhea. In some cases, only a few months of hormonal birth control is necessary to relieve dysmenorrhea.

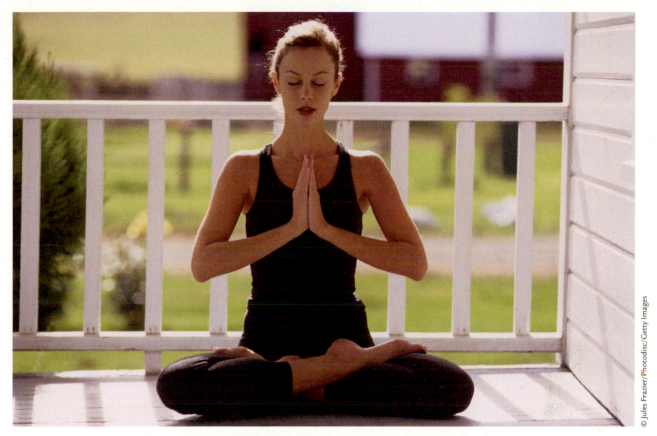

© Jules Frazier/Photodisc/Getty Images

FIGURE 5-2: Meditation and other relaxation techniques can be helpful in relieving dysmenorrhea.

In cases of severe dysmenorrhea, and when other methods have not been successful, there are surgical techniques that can be used to alleviate menstrual pain. One surgical procedure is presacral **neurectomy**, in which all the autonomic nerves to the uterus, both sensory and motor, are severed (Jedrzejczak et al., 2009). Such denervation of the uterus relieves dysmenorrhea, but this procedure permanently disrupts the normal functioning of the uterus and should only be considered for alleviation of pain if other methods are not effective.

Abnormal Uterine Bleeding

Variation in the normal pattern of menstrual cycles in terms of timing and amount of flow is called **abnormal uterine bleeding**. This condition is also called abnormal vaginal bleeding. Because abnormal

focus on

EXERCISE
Exercise to Relieve Dysmenorrhea

Exercising relieves menstrual cramps for many women. It has been noted that physically active women often suffer less menstrual distress. Few women would want to do push-ups or knee bends when having menstrual cramps, but a brisk walk can alleviate pain. Yoga uses meditation, controlled breathing and physical exercises to enhance fitness and relaxation. Several yoga postures focus specifically on the abdominal and lower back muscles and are recommended for women experiencing dysmenorrhea, both as a preventive measure and to relieve pain.

uterine bleeding can be a symptom of a serious underlying condition, it is important to determine why it is occurring. For example, bleeding in between what

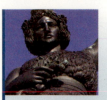

Historical Considerations
LYDIA PINKHAM'S VEGETABLE COMPOUND

One of the most successful patent medicines for "female complaints" was Lydia Pinkham's Vegetable Compound, first marketed in 1876. The compound contained a mixture of herbs in an 18 percent alcohol base and promised to cure "those painful complaints and weaknesses so common to our best female population" according to its advertising. Those complaints ranged from "ovarian troubles" to menstrual cramps, headache, "spinal weakness", fainting, and "the change of life". It was also considered by many to be a treatment for infertility, and some labels carried the slogan "a baby in every bottle". While the advertising stretched the truth, several of the herbs used in the formula are recognized as having bioactive properties that would have helped with some complaints. The original formula contained black cohosh (*Cimicifuga racemosea*), golden ragwort (*Senecio aureus*), unicorn root (*Aletris farinosa*), fenugreek (*Trigonella foenum-graecum*), and butterfly milkweed (*Asclepias tuberosa*). All of these herbs are used today by herbalists for treating reproductive issues and inflammation. Combined with the effects of the strong alcohol base, the compound was probably more effective and much less toxic than the mercury- and arsenic-based medicines commonly prescribed at the time. The elixir was so successful, that variations of this formula are still in production today.

would otherwise be regular periods may be of concern. However, light spotting that occurs just before or at the time of ovulation can be the result of the change in estrogen level that precedes the LH surge. Such mid-cycle bleeding is often accompanied by ovulatory pain, which is also called mittelschmerz, and is considered normal.

Some of the factors that contribute to dysmenorrhea can also cause abnormal uterine bleeding, including the presence of an IUD, benign uterine fibroids, endometriosis and hormonal imbalances. Abnormal bleeding may be the result of acute infection, a blood or liver disease which interferes with clotting factors, or a side effect of a medication. Malignant growths in the reproductive tract, such as endometrial or cervical cancer, can also cause abnormal bleeding (de Vries et al., 2008). Reproductive cancers will be discussed in detail in Chapter 7. These include complications of pregnancy such as miscarriage or ectopic pregnancy. There are circumstances when abnormal bleeding indicates a problem that requires immediate medical attention. If a woman has completed menopause (that is she has not had a period for 12 consecutive months) and she experiences vaginal bleeding, it may indicate endometrial

or cervical cancer. If a woman is soaking one or more menstrual pads or tampons per hour for more than a few hours, or if she is experiencing severe menstrual pain, she should seek medical attention.

Dysfunctional Uterine Bleeding

When a specific cause cannot be determined for abnormal uterine bleeding, the condition is frequently classified as **dysfunctional uterine bleeding (DUB)**. Dysfunctional uterine bleeding is believed to be due to hormonal abnormalities. Although DUB can occur during ovulatory cycles it is usually associated with menstrual cycles during which ovulation does not occur. These types of cycles are called anovulatory cycles. In an anovulatory cycle, the endometrium is not stimulated by progesterone because a corpus luteum has not formed. The endometrium remains in the proliferative phase and continues to thicken but never becomes secretory. This results in prolonged and heavy bleeding. The bleeding continues until new follicles in the ovary produces enough estrogen to stimulate new endometrial cell growth. New cell regeneration then stops the bleeding. Obese women are particularly prone to DUB because excess adipose tissue creates excess estrogen.

Anovulatory cycles and dysfunctional uterine bleeding are most frequent during the two transitional periods of a woman's life, just after menarche and just before menopause. About half of girls going through puberty do not ovulate during their initial menstrual cycles, and mild dysfunctional bleeding may occur and then resolve itself after several months to a year. Heavy and frequent menstruation is not unusual in premenopausal women because of the age related increased risk of endometrial cancer, it is especially important to seek medical evaluation for dysfunctional uterine bleeding.

Diagnosing Abnormal Uterine Bleeding

In the United States, it is estimated that 30 percent of women experience abnormal uterine bleeding at some time during their reproductive years. Some of the preliminary diagnostic tools that are used to determine the cause of abnormal uterine bleeding include:

- Physical examination including a review of a woman's medical history.
- Blood tests to check for anemia, thyroid hormone levels and blood clotting abnormalities. While blood clotting disorders affect only two percent of the general population, the incidence rises to 20 percent in women with DUB.
- Pap smear to test for cervical cancer.
- Endometrial biopsy to test for endometrial cancer. The risk of developing endometrial cancer increases with a woman's age.
- Ultrasound to check for uterine fibroids and other benign growths.
- Tests for STIs.

Additional tests may also be required. In some cases, a sonohystogram may be performed. With this test, an ultrasound probe is inserted into the uterus. The uterus is then examined using sterile saline solution, which makes fibroids, polyps, and other uterine abnormalities easier to identify. A hysteroscopy uses fiber optics inserted through the cervix and into the uterus, to visualize the endometrium. This procedure can be used to identify fibroids and polyps, and to obtain biopsies of the endometrium. A dilation and curettage (D and C) dilates the cervix and uses a tool called a curettage to scrape away sections of the endometrium for testing. Finally, transvaginal ultrasonography is used to determine the thickness of the endometrium and check for tumors or fibroids.

Treatments for Abnormal Uterine Bleeding

The decision about how or whether to treat abnormal uterine bleeding is determined by several factors including the severity of the bleeding, the woman's age, and whether or not she wants to have children in the future. Iron supplements may be prescribed if the condition is accompanied by anemia or if there is a potential to develop anemia.

Nonsteroidal anti-inflammatory drugs (NSAIDs) can be used to treat abnormal uterine bleeding. The nonsteroidal anti-inflammatory drugs are prostaglandin inhibitors. The antiprostaglandin effect may improve platelet aggregation which is responsible for blood clotting, and increases constriction of the blood vessels in the uterus, reducing blood flow. Hormonal treatments can also be used to treat abnormal uterine bleeding. Oral contraceptive pills containing estrogen and progestins mimic normal cycles and can reduce abnormal bleeding. In addition, progesterone releasing IUDs have also been shown to be effective for reducing menstrual bleeding and dysmenorrhea (Lethaby et al., 2005).

If uterine bleeding is severe and does not improve with other therapies, procedures such as endometrial ablation or endometrial resection may be used to

Critical Thinking

Risks Associated with Using Hormonal Forms of Birth Control to Treat Menstrual Irregularities

Hormonal forms of birth control such as oral contraceptives are often used to regulate the menstrual cycle and to treat abnormal menstrual symptoms. Scientific studies have shown that using hormonal forms of birth control can carry some serious health risks, and at the same time, may impart important health benefits. What are the factors that a woman would need to consider as she contemplates using hormonal birth control as a means for treating menstrual problems?

control this condition. In the case of endometrial ablation, the stratum functionalis is removed and the basal layer is coagulated using a laser, cautery, or ultrasound (Figure 5-3). Endometrial ablation usually prevents regeneration of the endometrium and the recurrence of DUB, at least temporarily. The treatment, which requires general anesthesia or a spinal block, results in amenorrhea or very scant flow. Because there is usually not enough endometrium left to allow implantation, this procedure can eliminate the possibility of future pregnancies. Endometrial ablation is an option for women who have DUB, but not large fibroids or polyps. Preliminary studies indicate that this procedure results in fewer complications than complete removal of the uterus, or hysterectomy. However, for about a quarter of women who have endometrial ablation, the endometrium grows back after two to four years and symptoms resume. They may then repeat the procedure or undergo hysterectomy to treat recurring DUB (Papadopoulos et al., 2010; Dickerson et al., 2007).

Endometrial resection is similar to endometrial ablation in that it removes the endometrial lining of the uterus. Like endometrial ablation, it is an option for women who do not have large uterine fibroids. This procedure also reduces a woman's chances of becoming pregnant. Another process, called operative hysteroscopy can be used to surgically remove small polyps which might be causing excessive bleeding from the inside of the uterus.

Hysterectomy

Hysterectomy, or removal of the uterus, is a permanent surgical treatment for treating DUB. The advantage of hysterectomy for treating DUB is that there is no risk of having to repeat the procedure. It should be noted however, that there are some serious potential drawbacks to hysterectomy. Although hysterectomy is a relatively safe surgery, there are risks, including blood clots, infection, adhesions, hemorrhage, bowel obstruction, and injury to the urinary tract. There is evidence that women who have undergone hysterectomy have an increased risk of developing urinary incontinence by age 60, compared to women who have an intact uterus (Allahdin et al., 2008; McPherson et al., 2005). The type of hysterectomy that is performed plays a role in the chances of developing incontinence, so it is important for women to be aware of all of their options before proceeding with this surgery (Ditto et al., 2010; Gimbel, 2007; Kato et al., 2007). In some cases, hysterectomy is associated with loss of sexual function, although some women have increased sex drive after hysterectomy (Pauls, 2010; McPherson et al., 2005). New, nerve-sparing surgeries may mitigate some of these problems (Pieterse et al., 2007). Some women experience feelings of depression after hysterectomy. Finally, having a hysterectomy eliminates a women's potential to become pregnant. Before hysterectomy, it is important that the cause of the excessive bleeding be investigated. A thorough diagnosis is important because correcting the problem with surgery can mask a symptom of an underlying condition that requires further attention.

Premenstrual Syndrome

It has been estimated that about seventy-five percent of menstruating women experience very mild to moderately uncomfortable symptoms during the days preceding their menstrual periods, a phenomenon called **premenstrual syndrome** or **PMS**. Women's

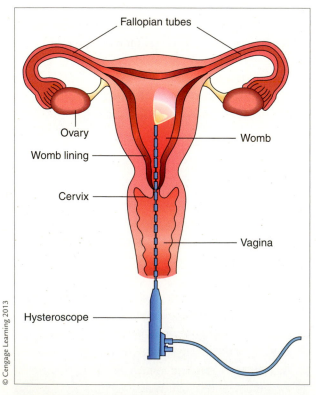

© Cengage Learning 2013

FIGURE 5-3: Endometrial ablation.

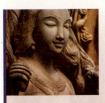

Social Considerations
CURRENT TRENDS IN HYSTERECTOMY

There is growing concern that hysterectomy may be overused as a treatment for DUB. In the United States, 30 percent, or one in every three women have a hysterectomy by the age of 60. In the UK 20 percent of women have one by the same age (El-Hemaidi et al., 2007). Between 50–70 percent of hysterectomies are performed to treat DUB, but in 50 percent of those hysterectomies, there is no evidence of cancer present. In some cases, hysterectomies are performed before other treatment options are explored. One of the reasons that hysterectomies are increasing in many countries may have to do with how the uterus is viewed by many in the medical community. In general, the uterus is viewed exclusively as a vessel for incubating a baby, and scant attention is paid to other functions that it may have. If a woman has passed her reproductive years, or does not want to become pregnant, it is often assumed that her uterus is no longer needed, and may in fact be a danger to her, since it has the potential to develop cancer. In some cases, the ovaries are viewed the same way and are removed with the uterus to eliminate the potential of developing ovarian cancer later in life.

Women who have a hysterectomy begin menopause an average of four years earlier, even if their ovaries are not removed. When a woman enters menopause, her risk of stroke and heart attack increase, and cardiovascular disease becomes a major cause of death for postmenopausal women. In fact, a woman's risk of dying from a heart attack after menopause is higher than her risk of dying from uterine or ovarian cancer. Having a hysterectomy also increases a woman's chance of developing osteoporosis (Ozdemir et al., 2009).

For some women whose lives are severely disrupted by DUB, hysterectomy may be the best solution to maintain their quality of life. However, it is important to consider that resorting to surgery for relief of symptoms can result in additional problems later in life. The tradeoffs must be considered and hysterectomy should be a last resort after other therapies have failed.

experience of PMS is highly variable. Premenstrual syndrome can sometimes be difficult to identify, but is generally thought to encompass a range of emotional and physical symptoms including anxiety, depression, irritability, fatigue, bloating, and joint and muscle pain during the days that precede menstruation. Not all women suffer from PMS, although many report some combination of symptoms of PMS days before the onset of menstruation. PMS has been the subject of much feminist critique, since PMS has been used as a way to dismiss women as unreliable or incompetent, overly emotional, and even mentally unstable. The physical and behavioral symptoms of PMS are outlined in Table 5-3. Most women experience only one or two of these, and a common characteristic of the symptoms is that they are clustered during the luteal phase of the menstrual cycle and disappear with the onset of menstruation. However, many of these symptoms can also occur independent of the hormonal fluctuations of the menstrual cycle. A smaller percentage of women suffer from a more severe and sometimes disabling form of PMS called **premenstrual dysphoric disorder (PMDD)**.

What Causes PMS?
Several factors have been proposed to explain the occurrence of premenstrual symptoms. Hormone fluctuations throughout the menstrual cycle can trigger many of the physiological and behavioral changes that women experience. Progesterone alters blood glucose levels, which may account for the carbohydrate cravings that some women experience,

Table 5-3   Symptoms of Premenstrual Syndrome.

Physical Symptoms of PMS	Emotional or Behavioral Symptoms of PMS
Breast Tenderness	Mood Swings
Edema and Weight Gain	Tension and Anxiety
Abdominal Bloating	Depressed Mood
Joint and Muscle Pain	Sleep Problems
Headache	Poor Concentration
Acne	Crying Spells
Constipation or Diarrhea	Appetite Changes and Food Cravings
Fatigue	

© Cengage Learning 2013

as well as headaches and mood swings. Interactions between reproductive hormones and neurotransmitters in the brain may also play a role. Insufficient levels of the neurotransmitter serotonin can cause feelings of depression, loss of sleep, fatigue and food cravings. PMS may also be linked with vitamin and mineral deficiencies, especially of calcium, vitamin D, vitamin B-6 and vitamin E (Khajehei et al., 2009; Bertone-Johnson et al., 2005). Duvan et al. (2010) have suggested that disturbances to the ratio of oxidants to antioxidants in the bloodstream may contribute to stress associated with PMS. Finally, in some women, PMS may also be a result of undiagnosed depression.

Diagnosing and Treating PMS

There are no laboratory tests available to diagnose PMS. Daily reporting of physical, behavioral and emotional changes in a journal for several months can be used to determine if symptoms are clustered around the luteal phase (last 14 days) of the menstrual cycle. Not everyone is equally convinced that PMS is a well-defined condition since it affects such a large proportion of the population. Some women's health advocates are concerned about the "medicalization" of menstrual symptoms and the labeling of PMS as another hormone-deficiency disease to be "cured" by prescription medications (Matusevich & Pierczanski, 2008). For many women, lifestyle changes can minimize the discomforts of PMS. The following is a list of recommendations to minimize symptoms of PMS:

- Get adequate exercise to reduce stress and to reduce symptoms of PMS.
- Eat healthy foods, including fruits, vegetables, and whole grains. These foods provide nutrients to maintain a healthy reproductive and nervous system, and they also provide fiber. Dietary fiber plays a role in maintaining healthy hormone balance by aiding in the removal of excess estrogen from the body. Take a daily multi-vitamin, and ensure adequate calcium and magnesium in the diet (Frackiewicz & Shiovitz, 2001).
- Consuming high glycemic index carbohydrates may increase the neurotransmitter serotonin in the brain. Increased levels of serotonin can moderate mood swings (Murakami et al., 2008).
- Avoid excess salt and increase water intake to reduce water retention and bloating.
- Avoid excess caffeine, alcohol, and high-sugar foods.
- Get enough sleep. Getting adequate rest helps to mitigate the effects of stress which can exacerbate PMS symptoms.
- Find healthy ways to cope with stress.

Medical treatments for symptoms of PMS include diuretics, hormonal contraceptives, and prescription antidepressants and anti-anxiety medications. Diuretics can be prescribed if reducing dietary salt intake is not

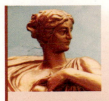

Cultural Considerations
PERCEPTIONS OF PMS

There is some evidence that cultural expectations can influence women's perception and reporting of PMS symptoms (Tscudin et al., 2010; Dennerstein et al., 2009; McMaster et al., 1997). A recent study has reported that women who are familiar with the phenomenon of PMS are likely to report more severe premenstrual symptoms than women who are not. Dr. Maria Marvan and her colleague at the Universidad de las Americas in Mexico (1999) showed a 10-minute videotape describing the negative aspects of PMS to half of a group of 86 Latina women and showed the other half (the control group) a videotape describing the menstrual cycle. The women in the study had no cultural preconceptions or prior knowledge about PMS. Both before and after viewing the tape, which they watched during the first week after menstruation, both groups were asked to report on symptoms they experienced in their premenstrual periods. Before viewing the videotape describing PMS, more than half of the experimental group reported no symptoms of pain, psychological distress, or other symptoms. Some reported mild symptoms, two percent reported moderate symptoms, and none reported severe symptoms. After viewing the tape, only two percent reported no symptoms, 37 percent reported mild symptoms, 54 percent reported moderate symptoms, and seven percent reported severe symptoms. In contrast, in women in the control group, there were no significant differences in premenstrual symptoms reported both before and after the women watched the videotape. None reported any severe symptoms.

effective for reducing premenstrual edema. Oral contraceptives prevent ovulation and stabilize extreme hormonal fluctuations. The hormone progesterone has been used to prevent symptoms of PMS, but its efficacy has recently been questioned (Ford et al., 2009). Some antidepressants are selective serotonin reuptake inhibitors (SSRIs). They enhance the amount of serotonin in the brain, potentially alleviating severe PMS (Brown et al., 2009). Anti-anxiety drugs can be effective when taken for a week to two weeks prior to menstruation. The benefits of these medications must be weighed against the potential negative side effects.

Premenstrual Dysphoric Disorder (PMDD)

Between five and eight percent of women suffer from a severe form of PMS called premenstrual dysphoric disorder or PMDD (Cunningham et al., 2009; Vigod et al., 2009). The symptoms of PMDD are similar to those of PMS, but are extreme enough to interfere with a woman's normal activities. PMDD was included in the research appendix of the revised edition (1987) of the American Psychiatric Association's *Diagnostic and Statistical Manual III (DSM-III-R)*

as a mental disorder, under the name late luteal phase dysphoric disorder. In the 1994 edition of the *DSM* (*DSM-IV*), the name was changed to premenstrual dysphoric disorder (PMDD). The word dysphoric means extreme discomfort, unpleasant, or ill at ease. Inclusion in the *Diagnostic and Statistical Manual* has important implications in the United States; if a diagnosis is in the *DSM*, health insurance companies are more likely to pay for treatment. To qualify for premenstrual dysphoric status, a woman must have at least five of 10 psychological and physical symptoms. These must occur during the week before and a few days after the onset of menstruation and include one or more of the following psychological symptoms: marked mood swings, persistent anger or irritability, marked anxiety or tension, or depression and feelings of hopelessness (Rapkin & Winer, 2009). Box 5-2 outlines the symptoms of PMDD.

Originally, it was proposed that PMDD was caused by hormonal imbalances occurring during the menstrual cycle. However, it is now believed that PMDD is more likely an abnormal response to normal reproductive hormone fluctuations (Cunningham

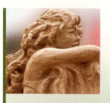

Economic Considerations
THE SELLING OF PMDD

Premenstrual dysphoric disorder (PMDD) is described as an extreme form of PMS, although many health professionals are reluctant to accept PMDD as a distinct diagnosis from PMS. Work by Gehlert et al. (2009) found just over one percent of women meet the clinical criteria of the condition, far lower than 20–30 percent cited by some authors (Steiner et al., 2011). Some psychologists note that what is thought to be PMDD can easily be confused with mental health disorders, most notably depression (Zukov et al., 2010). A 2002 article appearing in the *Monitor on Psychology* of the American Psychological Association posed the question "Is PMDD Real?" and noted the following critiques from two prominent feminist scholars:

> "PMS and PMDD are both 'culture-bound' syndromes," says Joan Chrisler, PhD, a psychology professor at Connecticut College and president of the Society for Menstrual Cycle Research. "There is no evidence [that PMDD exists], though

people have to find such evidence," says Paula Caplan, PhD, author of "They Say You're Crazy" (Perseus Books, 1995). "It is really appalling that using PMDD for women who want recognition for discomfort is a very clear message that goes something like: 'OK, OK, we'll believe you are feeling bad if we get to call you mentally ill for feeling bad.' " (Daw, 2002. p 58).

Daw argued that PMDD was used as a marketing tool to extend the patent protection of specific antidepressants. It was reported that the manufacturer of the antidepressant spent more than $33 million promoting the drug specifically to treat PMDD and that several of the studies identifying PMDD were funded by the same manufacturer (Daw, 2002). While PMDD is a serious condition for a small percentage of women, using the disorder to promote medication for a large population of women who are experiencing significantly milder symptoms of PMS can be seen as an example of the "medicalization" of menstruation.

BOX 5-2

Symptoms of Premenstrual Dysphoric Disorder

The symptoms of PMDD, as outlined by the United States Office on Women's Health in the Department of Health and Human Services include:

- feelings of sadness or despair, or possibly suicidal thoughts
- feelings of tension or anxiety
- panic attacks
- mood swings, crying
- lasting irritability or anger that affects other people

- disinterest in daily activities and relationships
- trouble thinking or focusing
- tiredness or low energy
- food cravings or binge eating
- feeling out of control
- physical symptoms, such as bloating, breast tenderness, headaches, and joint or muscle pain

---

et al., 2009). As with PMS, some lifestyle changes may help ease PMDD symptoms. In fact, the same lifestyle changes that can alleviate PMS can be helpful in managing PMDD. Medical treatments for PMS are also used to treat PMDD (Steiner, 2000), including

hormonal contraceptives to regulate hormones and reduce symptoms. Antidepressants called selective serotonin reuptake inhibitors (SSRIs) increase serotonin levels in the brain and have also been shown to help some women with PMDD.

CONCLUSION

In conclusion, characteristics of the menstrual cycle can be highly variable between women and throughout an individual woman's lifetime. This is not surprising considering the complex hormonal and physiological interactions that orchestrate the female reproductive cycle. In some cases, uncomfortable changes in a woman's cycle are benign and simply require lifestyle adjustments to alleviate them. Others can be symptoms of more dangerous underlying conditions that require medical attention. A woman's own experience of what is normal for her is important for distinguishing between harmless changes and signs of a problem that should be investigated.

REVIEW QUESTIONS

1. What are the differences between primary and secondary amenorrhea?

2. What are some potential causes of primary amenorrhea?

3. What are some potential causes of secondary amenorrhea?

4. What is meant by dysfunctional uterine bleeding?

5. What are the current treatment options for dysfunctional uterine bleeding?

6. Which chemicals in the body are responsible for producing dysmenorrhea?

7. What is the difference between PMS and premenstrual dysphoric syndrome?

CRITICAL THINKING QUESTIONS

1. Why is amenorrhea of potential concern in young women?

2. What are the factors that a woman must consider when choosing a treatment option for menstrual irregularities?

WEBLINKS

National Institute of Mental Health (NIMH), NIH, HHS
www.nimh.nih.gov
American College of Obstetricians and Gynecologists (ACOG)
www.acog.org

The Hormone Foundation
www.hormone.org

REFERENCES

Abraham, S. F., Beaumont, P. J., Fraser, I. S., & Llewellyn-Jones, D. (1982). Body weight, exercise and menstrual status among ballet dancers in training. *British Journal of Obstetrics and Gynaecology, 89*(7), 507–510.

Allahdin, S., Harrild, K., Warraich, Q. A., & Bain, C. (2008). Comparison of the long-term effects of simple total abdominal hysterectomy with transcervical endometrial resection on urinary incontinence. *British Journal of Obstetrics and Gynaecology, 115*(2),199–204.

American Psychiatric Association. (1987). *Diagnostic and statistical manual of mental disorders* (3rd ed. rev.). Washington, DC: Author.

American Psychiatric Association. (1994). *Diagnostic and statistical manual of mental disorders* (4th ed.). Washington, DC: Author.

Andersen, A. E., & Ryan, G. L. (2009). Eating disorders in the obstetric and gynecologic patient population. *Obstetrics & Gynecology, 114*(6), 1353–1367.

Bertone-Johnson, E. R., Hankinson, S. E., Bendich, A., Johnson, S. R., Willett, W. C., & Hanon, J. E. (2005). Calcium and vitamin D intake and risk of incident premenstrual syndrome. *Archives of Internal Medicine, 165*(11), 1246–1252.

Brown, J., O'Brien, P. M., Majorbanks, J., & Wyatt, K. (2009). Selective serotonin reuptake inhibitors for premenstrual syndrome. *Cochrane Database Systemic Review, 15*(2), CD001396.

Chrisler, J. C., & Levy, K. B. (1990). The media construct a menstrual monster: A content analysis of PMS articles in the popular press. *Women and Health, 16*(2), 89–105.

Cumming, D. C., Vickovic, M. M., Wall, S. R., & Fluker, M. R. (1985). Defects in pulsatile LH release in normally menstruating runners. *Journal of Clinical Endocrinology and Metabolism, 60,* 810–812.

Cunningham, J., Yonkers, K. A., O'Brien, S., & Erikson, E. (2009). Update on research and treatment of premenstrual dysphoric disorder. *Harvard Review of Psychiatry, 17*(2), 120–137.

Dalton, K. (1984). *The premenstrual syndrome and progesterone therapy* (2nd ed.). Chicago, IL: Year Book Medical Publishers.

Davis, J. P., Chesney, P. J., Wand, P. J., et al. (1980). Toxic shock syndrome. *New England Journal of Medicine, 303*(25), 1429–1435.

Daw, J. (2002). Is PMDD real? *Monitor on Psychology, 33,* 58.

De Souza, M. J., Toombs, R. J., Scheid, J. L., O'Donnel, E., West, S. L., & Williams, N. I. (2010). High prevalence of subtle and severe menstrual disturbances in exercising women: Confirmation using daily hormone measures. *Human Reproduction, 25*(2), 491–503.

Dennerstein, L., Lehert, P., Backstrom, T. C., & Heinemann, K. (2009). Premenstrual symptoms—severity, duration and typology: An international cross-sectional study. *Menopause International, 15*(3), 120–126.

deVries, C. J., Wieringae-de Waard, M., Vervoort, C. L., Ankum, W. M., & Bindeis, P. J. (2008). Abnormal vaginal bleeding in women of reproductive age: A descriptive study of initial management in general practice. *BMC Women's Health, 8*(1), 7.

Dickerson, K., Munro, M. G., Clark, M., Langenberg, P., Scherer, R., Frick, K., Zhu, Q., Hallock, L., Nichols, J., & Yalcinkaya, T. M. (2007). Surgical Treatment Outcomes Project for Dysfunctional Uterine Bleeding (STOP-DUB) Research Group. Hysterectomy compared with endometrial ablation for dysfunctional uterine bleeding: A randomized controlled trial. *Obstetrics and Gynecology, 11*(6), 1279–1289.

Ditto, A., Martinelli, F., Borreani, C., Kusamura, S., Hanozet, F., Brunelli, C., Rossi, G., Solima, E., Fortanelli, R., Zanaboni, F., Grijuela, B., & Raspagliesi, F. (2009). Quality of life and sexual, bladder, and intestinal dysfunctions after class III nerve sparing and class II radical hysterectomies: A questionnaire-based study. *International Journal of Gynecological Cancer, 19*(5), 953–957.

Drinkwater, B., Johnson, M., Loucks, A., et al. (1997). The female athlete triad. *Medical Science and Sports Exercise, 29,* 1–16.

Duvan, C. L., Curmaoglu, A., Turhan, N. O., Karasu, C., & Kafali, H. (2011). Oxidant/antioxidant status in premenstrual syndrome. *Archives of Gynecology and Obstetrics, 283*(2), 299–304.

El-Hemaidi, I., Gharaibeh, A., & Shehata, H. (2007). Menorrhagia and bleeding disorders. *Current Opinion in Obstetrics and Gynecology, 19*(6), 513–520.

Fenichel, R. M., & Warren, M. P. (2007). Anorexia, bulimia, and the athletic triad: Evaluation and management. *Current Osteoporosis Report, 5*(4), 160–164.

Ford, O., Lethaby, A., Roberts, H., & Mol, B. W. (2006). Progesterone for premenstrual syndrome. *Cochrane Database Systemic Review, 15*(2), CD003415.

Frackiewicz, E. J., & Shiovitz, T. M. (2001). Evaluation and management of premenstrual syndrome and premenstrual dysphoric disorder. *Journal of the American Pharmaceutical Association (Washington), 41*(3), 437–447.

Frank, R. T. (1931). The hormonal causes of premenstrual tension. *Archives of Neurology and Psychiatry, 26,* 1053–1057.

Fraser, I. S., Critchley, H. O., & Munro, M. G. (2007). Abnormal uterine bleeding: Getting our terminology straight. *Current Opinion in Obstetrics and Gynecology, 19*(6), 591–595.

Frisch, R. E. (1987). Body fat, menarche, fitness and fertility. *Human Reproduction, 2*(6), 521–522.

Frisch, R. E. (1993). Critical fat. *Science, 261*(5125), 1103–1104.

Frisch, R. E. (1996). The right weight: Body fat, menarche, and fertility. *Nutrition, 12*(6), 452–453.

Frisch, R. E. (1997). Critical fatness hypothesis. *American Journal of Physiology, 273*(1 Pt. 1), E231–232.

Frisch, R. E., Wyshak, G., Albright, N. L., Albright, T. E., & Schiff, I. (1989). Lower prevalence of non-reproductive system cancers among female former college athletes. *Medical Science and Sports Exercise, 21*(3), 250–253.

Furia, J. (1999). The female athlete triad. *Medscape Orthopedics and Sports Medicine, 3*(1), 1–7.

Gehlert, S., Song, I. H., Chang, C. H., & Hartlage, S. A. (2009). The prevalence of premenstrual dysphoric disorder in a randomly selected group of urban and rural women. *Psychological Medicine, 39*(1), 129–136.

Gimble, H. (2007). Total and subtotal hysterectomy for benign uterine diseases? A meta–analysis. *Acta Obstetricia et Gynecologica Scandinavica, d86*(2),133–144.

Grgic, V. (2009). Dysmenorrhea induced by lumbro-sacral spine disorders. Pathogenesis, diagnosis and therapy with special emphasis on spinal manipulative therapy. *Lijec Vjesn, 131*(9–10), 275–279.

Hoch, A. Z., Pajewski, N. M., Maraski, L., Carrera, G. F., Wilson, C. R., Hoffmann, R. G., Schimke, J. E., & Gutterman, D. D. (2009). Prevalence of the female athlete triad in high school athletes and sedentary students. *Clinical Journal of Sport Medicine, 19*(5), 421–428.

Jedrzejczak, P., Sokaiska, A., Spaczynski, R. Z., Duleba, A. J., & Pawelczyk L. (2009). Effects of presacral neurectomy on pelvic pain in women with and without endometriosis. *Ginekologia Polska, 80*(3),172–178.

Kato, K., Suzuka, L., Osaki, T., & Tanaka, N. (2007). Unilateral or bilateral nerve–sparing radical hysterectomy: A surgical technique to preserve the pelvic autonomic nerves while increasing radicality. *International Journal of Gynecological Cancer, 17*(5), 1172–1178.

Khajehei, M., Abdali, K., Parsanezhad, M.E., & Tabatabaee, H.R. (2009). Effect of treatment with dydrogesterone or calcium plus vitamin D on the severity of premenstrual syndrome. *International Journal of Gynecology, 105*(2), 158–161.

Lambrinoudaki, I., & Papadimitriou, D. (2010). Pathophysiology of bone loss in the female athlete. *Annals of the New York Academy of Sciences, 1205*(1), 45–50. *doi: 10.1111/j.1749-6632.2010.05681.x.*

Lethaby, A. E., Cooke, I., & Rees, M. (2005). Progesterone or progesterone-releasing intra-uterine systems for heavy menstrual bleeding. *Cochrane Database Systematic Review, Oct 19* (4), CD002126.

Majoribanks, J., Proctor, M., Farquhar, C., & Derks, R. S. (2010). Nonsteroidal anti-inflammatory drugs for dysmenorrhea. *Cochrane Database Systematic Review, Jan 20*(1), CD001751.

Marvan, M. L., & Escobedo, C. (1999). Premenstrual symptomatology: Role of prior knowledge about premenstrual syndrome. *Psychosomatic Medicine, 61*(2), 163–167.

Master-Hunter, T., & Heiman, D. L. (2006). Amenorrhea: Evaluation and treatment. *American Family Physician, 73*(8), 1374–1382.

Matusevich, D., & Pieczanski, P. (2008). The medicalization of feminine suffering: Premenstrual dysphoric disorder. *Vertex, 19*(81), 280–291.

Mayo Clinic. (2008). Amenorrhea. Retrieved April 5, 2010 from http://www.mayoclinic.com/ amenorrhea/DS00581.

Mayo Clinic. Menorrhagia (heavy menstrual bleeding). (2009). Retrieved April 5, 2010 from http://mayoclinic.com/print/menorrhagia/DS00394.

Mayo Clinic. Premenstrual dysphoric disorder (PMDD): A severe form of PMS. (2008). Retrieved April 5, 2010 from http://www.mayoclinic.com/pmdd/AN01372.

McMaster, J., Cormie, K., & Pitts, M. (1997). Menstrual and premenstrual experiences of women in a developing country. *Health care for Women International, 18*(6), 533–541.

McPherson, K., Herbert, A., Judge, A., Clarke, A., Bridgman, S., Maresh, M., & Overton, C. (2005). Psychosexual health 5 years after hysterectomy: Population-based comparison with endometrial ablation for dysfunctional uterine bleeding. *Health Expect, 8*(3), 234–243.

McPherson, K., Herbert, A., Judge, A., Clarke, A., Bridgman, S., Maresh, M., & Overton, C. (2005). Self-reported bladder function five years post-hysterectomy. *Journal of Obstetrics and Gynaecology, 25*(5), 469–475.

Murakami, K., Sasaki, S., Takahashi, Y., Uenishi, K., Watanabe, T., Kohri, T., Yamasaki, M., Watanabe, R., Baba, K., Shibata, K., Takahashi, T., Hayabuchi, H., Ohki, K., & Suzuki, J. (2008). Dietary glycemic index is associated with decreased premenstrual symptoms in young Japanese women. *Nutrition, 24*(6), 554–561.

Nagata, C., Hirokawa, K., Shimizu, N., & Shimizu, H. (2005). Associations of menstrual pain with intake of soy, fat, and dietary fiber in Japanese women. *European Journal of Clinical Nutrition, 59*(1), 88–92.

Nagata, C., Oba, S., & Shimizu, H. (2006). Associations of menstrual cycle length with intake of soy, fat, and dietary fiber in Japanese women. *Nutrition Cancer Journal, 54*(2), 166–170.

Nagata, C., Hirokawa, K., Shimizu, N., & Shimizu, H. (2004). Associations of premenstrual symptoms with intake of soy, fat, and dietary fiber in Japanese women. *BJOG, 111*(6), 594–599.

Nattiv, A., Loucks, A. B., Manore, M. M., Sanborn, C. F., Sundgot-Borgen, J., & Warren, M. P. (2007). American College of Sports Medicine position stand. The female athlete triad. *Medicine & Science in Sports & Exercise, 39*(10), 1867–1882.

Ozdemir, S., Celik, C., Gorkemil, H., Kiyici, A., & Kaya, B. (2009). Compared effects of surgical and natural menopause on climacteric symptoms, osteoporosis, and metabolic syndrome. *International Journal of Gynecology & Obstetrics, 106*(1), 57–61.

Papadopoulos, M. S., Tolikas, A. C., & Miliaras, D. E. (2010). Hysterectomy—Current methods and alternatives for benign indications. *Obstetrics and Gynecology International, 2010,* 356740. doi:10.1155/2010/356740

Pauli, S. A., & Berga, S. L. (2010). Athletic amenorrhea: Energy deficit or psychogenic challenge? *Annals of the New York Academy of Sciences, 1205*(1), 33–38. doi: 10.1111/j.1749–6632.2010.05663.x.

Pauls, R. N. (2010). Impact of gynecological surgery on female sexual function. *International Journal of Impotence Research, 22,* 105–114. doi:10.1038/ijir.2009.63

Pieterse, Q. D., Ter Kuile, M. M., Deruiter, M. C., Trimbos, J. B., Kenter, G. G., & Maas, C. P. (2008). Vaginal blood flow after hysterectomy with and without nerve sparing. A preliminary report. *International Journal of Gynecological Cancer, 18*(3), 576–583. doi: 10.1111/j.1525–1438.2007.01046.x

Proctor, M. L., & Farquhar, C. M. (2007). Dysmenorrhoea. *Clinical Evidence,* (2007, March 1), 0813.

Rapkin, A. J., & Winer, S. A. (2009). Premenstrual syndrome and premenstrual dysphoric disorder: Quality of life and burden of illness. *Expert Review of Pharmacoeconomics & Outcomes Research, 9*(2), 157–170.

Reame, N. E., Sauder, S. E., Case, G. D., et al. (1985). Pulsatile gonadotropin secretion in women with hypothalamic amenorrhea: Evidence that reduced frequency of gonadotropin-releasing hormone secretion is the mechanism of persistent anovulation. *Journal of Clinical Endocrinology and Metabolism, 61*(5), 851–858.

Reid, R. L., & Van Vugt, M. A. (1987). Weight-related changes in reproductive function. *Fertility and Sterility, 48*(6), 905–913.

Singh, A., Kiran, D., Singh, H., Nel, B., Singh, P., & Tiwari, P. (2008) Prevalence and severity of dysmenorrheal: A problem related to menstruation, among first and second year female medical students. *Indian Journal of Physiology and Pharmacology, 52*(4), 389–397.

Steiner, M., Peer, M., Palova, E., Freeman, E. W., Macdougall, M., & Soares, C. N. (2010). The premenstrual symptoms screening tool revised for adolescents (PSST-A): Prevalence of severe

PMS and premenstrual dysphoric disorder in adolescents. *Archives of Women's Mental Health, 14*(1), 77–81.

Steiner, M. (2000). Premenstrual syndrome and premenstrual dysphoric disorder: Guidelines for management. *Journal of Psychiatry & Neuroscience, 25*(5), 459–468.

Stokic, E., Srdic, B., & Barak, O. (2005). Body mass and the occurrence of amenorrhea in ballet dancers. *Gynecological Endocrinology, 20*(4), 195–199.

Szeverenyi, P., & Torok, Z. (2008). The relationship between hysterectomy and sexual life according to the latest research. *Orv Hetil, 149*(13), 589–595.

Tschudin, S., Bertea, P. C., & Zemp, E. (2010). Prevalence and predictors of premenstrual syndrome and premenstrual dysphoric disorder in a population-based sample. *Archives of Women's Mental Health, 13*(6), 485–494.

Vigood, S. N., Ross, L. E., & Steiner, M. (2009). Understanding and treating premenstrual dysphoric disorder: An update for the women's health practitioner. *Obstetrics & Gynecology Clinics of North America, 36*(4), 907–924.

Warren, M. P. (1985). Effect of exercise and physical training on-menarche. *Seminars in Reproductive Endocrinology, 3,* 17–25.

Warren, M. P., Voussoughian, F., Greer, E. B., et al. (1999). Functional hypothalamic amenorrhea: Hypoleptinemia and disordered eating. *Journal of Clinical Endocrinology and Metabolism, 84*(3), 873–877.

Woolcock, J. G., Critchley, H. O., Munro, M. G., Broder, M. S., & Fraser, I. S. (2008). Review of the confusion in current and historical terminology and definitions for disturbances of menstrual bleeding. *Fertility and Sterility, 90*(6), 2269–2280.

Zegeye, D. T., Megabiaw, B., & Mulu, A. (2009). Age of menarche and the menstrual pattern of secondary school adolescents in northwest Ethiopia. *BMC Women's Health, Oct 5*(9), 29.

Zukov, I., Ptácek, R., Raboch, J., Domluvilová, D., Kuzelová, H., Fischer, S., & Kozelek, P. (2010). Premenstrual dysphoric disorder—Review of actual findings about mental disorders related to menstrual cycle and possibilities of their therapy. *Prague Medical Report, 111*(1), 12–24.

chapter 6

REPRODUCTIVE TRACT INFECTIONS

CHAPTER COMPETENCIES

Upon completion of this chapter, the reader will be able to:

- Identify the role of normal flora
- Identify the causes and symptoms of urinary tract infections
- Identify the causes and symptoms of vaginosis

- Identify the common STIs
- Discuss the risks of specific STIs
- Explain how to prevent transmission of STIs

KEY TERMS

acquired immuno-
deficiency syndrome
(AIDS)
bacterial vaginosis (BV)
Candida albicans
candidiasis
CD4 receptor
Chlamydia trachomatis

expedited partner
therapy (EPT)
genital warts
herpes virus
human immuno-
deficiency virus (HIV)
human papillomavirus
(HPV)

Lactobacillus
microbiocides
Neisseria gonorrhoeae
normal flora
pathogen
pelvic inflammatory
disease (PID)
probotics

Staphylococcus aureus
T-helper lymphocytes
toxic shock syndrome
(TSS)
Treponema pallidum
Trichomonas vaginalis
vaginitis

The body is populated by a vast collection of normally benign microbes—the **normal flora**—that live on the skin, in the digestive tract, in the respiratory tract, and in the reproductive tract (Figure 6-1). These "good microbes" work to counter the **pathogens**, microbes which cause disease in the majority of people infected by them. In the reproductive system, those pathogens are often sexually-transmitted infections (STIs).

COMPETITION BETWEEN NORMAL FLORA AND PATHOGENS

Normal flora protect the body by secreting chemicals that limit the growth of the pathogens and by competing for nutrients and space. The role of normal flora in protecting the reproductive tract demonstrates both how beneficial these organisms are and the delicate balancing act which keeps the reproductive tract healthy.

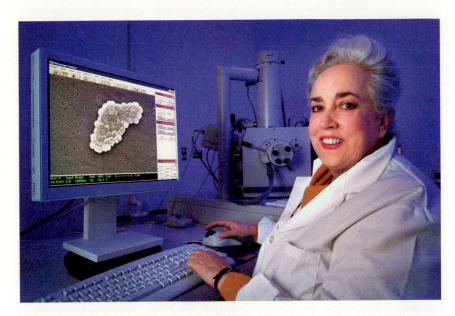

FIGURE 6-1: Janice Carr, a CDC microbiologist and electron microsopist, is scanning a specimen of *Acinetobacter baumannii* bacteria. This bacteria is widely distributed in nature and is among normal flora found on human skin. *(Courtesy of CDC/Photo by James Gathany and Jana Swenson)*

For example, the warm, moist conditions in a woman's vagina make it an ideal location for many microorganisms. The secretions and shed cells provide a nutrient-rich environment for both normal flora and pathogens. The vaginal opening provides access for a variety of microbes. Vaginal normal flora, especially bacteria from the genus **Lactobacillus**, feed on carbohydrates secreted by the vaginal cells and produce lactic acid and hydrogen peroxide (H_2O_2) (Elkins et al., 2008). These lactic acid–producing *Lactobacillus* are responsible for the acidic pH that provides some protection against colonization by pathogens or overgrowth of other normal flora such as the fungus **Candida albicans**, another resident of the reproductive tract. The peroxide also inhibits the growth of a variety of pathogenic species (Kaewsrichan et al., 2006; Mijač et al., 2006). Research has shown that women with stable microbial populations in the vagina are less likely to develop gynecological infections (Biaga et al., 2009). These infections fall under two main categories—those primarily caused by overgrowth or irritation by normal flora and those primarily caused by pathogens that are usually sexually transmitted.

Anything that disrupts the balance of normal vaginal flora can result in a vaginal inflammation, or **vaginitis**. Disruptions include hormonal changes which alter carbohydrate secretions, changes in vaginal pH, antibiotics which may inhibit *Lactobacillus*, or even physical irritation to the mucus membranes of the reproductive tract. Typical signs of a gynecological infection, whether due to a simple disruption of the normal flora or more severe STIs, are irritation of the vulva, discolored and excessive vaginal discharge, and discomfort in the pelvic cavity.

PELVIC INFLAMMATORY DISEASE

An infection of the upper reproductive tract is generally referred to as **pelvic inflammatory disease** (**PID**). The CDC (2008) estimates that more than a million women a year develop PID. The term PID can be used to describe any infection of the pelvic cavity ranging from infection of the fallopian tubes (salpingitis) to full involvement of the peritoneal cavity (peritonitis). As described previously, the ends of the fallopian tube are open, not sealed around the ovary. This opening acts as a conduit that may allow microbes to move from the vagina, through the uterus and fallopian tubes and into the pelvic cavity. Factors that increase the risk for developing PID include having multiple sexual partners, an untreated STI, and douching (CDC, 2008). However, a woman can develop PID without ever having been sexually active. Potentially, though rarely, any of the vaginal normal flora can migrate through the uterus and into the pelvic cavity, causing infection. Despite public perceptions of intrauterine devices (IUDs) as a primary cause of PID, the use of an IUD increases the risk of PID by only 0.15 percent (Shelton, 2001). The majority of PID cases appear to be caused by untreated sexually transmitted infections, especially gonorrhea and chlamydia (CDC, 2008).

One symptom of an acute pelvic infection is lower abdominal tenderness or pain, usually localized in an area above the pubic bone. Other symptoms may mimic those of a urinary tract infection (UTI). The infection may begin with intermittent pain which progresses to a constant discomfort. It is accompanied by fever, sometimes by nausea and vomiting, and malaise. Left untreated, PID can lead to chronic pelvic pain, infertility, tubal ulcerations, and an increased risk of ectopic pregnancy due to scarring of the fallopian tube (Crossman, 2006). Once formed, scar tissue remains even after the infection is treated. Scar tissue may partially block the tube, narrowing it enough that the tiny sperm can move through, but the much larger fertilized egg becomes trapped and can implant in the tube, resulting in an ectopic pregnancy. A single incidence of PID produces complications in up to 25 percent of women (Huether & McCance, 2008).

FACTORS INFLUENCING GYNECOLOGICAL INFECTIONS

Each woman's susceptibility to gynecological infection depends on a number of factors. Genetics may play a role, causing some women to produce altered cell surface markers which increase susceptibility to specific microbes (Bouckaert et al., 2006). Behaviors may increase exposure to pathogens or alter the population of normal flora. Even within a population of microbes, some are more virulent than others. Coinfections with STIs are common; having one STI can predispose an individual to infection with another (Fleming & Wasserheit, 1999). Damage to the normal barriers of the reproductive system's mucus membrane allows other organisms access. With a basic understanding of the organisms that cause them, most STIs can be treated and their transmission controlled.

Historically, treatments of gynecological infections involved administering heavy metals such as mercury and arsenic and were usually unsuccessful. In addition, societal attitudes toward STIs prevented many individuals, especially women, from seeking treatment (Hayes, 1869). The development of penicillin offered the first successful treatment option for bacterial infections, but did not treat viral or fungal infections. After an antibiotic has killed a bacterial pathogen, the damage it caused remains. STI infec-

tions are a common cause of infertility with scar tissue blocking the fallopian tubes or the vas deferens. Viral STIs bring their own set of problems. Antiviral medications usually do not cure viral STIs, but can limit the symptoms and lower transmission rates.

The over-prescription and misuse of antibiotics has led to the development of antibiotic-resistant strains of many bacteria. As this resistance is transferred from one bacterium to another, current treatments no longer work. A similar pattern is seen with treatment of viral infections. Viruses can evolve resistance to the current antiviral medication. The rapidly changing microbial landscape and the development of new medications lead to frequent development of new treatment regimes. The World Health Organization (WHO) and the Centers for Disease Control (CDC) publish up-to-date information on treatments for most gynecological infections.

PREVENTING TRANSMISSION OF GYNECOLOGICAL INFECTIONS

It is important to recognize that gynecological infections can affect anyone. They are contagious illnesses, communicated by people, and differ from other communicable diseases only by the parts of the body that they affect. These infections are not spread via air or water; instead are transmitted through very intimate skin to skin contact or by the exchange of body fluids. Anyone who is sexually active—whether by choice or as a result of rape or abuse—is at risk of becoming infected with an STI.

While many of the gynecological infections are caused by sexually-transmitted organisms, virulent strains of normal flora can be passed between partners during intercourse, producing infections as well. This transmission back and forth between partners can complicate treatment. Preventing an infection is usually preferable to coping with the consequences of the infection (Figure 6-2). The anxiety and lack of knowledge that sometimes surround gynecological infections can hamper effective treatment and support the spread of these infections.

While microbes may initially gain access through the reproductive tract, infections of the reproductive tract have the potential to invade the pelvic cavity, urinary tract, and other body systems. The mucus membranes of the digestive and respiratory tracts are similar to those of the reproductive tract and can also

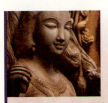

Social Considerations
CAN HEALTH PRACTITIONERS LESSEN THE STIGMA OF STIS?

A woman's experience of being diagnosed with an STI can be heavily influenced by cultural, religious, and social factors (Nack, 2000; Nack, 2002; Rusch et al., 2008). In North America, there is a bias to view multiple sexual experiences as a more acceptable behavior for men than for women. This "double standard" plays an important role in the way a woman makes sense of an STI diagnosis (Nack, 2002). Canadian researchers discovered that a woman's race, ethnicity, and age impact how she responds to being diagnosed with an STI (Rusch et al., 2008). Nack's research reveals that many women experience a sort of crisis when they are faced with a diagnosis which they've previously associated only with promiscuous "bad" women and must decide "whether to revise their actual social identities into that of fallen women"

(Nack, 2002). The way in which the health practitioner informs a woman of the diagnosis and interacts with her makes a difference. Healthcare workers who are nonjudgmental and who provided good medical advice tend to lessen the crisis for women while practitioners who express revulsion or whose use of language reinforce stereotypes of the "bad woman" tend to further negative perceptions.

One of the potential management strategies adopted by some women was to transfer the blame to their partners, viewing them as contagious and dangerous. This was more prevalent when the woman felt betrayed by her partner (Nack, 2000). The strategy of blaming someone else was clearly a coping mechanism, and all of the women in Nack's study eventually moved from denial or deflection to acceptance.

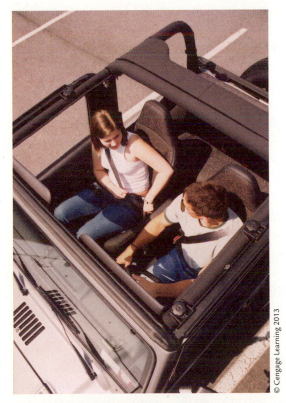

FIGURE 6-2: Just as safety belts are used to prevent physical injury in a motor vehicle accident, preventing an STI is preferable to dealing with its consequences.

© Cengage Learning 2013

serve as entry points for STIs. A 2004 report on syphilis in Chicago, IL, found that between the years 2000 and 2002, 13.7 percent of syphilis cases involved individuals engaging only in oral sex (CDC, 2004). In these individuals, the bacteria colonized the oral and respiratory mucosa. Other STIs transmittable via oral sex include *Chlamydia*, human immunodeficiency virus (AIDS), human papilloma virus (HPV), hepatitis, herpes, and gonorrhea (CDC, 2009).

The chances of acquiring a sexually transmitted gynecological infection can be substantially reduced by practicing safer sexual behaviors. Abstinence and limiting the number of sexual partners reduces the risk. People who have active sex lives with several partners must take responsibility for their own health and for the health of their partners to prevent infection. It is difficult to regard a sexual partner as a potential threat, but any sexual contact poses a potential infection risk.

Barriers and Biocides

The use of a latex condom may be a barrier against transmission of disease but cannot be relied upon to provide infallible protection. In theory, a condom, either male (Figure 6-3) or female (Figure 6-4),

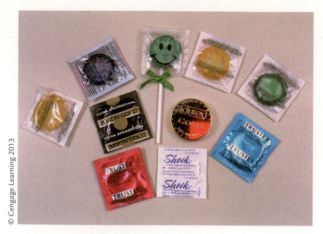

© Cengage Learning 2013

FIGURE 6-3: Male condoms can act as a barrier against disease transmission, but it is important to note that most novelty condoms are not designed to prevent transmission of STIs.

will prevent skin-to-skin and fluid-to-skin contact between partners. However, small tears and punctures in a condom can allow microbes through. Leakage and contact with body fluids will also allow for potential infections. In addition, many novelty condoms are not designed to prevent transmission of STIs. Other contraceptive methods (Chapter 13) are not effective in preventing the transmission of STI's. Barrier contraceptives like a diaphragm or cervical cap, hormonal contraceptives, and IUDs provide no protection because there is still contact with body fluids which may contain pathogens and may infect either partner.

Microbiocides, topical treatments applied to the vagina to prevent infections with STIs, represent a new and still experimental method of preventing transmission. Research shows that one microbiocide, terameprocol, when used as a vaginal ointment prevents transmission of several sexually transmitted viruses (Khanna et al., 2008). For women whose partners refuse to use condoms, microbiocides can provide a method of protection that does not require a partner's active participation or knowledge.

Teens at High Risk for STI

Teenagers are at an especially high risk for contracting STIs. The 2007 Youth Risk Behavior Survey found that 48 percent of the high school students surveyed had had sex at least once, yet 39 percent of those students had failed to use a condom. Of those students, 7.1 percent had their first intercourse before age 13 (Eaton et al., 2008). Many teens are unwilling or unable to access reproductive health services. Compounding the problem is the collection of misin-

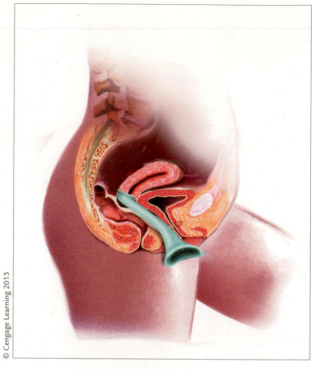

© Cengage Learning 2013

FIGURE 6-4: Proper insertion of a female condom.

formation teens often gather concerning sexual behavior and safer sex practices. This set of circumstances creates a situation in which STIs can spread easily.

Expedited Partner Therapy (EPT)

If someone is diagnosed with an STI, **expedited partner therapy (EPT)** is often used to provide prompt treatment to all of the individuals involved. With EPT, individuals diagnosed with an STI are given medications for treatment along with doses for their potentially infected partner or partners. Current guidelines recommend EPT for gonorrhea and chlamydia infections (CDC, 2006). While it is recommended that all individuals who might be infected see a health professional for evaluation, EPT does provide treatment for those either unwilling or unable to seek treatment for themselves. Not all states allow EPT. A chart of the current status of EPT in the United States is shown in Figure 6-5.

INFECTIONS CAUSED BY NORMAL FLORA

Not all infections associated with the reproductive system are sexually transmitted. Despite their normally beneficial roles, either an imbalance in the normal flora or misplacement of the normal flora can produce uncomfortable, painful, and potentially

Critical Thinking

Abstinence-Only Sex Education

A recently released report from the CDC finds that one in four teenage girls in the United States is infected with an STI (CDC, 2008), despite the promotion of abstinence-only sex education programs across the country between the years 2000 and 2008. Clearly something failed with regard to educating America's young girls about preventing transmission of STIs. A study by Kohler, Manhart, & Lafferty (2008) found that teens who received comprehensive sexual education had significantly fewer pregnancies than those who received abstinence–only sex education, although the study did not show any difference in rates of STI within this study group. However, another study found that teens who received a comprehensive program were more likely to use condoms and did experience fewer STIs (Shafii et al., 2007). The CDC recommendations support a comprehensive approach to sexual education that promotes consistent condom use as well as abstinence as effective methods to prevent STIs.

Why continue abstinence-only programs when the research does not demonstrate they work? Are there situations in which they could be effective? In addition to STI infections, what other issues could abstinence-only programs contribute to?

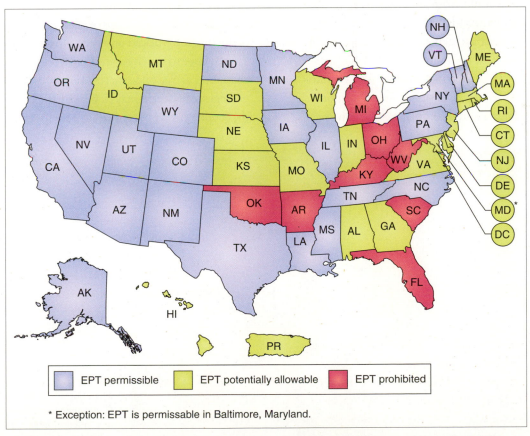

EPT permissible   EPT potentially allowable   EPT prohibited

* Exception: EPT is permissable in Baltimore, Maryland.

FIGURE 6-5: Legal Status of Expedited Partner Therapy (EPT). *(Courtesy of CDC/Division of STD Prevention; National Center for HIV/AIDS, Viral Hepatitis, STD, and TB Prevention. www.cdc.gov/std/ept/legal/default.htm.)*

dangerous infections. These infections can occur at any point in a woman's life, but are more common in sexually active women due to the introduction of a partner's normal flora and the potential of physical irritation. Common gynecological infections associated with normal flora include urinary tract infections, vaginitis, and pelvic inflammatory disease.

Vaginitis

Vaginitis is the generic term for inflammation and infection of the vagina. Symptoms include itching and inflammation of the vulva and the vaginal opening often associated with an abnormal vaginal discharge. Pain during sexual intercourse, pain and burning during urination, and local swelling (edema) may also occur to varying degrees. The normal vaginal discharge varies in consistency and amount depending on the stage of the reproductive cycle, but it is normally clear and odorless. Changes in vaginal discharge are often the first indicator of vaginitis.

There is no single cause for vaginitis. In some women, it may result from an allergic reaction to laundry detergent, bath and body products, or spermicides. If an allergen can be identified, it can be eliminated, and the vaginitis should disappear. However, in the majority of women with vaginitis, the cause is infection by a yeast (most commonly *Cancidia albicans*), or other organisms such as *Trichomonas, Gardnerella vaginalis, Mycoplasma hominis, Prevotella,* or *Mobiluncus* (CDC, 2006).

Yeast Infections – Vulvovaginal Candidiasis

Vulvovaginal candidiasis (VVC), fungus infection, and yeast infection are all names for vaginitis caused by members of the fungal genus *Candida*. These infections are primarily caused by the species *Candida albicans*. *Candida* is part of the body's normal flora, but an imbalance in the normal flora of the vagina may allow overgrowth of *Candida,* resulting in VVC. The symptoms of VVC include intense itching of the vulva, burning sensations, especially after urinating, and changes in vaginal discharge. The vaginal discharge may be light and watery, but it may also be quite heavy, white, and have a cheese curd–like consistency. Generally, the discharge is odorless. Both T-cell and cytokine levels rise during the infection and are responsible for many of the allergy-like symptoms (Fan et al., 2008). Examination of the vagina may reveal white plaques located on the vaginal walls. The definitive diagnosis is made by a wet smear technique. A cotton swab is used to remove some of the discharge, which is then mixed with a few drops of saline solution. One drop of this mixture is placed on a slide, which is viewed under a microscope to search for the fungal cells. *Candida* species appear as oval budding cells (Figure 6-6); other non-pathogenic yeast cells may be present as spores only. Over the counter test strips for yeast infections are also now

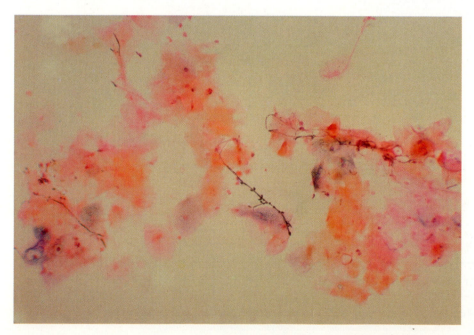

FIGURE 6-6: A photomicrograph of a vaginal smear identifying *Candida albicans* using gram-stain technique. *Candida albicans* lives in numerous parts of the body as normal flora. However, when an imbalance occurs, such as when hormonal balances change, *C. albicans* can multiply, resulting in a mucosal or skin infection called **candidiasis**. *(Courtesy of CDC/Dr. Stuart Brown)*

available. Systemic candidiasis—affecting the entire body—is rare and usually limited to severely immunocompromised individuals (Pappas, 2006).

Taking antibiotics can suppress the normal bacteria of the vagina that ordinarily keep *Candida* in check. *Lactobacillus* bacteria are especially sensitive to antibiotics, whereas fungi are not. In order to prevent a yeast infection, some physicians advise taking **probiotics** such as acidophilus capsules or eating yogurt with active cultures to restore the natural intestinal bacteria to the digestive tract. Both contain live *Lactobacillus* cultures and are said to be useful in avoiding or treating the symptoms produced by an antibiotic's destruction of the intestinal and vaginal normal flora. A 2007 review of the literature on the use of probiotics found mixed results with studies both supporting the effectiveness of *Lactobacillus* and others finding no benefits (Falagas, Betsi, & Athanasiou).

In addition to the influence of antibiotics, several other factors have been implicated in VVC. The changes in hormone levels during pregnancy increase the amount of simple sugars in vaginal secretions, providing additional food for the fungus, and predisposing a woman to the development of *Candida* infections. A woman's choice of contraceptive can increase her risk of infection. *Candida* biofilms, which are thin layers of microbes, have been found colonizing both contraceptive vaginal rings (Camacho et al., 2007) and IUDs (Chassot et al., 2008). The fungi can then transfer and adhere to the vaginal mucosa, a necessity for colonization and infection (Taguti Irie et al., 2006). Diabetes creates conditions in the body that favor certain species of *Candida*, and the CDC lists diabetes as a risk factor for *Candida* infections. Goswami et al., (2006) found a second species, *Candida glabrata,* caused the majority of cases of VVC in diabetic women rather than *C. albicans.* Other risk factors for VVC include HIV infection, corticosteroid therapy, and immunosuppressive medications.

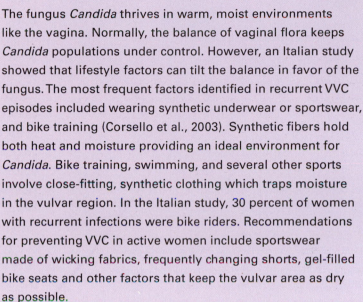

focus on

EXERCISE
Exercise and VVC

The fungus *Candida* thrives in warm, moist environments like the vagina. Normally, the balance of vaginal flora keeps *Candida* populations under control. However, an Italian study showed that lifestyle factors can tilt the balance in favor of the fungus. The most frequent factors identified in recurrent VVC episodes included wearing synthetic underwear or sportswear, and bike training (Corsello et al., 2003). Synthetic fibers hold both heat and moisture providing an ideal environment for *Candida*. Bike training, swimming, and several other sports involve close-fitting, synthetic clothing which traps moisture in the vulvar region. In the Italian study, 30 percent of women with recurrent infections were bike riders. Recommendations for preventing VVC in active women include sportswear made of wicking fabrics, frequently changing shorts, gel-filled bike seats and other factors that keep the vulvar area as dry as possible.

Trichomonas vaginalis

Trichomonas vaginalis is a parasitic protist, a single-celled animal that moves by means of four whip-like flagella (Figure 6-7). Trichomonas is considered to be the most common reproductive system infection globally (Johnston & Mabey, 2008). In the United States, the CDC estimates there are 7.4 million new trichomoniasis diagnoses annually (2007). The exact number of individuals carrying *Trichomonas* is unknown. Reporting of an infection to the CDC is not required, and the high number of asymptomatic individuals, both male and female, further clouds the issue. Diagnosis of a *Trichomonas* infection is most commonly done by examining fresh samples of vaginal discharge under the microscope. However, many physicians prefer to use culture methods or DNA analysis for more accurate diagnosis (Schwebke & Lawing, 2002). Reinfection with *Trichomonas* is common after treatment, and it is recommended that partners be treated as well to avoid passing the microbe back and forth.

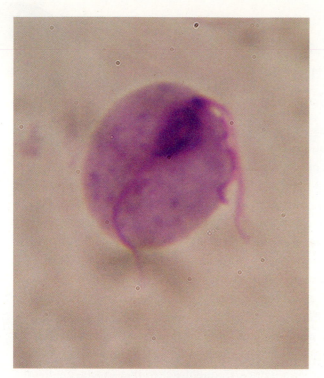

FIGURE 6-7: The flagellated protist *Trichomonas vaginalis*, a cause of vaginitis. *(Courtesy of Theresa Hornstein)*

Trichomonas vaginalis is normal flora for many people, but the more virulent strains are often sexually transmitted. The organisms can remain dormant in the vagina for years. Normal vaginal pH appears unfavorable for growth of this organism, and circumstances that reduce the vaginal acidity allow the organism to multiply. One factor that can reduce vaginal acidity is a reduction in the number of *Lactobacillus*. A study found vaginal *Lactobacillus* populations to be 15 percent lower in women with trichomoniasis than in uninfected women (Mijac et al., 2006). Other factors that may result in symptoms of trichomoniasis include pregnancy, trauma to the vaginal walls, increased vaginal secretions, and coinfection with another microbe. Pregnant women with active *Trichomonas* can, rarely, transmit the organism to their infants (Schwandt, Williams, & Beigi, 2008).

Almost three-quarters of the women harboring *Trichomonas* in their vaginas never have any symptoms. When present, those symptoms vary dramatically. The most severe symptoms include profuse, frothy, gray malodorous discharge with severe itching, redness and swelling of the vulva and vaginal opening, pain during intercourse and pain when urinating. In most women, the symptoms are less severe. Current research indicates that symptomatic infections are dependent on both vaginal pH and the surface markers of the parasite (Malla et al., 2008).

Bacterial Vaginosis

The most common cause of unusual vaginal discharge is **bacterial vaginosis (BV)**. While originally linked by Gardner and Dukes (1955) with overgrowth of the bacterium *Gardnerella*, further studies have indicated a more complicated picture that involves a disruption of the normal flora (Pirotta et al., 2009). BV is characterized by an increasing overgrowth of anaerobic bacteria and a corresponding decrease in levels of lactobacilli (Mastromarino et al., 2009). Women who lacked H_2O_2-producing *Lactobacillus* tend to have increased rates of BV (Mijac et al., 2006).

A watery, whitish discharge and a characteristic "stale-fish" odor are classic symptoms of BV. The bacteria do not ordinarily cause an inflammatory response in the vagina so itching and burning are usually absent. Diagnosis is based on examination of a stained smear of the vaginal secretions under a microscope and visual identification of the bacteria. A higher than normal vaginal pH is common with this infection but not diagnostic. The CDC does not recommend attempting to grow the suspected bacteria for diagnostic purposes (CDC, 2007).

Urinary Tract Infections

Urinary tract infections (UTIs) affect more than 12 million women in the United States each year (Griebling, 2007). The term urinary tract infection is an inclusive term used to describe a collection of conditions infecting the urinary system including cystitis (bladder infection) and urethritis (inflammation of the urethra). Nearly 50 percent of women will develop a UTI at some point during their lifetime (Griebling, 2005). The female urethra is shorter, only about 4 cm in length, when compared to the male urethra, which is 18–20 cm long. This anatomical difference makes it easier for motile bacteria to migrate through the urethra of a woman and colonize the bladder. The external opening of the urethra is exposed to vaginal discharges containing bacteria, as well as organisms like *Escherichia coli*, *Proteus*,

Citrobacter and other intestinal normal flora from the colon that may also colonize the bladder.

Sexual activity is associated with an increased risk of UTIs. The use of barrier contraceptives, such as a cervical cap, diaphragm, or condom, can produce irritation. Spermicides can alter the vaginal normal flora (Gupta, 1998; Valdevenito, 2008) and disruptions of the vaginal normal flora may provide fertile ground for pathogens that can then easily migrate to the urethra causing infection.

Why some women experience recurrent bladder infections while others do not is unknown, but there are several theories. Some women appear to be genetically susceptible to a specific type of the bacteria *E. coli* which attaches to glycoproteins in the bladder wall (Bouckaert et al., 2006). An experimental oral vaccine against *E. coli* was found to reduce the rate of recurrence (Valdevenito, 2008). Many of the *E. coli* which cause recurrent bladder infections are highly sensitive to H_2O_2 (hydrogen peroxide). The vaginal normal flora that produce trace amounts of H_2O_2 as part of their normal metabolic processes appear to be especially important in preventing UTIs. Several studies found reduced numbers of H_2O_2-producing normal flora in the vaginas of women with recurrent UTIs (Gupta et al., 1998; Kirjavainen et al., 2009; Reid & Bruce, 2006; Uehara, 2006; Anderson et al., 2006). Any factor which inhibits the growth of these protective, H_2O_2-producing bacteria potentially increases a woman's chance of developing a UTI. Injury or muscle weakness in the pelvis is often associated with stress incontinence and may allow contaminated urine to remain within the bladder. While urine is normally sterile, it is a nutrient-rich medium that will readily support the growth of bacteria that may colonize the bladder.

Symptoms of cystitis are burning pain on urination, and an urge to urinate frequently The urine appears cloudy and dark due to phagocytic WBCs, red blood cells, and bacteria, and trace amounts of blood may be visible. There may also be fever, backache, and lower abdominal pain. Urethritis and cystitis are lower UTIs; they produce pain but usually respond to treatment and rarely cause complications. If a bladder infection is not treated, it can spread through the ureters to the kidneys and cause a kidney infection, resulting in an upper UTI that is a potentially far more serious disease. Kidney infections present with a broad range of symptoms including chills followed by a fever higher than 101°F,

focus on NUTRITION
Berries and Health

Folk medicine has long held that berries are beneficial for health. New studies are supporting that belief with research. While cranberries have been the major focus due to their ethnographic use to treat recurrent UTIs (Jepson & Craig, 2008), further research demonstrates that other berries also have potent health benefits. Finnish studies of both blueberries and black currents show the tannin-rich berries have strong antimicrobial activity (Heinonen, 2007), indicating these fruits may be useful for both treating and preventing infection by a range of microbes. Berry phenol extracts demonstrate strong antimicrobial activity against *Helicobacter pylori*, *E. coli*, *Candida albicans*, and some strains of *Salmonella* (Nohynek et al., 2006). Cranberry juice contains hippuric acid which acidifies the urine and makes the bladder less hospitable to bacteria. While it has been theorized that a pH drop is responsible for cranberry juice's reputation for fighting bladder infections, new research indicates that proanthocyanidins, pigment molecules found in cranberries, are responsible for preventing *E. coli* from attaching to the bladder wall (Howell, 2005). The results of a review of 10 studies indicate that cranberry juice can significantly reduce the rate of recurrent UTIs over a 12-month period in women who suffer from recurrent UTIs (Jepson & Craig, 2008).

Berries appear to provide more than just protection from microbes. Research by Shukitt-Hale et al. (2008) indicates that the polyphenolic compounds found in berries have strong antioxidant and anti-inflammatory properties which may, also, protect the body from age-related neurological problems.

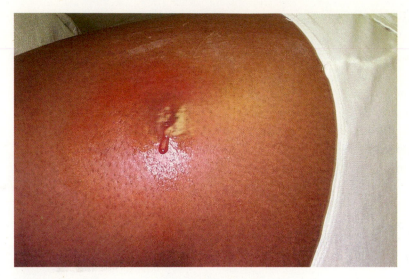

FIGURE 6-8: Methicillin-resistant *Staphylococcus aureus* bacteria (MRSA) caused this cutaneous abscess located on the hip, which had begun to spontaneously drain, releasing its purulent contents. *(Courtesy of CDC/Bruno Coignard, M.D.; Jeff Hageman, M.H.S.)*

pain and tenderness in the lower back, nausea and vomiting. In severe cases, permanent damage to the kidneys and septicemia, an infection of the blood, can occur (CDC, 2005). The damaged kidneys cannot maintain the proper fluid and electrolyte balance in the body, resulting in symptoms ranging from edema to muscle cramps and heart failure. Depending on the microbes involved, septicemia may result in fever, blood clots, vessel damage, or ruptured red blood cells.

Toxic Shock Syndrome

Toxic shock syndrome (TSS) made headlines in the United States during the 1980s as a novel disease that primarily targeted menstruating women who used tampons. Despite common beliefs, TSS is not a new disease, not necessarily a tampon-related disease, and not associated exclusively with menstruation. Originally identified in 1927 as staphylococcal scarlet fever in children, TSS is caused by ***Staphylococcus aureus***, a common bacterium found living as normal flora in many people. TSS presents with a sudden onset of high fever, sore throat, diarrhea, a sunburn-like skin rash, kidney failure, liver abnormalities, and a rapid drop in blood pressure leading to shock. A variation of the infection, menstrual toxic shock syndrome (mTSS), is linked with the use of high-absorbency tampons. In the United States, the printed insert in tampon packages now contains information about methods to minimize the risk of developing mTSS. Cases of mTSS are quite rare. In 2006, only100 cases were reported in the United States (MMWR, 2008). Although mTSS is uncommon, women should be aware that any sudden onset of fever, nausea, and vomiting during or just after a menstrual period merits immediate medical assistance, particularly if tampons are being used.

In recent years, a virulent strain of the bacterium, methicillin-resistant *Staphylococcus aureus* (MRSA), has claimed public attention, not specifically as the causative agent of mTSS but in association with severe infections in a general community (Figure 6-8). Both men and women have developed TSS from MRSA infections of burns, skin abrasions, surgical incisions, and insect bites. Women have contracted the disease after childbirth, either by vaginal delivery or cesarean section. The toxins produced appear to be the same whether the infection is associated with menstruation or not, and the clinical symptoms are the same (Descloux et al., 2008). Strains of MRSA have been found circulating throughout France (Durand et al., 2006), Australia (Nimmo et al., 2006) and Asia (Tekerekoglu et al., 2007). A study in Turkey expressed concerns about unidentified outbreaks, especially with regard to hospital-acquired infections (Tekerekoglu et al., 2007).

INFECTIONS THAT ARE PRIMARILY SEXUALLY TRANSMITTED

Humans have dealt with sexually transmitted infections for millennia. Ancient Greek and Roman literature both contain references to STIs, and thirteenth-century Crusaders returned to Europe with treatments for a condition identified as venereal leprosy (Rose, 1997). While diagnosis for many STIs was highly questionable historically, a condition assumed to be syphilis was reported as early as 1495 (Hayes, 1869). Historically, STIs have been blamed on a variety of causes ranging from sexual excess to punishments from a deity. Modern science has countered much of the early mythology concerning the causes of STIs, but new myths continue to appear concerning treatments and transmission.

Bacterial Infections

Most of the bacterial infections that cause STIs are mucus membrane parasites, feeding on the lining of the reproductive system and other mucus membranes throughout the body. STIs caused by bacteria will usually respond to antibiotic treatment. The three most common bacterial STIs are chlamydia, gonorrhea, and syphilis.

Chlamydia

Chlamydia trachomatis has earned the dubious title of the most prevalent STI in the United States. The CDC estimates 2.2 million people between the ages of 14 and 39 are currently infected in the United States (CDC, 2010). Reporting of *Chlamydia* infections increased 57 percent between 2001 and 2006 (Shepard, 2008), although the increase may be a result of more testing and better reporting rather than an actual increase in the number of infections. Teenagers have a higher infection rate than any other age group, with one out of four in some populations harboring *Chlamydia*. The typical high-risk patient is under 20 years of age, is sexually active with more than one partner, has had a history of STIs, and does not regularly use condoms. Primary infections of the reproductive tract are often asymptomatic. When symptoms are present, they include abnormal vaginal discharge and pain when urinating. Untreated *Chlamydia* infections can produce PID, vaginitis, and an increased risk of ectopic pregnancy.

An infant delivered vaginally by a woman with a *Chlamydia* infection has a 50–70 percent risk of acquiring the infection from its mother. More than 100,000 newborns are infected annually. About 15–25 percent of these exposed children develop an acute eye infection called inclusion conjunctivitis within the first two weeks of life, and 20 percent develop pneumonia within two to three months. Conjunctivitis and pneumonia are the two well-established consequences of neonatal infection, but there is some evidence that *Chlamydia* can contribute to middle ear infections, nasal passage obstruction, and inflammation of the bronchioles.

Because the majority of women who harbor *Chlamydia* are asymptomatic and frequently untreated, the disease is a potential risk to their health and to the health of any children they may have. Lab tests, such as gram staining which is used to confirm many kinds of infections, are only 40 percent accurate in identifying *Chlamydia*. In the past, the only certain method of verification was by special tissue culture techniques that were both expensive and time consuming. Newer nucleic acid amplification tests have proven more effective than cultures for diagnosing infections (Schachter et al., 2008). It is not required that cases of *Chlamydia* infection be reported to local health officials. The infection responds to antibiotic treatment, however, partners frequently reinfect each other. *Chlamydia* infections are candidates for EPT.

Gonorrhea

Gonorrhea is caused by the bacterium **Neisseria gonorrhoea** (Figure 6-9). It grows well only in the moist mucous membranes of the body. Away from the body, the bacteria are very susceptible to drying and lower temperatures, and will die within seconds.

By law, in the United States, all cases of gonorrhea must be reported to local health officials making gonorrhea the second most frequently reported communicable disease in the United States today, following chlamydia. In 2006, more than 350,000 cases were reported, but the CDC estimates that only about half of all cases are actually reported (CDC, 2008). One probable reason for the low number of reported cases is that more than half of women who are infected with gonorrhea do not show symptoms. In women who present with symptoms, vaginal discharge and painful and frequent urination may occur. The discharge is distinctively green or yellow in color with an unpleasant odor, but only a small amount of discharge is produced and so may go unnoticed. If the Skene's glands are invaded, pushing up on the urethra will result in a pus-filled discharge from their ducts. Bartholin's glands may also become infected and the

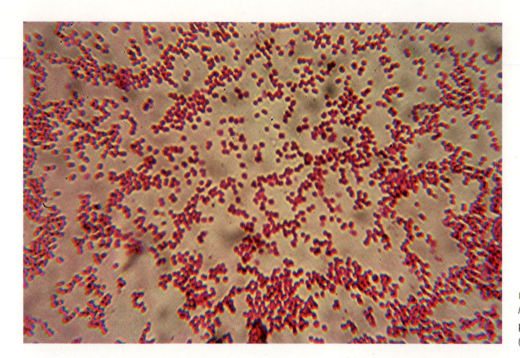

FIGURE 6-9: The bacteria *Neisseria gonorrhoea* which produces gonorrhea. *(Courtesy of Theresa Hornstein)*

ducts of this gland may be obstructed. In a small percentage of women, the gland may become abscessed and produce tenderness that makes walking or sitting extremely painful.

Sometimes, a local gonorrhea infection is self-limiting. The bacterium is destroyed by the immune system, or a woman can become an asymptomatic carrier. However, some women can develop additional symptoms later as the organism spreads to the upper reproductive tract and causes further complications. Undiagnosed and untreated, or inadequately treated, gonorrhea is one of the leading causes of PID. In about one percent of untreated gonorrhea cases, the bacteria enter the bloodstream, a condition called a disseminated infection. Occurring predominantly in women, a disseminated infection produces a characteristic skin rash, chills, fever, and arthritic joint pains in the wrist, ankles, knees, and feet. If a disseminated infection is untreated, or if treatment is delayed, joints can become permanently damaged. Occasionally, the gonorrhea bacteria can also invade the heart (endocarditis), the brain (meningitis), and the liver (toxic hepatitis), causing severe damage. If a pregnant woman has gonorrhea when she delivers her baby, the infection is transmitted to the infant's eyes as it travels through the cervix and vagina. This eye infection can cause blindness. It is prevented by treating the baby's eyes immediately after delivery with an antibiotic ointment.

In men, the symptoms of a gonorrhea infection are much more obvious. They include a thick, pus-laden discharge from the urethra (Figure 6-10) and

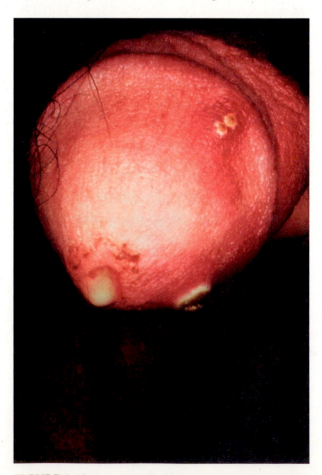

FIGURE 6-10: Gonorrhea discharge in males. *(Courtesy of CDC)*

Oral Gonorrhea

Lizzie goes to the clinic on campus for a sore throat, a fever, and aching joints. She thinks she's coming down with strep throat. The clinic takes a throat swab for testing. Testing shows the organism is not the bacteria which cause strep. When called to come back for further testing, Lizzie says that her boyfriend had been in earlier that month for treatment of what he thought was a bladder infection.

Lizzie says that she and Troy had oral sex without using a condom. Lizzie has developed a gonorrhea infection of the throat which has spread to the bloodstream producing fever and joint pain.

1. Why can the bacteria grow in the throat?

2. How could they have prevented transmission from Troy to Lizzie?

extremely painful urination. The urine is cloudy with pus and sometimes bloody. Many infected men will also have enlarged and tender lymph nodes in the groin and inflammation of the testicles.

Anal intercourse may result in inoculation of the bacteria into the anus and rectum, and oral-genital contact can result in gonorrheal pharyngitis or tonsillitis. Although nonvenereal transmission of gonorrhea infections has been known to occur in infants through contact with the bacteria on a mother's hands, it would be extremely difficult to catch the disease from non-sexual contact.

The presence of a gonorrhea infection can be diagnosed by a microscopic examination of a stained sample of secretions from the patient. This method is more accurate for men but not very sensitive for women—only one in two women with gonorrhea have a positive test. Other testing methods involve growing the bacteria and testing for bacterial DNA. The DNA test is combined with culture methods to produce the most accurate test results (Whiley et al., 2008). Currently, resistance of some strains of gonorrhea to antibiotics has become a major problem throughout the world as strains resistant to most common antibiotics spread (Lewis, 2007). Several kinds of gonorrhea vaccines are being tested in the laboratory and clinically, but currently there are none in commercial production.

Syphilis

Syphilis is caused by the thread-like, spiral bacterium **Treponema pallidum**. This type of spiral bacterium is called a spirochete. Its length is about the diam-

eter of the largest white blood cell, but it is so thin it is almost undetectable using a typical microscope (Figure 6-11). The syphilis bacterium is an extremely delicate organism, very sensitive to drying and temperature changes, so it does not survive long outside the body, making transmission via inanimate objects virtually impossible. An open lesion on an infected individual is highly infectious, and there have been instances in which doctors, dentists, or nurses in their professional work have contracted the disease through a break in the skin. The usual transfer of the spirochete, however, results from vaginal, anal, or oral-genital sexual intercourse.

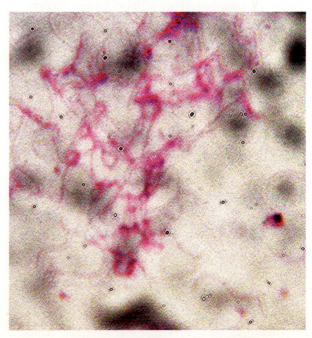

FIGURE 6-11: The bacteria *Treponema pallidum* which causes syphilis. (*Courtesy of Theresa Hornstein*)

By 1950, most states had passed laws requiring syphilis cases to be reported to health officials, and the disease was thought to have been brought under control through education and the tracing of sexual contacts of reported cases. Once nearly defeated in the United States, syphilis has made a dangerous comeback nationwide, with over 46,000 cases reported in 2008 (CDC). Between 2007 and 2008, cases of syphilis rose 13 percent. Untreated, syphilis can affect the central nervous system to produce blindness, deafness, insanity, and ultimately, death.

Treponema can invade any moist mucosal surface, although they can also enter through a minute break in intact skin, and travel to the bloodstream. After an incubation period averaging about three weeks, a primary lesion called a chancre appears at the site of contact. The chancre is a hard, painless ulcer (Figure 6-12). Treated or not, the primary lesion will spontaneously heal, leaving no evidence that it had been there, but the blood is still infectious. If the chancre is on the vagina or cervix and a woman has had no other reason to see a gynecologist, the disease will most likely remain undetected and untreated.

Secondary syphilis appears two to six months after the initial exposure, sometimes occurring at the same time the primary chancre is subsiding. During the secondary stage, syphilis may mimic allergic reactions, flu, and strep throat. In addition, there may be a pale skin rash on the body, most noticeable on the palms and the soles of the feet. Less common manifestations are hair loss

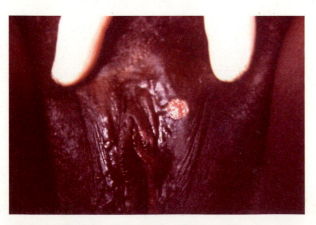

FIGURE 6-12: Primary syphilis lesion. *(Courtesy of CDC)*

and the presence of grayish-white lesions in the mucous membrane of the mouth and throat. If there are lesions on the mouth, any oral contact may be contagious. Untreated, the symptoms of the secondary stage will subside, although they may recur. The disease may then progresses to the latent stage.

In 15 percent of untreated latent syphilitics, the disease progresses to the tertiary or late syphilis stage (CDC, 2009). The complications of late syphilis can affect any part of the body. They may be benign, producing only a skin lesion, called a gumma, with no further disability, or they may include a systemic reaction that involves the brain and spinal cord (neurosyphilis), the heart and lungs, or other systems of the body. Neurosyphilis often mimics Alzheimer's disease (van Eijsden et al., 2008). For 10 percent of individuals affected with tertiary syphilis, the disease is fatal. There is no way of knowing which cases of latent syphilis will progress to tertiary syphilis or how severe and extensive the complications will be.

In an untreated pregnant woman, the spirochetes in maternal blood can pass to the unborn child. Syphilis during pregnancy contributes to spontaneous abortion (miscarriage) and stillbirths. If the pregnancy continues to completion, most full-term deliveries result in a baby with congenital syphilis, having marked and severe deformities. Unfortunately, the incidence of congenital syphilis is far greater than in the relatively recent past. In 2007, the rate was 10.5 cases per 1,000,000 live births, an increase of 15 percent from 2006 (CDC, 2009). Blood tests for syphilis are a routine part of most prenatal examinations, and if the infection is discovered early enough, treatment produces protection for the infant. Even if the fetus is already infected, control of the disease is possible, and further damage can be prevented.

Syphilis can be diagnosed by examining the fluid from a lesion for spirochetes under a darkfield microscope. The lab tests are based on the presence of antibodies produced to *Treponema*. Two tests, the immunochromatographic strip test and the rapid test device, produce correct results in 94 percent of cases (Nessa et al., 2008). In the early stages, syphilis responds well to antibiotics although some resistant strains of the bacteria have recently appeared (Stoner, 2007). Currently there is no vaccine for syphilis.

Historical Considerations

WHOSE POX IS IT?

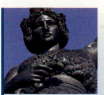

The origins of syphilis have been debated for centuries. Early theories held the disease was brought back to Europe by members of Columbus' crew in 1492 from Haiti. The French blamed Spanish sailors for spreading the "Spanish pox". In England, the spread of syphilis was blamed on the French and the disease was called the "French pox".

New analysis of both New and Old World remains indicate the disease was widespread long before the voyage of Columbus. Skeletons from the Hull Magistrates Court friary in England, dating from before 1450, show syphilitic changes in the sinuses and leg bones (Von Hunnius et al., 2006). Analysis of pre-Columbian skeletons from Pompeii and Naples also show syphilis-related changes to the bone, indicating the disease was in Europe long before Columbus (Roberts, 2002). Skeletons from what is now New Mexico, Florida, and Ecuador indicate the disease was present there as long as 6,000 years ago (Rose, 1997).

Viral Infections

Viruses are minute infectious agents that are composed of nucleic acid, either DNA or RNA but not both, and a protein. Viruses reproduce only inside living cells. These organisms invade the host cells and take over, hijacking the cell's normal functions. Once a virus has invaded, the viral genes use the host cell to make more copies of the virus. The new viruses then escape from the host cells to infect others. Unlike bacterial infections, viral infections cannot be treated with antibiotics. Viral STIs include herpes, HPV, hepatitis B and C, and HIV.

Herpes

Members of the **herpes virus** family have an affinity for attacking the skin surfaces and mucous membranes of the body producing oozing blisters. These disappear during periods of remission when the virus hides in nerves. Recurrent outbreaks can be triggered by any number of factors—a cold, a fever, a gastrointestinal upset, a severe case of sunburn, menstruation, or emotional stress. Herpes simplex virus 1 (HSV-1) is best known for causing the common cold sore and is rarely sexually transmitted. HSV-2 is most commonly associated with genital herpes and transmission is almost exclusively through sexual contact. Women are more likely to be infected than men; the CDC (2008) estimates that one in four women are infected with HSV-2. However, the exact number of cases is uncertain because many people are asymptomatic. The virus is transmitted through mucus membrane contact. Individuals can still shed the virus and infect their partners without showing blisters. The virus can be passed during intercourse or by oral sex. Transmission to other mucus membranes, including those surrounding the eyes, is also possible.

The first episode or primary attack of genital herpes is usually the most extensive and most painful. The incubation period after initial contact for the first outbreak may be up to two weeks. Initial symptoms are pain and itching, fever, muscle aches, and swollen glands. Blisters will appear after a few days at the infection site, and, then, rupture, releasing highly infectious fluid (Figure 6-13). After a week to 10 days, the blisters heal spontaneously, leaving no scars unless they have become secondarily infected.

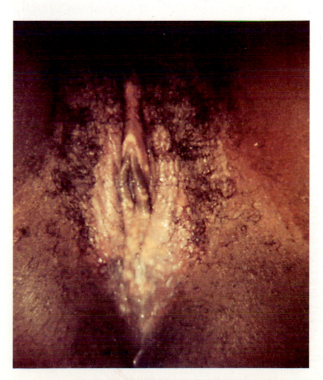

FIGURE 6-13: Herpes blisters. *(Courtesy of CDC/Susan Lindsley)*

After the blisters have healed, the initial active phase of the infection is over, but the virus is still present in the body and enters a latent phase in the nervous system. With oral herpes, the virus lies dormant in a large group of sensory nerves located near the cheekbone. With a genital infection, the virus invades nerves that lie next to the lower spinal cord. If the latent virus is reactivated, it takes the same nerve pathway back to skin supplied by the sensory nerve endings. Recurrent infections are usually of shorter duration and have much milder symptoms.

An active genital herpes infection during pregnancy can increase likelihood of miscarriage, and an outbreak late in a pregnancy increases the risk of premature delivery. Newborns can become infected during delivery. In 1999, the American College of Obstetricians and Gynecologists (ACOG) determined that women with active herpes infection should have cesarean deliveries, although those without an active outbreak can deliver vaginally with a low risk of infecting the baby. They also concluded that antiviral therapy to prevent an active outbreak was warranted for women past 36 weeks gestation who have a history of recurrent herpes infections. There are several drugs which can control the frequency of herpes outbreaks and shorten the duration of outbreaks, but none of the current antiviral medications can cure the condition nor clear the virus from the body. Even with treatment, infected individuals can continue to shed the virus, acting as a reservoir and infecting other individuals.

Viral Hepatitis

Hepatitis (liver inflammation) can have a number of causes, but the most common cause is infection by one of many different groups of hepatitis viruses. Hepatitis infections do not directly affect the reproductive system. Instead, they cause problems because they interfere with liver function. Classic symptoms include jaundice, swollen and painful abdomen, and metabolic problems. Blood clotting factors are made in the liver, and a hepatitis infection can interfere with their production leading to bruising, excessive bleeding, and spontaneous nose bleeds. Bile production decreases as the liver cells are damaged, and digestion of lipids decreases. In severe cases, hepatitis can lead to liver failure and death.

Hepatitis A, B, and C are the most common types in the United States. Hepatitis A is usually a self-limiting, short-term infection transmitted though contaminated food or water. It is not sexually transmitted nor does it appear to cross the placenta. Hepatitis B and C are transmitted through contaminated body fluids including semen, vaginal secretions, and blood. Both frequently produce chronic carriers, people who shed the virus without showing symptoms of the illness. Chronic Hepatitis B or C infections can lead to long-term liver damage, and chronic infections are a leading cause of liver cancer. In 1991, a vaccine for Hepatitis B was developed. Many states now require all school children to be vaccinated against Hepatitis B. This requirement has led to a dramatic reduction in the number of new cases of Hepatitis B.

Hepatitis infections during pregnancy pose serious threats to both mother and child. In the United States, a pregnant woman with untreated Hepatitis B runs a 40 percent chance of passing the virus to her baby. Hepatitis B can also be transmitted in breast milk. Approximately a quarter of those cases result in fatal liver disease in the child (CDC, 2008). Hepatitis C can be transmitted from mother to child during pregnancy, although not through breast-feeding. Another strain contracted through contaminated water, Hepatitis E, is uncommon in the United States. The virus is more common in southern Asia, Africa, and Mexico. While most people who contract Hepatitis E recover, the infection is fatal in up to one third of pregnant women, particularly if they contract the infection during the third trimester (CDC, 2009).

Human Papilloma Virus (HPV)

Human papillomavirus (HPV) is a sexually transmitted member of a large group of viruses that produce warts. Because HPV infections are not required to be reported to federal health officials, no one knows the real prevalence of this disease. The CDC estimates 20 million people in the United States have genital HPV infections that can be transmitted to others, and every year, about 6.2 million people become infected (CDC, 2009).

In men, **genital warts** occur most commonly on the glans and urethral opening on the tip of the penis, on the shaft of the penis, and on the scrotum. In women, the most common site is the perineum, but they may also be scattered over the vulva, the vaginal opening, and the skin of the thighs. Genital warts can also occur within the vagina and on the cervix (Figure 6-14). If the virus invades the throat, the warts can grow in the respiratory system causing a rare recurrent respiratory papillomatosis or RRP (CDC, 2009). HPV has also been linked to several cancers including cervical cancer.

There are more than 100 different HPV types, but only six have been associated with cervical cancer (Vonka & Hamsíková, 2007). Types 6 and 11 are most frequently associated with the typical soft, cauliflower-like, fleshy genital warts that grow in or around the vagina, anus, or perineum. Cervical cancer is most often associated with HPV types 16 and 18. Other malignancies associated with HPV include cancers of the anus, vulva, vagina, and penis (Louchini, Goggin & Steben, 2008).

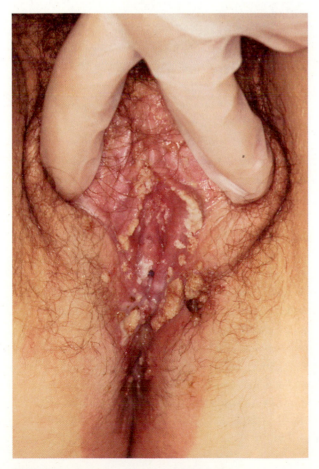

FIGURE 6-14: Genital warts. *(Courtesy of CDC/Joe Millar)*

There are currently two vaccines approved in the United States for preventing HPV infections. Gardasil is a quadrivalent vaccine which provides protections against HPV types 6, 11, 16, and 18. Cervarix is a bivalent vaccine which provides protection against HPV types 16 and 18. These vaccines are designed to prevent HPV and are most effective if the three dose series is given before an individual becomes sexually active. In December of 2009, the Advisory Committee on Immunization Practices (ACIP) issued new provisional recommendations for HPV vaccinations. Vaccination is recommended for females ages 9-26. Only the quadrivalent vaccine is recommended for males ages 9-26. These vaccines are not designed to treat HPV.

Human Immunodeficiency Virus (HIV)

On June 5, 1981, the Centers for Disease Control (CDC) published a brief report on an outbreak of a mysterious illness affecting five gay men in Los Angeles. The disease was *Pneumocystis carinii* pneumonia, a type of pneumonia previously seen only in cancer patients with profoundly suppressed immune systems. This short article marked the beginning of the **acquired immunodeficiency syndrome (AIDS)** epidemic. The cause of the disease has been identified as **human immunodeficiency virus (HIV)**. The Joint United Nations Programme on HIV/AIDS (UNAIDS) estimates that 60 million people have become infected with HIV since it was first identified. Of those, nearly 25 million have died (2009). The epidemic has spread to all corners of the globe. Sixty-seven percent of individuals living with HIV live in sub-Saharan Africa (UNAIDS, 2009). In Central Asia and Eastern Europe, HIV rates have increased by 50 percent since 2004 (UNAIDS Update, 2007). In the United States, women constituted the fastest-rising group at risk for contracting AIDS and make up 26 percent of HIV cases (CDC, 2007). At the beginning of the epidemic homosexual or bisexual men and people with a history of injecting drugs accounted for the largest number of AIDS cases. However in recent years, there has been a steady increase in heterosexuals affected, especially within racial and ethnic minority populations. In the United States, African Americans account for 49 percent of new infections (CDC, 2007).

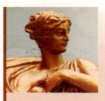

Cultural Considerations
MARRIAGE AND HIV

According to the latest global estimates provided by the World Health Organization and UNAIDS, women comprise 50 percent of people living with HIV. While the numbers are equitable, the situation for women is far from it, and the fight for gender equality is increasingly understood as one of the vital components of an effective fight against this pandemic. As the Global Coalition on Women and AIDS has noted: "In some parts of the world, women and girls are infected with HIV almost as soon as they start having sex. Almost everywhere, traditions tolerate and even encourage men to have multiple sexual partners. Women, on the other hand, are expected to abstain or be faithful. In many places, they are expected to know little about sex or sexuality, and remain dangerously uninformed" (GCWA, 2009).

The traditional 'ABC strategy' of HIV prevention (**A**bstinence from sexual activity, **B**eing faithful to a single partner, and correct and consistent **C**ondom use) has been criticized because it does not take into account the particular needs of women and girls, and as such has proven only partially successful in practice. In places where sexual violence is high, abstinence is often simply not an option for women and girls. However, it is not just young women coerced into sex outside of marriage who are at risk. Women are also often exposed to HIV regardless of whether they themselves are faithful because where men are unfaithful, female monogamy does not prevent a woman from becoming infected. A married woman engaging in monogamous heterosexual sex with her husband can still be at risk if her husband is being unfaithful to her (Osagbemi et al., 2007). Physical and sexual violence within a married relationship can add to this problem, making it harder for women to maintain sexual autonomy. In addition, women who fear or experience violence lack the power to ask their partners to use condoms or to refuse unprotected sex.

In Cambodia, which has the highest proportion of HIV-positive adults in Southeast Asia, married women now account for almost half of all new HIV infections in the country (Kaiser, 2005). In Zambia, only 11 percent of women believe that a woman has the right to ask her husband to use a condom—even if he has proven himself to be unfaithful and is HIV-positive (GCWA, 2009). In Zimbabwe, researchers revealed that the majority of HIV positive women were infected by their husbands (GCWA, 2009). Furthermore, married women who suspect their husbands are HIV positive do not always have many options to change their situations. According to one woman interviewed as part of the study, "We see our husbands with wives of men who have died of AIDS. What can we do? If we say no to sex, they'll say pack and go. If we do, where do we go to?" (GCWA, 2009). The study found that being married, or having been married, was itself a risk factor for women in contracting HIV (GCWA, 2009).

The high incidence of non-consensual sex, women's inability to negotiate safer sex, and in many cases fear of abandonment or eviction from homes and communities, present extreme challenges—particularly for the world's poorest women. To address these realities, HIV prevention strategies must be developed which take into account women's particular needs, and their unequal position in many societies. Today, HIV/AIDS programs are increasingly addressing harmful gender norms and stereotypes, including working with men and boys to change norms related to fatherhood, sexual responsibility, decision making and violence, and by providing comprehensive, age-appropriate HIV/AIDS education for young people that addresses gender norms.

AIDS is the most advanced stage in a continuum of effects of HIV infection. After initial infection, an individual begins producing antibodies to HIV. Generally, there are few initial signs of illness. Some infected people develop fever, malaise, and swollen glands similar to the symptoms of mononucleosis, but many remain asymptomatic for an average of 9–11 years. During the asymptomatic period, a person may be totally unaware of the infection but can spread the virus to others because their body fluids contain HIV and are infective. Less than 40 percent of people infected with HIV are aware that they have it (UNAIDS, 2009). With the passage of time, other symptoms may occur including swollen lymph nodes, unexplained weight loss, bumps or a rash on the skin, chronic fatigue, fever, night sweats, diarrhea, cough, and shortness of breath.

HIV targets those that have a cell surface receptor molecule called CD4. The virus binds to the **CD4 receptor**, merges with the host cell's membranes, and invades the cell. CD4 receptor protein is present on certain white blood cells, namely a lymphocyte population known as **T-helper lymphocytes**. T-helper cells help other lymphocytes combat foreign antigens. CD4 receptors are also found on macrophages, blood cells that attack and engulf cells infected by viruses and bacteria. By damaging these immune cells, the virus has the ability to severely depress the immune system. HIV may also infect some other types of cells, including supporting cells in the nervous system, cells lining the digestive tract, and certain bone marrow cells. Infection of these target cells may account for the mental deterioration, diarrhea, and various blood abnormalities that are associated with full-blown AIDS.

With the continued depletion of the T-helper lymphocytes and immune system failure, opportunistic infections—those caused by organisms that ordinarily would be unable to produce disease in healthy individuals—can take hold in the immunosuppressed with life-threatening effects. Key opportunistic infections associated with AIDS include *Pneumocystis carinii* pneumonia, herpes simplex, toxoplasmosis, cytomegalovirus, candidiasis, and tuberculosis. Tuberculosis infects roughly 33 percent of people living with HIV (UNAIDS, 2009). Because the immune system also defends the body against cancer,

AIDS patients may develop malignancies such as Kaposi's sarcoma and non-Hodgkin's lymphoma, and abnormal Pap smears indicating cervical disease in women. AIDS patients can also suffer from weight loss, persistent and relentless diarrhea, fever, and an AIDS-related dementia that impairs mental function.

HIV is transmitted through contact with contaminated body fluids including blood, semen, and vaginal secretions. Transmission is enhanced by concurrent infection with other sexually transmitted diseases, particularly those that cause open sores or ulcers. STIs also increase the number of white blood cells in the genital tract and provide additional opportunity for infection. Uncircumcised men are more likely to contract infection than circumcised men. Women who have sex with infected men are about 10–14 times more likely to catch HIV than are men who have sex with infected women because the virus is more concentrated in semen than in vaginal fluid (Hurtado Navarro et al., 2008). Cases of mother-to-infant transmission at the time of birth have steadily increased and, in some locations, have become a major cause of death among infants and young children. Ninety-one percent of the new infections in children are occurring in sub-Saharan Africa (UNAIDS, 2009) either from transmission during pregnancy or from breast milk contaminated with the virus.

There is no cure for HIV. Antiretroviral drug therapy does not totally eradicate the virus, which persists in the lymphocytes, and could become reactivated despite intensive treatment. HIV therapy in pregnant women has proven successful in limiting transmission to newborns (WHO, 2007). Attempts to develop an HIV vaccine have been unsuccessful, although a recent vaccine trial in Thailand did demonstrate some success (Bansal et al., 2010).

CONCLUSION

Despite its protective mechanisms, a woman's reproductive system is a prime site for the growth of microbes. Changes in the normal floral population in the vagina can lead to infections throughout the body. In addition, pathogenic STIs can enter the body causing discomfort, infertility, live-threatening illnesses, and, in pregnant women, potential damage to the fetus. While treatment options exist for some STIs, prevention is the better option.

REVIEW QUESTIONS

1. What is normal flora?

2. How do normal flora differ from pathogens?

3. What causes vaginitis?

4. How can STIs be prevented?

5. What are the consequences of untreated STI's?

CRITICAL THINKING QUESTIONS

1. How are viral infections different from bacterial infections?

2. What advantages are there to EPT?

3. If STIs pose such health risks why not just dose everyone with antibiotics?

4. Which is better—abstinence only sex education or comprehensive sex educations? Why?

REFERENCES

Anderson, N., Conly, J., Mainprize, T. C., Meuser, J., Nickel, J. C., Senikas, V. M., & Zhanel, G. G. (2006). Uncomplicated urinary tract infection in women. Current practice and the effect of antibiotic resistance on empiric treatment. *Canadian Family Physician, 52*, 612–618.

Bansal, G. P., Malaspina, A., & Flores, J. (2010). Future paths for HIV vaccine research: Exploiting results from recent clinical trials and current scientific advances. *Current Opinion in Molecular Therapeutics, 12*(1), 39–46.

Biagi, E., Vitali, B., Pugliese, C., Candela, M., Donders, G. G., & Brigidi, P. (2009). Quantitative variations in the vaginal bacterial population associated with asymptomatic infections: A real-time polymerase chain reaction study. *European Journal of Clinical Microbiology & Infectious Diseases, 28*(3), 281–285.

Bouckaert, J., Mackenzie, J., de Paz, J. L., Chipwaza, B., Choudhury, D., Zavialov, A., Mannerstedt, K., Anderson, J., Piérard, D., Wyns, L., Seeberger, P. H., Oscarson, S., De Greve, H., & Knight, S. D. (2006). The affinity of the FimH fimbrial adhesin is receptor-driven and quasi-independent of *Escherichia coli* pathotypes. *Molecular Microbiology, 61*(6), 1556–1568.

Camacho, D. P., Consolaro, M. E., Patussi, E. V., Donatti, L., Gasparetto, A., & Svidzinski, T. I. (2007). Vaginal yeast adherence to the combined contraceptive vaginal ring (CCVR). *Contraception, 76*(6), 439–443.

Centers for Disease Control. (2004, October 22). *Morbidity and mortality weekly report, 53*(41).

Centers for Disease Control. (2006, August 4). Sexually transmitted disease guidelines, 2006. *Morbidity and mortality weekly report, 55*(No. RR–11).Retrieved April 2008 from http://www.cdc.gov/ncidod/dbmd/diseaseinfo/urinarytractinfections.htm.

Centers for Disease Control. (2008, April 7). Pelvic inflammatory disease. Fact sheet. Retrieved April 10, 2008 from http://www.cdc.gov/STI/PID/STIFact-PID.htm.

Centers for Disease Control. (2009, June). Oral sex and HIV risk HIV/AIDS fact sheet. Retrieved July 1, 2009 from http://www.cdc.gov/hiv/resources/factsheets/pdf/oralsex.pdf.

Centers for Disease Control, Division of STD Prevention, National Center for HIV/AIDS, Viral Hepatitis, STD, and TB Prevention. (2009, November). Sexually transmitted diseases in the United States, 2008: National surveillance data for chlamydia, gonorrhea, and syphilis.

Centers for Disease Control. (2009, December). ACIP provisional recommendations for HPV vaccine. Retrieved January 2010 from http://www.cdc.gov/vaccines/recs/provisional/downloads/hpv-vac-dec2009-508.pdf.

Chassot, F., Negri, M. F., Svidzinski, A. E., Donatti, L., Peralta, R. M., Svidzinski, T. I., & Consolaro, M. E. (2008). Can intrauterine contraceptive devices be a *Candida albicans* reservoir? *Contraception, 77*(5), 355–359.

Corsello, S., Spinillo, A., Osnengo, G., Penna, C., Guaschino, S., Beltrame, A., Blasi, N., & Festa, A. (2003). An epidemiological survey of vulvo-vaginal candidiasis in Italy. *European Journal of Obstetrics, Gynecology and Reproductive Biology, 110*(1), 66–72.

Crossman, S. H. (2006). The challenge of pelvic inflammatory disease. *American Family Physician, 73*(5), 859–864.

Descloux, E., Perpoint, T., Ferry, T., Lina, G., Bes, M., Vandenesch, F., Mohammedi, I., & Etienne, J. (2008). One in five mortality in non-menstrual toxic shock syndrome versus no mortality in menstrual cases in a balanced French series of 55 cases. *European Journal of Clinical Microbiology & Infectious Diseases. 27*(1), 37–43.

Durand, G., Bes, M., Meugnier, H., Enright, M. C., Forey, F., Liassine, N., Wenger, A., Kikuchi, K., Lina, G., Vandenesch, F., & Etienne, J. (2006). Detection of new methicillin-resistant *Staphylococcus aureus* clones containing the toxic shock syndrome toxin 1 gene responsible for hospital- and community-acquired infections in France. *Journal of Clinical Microbiology, 44*(3), 847–853.

Eaton, D., Kann, L., Kinchen, S., Shanklin, S., Ross, J., Hawkins, J., Harris, W., Lowry, R., McManus, T., Chyen, D., Lim, C., Brener, N., Wechsler, H., (2008). Youth risk behavior surveillance: United States, 2007. *Morbidity and Mortality Weekly Report, 57*(SS04), 1–131.

Elkins, C., Muñoz, M., Mullis, L., Stingley, R., & Hart, M. (2008). *Lactobacillus*-mediated inhibition of clinical toxic shock syndrome *Staphylococcus aureus* strains and its relation to acid and peroxide production. *Anaerobe, 14*(5), 261–267.

Falagas, M. E., Betsi, G. I., & Athanasiou, S. (2007). Probiotics for the treatment of women with bacterial vaginosis. *Clinical Microbiology and Infection, 13*(7), 657–664.

Fan, S. R., Liu, X. P., & Li, J. W. (2008). Clinical characteristics of vulvovaginal candidiasis and antifungal susceptibilities of Candida species isolates among patients in southern China from 2003 to 2006. *Journal of Obstetrics & Gynaecology Research, 34*(4), 561–566.

Fleming, D. T., & Wasserheit, J. N. (1999). From epidemiological synergy to public health policy and practice: The contribution of other sexually transmitted diseases to sexual transmission of HIV infection. *Sexually Transmitted Infections, 75*(1), 3–17.

Gardner, H. L., & Dukes, C. D. (1955). *Hemophilus vaginalis* vaginitis. *American Journal of Obstetrics and Gynecology, 69*(5), 962–975.

Global Coalition on Women and AIDS. (2004, February 2). HIV protection and prevention efforts are failing women and girls. Press release.

Goswami, D., Goswami, R., Banerjee, U., Dadhwal, V., Miglani, S., Lattif, A. A., & Kochupillai, N. (2006). Pattern of *Candida* species isolated from patients with diabetes mellitus and vulvovaginal candidiasis and their response to single dose oral fluconazole therapy. *Journal of Infection, 52*(2), 111–117.

Griebling, T. L. (2005). Urological diseases in America project: Trends in resource use for urinary tract infections in women. *Journal of Urology, 173*(4), 1281–1287.

Griebling, T. L. (2007). Urinary tract infection in women. In Litwin, M. S., & Saigal, C. S. (Eds.), *Urologic diseases in America*. DHHS, PHS, NIH, NIDDK. Washington, DC: Government Printing Office (NIH Publication No. 07-5512:587–619).

Gupta, K., Stapleton, A. E., Hooton, T. M., Roberts, P. L., Fennell, C. L., & Stamm, W. E. (1998). Inverse association of H_2O_2-producing lactobacilli and vaginal *Escherichia coli* colonization in women with recurrent urinary tract infections. *Journal of Infectious Diseases, 178*(2), 446–450.

Hayes, A. H. (1869). *Sexual physiology of woman, and her diseases.* Boston, MA: Peabody Medical Institute.

Heinonen, M. (2007). Antioxidant activity and antimicrobial effect of berry phenolics—A Finnish perspective. *Molecular Nutrition & Food Research, 51*(6), 684–691. DOI: 10.1002/mnfr.200700006

HIV cases increasing among married women in Cambodia, 'The World' reports. (2005, March 1). Retrieved March 31, 2009, from http://news.bbc.co.uk/2/hi/asia-pacific/3872773.stm.

Howell, A. B., Reed, J. D., Krueger, C. G., Winterbottom, R., Cunningham, D. G., & Leahy, M. (2005). A-type cranberry proanthocy-anidins and uropathogenic bacterial anti-adhe-sion activity. *Phytochemistry, 66*(18), 2281–2291.

Huether, S. E., & McCance, K. L. (2008). *Understanding pathophysiology.* St. Louis, MO: Mosby, Inc.

Hurtado Navarro, I., Alastrue, I., Del Amo, J., Santos, C., Ferreros, I., Tasa, T., & Pérez-Hoyos, S. (2008). Differences between women and men in serial HIV prevalence and incidence trends. *European Journal of Epidemiology, 23*(6), 435–450. doi: 10.1007/s10654-008-9246-2

Jepson, R. G., & Craig, J. C. (2008). Cranberries for preventing urinary tract infections. *Cochrane Database of Systematic Reviews, 23*(1), CD001321.

Johnston, V. J., & Mabey, D. C. (2008). Global epi-demiology and control of *Trichomonas vaginalis. Current Opinion in Infectious Diseases, 21*(1), 56–64.

Joint United Nations Programme on HIV/AIDS. (2009, December). AIDS epidemic update.

Kaewsrichan, J., Peeyananjarassri, K., & Kong-prasertkit, J. (2006). Selection and identification of anaerobic lactobacilli producing inhibitory compounds against vaginal pathogen. *FEMS Immunology and Medical Microbiology,. 48*(1), 75–83.

Kaiser Daily HIV/AIDS Report. (2005, March 1). HIV cases increasing among married women in Cambodia, 'The World' reports. Retrieved March 31, 2009, from http://www.kai-sernetwork.org/daily_reports/rep_index.cfm?DR_ID=28381.

Khanna, N., Dalby, R., Connor, A., Church, A., Stern, J., & Frazer, N. (2008). Phase I clinical trial of repeat dose terameprocol vaginal ointment in healthy female volunteers. *Sexually Transmitted Diseases, 35*(6), 577–582.

Kirjavainen, P. V., Pautler, S., Baroja, M. L., Anukam, K., Crowley, K., Carter, K., & Reid, G. (2009).

Abnormal immunological profile and vaginal microbiota in women prone to urinary tract infec-tions. *Clinical Vaccine Immunology, 16*(1), 29–36.

Kohler, P. K., Manhart, L. E., & Lafferty, W. E. (2008). Abstinence-only and comprehensive sex education and the initiation of sexual activity and teen pregnancy. *Journal of Adolescent Health, 42*(4), 344–351.

Lewis, D. A. (2007). Antibiotic-resistant gonococci—Past, present and future. *South African Medical Journal, 97*(11), 1146–1150.

Louchini, R., Goggin, P., & Steben, M. (2008). The evolution of HPV-related anogenital cancers reported in Quebec: Incidence rates and survival probabilities. *Chronic Diseases in Canada, 28*(3), 99–106.

Malla, N., Kaul, P., Sehgal, R., & Gupta, I. (2008). In vitro haemolytic and cytotoxic activity of soluble extract antigen of *T. vaginalis* isolates from symp-tomatic and asymptomatic women. *Parasitology Research, 102*(6), 1375–1378.

Mastromarino, P., Macchia, S., Meggiorini, L., Trinchieri, V., Mosca, L., Perluigi, M., & Midulla, C. (2009). Effectiveness of lactobacillus-containing vaginal tablets in the treatment of symptomatic bacterial vaginosis. *Clinical Microbiology and Infection,15*(1), 67–74.

Mijac, V. D., Dukić, S. V., Opavski, N. Z., Dukić, M. K., & Ranin, L. T. (2006). Hydrogen peroxide pro-ducing lactobacilli in women with vaginal infec-tions. *European Journal of Obstetrics & Gynecology and Reproductive Biology, 129*(1), 69–76.

Nack, A. (2000). Damaged goods: Women manag-ing the stigma of STIs. *Deviant Behavior, 21*(2), 95–121.

Nack, A. (2002). Bad girls and fallen women: Chronic STI diagnoses as gateways to tribal stigma. *Symbolic Interaction, 25*(4), 463–485.

Nessa, K., Alam, A., Chawdhury, F. A., Huq, M., Nahar, S., Salauddin, G., Khursheed, S., Rahman, S., Gurley, E., Breiman, R. F., & Rahman, M. (2008). Field evaluation of simple rapid tests in the diagnosis of syphilis. *International Journal of STD and AIDS, 19*(5), 316–320.

Nimmo, G. R., Coombs, G. W., Pearson, J. C., O'Brien, F. G., Christiansen, K. J., Turnidge, J. D., Gosbell, I. B., Collignon, P., & McLaws, M. L. (2006).

Methicillin-resistant *Staphylococcus aureus* in the Australian community: An evolving epidemic. *Medical Journal of Australia, 184*(8), 384–388.

Nohynek, L. J., Alakomi, H. L., Kähkönen, M. P., Heinonen, M., Helander, I. M., Oksman-Caldentey, K. M., & Puupponen-Pimiä, R. H. (2006). Berry phenolics: Antimicrobial properties and mechanisms of action against severe human pathogens. *Nutrition and Cancer, 54*(1), 18–32.

Osagbemi, M. O., Joseph, B., Adepetu, A. A., Nyong, A. O., & Jegede, A. S. (2007). Culture and HIV/AIDS in Africa: Promoting reproductive health in light of spouse-sharing practice among the Okun people, Nigeria. *World Health & Population*, *9*(2), 14–25.

Pappas, P. G. (2006). Invasive candidiasis. *Infectious Disease Clinics of North America, 20*(3), 485–506.

Pirotta, M., Fethers, K., & Bradshaw, C. (2009). Bacterial vaginosis—More questions than answers. *Australian Family Physician, 38*(6), 394–397.

Reid, G., & Bruce, A. W. (2006). Probiotics to prevent urinary tract infections: The rationale and evidence. *World Journal of Urology, 24*(1), 28–32.

Roberts, C. (2002). Secrets of the dead. New York, NY : Thirteen/WNET. Educational Broadcasting Corporation. Retrieved from http://www.pbs.org/wnet/secrets/previous_seasons/case_syphilis/interview.html.

Rose, M. (1997, January-February). Origins of syphilis. *Archaeology, 50*, 1, 24-25. Retrieved from http://www.archaeology.org/9701/newsbriefs/syphilis.html "*Origins of Syphilis*" 50:1.24–25.

Rusch, M. L. A., Shoveller, J., Burgess, S., Stancer, K., Patrick, D. M., & Tyndall, M. W. (2008). Preliminary development of a scale to measure stigma relating to sexually transmitted infections among women in a high risk neighborhood. *BMC Women's Health, 8.* Retrieved May 27, 2009, from http://www.pubmedcentral.nih.gov/articlerender.fcgi?artid=2610028.

Schachter, J., Moncada, J., Liska, S., Shayevich, C., & Klausner, J. D. (2008). Nucleic acid amplification tests in the diagnosis of chlamydial and gonococcal infections of the oropharynx and rectum in men who have sex with men. *Sexually Transmitted Diseases, 35*(7), 637–642.

Schwandt, A., Williams, C., & Beigi, R. H. (2008). Perinatal transmission of *Trichomonas vaginalis:* a case report. *Journal of Reproductive Medicine, 53*(1), 59–61.

Schwebke, J. R., & Lawing, L. F. (2002). Improved detection by DNA amplification of *Trichomonas vaginalis* in males. *Journal of Clinical Microbiology, 40*(10), 3681–3683.

Shafii, T., Stovel, K., & Holmes, K. (2007). Association between condom use at sexual debut and subsequent sexual trajectories: A longitudinal study using biomarkers. *American Journal of Public Health, 97*(6), 1090–1095.

Shelton, J. D. (2001). Risk of clinical pelvic inflammatory disease attributable to an intrauterine device. *Lancet, 357*(9254), 443.

Shepherd, S. (2008). A plea for protection. *Health Services Journal, 1,* 22–24.

Shukitt-Hale, B., Lau, F. C., & Joseph, J. A. (2008). Berry fruit supplementation and the aging brain. *Journal of Agricultural and Food Chemistry, 56*(3), 636–641.

Stoner, B. P. (2007). Current controversies in the management of adult syphilis. *Clinical Infectious Diseases, 44* Suppl 3, S130–146.

Swan, J., Breen, N., Coates, R. J., Rimer, B. K., & Lee, N. C. (2003). Progress in cancer screening practices in the United States: Results from the 2000 National Health Interview Survey. *Cancer, 97*(6), 1528–1540.

Taguti Irie, M. M., Lopes Consolaro, M. E., Aparecida Guedes, T., Donatti, L., Valéria Patussi, E., & Estivalet Svidzinski, T. I. (2006). A simplified technique for evaluating the adherence of yeasts to human vaginal epithelial cells. *Journal of Clinical Laboratory Analysis, 20*(5), 195–203.

Tekerekoglu, M. S., Ay, S., Otlu, B., Ciçek, A., Kayabaş, U., & Durmaz, R. (2007). Molecular epidemiology of methicillin-resistant *Staphylococcus aureus* isolates from clinical specimens of patients with nosocomial infection: Are there unnoticed silent outbreaks? *New Microbiology, 30*(2), 131–137.

Uehara, S., Monden, K., Nomoto, K., Seno, Y., Kariyama, R., & Kumon, H. (2006). A pilot study evaluating the safety and effectiveness of Lactobacillus vaginal suppositories in patients with recurrent urinary tract infection. *International Journal of Antimicrobial Agents, 28,* Suppl 1, S30–34.

UNAIDS. (2009). AIDS epidemic update. Retrieved December 20, 2009 from www.unaids.org/en/dataanalysis/epidemiology/2009aidsepidemicupdate/.

Valdevenito, S. J. P. (2008). Recurrent urinary tract infection in women. *Revista Chilena de Infectología. 25*(4), 268–276.

van Eijsden, P., Veldink, J. H., Linn, F .H., Scheltens, P., & Biessels, G. J. (2008). Progressive dementia and mesiotemporal atrophy on brain MRI: Neurosyphilis mimicking pre-senile Alzheimer's disease? *European Journal of Neurology, 15*(2), e14–15.

Von Hummius, T., Roberts, C., Saunders, D., & Boylston, A. (2006). Histological identification of syphilis in pre-Columbian England. *American Journal of Physical Anthropology, 129*(4), 559–566.

Vonka, V., & Hamsíková, E. (2007). Vaccines against human papillomaviruses—A major breakthrough in cancer prevention. *Central European Journal of Public Health, 15*(4), 131–139.

Vonka, V., Kaňka, J., Jelínek, J., Šubrt, I., Suchánek, A., Havránková, A., Váchal, M., Hirsch, I., Domorázková, E., Závadová, H., Richterová, V., Náprstková, J., Dvořáková, V., Svoboda, B. (1984). A prospective study of the relationship between cervical neoplasia and herpes simplex type-2 virus. *International Journal of Cancer, 33,* 61–70.

Whiley, D. M., Garland, S. M., Harnett, G., Lum, G., Smith, D. W., Tabrizi, S. N, Sloots, T. P., & Tapsall, J. W. (2008). 'Exploring 'best practice' for nucleic acid detection of *Neisseria gonorrhoeae. Sex Health, 5*(1), 17–23.

World Health Organization. (2007). *Guidance on global scale-up of the prevention of mother-to-child transmission of HIV.* Geneva, Switzerland: Author.

BREAST HEALTH

INTRODUCTION

Human beings belong to the taxonomic class Mammalia and, like other mammals, have mammary glands which secrete milk to nourish their offspring, a process called **lactation**. Baby mammals are born in a relatively immature and highly dependent state, unable to forage for their own food or even to digest and assimilate an adult diet. Instead, newborn mammals subsist on milk, produced by the mammary glands of their mothers. The number of pairs of mammary glands present is related to the number of young per birth. Mammals like cats or dogs that produce large litters of offspring, commonly have

six or seven pairs of breasts (Figure 7-1). In humans and other primates who usually produce one or two offspring at a time, there is only a single functional pair of nipples, each associated with mammary glands that produce milk. Human males have mammary glands just as females do, but usually lack the hormonal stimulation to produce milk.

Unlike other mammals, the breasts of primates are located on the chest and not the abdomen. Unlike other primates, who have flat breasts even during pregnancy and lactation, the human female has comparatively large mammary glands. Sexual interest in breasts seems to be peculiar to humans,

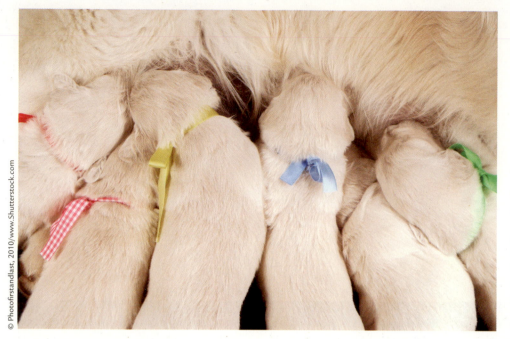

© Photofirstandlast, 2010/www.Shutterstock.com

FIGURE 7-1: Mammals that produce large litters, such as dogs, need six or seven pairs of breasts to nourish their newborn offspring. Humans have only one pair of breasts to feed the one or two children produced with a typical birth.

although the erotic importance of breasts varies among human cultures. The roles that breasts play as a source of eroticism, as a symbol of femininity, and as a measure of beauty has little to do with their biological function and much to do with the aesthetic ideals of specific cultures.

ANATOMY OF THE BREASTS

The breast is a modified sweat gland, lying over the pectoralis major muscles of the chest wall (Figure 7-2 A). Each breast extends approximately from the second to the sixth or seventh rib and from the lateral border of the sternum to the axilla, or armpit. The upper, outer portion of the breast is thicker and primarily composed of glandular tissue. It extends toward the armpit as the axillary tail, an anatomical feature significant in the spread of breast cancer.

The glandular tissue itself consists of up to 15 lobes, each with its own lactiferous duct, that converge like the spokes of a wheel on the nipple (Figure 7-2B). The major lobes of glandular tissue in each breast are further subdivided into smaller lobules which terminate in pockets called alveoli lobules. The alveolar cells, under hormonal influence, synthesize and secrete milk. During pregnancy, the increased levels of estrogen and progesterone stimulate the alveoli of both mother and child. Newborn babies of both sexes often have slightly enlarged breasts that can secrete milky fluid for several days.

The lobes, lobules, and their ducts are surrounded and separated from each other by bundles of connective tissue. The largest of these partitions are called the **Cooper's ligaments**, and they extend from the layer of connective tissue, or deep fascia, over the muscles of the chest wall to the layer of superficial fascia just under the skin. Fat accumulates in these ligaments and in all the connective tissue of the breast, producing a fat layer overlying the breast just under the breast skin. The only muscle tissue in the breasts surrounds the alveoli and ducts.

The **lactiferous ducts** enlarge slightly into a lactiferous sinus before reaching the nipple. The nipple itself is then perforated by tiny openings. The characteristic pigmented skin of the nipple extends out onto the breast for approximately 1–2 cm to form the **areola**. The pigmentation of the areola is influenced by skin pigmentation and the level of reproductive hormones present. The areola contains modified glands, called Montgomery's glands, which enlarge or regress in response to hormonal changes. Their number increases during pregnancy and lactation, secreting fluids to lubricate the nipples. Along the margin of the areola are other large sweat and sebaceous glands, some associated with hair follicles. The skin of the areola and the

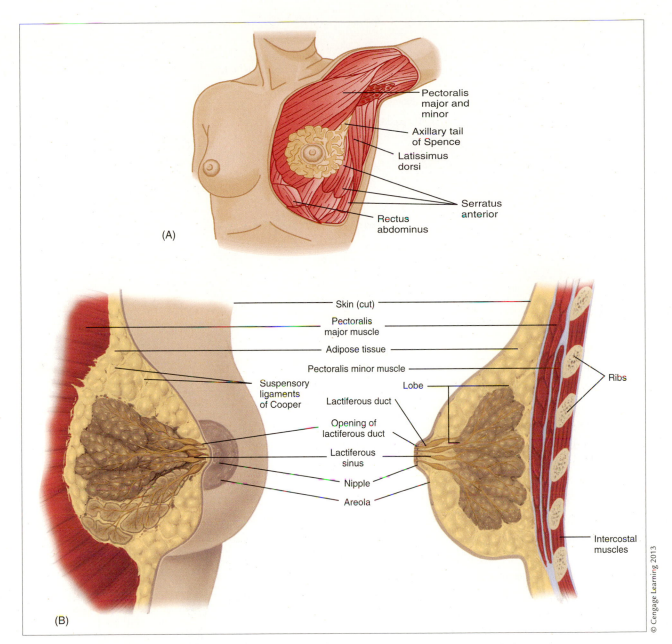

FIGURE 7-2: A. Position of the Breasts in relation to the thoracic muscles. B. The internal structures of the breast.

nipples contains bands of smooth muscle fibers that are responsible for erection of the nipples when they are stimulated.

Differences in breast size and shape are determined by the relative amounts of fatty and connective tissue, dependent on genetic and endocrine factors, or as a result of how much body fat the woman has. All women have approximately the same amount of mammary gland tissue, about five milliliters. The actual size of the breasts has no relationship to a woman's ability to produce milk.

Blood Supply to the Breasts

The primary blood supply to the breasts is from a branch of the subclavian artery called the internal mammary, with additional contributions from the thoracic branch of the axillary artery (Figure 7-3). The veins that drain the blood from the breasts follow a pathway that quickly leads into the large vein, the superior vena cava, which enters the right side of the heart. From there the blood is pumped directly to the lungs to be oxygenated before it is returned to the left side of the heart for distribution throughout

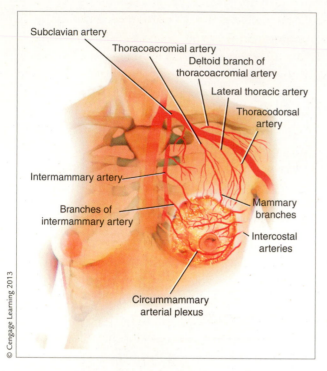

FIGURE 7-3: Blood supply to the breast.

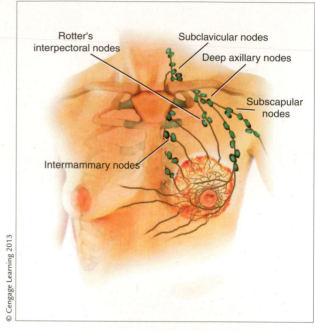

FIGURE 7-4: Lymphatic drainage of the breast.

the body. The ather direct route from the breasts to the lung capillaries may be significant in the spread of breast cancer.

Lymphatic Drainage of the Breasts

All cells of the body are bathed in a fluid which leaks from the capillaries. Some of this fluid eventually drains into the lymph vessels, where it is filtered by lymph nodes before it returns to the circulatory system. From the breasts, most of the lymph drains toward the underarm, through a series of nodes (Figure 7-4). The first nodes encountered are the four to six anterior pectoral nodes, also called the low axillary nodes. From there the lymph passes to the central axillary nodes embedded in a fat pad in the center of the armpit. The lymph then proceeds to the upper part of the axilla into the lateral nodes along the axillary vein, and then to the deep axillary or subclavicular nodes (Figure 7-5).

If cancer develops in the breasts, malignant cells can invade the lymph system or other tissues in a process known as metastasis. The lymph nodes contain white blood cells, which can destroy the cancer cells before they spread. Because most of the breast lymph (75 percent) drains into the axillary nodes, it is

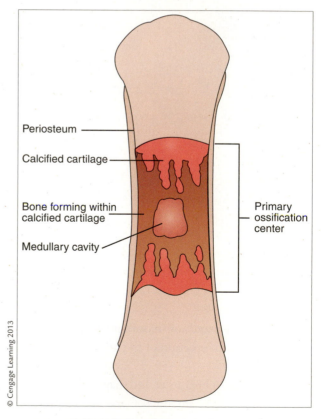

FIGURE 7-5: Pathways of lymphatic drainage from the breast.

common to remove the primary tumor in the breast and the axillary lymph nodes to eradicate the cancer. This may not always be successful because of the secondary lymph channels that pass to the internal mammary nodes or through other channels. When lymph nodes have been invaded by cancer cells, they are said to be "positive" nodes.

CHANGES IN THE BREASTS THROUGHOUT THE LIFESPAN

Breast tissue has receptors for the reproductive hormones estrogen and progesterone and is subject to changes in response to fluctuations in reproductive hormone concentrations throughout the lifespan. Puberty, the menstrual cycle, pregnancy, and menopause all have an impact on breast morphology and function.

Breast Development and Puberty

Before menarche, the **mammary glands** of both males and females consist only of a few ducts surrounded by connective tissue. For females, with the onset of puberty, the duct tissue are stimulated by estrogen and begin to branch, forming the buds of the future lobules and alveoli. The connective tissue also proliferates and becomes infiltrated with fat, and the breast begins to assume their mature shape. When ovulatory cycles begin to occur and the corpus luteum secretes progesterone, the characteristic structure of the breast during the childbearing years is developed.

Breast Changes and the Menstrual Cycle

Throughout her reproductive years, a woman's breasts undergo cyclical changes in response to changing levels of estrogen and progesterone during the menstrual cycle. During the proliferative phase of the cycle, the high levels of estrogens stimulate the proliferation of cells in the ducts and the alveoli. This increase continues into the postovulatory or secretory phase of the cycle, when the increasing levels of progesterone result in the dilation of the ducts and the differentiation of the alveolar cells into secretory cells. After ovulation, there is also an increased blood flow to the breasts and, in the week before menstruation, some women experience fluid retention and slight enlargement of their breasts.

When menstruation starts, there is some secretion of droplets by alveolar cells but it is usually not noticeable. Toward the end of menstruation, and if conception has not occurred, the proliferated tissues begin to regress and are reabsorbed. The ducts become narrower, the lobules and alveoli become smaller, and the tissue edema disappears. But, before the tissue can totally regress, a new cycle starts and the estrogen again induces more proliferation. The ducts and alveoli never have a chance to completely return to the way they were before the preceding cycle, and each additional ovulatory cycle, therefore, results in a little more mammary tissue development. This process continues until approximately age 35.

Breast Changes during Pregnancy

Throughout the nine months of pregnancy, the breasts are preparing for nursing. Within the first three to four weeks of gestation, the ducts of the mammary glands sprout branches, and more lobules and alveoli are formed. These changes are much greater than those that occur each menstrual cycle, and as a result, the breasts become larger and become heavier and more tender as pregnancy progresses. Each breast gains nearly a pound in weight by the end of pregnancy. These changes can put strain on the Cooper's ligaments causing the breasts to become more pendulous after pregnancy.

Changes in the Breasts with Age

Over time, the Cooper's ligaments in the breasts can stretch causing a condition called ptosis, or sagging breasts. The weakening of the Cooper's ligaments is also called Cooper's droop. Opinions vary as to whether going braless contributes to sagging breasts. It seems logical that supporting the weight of the breasts against gravity with a well fitting bra diminishes the stress on the network of connective tissues that supports the fat and glandular components of the breasts. Shifts in body fat, decreased levels of reproductive hormones with menopause, and changes in elasticity all contribute to the age-related changes in the breast.

LACTATION AND BREAST FEEDING

Lactation is the production of milk to feed a baby. The World Health Organization (2007) has recommended that breastfeeding should be the first choice

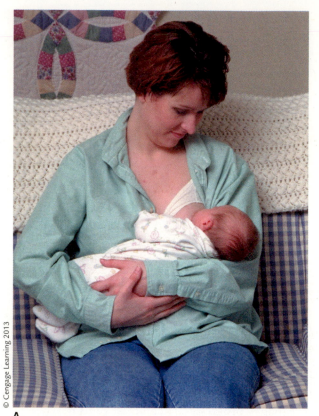

A.

© Cengage Learning 2013

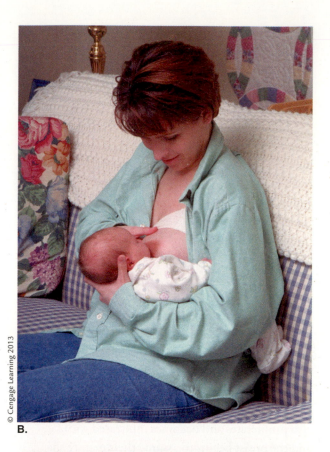

B.

© Cengage Learning 2013

for nourishing newborns and babies (WHO, 2007) (Figure 7-6). They recommend that feeding be initiated within the first hour after birth. Exclusive breastfeeding is recommended up to six months of age, and breast feeding, supplemented with other foods, should continue until the child is two years old. The American Academy of Pediatrics (AAP), the American Academy of Family Practice (AAFP), and the American Dietetic Association (ADA) also advocate breastfeeding for all full-term newborns and maintaining that breast milk should be the sole nutrient for the first six months of life, and continue for at least one year (Gartner et al., 2005; James et al., 2009). Fewer than 25 percent of women in the United States were breastfeeding their babies in 1971; currently, about 74 percent of women initiate breastfeeding, but only 31.5 percent are exclusively breastfeeding. By six months, the percentage has dropped to 11.9 percent (Stuebe, 2009).

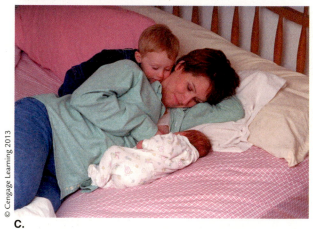

C.

© Cengage Learning 2013

FIGURE 7-6: Breastfeeding is the widely recommended first choice for nourishing newborns and babies. There are several different holds a mother can use to feed her baby: A. Cradle hold; B. Football hold; and C. Side-lying hold.

Composition of Breast Milk

Human breast milk is the ideal food for human babies. In contrast with cow's milk and formula, the proteins found in human milk are more digestible by babies

and provide all the essential amino acids and other nutrients needed for a newborn. Moreover, the proteins in cow's milk can cause allergic reactions, and circulating antibodies to these proteins have been found in a majority of formula-fed babies even when they show no evidence of allergy. Instances of unexplained crib deaths have been linked to severe allergic reactions to cow's milk (McLaughlan & Coombs, 1983). The fat content in human milk is also more digestible and allows greater uptake of fat-soluble vitamins A and D from the intestine. In addition, there is evidence that nucleotides found in breast milk that are not found in formula support early infant growth and brain development (Singhal et al., 2010).

Breast milk is rich in antibodies to the microbes that the mother has immunity to. These antibodies provide protection as the child begins to establish its own normal flora and builds its own immune system. The level of immune factors is highest in colostrum and milk produced in the first weeks of nursing. **Colostrum** is a fluid containing protein and carbohydrates but lacking milk fat, and it is an important source of antibodies for the newborn. Colostrum is recommended by WHO (2007) as the perfect food for the newborn.

The Physiology of Lactation

Many of the body's hormones play an important role in establishing and maintaining lactation (Figure 7-7). Two hormones that are involved in stimulating the breasts for lactation are estrogen and progesterone. Other important hormones include prolactin and growth hormone from the pituitary, and placental lactogen and human chorionic gonadotropin from the placenta. Additional hormones also play a role. Adrenal corticosteroids, insulin, thyroid hormone, and parathyroid hormones all contribute to the duct and alveolar growth and differentiation of secreting cells.

Prolactin, secreted by the anterior pituitary in increasing levels throughout pregnancy, triggers the synthesis and secretion of milk after the birth of a baby. This hormone causes the cells of the glandular alveoli of the breasts to utilize the nutrients brought to the gland in the circulating blood, including amino acids, fatty acids, and glucose. From those building blocks, the gland synthesizes milk protein, milk fat, and milk sugar; adds ions, vitamins, and water; and secretes them as milk. During the last weeks of pregnancy, the presence of large amounts of estrogens and progesterone alters the effects of prolactin and causes the synthesis and secretion of colostrum instead of milk. Within two to three days after birth, the high levels of estrogens and progesterone in the mother's body drop, and prolactin

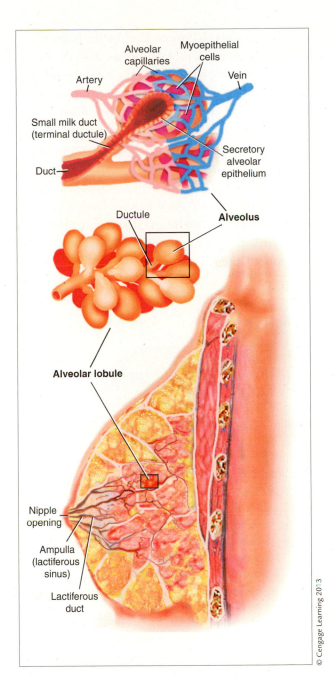

FIGURE 7-7: Physiology of lactation.

then stimulates the production and secretion of milk instead of colostrum.

While prolactin is required for stimulating the production and secretion of milk in the alveoli, the hormone oxytocin must be present so that the milk can be ejected from the alveoli to the nipples. The stimulus of suckling on the nipple causes oxytocin to be released from the posterior pituitary gland. Oxytocin induces smooth muscle surrounding the alveoli to contract, a process known as a milk letdown reaction (Figure 7-8). The milk enters the ducts and begins to flow easily from the breasts. In a nursing mother, milk letdown can be elicited merely by hearing a baby cry or by thinking about a baby. As long as the mother continues to nurse, the milk will continue to be produced, potentially for several years. The presence of prolactin and oxytocin result in milk production under the stimulus of sucking. The nursing mother requires an additional 500 calories a day to support milk production (Figure 7-9). When the baby is weaned and the nipples are no longer stimulated, prolactin and oxytocin secretion stops, and milk is no longer synthesized and released.

The Mechanics of Breast Feeding

While breastfeeding is a natural process, there are some techniques that can be learned to increase a mother and her infant's success at breastfeeding. Positioning the infant correctly is important, especially when initiating breastfeeding. For breastfeeding to take place, the infant must "latch on" by taking the nipple and areola into its mouth and beginning to suckle. A position called the C-hold will support both the breast and the baby, making it easier for the infant to latch on. Figure 7-10 shows a nursing mother supporting her breast with one hand and her infant with the other in the C-hold technique. From

FIGURE 7-8: Physiology of the letdown reflex.

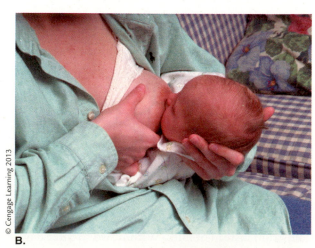

A.

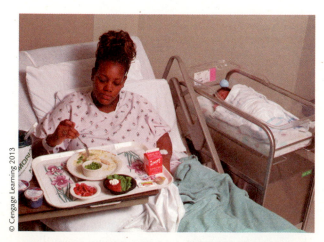

FIGURE 7-9: Breastfeeding mothers require an extra 500 calories a day.

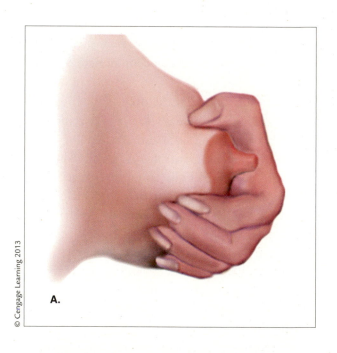

B.

FIGURE 7-10: C-hold technique for initiating breastfeeding. A. Hand placement. B. Position of the infant.

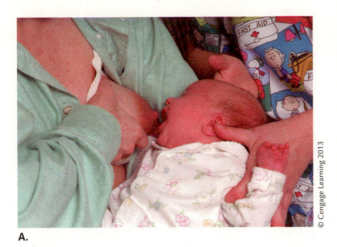

A.

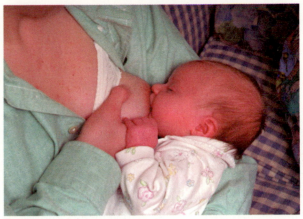

B.

© Cengage Learning 2013

FIGURE 7-11: Stimulating the baby to latch on. A. Touching the baby's mouth with the nipple or with a finger stimulates the rooting reflex. B. When the baby opens its mouth as part of the rooting reflex, the mother can put the baby's mouth on her nipple.

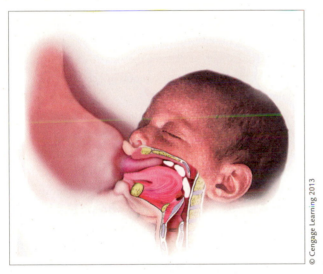

© Cengage Learning 2013

FIGURE 7-12: When the baby latches on, the entire nipple will be drawn into its mouth for nursing.

this position, the mother can hold the infant close to her nipple and brush the baby's lower lip with the nipple. This will elicit the rooting reflex in the baby and it will open its mouth wide. Once the infant has opened its mouth, the mother can guide her nipple to the infant's mouth (Figure 7-11). When the infant begins to suckle, the mother may experience some discomfort for the first few seconds, but this usually diminishes quickly (Figure 7-12). Nipple soreness can be avoided by inserting a finger into the corner of the infant's mouth to break the suction. It is recommended that both breasts be nursed at each feeding to stimulate milk production.

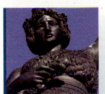

Historical Considerations
SUPPORT FOR BREASTFEEDING

In 1956, Mary White and Marion Thompson, together with some of their friends, had the idea of forming an organization that would provide new mothers with support and information that they needed to successfully breastfeed their babies. The organization was called the La Leche League. In this organization, women who were experienced in nursing informed and advised other nursing mothers. The League today has grown to more than 3,000 chapters throughout the world. In its manual, *The Womanly Art of Breastfeeding*, interested women can obtain practical knowledge about breastfeeding. The La Leche League provides group meetings and individual counseling for both support and personal instruction. La Leche League chapters are listed in the telephone book or on the Internet.

Benefits of Breastfeeding

The benefits of breastfeeding are many, for both the mother and the infant. In fact, it is reasonable to consider that by not breastfeeding both mother and infant are at increased risk for disease (Stuebe, 2009). In the United States, the postnatal infant mortality rate is estimated to be 21 percent higher in formula-fed infants (Gartner et al., 2005, Chen & Rogan, 2004). Breastfed newborns have a greater resistance to gastrointestinal disorders and to respiratory and ear infections, than formula-fed infants (Kramer & Kakuma, 2002; Ip et al., 2007; Gartner et al., 2005). In addition, the length of time that an infant is breastfed is inversely related to their chances of developing obesity later in life (Ip et al., 2007; Krebs & Jacobson, 2003). Research has indicated that breastfed babies are less likely to develop asthma, type 1 and 2 diabetes, and childhood leukemia than are formula-fed infants. Premature infants who are breastfed are less likely to develop potentially fatal necrotizing enterocolitis.

Breastfeeding imparts benefits to the mother as well. The uterus, under the influence of oxytocin produced by nursing, returns to its pre-pregnancy size more easily and rapidly after childbirth, and there are fewer problems with uterine infection post delivery. It may be easier to return to pre-pregnancy weight if a woman is nursing since calories are expended to produce milk. Breastfeeding also reduces a woman's lifetime chances of developing type 2 diabetes and obesity (Stuebe, 2009). Women who breastfeed also have a reduced chance of developing breast and ovarian cancer (Ip et al., 2007). For many women, the successful breastfeeding of their babies provides a secure, gratifying, and satisfying experience that contributes to the quality of the mother–child interaction (Ekstrom & Nissen, 2006). Breastfeeding is also associated with a reduced risk of developing postpartum depression (Ip et al., 2007). Breast milk is always ready, at the right temperature, does not have to be pasteurized, and is not subject to the bacterial contamination that can occur with formula. In addition, breast milk, unlike formula, is free.

Nursing mothers are relatively infertile, since ovulation and menstruation return more slowly in women who lactate. The frequency and amount of nursing prolongs the amenorrhea, but it is also affected by body weight, being of shorter duration in heavier women. In many parts of the world where women are poorly nourished, breastfeeding prevents a significant number of pregnancies. Half of the women who breastfeed are able to conceive within the first six months postpartum, while the other half seem to be

protected, but because there is no way of knowing in which 50 percent a woman may fall, lactation is not a substitute for contraception.

Obstacles to Breastfeeding

There are several factors that can interfere with a woman's decision to breastfeed her baby. These factors include characteristics of the woman's breasts that prevent successful breastfeeding, the presence of microbes or chemicals in the mother's milk that could be harmful to the baby, and lack of social support. Some chronic diseases can also interfere with breastfeeding. Certain infections, including HIV, can pass from mother to infant through breastfeeding (Mofenson, 2010). Hepatitis B virus is detectable in human breast milk, but does not seem to contribute to infants developing the disease. Women who are receiving radiation, chemotherapy or tamoxifin therapy for cancer, or certain medications for lupus should not breastfeed while receiving treatments (Helewa et al., 2002).

Pain killing medications used during labor and delivery cross from the mother to the infant through the placenta, and reduce the infant's alertness for hours after it is born. These effects can interfere with the successful establishment of breastfeeding (Reynolds, 2010). Many women who are highly motivated to breastfeed can still have trouble with lactation unless they recieve instruction and encouragement. If they have initial difficulty getting breastfeeding started or develop problems with engorged breasts, leaking, or sore nipples, they may give up and switch to bottle-feeding. Anxiety about breastfeeding, especially when accompanied by inadequate instruction and a lack of support can inhibit oxytocin levels and the milk letdown reflex. Hospital practices, such as separating new mothers from their infants and providing formula, can interrupt the successful establishment of breastfeeding. Providing instruction and allowing feeding on demand, on the other hand, can promote successful breastfeeding.

Any chemicals in a woman's blood have the potential to get into her breast milk (American Academy of Pediatrics, 2005). These include medications, drugs, and alcohol. The baby, smaller in size and with immature kidneys and liver, is not able to detoxify substances as well as an adult. Some drugs are definitely known to cause health problems; others, such as alcohol and caffeine, are considered safe in moderate amounts for nursing mothers. Large quantities, however, can result in responses in babies similar to those in adults. Alcohol becomes concentrated in breast milk and interferes with milk production. Because alcohol is passed to the infant, breastfeeding mothers should limit their consumption and avoid breastfeeding for two hours after drinking (Gartner et al., 2005). Nicotine and other components of cigarette smoke are present in breast milk, and in the case of nicotine, its concentration is one-and-a-half to three times the concentration found in the mother's blood. Although infants of mothers who smoke are more likely to develop respiratory problems than non-smoker's infants, there is evidence that infants of mothers who smoke and who are breastfed are less likely to develop respiratory problems than are smoker's infants who are bottle-fed (APA, 2005).

Psychotropic drugs used to treat anxiety and depression can also pass from the mother to her infant in breast milk. These drugs have a fairly long half life in the body and may accumulate in the tissues of infants, particularly in their brains. It is not known how these drugs may affect long term development of the nervous system. Researchers suggest that infants who are being breastfed by mothers who are taking antidepressants should be monitored for possible effects from the medications such as irritability and changes in sleep or feeding patterns. They also suggest that mothers should breastfeed before taking their medications and avoid breast-feeding during hours of the day when the medications are at peak levels in their milk. These peak times will vary depending on the medications that are prescribed (Pearlstein, 2008).

The ability to breastfeed may be reduced or impossible if the mother has undergone a mastectomy, breast reduction surgery, or breast augmentation. Breast biopsies, depending on the location of the incision can also interfere with milk production and flow. Underdeveloped breasts and inverted or flat nipples can reduce a women's ability to breastfeed. If a woman has pierced nipples, she will probably still be able to breastfeed, but she should remove any breast jewelry while nursing to eliminate the possibility of the baby choking.

There has been some concerns raised that silicone from silicone breast implants can leak and appear in human breast milk, raising questions about effects on the nursing infant (Zoccali et al., 2008). The chemistry of silicon is complex, and, at present, there is no definitive verdict about the effects of leaking silicone implants on nursing babies (Semple, 2007; Lee & Zuckerman, 2002). In addition to silicone, recent studies have detected increased levels of the metal platinum in the tissues of women, including the breast milk, who have silicone implants (Lykissa & Maharaj, 2006). Platinum is used to create the silicone gel that fills implants. So far, platinum from the implants has been linked to neurological problems in the women exposed to it (Maharaj, 2007; Brook, 2006).

Breastfeeding while working outside the home provides additional challenges. Mothers have to express their milk with a breast pump before they leave or use one at the workplace and may have to get the milk back home to the baby during the day (Figure 7-13). Women frequently face public resistance when attempting to breastfeed in public, even though public breastfeeding is legal. In the United States, 20 states have passed legislation protecting a woman's right to breastfeed in public.

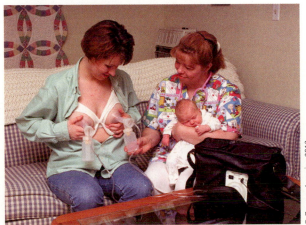

© Cengage Learning 2013

FIGURE 7-13: Breast pumps allow mothers to express milk for feeding to their infant when they cannot breastfeed.

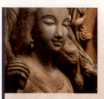

Social Considerations
SUPPORT FOR BREASTFEEDING MOTHERS IN THE WORKPLACE

Women have always worked and breastfed, balancing their responsibilities of caring for an infant with all of the other responsibilities in their lives. While the concept is not new, the modern workplace can present moms with new challenges when it comes to breastfeeding. While many women know that breastfeeding is best, many find it difficult to accommodate breastfeeding once they return to work. Today, women with infants and children are a fast growing segment of the United States labor force. To date, no federal law establishes or protects a right to pump breast milk in the workplace, but a few states have adopted legislation to this effect (Marcus, 2008). Fortunately, many employers are trying to be more sensitive to the needs of breastfeeding mothers in the workplace, allowing women space in the office to pump and store milk (some designating a breastfeeding mothers break room), or giving mothers extended breaks to go back home or to the daycare to breastfeed their child. Depending on the kind of work, other employers don't mind if new mothers take their babies to work with them so that they can care for their infants and breastfeed while on the job.

New mothers may find it helpful to take a practice day before they start work to experiment with new routines for going back to work. Sometimes it can help to ease into work gradually, if that is something that can be worked out with one's employer. It may also be helpful to talk to other working mothers, and see what strategies have worked best for them. Some employers also provide other options to new mothers including part-time work, job sharing, individualized scheduling of work hours or flex time, phase-back, a compressed work week, or telecommuting. These alternatives can be worth looking into if they make it easier to breastfeed. Employers that allow flexibility have noticed positive results for their companies. In particular, women who are accommodated to breastfeed their babies have fewer missed days of work to take care of sick infants, lower healthcare costs and increased job satisfaction and worker productivity.

Environmental Toxins Found in Breast Milk

Environmental pollutants can be a source of contamination of mother's milk. Pesticides, heavy metals, antibiotics, and all sorts of organic industrial wastes eventually find their way into food and breast milk (Denham et al., 2005). Organic toxins are stored in the body fat, resist breakdown by usual body detoxifying enzymes, and can be excreted through breast milk. Pan et al. (2010) found PCBs, DDT, and other endocrine disruptors in breast milk but found no effect on infant growth during the first 12 months of life. Additional long term studies are needed.

The role of such environmental contaminants in producing harmful effects in children is still unknown, but recent concerns about endocrine disruptors such as BPA have led to new regulation aimed at reducing exposure. Lactating women can consider having their breast milk analyzed for PCBs and PBBs if they work on a farm, have frequently eaten large quantities of fish from contaminated lakes or rivers, or are otherwise exposed occupationally to these chemicals. Most women should not avoid breastfeeding solely because of toxins found in their food and water supply. Cow's milk and formula have been shown to contain many of the same environmental pollutants, sometimes in even higher concentrations.

Induced Lactation

Induced lactation, also called relactation, is the ability to produce breast milk in response to sucking stimulation when there has been no preceding pregnancy. In 1977, Elizabeth Hormann, a pioneer of the relactation movement, reported the results of a survey of 65 women who wanted to provide the psychological and physiological benefits of breastfeeding to their adopted babies. Eighteen of the women had never been pregnant, seven had been pregnant but had not nursed, and 40 had been pregnant and had lactated before. The majority of infants received by the adoptive mothers were under one month of age, but some of them were already receiving some type of solid food as well as formula when they arrived. All 65 women were successful in producing milk, although all but one had to supplement with formula because milk production was not adequate to fully sustain the baby. In spite of the need for supplementation, the women in the study reported satisfaction in the emotional bonding they experienced nursing their adopted babies.

In humans, it has been shown that when the breasts and nipples are manually stimulated, or sometimes as a result of chest injury, surgery, or shingles (herpes zoster), lactation can result. Sensory nerve impulses from the breasts are relayed to the spinal cord and then up to the hypothalamus of the brain. The prolactin-inhibiting factor that ordinarily keeps lactation from occurring is suppressed, and the prolactin can then be released resulting in milk production. Women who want to nurse adopted babies require a month or more of preparation through breast stimulation to increase serum prolactin levels.

NON-CANCEROUS CONDITIONS OF THE BREAST

There are several conditions that can cause lumps, inflammation, or other changes in the breast that are not cancerous. However, it is important to have unusual breast changes evaluated by a healthcare provider as soon as possible in order to make sure that they are not malignant. The good news is that most lumps found in the breasts are not cancerous. Breast cancer is discussed in detail in Chapter 8.

Fibrocystic Changes in the Breasts

Most women are aware of some feelings of fullness and lumpiness in their breasts just before or during menstruation, with a large number of tender nodules. This increased nodularity usually appears in both breasts in approximately the same location each cycle and disappears after menstruation. These monthly changes are collectively called **fibrocystic changes in the breast**; formerly fibrocystic breast disease. These changes are also called chronic cystic

mastitis, mammary dysplasia, cystic mastalgia, benign breast disease, and a variety of other designations (American Cancer Society, 2010). A woman who regularly performs monthly breast self-examination learns to distinguish her own normal thickenings and lumpiness from changes that are new. Any one lump, however, that begins to grow out of line with the rest is suspicious.

Fibrocystic changes in the breasts are caused by an overgrowth of fibrous tissues in the connective tissues supporting the breasts. This fibrosis is often accompanied by the presence of fluid-filled cysts, which contribute to the lumpy feeling of fibrocystic breasts. Fluctuations in hormone levels during the menstrual cycle and as women approach menopause can cause fibrocystic changes in the breasts. When such overgrowth blocks ducts and prevents normal drainage of secretions from the breasts, cysts can result. In contrast to malignant breast cancer lumps, the cysts that develop move freely when pressed and do not exhibit sharply defined edges. Symptoms often decline after menopause when levels of estrogen and progesterone drop.

Fibrocystic changes to the breasts are not a disease, and there are no specific treatments suggested for this condition. For some women, diet and lifestyle changes help to reduce discomfort. Some research suggests that fibrocystic changes are linked to caffeine consumption, which promotes fluid retention, and avoiding caffeine may be effective in preventing symptoms. However, studies show mixed results regarding the effectiveness of limiting caffeine. (Rosolowich et al., 2006; Norlock, 2002).

Other options to reduce discomfort include wearing a supportive bra, taking over-the-counter pain relievers, and limiting salt consumption which can encourage fluid retention. An under functioning thyroid gland has been associated with fibrocystic changes, and, possibly, hypothyroidism should be investigated in women who suffer from breast lumps (Mardaleishvili et al., 2006). One current theory hypothesizes that these changes are caused by an imbalanced estrogen/progesterone ratio, or an inappropriate breast tissue response to the normal variations in ovarian hormones. For the most part, experiencing fibrocystic changes to the breast does not make a woman more likely

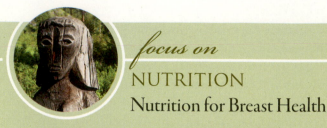

focus on
NUTRITION
Nutrition for Breast Health

What role does diet play in maintaining breast health and preventing breast cancer? Scientific research has shown that some of the nutrients and other substances found in foods can reduce a woman's risk of developing breast cancer. Vitamin D, for example, has been shown to have a positive effect on preventing reproductive cancers, including breast cancer (Lin et al., 2007; Abbas et al., 2007; McCullough et al., 2005). There is also increasing evidence that a diet rich in phytoestrogens can play an important role in reducing a woman's chances of developing breast cancer. Phytoestrogens are chemical components found in some plants that can act as weak estrogens in the human body. There are many phytoestrogens including soy isoflavonoids, lignans, and coumestrol, and the effects of individual types of phytoestrogens are variable (Hedelin et al., 2008). For example, there is some evidence that soy isoflavones may reduce the symptoms of fibrocystic changes to the breasts (Fleming, 2003), but in some cases these same isoflavones can stimulate breast cancer tumor cells to grow (Power & Thompson et al., 2007).

to develop breast cancer later in life. Only women who have been diagnosed with one form of fibrocystic changes, called atypical **hyperplasia**, face an increased risk of developing breast cancer (Habor et al., 2010).

Mastitis

Mastitis is an inflammation of the breasts that can occur if the lactiferous ducts become infected. This condition is most likely to develop in women who are breastfeeding. The infection can cause a lump or an area of thickened skin to develop around the infection. For breastfeeding women who develop mastitis, antibiotics are the most likely treatment, although surgery may be needed if the infection has become an abscess. A second form of mastitis, called periductal mastitis, is more likely to develop in postmenopausal women. Periductal mastitis can lead to scarring of the milk ducts, breast lumps, pain, nipple discharge, and nipple retraction. If periductal mastitis does not respond to antibiotics, it needs further

evaluation to distinguish it from inflammatory breast cancer, which has similar symptoms.

Non-fibrocystic Breast Cysts

Breast cysts can develop without the fibrosis that characterizes fibrocystic changes to the breasts. These cysts are caused by dilated ducts, and they often appear during the two weeks before menstruation and can disappear spontaneously after menses. Most cysts are oval or round in shape and feel smooth and firm. They usually move slightly when pressed. In contrast to breast lumps caused by cancer, cysts often feel painful or tender to the touch. These cysts seem to be associated with fluctuating hormone levels during a woman's menstrual cycle.

Fibroadenoma

Fibroadenomas are a specific type of cyst, most commonly found in young women in their 20s or 30s, although they can occur in women of any age. Fibroadenomas are round and feel more solid than a fluid filled cyst. They have a rubbery texture. These masses can grow quite large, some reaching the size of a small plum, and they often bounce or move slightly when pressure is applied to them. These cysts are not malignant and are usually painless. Fibroadenomas, like most cysts, respond to hormonal changes. They are the result of excess growth of glandular and connective tissue of the breast. Because they respond to changes in hormone levels, they can enlarge during pregnancy and tend to disappear after menopause. Mammography and ultrasound are used to diagnosis a fibroadenoma and distinguish it from breast cancer or other types of cysts. Often times a biopsy is required to make a clear diagnosis. Like other types of cysts, fibroadenomas sometimes disappear on their own, but may have to be surgically removed if they persist or cause discomfort. Table 7-1 shows characteristics of common breast masses, including fibroadenomas.

Table 7-1   Characteristics of Common Breast Masses.

	Gross Cyst	Fibroadenoma	Carcinoma
Age	30–60; diminishes after menopause	puberty to menopause	most common after 50 years
Shape	round	round, lobular, or ovoid	irregular, stellate, or crab-like
Consistency	soft to firm	usually firm	firm to hard
Discreteness	well defined	well defined	not clearly defined
Number	single or grouped	most often single	usually single
Mobility	mobile	very mobile	may be mobile or fixed to skin, underlying tissue or chest wall
Tenderness	tender	nontender	usually nontender
Erythema	no erythema	no erythema	may be present
Retraction/dimpling	not present	not present	often present

Courtesy of Littleton, L.Y., and Engebretson, J.C. (2002). *Maternal, Neonatal and Women's Health Nursing.* Clifton Park, NY: Cengage Learning.

Phyllodes Tumor

Another type of lump, which is similar in many ways to a fibroadenoma, is a phyllodes tumor. These tumors are less common than fibroadenomas, and are distinguished from fibroadenomas by their rapid growth. They are usually benign, but in some cases they can be cancerous. Even after a biopsy, it may be difficult to distinguish a fibroadenoma from a phyllodes tumor. The most common treatment for a phyllodes tumor is to remove it surgically. These tumors have a tendency to recur.

Intraductal Papilloma

A noncancerous mass that develops in a milk duct is called an intraductal papilloma. These are often felt as small lumps near the edge of the areola. Intraductal papillomas can be alarming, because they often cause a bloody discharge from the nipple. Mammograms and ultrasound are usually used to diagnose these lumps, and surgery to remove the affected duct is the usual treatment. After surgery, the removed tissue is examined for cancer cells.

SCREENING FOR BREAST CONDITIONS

The primary purpose of screening is to distinguish benign conditions of the breasts from breast cancer. Breast self-exams, clinical breast exams, and mammography can identify abnormal breast conditions. Of these, **mammograms** are the most effective at detecting the smallest and earliest breast cancer tumors. MRI, sonography, and biopsies are also used to identify abnormal conditions and distinguish benign conditions from breast cancer. In addition to any unusual and persistent breast lumps, the following symptoms should be examined by a doctor because they can indicate breast cancer:

- Dimpled skin or pitting of skin on the breast, resembling the skin of an orange
- Redness
- Spontaneous clear or bloody discharge from the nipple
- Changes in the contour or shape of a breast
- Changes in the size of a breast
- Retraction or indentation of a nipple
- Any flattening or indentation of the skin over the breast

Breast Self Examination

Breast self examination (BSE) has been criticized as being unreliable for the detection of breast cancer (Nelson et al., 2009). The reason that BSE has been criticized is that, on average, by the time a tumor is large enough to be detected by touch, it is already large enough to have metastasized to other parts of the body, and treatment is much more difficult. Mammograms, which can detect significantly smaller breast lumps, are recommended instead to detect early breast cancer. However, for younger women, who do not yet qualify for insurance reimbursement for mammograms and for other women who do not have ready access to mammograms, BSE can be an important way to find out if something is amiss. BSE does not just involve feeling the breasts for lumps. It also involves a visual inspection of the breasts which can alert a woman to several of the symptoms of breast cancer which may appear before a lump is palpable. This awareness can potentially save her life. Finally, BSE is easy to do and it is done without any risk or cost to a woman.

Between menarche and menopause, BSE should become a regular monthly health habit as soon as the menstrual period is over. At that time, levels of ovarian hormones are low, and the breasts are less likely to be tender and swollen. Women who are no longer menstruating should identify a specific date each month to perform their BSE.

Technique of BSE

A **breast self-examination** consists of three steps-feeling the breast while wet, inspection in front of a mirror, and palpation while lying down. Figure 7-14 provides a guide for performing this important self-examination.

While taking a shower or a bath, move gently over every part of the wet breasts with a soapy hand. Raise the left arm behind the head and, with the flat fingers of the relaxed right hand, feel the entire left breast, beginning at the outermost top and moving in decreasing concentric circles, finishing at the nipple. Move high into the armpit and all the way over onto the breastbone. Then repeat the procedure for the right breast, using the flat fingers of the left hand and raising the right arm behind the head.

Before getting dressed, sit or stand in front of a mirror with the breasts exposed. There should be a good, strong light, and the mirror should be large enough to allow inspection of the breasts while facing it directly. With arms at the sides, look at the breasts for bulges, asymmetry, or areas of surface flattening. Many women have unequal-sized breasts. As long as the contours of the breasts are symmetrical, inequality in size is perfectly normal.

Continue the inspection, looking for any deviation of a nipple, which could mean that it is being pulled toward an underlying tumor. Check for retraction of the nipple, the areola, or the skin. Examine the breasts for redness, any sore or ulceration of the skin, and for edema of the skin, which can exaggerate the pores so the skin looks like an orange peel. Make certain there has been no change from the previous examination.

Next, raise the arms high above the head to expose the sides and undersurfaces of the breasts and repeat the same observations. Cancer can produce retraction of the skin, manifested by anything from a small skin dimple or puckering to shrinkage of the entire breast. Raising the arms moves the muscles under the breast and may cause skin retraction or nipple deviation that may not have been apparent before.

Then, place the palms on the hips and press down to contract the pectoral muscles. Again, changes that are not visible in other positions may become

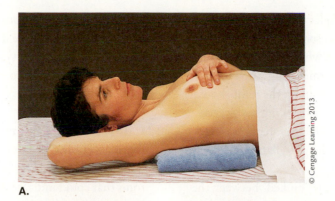

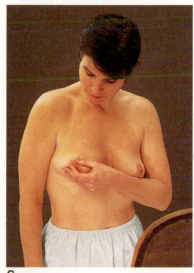

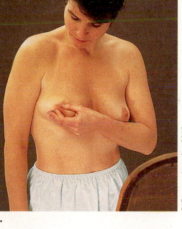

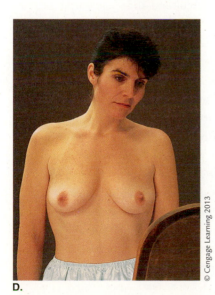

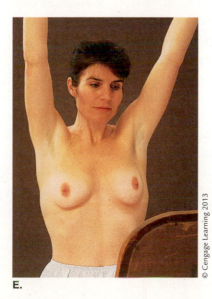

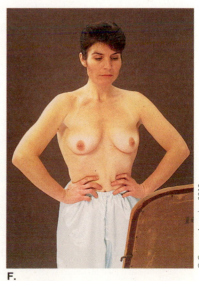

FIGURE 7-14: Breast self-examination. A. Palpitating the breasts while lying down. B. Palpitating the breasts while standing C. Compression of the nipples. D. Visual Examination before a mirror: arms at the sides. E. Visual Examination before a mirror: arms overhead. F. Visual Examination before a mirror: hands pressed into hips.

apparent. Bend forward to let the breasts hang free and check for anything unusual.

Repeat the palpitation while lying down. To examine the right breast, a small pillow or a folded bath towel should be placed under the right shoulder. This maneuver flattens and spreads out the breast evenly over the chest wall. The right hand is placed behind the neck. This also helps to flatten the breast into a thin layer.

The nipple is then gently "milked" between the thumb and forefinger. Most types of discharge that come from both breasts are nothing to worry about. If a discharge is watery, yellow or pink, or bloody, and occurs only on one side, it is suspicious and should be investigated. A slight scaling on the nipple associated with the menstrual period is not unusual.

Repeat the procedure on the left breast. If a lump or skin dimple or nipple discharge is discovered during BSE, the abnormality should be investigated by a healthcare provider as soon as possible to identify the cause.

Clinical Breast Exam

During a **clinical breast exam** a healthcare provider examines the breasts for lumps or other visible symptoms that could indicate cancer. Usually the auxiliary lymph nodes will also be palpitated to check for swelling or lumps. The American Cancer Society suggests that all women have clinical breast exams every three years until age 40 and once every year after age 40. Research concerning the effectiveness of clinical breast exams for reducing mortality due to breast

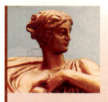

Cultural Considerations
WORLDWIDE PATTERNS IN BREAST CANCER

There are worldwide geographic differences in breast cancer as well as ethnic and religious differences that have been postulated, in the absence of other known reasons, to be due to differences in dietary practices. The amount of fat and fiber eaten could be a factor explaining the high risk of breast cancer in Western countries where a diet high in fat and animal protein is consumed, and the much lower risk of breast cancer in less developed countries where women eat vegetarian or semi vegetarian, low-protein, high-fiber diets. Incidence rates are five to six times higher in North America and Europe than in Asia and Africa, and Caucasians have a much higher rate. Eskimo and Yemenite women almost never get breast cancer; the incidence is also very low in women of Asian descent. For example, Japan has a low breast cancer rate and a low average fat intake, and the United States has a high breast cancer rate and an average diet in which 40 percent of the calories are derived from fat. But if Asians migrate to the West, their incidence rate becomes that of the local population in a few generations.

The mortality from breast cancer is very high in Western Europe, particularly in the Netherlands;

in the United States it is highest in the northern states. For unknown and puzzling reasons, lower mortality rates occur in the southern or southwestern states, and the lowest rate is in Hawaii. Although the curious cultural and sociological factors that appear to be involved in the incidence of breast cancer must be acting through some biological mechanisms, they have not as yet been identified. What underlies the relationship of breast cancer to diet, or to stress, or to lifestyle? There are no definitive answers, but it is known that breast cancer occurs more frequently in affluent women than in poor women. In one group of Indian women, the Parsis of Bombay, the incidence of breast cancer is three times what it is in the Hindu, Muslim, Christian, and Jewish women in India. Parsi women are wealthier and better educated than the rest of the Indian population. When certain groups, such as the Parsi, have a greatly increased incidence, or the Native Americans have a much lower incidence, it would appear that a genetic predisposition or innate resistance to the development of breast cancer may be operating.

cancer have had mixed results so far (Nelson et al., 2009; Humphrey et al., 2002).

Mammography

Mammography is currently the most important diagnostic tool for the early detection of breast cancer (Figure 7-15). Early detection of breast cancer by

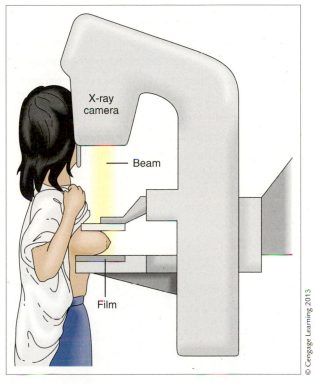

FIGURE 7-15: A mammogram is an X-ray of the breast.

© Cengage Learning 2013

mammograms has reduced the number of deaths in the United States caused by this cancer by 30 percent since 1990 (Kopans, 2010; Margolis, 2010). Mammograms play a major role in the reduction of mortality by detecting a substantial proportion of breast cancers that are too small to be detectable by palpation. The smallest mass or lump that can be felt by palpation during BSE or a clinical breast examination is about 1 cm in diameter. At this small size, a cancer may have been present in the breast for many months or even for several years. Some of these breast cancers are capable of metastasizing to the lymph nodes or to other organs making treatment more difficult. Mammograms can detect smaller tumors at an extremely early stage, when treatment is much more likely to be successful. Mammograms can also be used to determine the exact location of a mass for biopsy or for surgery (Figure 7-16).

A screening mammogram is one used to detect breast changes in women who have no sign of breast cancer. A diagnostic mammogram is used to diagnose a breast change such as a lump, pain, nipple discharge, or change in shape or size of the breast. The American Cancer Society's current recommendations (Smith et al., 2010) for the use of screening mammograms in asymptomatic, apparently healthy women are as follows:

- The basic detection methods for breast cancer are breast self-examination, clinical examination by a healthcare professional, and mammography.

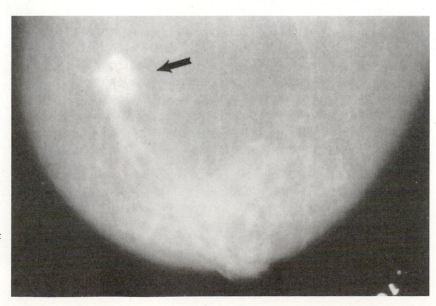

FIGURE 7-16: A film screen mammographic image of a breast with a cancer tumor. *(Courtesy of Dr. John Milbrath, Breast Diagnostic Clinic & Treatment Center, S.C., Milwaukee, WI.)*

- Women 20 years of age and older should perform breast self-examination every month, and women between the ages of 20 and 39 should have a physical examination of the breast by a healthcare professional every 3 years.
- Women 40 years and older should practice breast self-examination, have a clinical breast examination, and have a mammogram annually.

Women with a family history of breast cancer, especially in a mother or sister, have a higher risk and should discuss more frequent screening with their healthcare providers. They may benefit from beginning screening at age 30 instead of age 40 (Lee et al., 2010). Women who have had a previous history of breast cancer and have remaining breast tissue are also at increased risk and should discuss screening schedules with their physician.

Mammography, while valuable, has its limitations. Detecting even a very tiny tumor (less than 1 mm) may not always mean that removing it can result in a cure. A fast-growing or very aggressive cancer may already have spread to other parts of the body such as the bone or lung and be undetectable. Fortunately, this is not usually the case; the earlier the detection, the more likely the survival. A mammogram fails to reveal a breast cancer 10–15 percent of the time, especially in women under age 40, whose denser breasts are harder to evaluate by x-ray (Figure 7-17). Such false-negative reports can lead a woman (and her doctor) to be falsely reassured, even if she has found a lump by BSE.

A false positive occurs when a mammogram is read as abnormal but no cancer is detected with follow up procedures such as additional mammograms, ultrasound, or a biopsy. False positives are

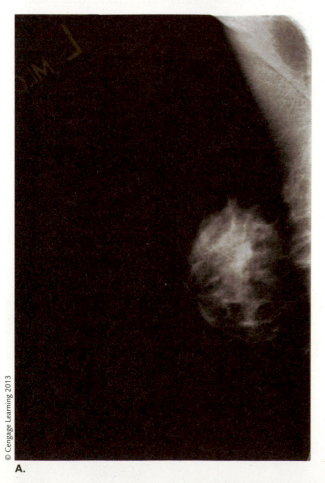

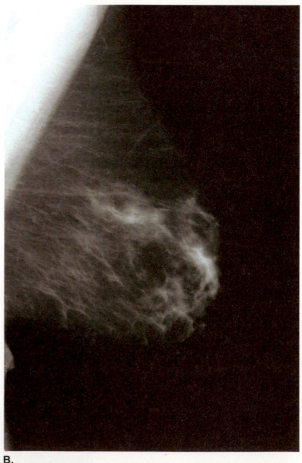

© Cengage Learning 2013

A.

B.

FIGURE 7-17: A. Mammogram of premenstrual breast tissue. B. Mammogram of postmenstrual breast tissue.

Critical Thinking

If it was possible to design an ideal lifetime strategy for maintaining breast health, what would it look like? What factors, considerations, and advice should be included?

more common in younger women. According to the National Cancer Institute, about 97 percent of women between 40 and 49 who have abnormal mammograms do not have cancer, and 86 percent of women age 50 and older with abnormal mammograms do not have cancer. They all undergo follow-up procedures, of course, which can potentially be anxiety provoking and expensive. Some have suggested that routine screening mammograms be postponed until age 50 to avoid false positives and the follow up that they entail (US Preventive Services Task Force, 2009), but these recommendations have not been adopted by the American Cancer Society, and the United States Department of Health and Human Services because postponing mammograms until age 50 would result in an increase in breast cancer deaths. In addition, there is growing concern that the recommendations of the task force were not based on sound scientific evaluation of the available data concerning mammograms and breast cancer (Kopans, 2010).

Ultrasound

With ultrasound, reflected high-frequency sound waves bounce off the various fatty and fibrous tissues of the breast, and are converted electronically for display as images. Sonography is often used to distinguish between a simple fluid-filled benign cyst and a solid tumorous lump (Figure 7-18). Mammograms cannot distinguish between these two types of lumps. In most cases, fluid-filled cysts are not cancerous. However, the cyst may have to be aspirated or drained to see if it contains bloody fluid, which can be a sign of malignancy. Ultrasound can also be used to visualize a lump in the typically denser breast tissues of younger women. A disadvantage of sonography as a screening tool is its inability to find masses smaller than 2 mm, so it is not as sensitive as mammograms. In addition, small calcium deposits, an early sign of cancer on a mammogram, are not visible with ultrasound. Future improvements in equipment may make sonograms more useful as a screening method, as researchers in ultrasound claim that the technique could theoretically pick up very tiny abnormalities.

Biopsy

A biopsy is a tissue or cell sample removed from the suspicious area or lump for a microscopic examination by a pathologist. A surgical biopsy requires a skin incision and removal of the entire lesion together with a zone of normal tissue around it.

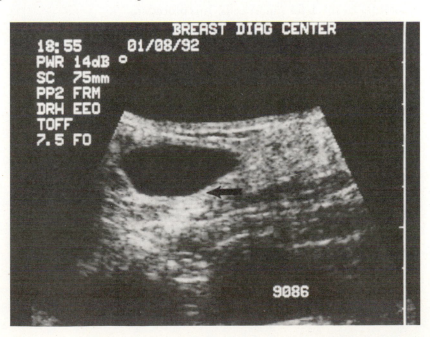

FIGURE 7-18: Ultrasound image of a benign fluid-filled breast cyst. (Courtesy of Dr. John Milbrath, Breast Diagnostic Clinic and Treatment Center, S.C., Milwaukee, WI.)

Case Study

Breast Cancer

Desta is 23 years old. She and her family are recent immigrants from Ethiopia. She is currently enrolled at a community college where she is taking a Biology of Women class. After studying breast cancer, Desta decides to start doing monthly BSE even though she has none of the risk factors. After a few months, she notices a small, irregularly shaped lump that does not move when she presses on it. She would not have noticed this lump if she was not doing BSE because the lump is painless. Desta made an appointment at her local community health clinic to see a nurse practitioner. The nurse practitioner performs a clinical breast exam and orders a mammogram, which reveals an abnormality in Desta's breast. The mammogram cannot determine whether the lump is a cyst or something else, so an ultrasound is ordered. The ultrasound reveals the mass is not a cyst, and Desta is scheduled for a biopsy. Additional testing identifies an aggressive cancer, but one still in the early stages. Desta is frightened about the next steps but acknowledges BSE may have saved her life.

1. What characteristics of the tumor would lead to the suspicion it was cancerous?

2. Why is BSE especially important for younger women?

Biopsies are used to determine whether the tissue is malignant, and if surgery will be needed. A biopsy can also indicate what type of surgery will be required. There are several types of biopsies that can be performed on the breasts (Figure 7-19). A fine-needle aspiration biopsy is performed with a very thin needle to remove a small section of tissue or fluid from a cyst, which will then be examined in a laboratory to check for cancer cells. This procedure is usually performed to distinguish a fluid-filled cyst from a solid mass. Core needle biopsy uses a needle slightly larger in diameter to remove a cylinder of tissue roughly the size of a grain of rice. A stereotactic biopsy is used to take tissues from micro calcifications that show up on a mammogram, but cannot be felt or detected using ultrasound. Biopsies require local anesthesia and often use a mammogram to guide the needle. Surgical biopsy involves removing all or part of a breast lump to determine if it is cancerous. Surgical biopsy is usually performed on an outpatient basis. The accuracy rates for surgical biopsies and needle biopsies are the same, and each has advantages and disadvantages that should be discussed with the doctor. There are a number of factors to be considered—the size of the breast abnormality, its location, and how likely it is to be cancer.

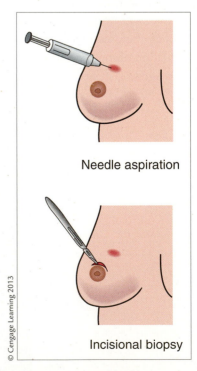

Needle aspiration

Incisional biopsy

© Cengage Learning 2013

FIGURE 7-19: Breast biopsy.

Magnetic Resonance Imaging (MRI)

With magnetic resonance imaging (MRI), a patient lies within a strong magnetic field that creates a composite picture of the interior of the body. Any change from the normal resonance in an organ can then be detected. Breast MRI equipment is specialized and produces higher-quality images than MRI designed for the rest of body scanning. MRI can be used when conventional mammograms are difficult to interpret, and when additional information about the state of a breast is required. It can detect tumors that are too small to be detected by physical exams or mammograms. This method is expensive and creates a large number of false positives, so it is not used for routine screening. The American Cancer Society recommends that women who have a lifetime breast cancer risk of 20 percent or higher have a yearly MRI screening. This would include women who received chest radiation between the ages of 10 and 30, and women with a strong family history of breast cancer. In some cases, women who have recently been diagnosed with breast cancer have an MRI done to check for additional tumors in the breast with the diagnosed lump or in the opposite breast. Several studies have shown that MRI is more sensitive at detecting breast cancer, particularly in women at high risk (Sardanelli et al., 2010; Ravert & Hoffaker, 2010).

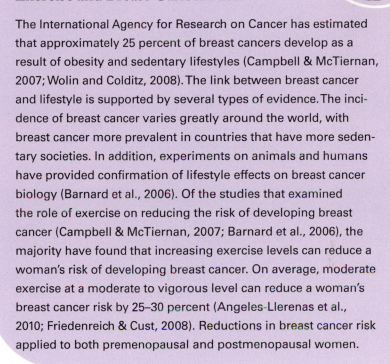

focus on

EXERCISE
Exercise and Breast Cancer Risk

The International Agency for Research on Cancer has estimated that approximately 25 percent of breast cancers develop as a result of obesity and sedentary lifestyles (Campbell & McTiernan, 2007; Wolin and Colditz, 2008). The link between breast cancer and lifestyle is supported by several types of evidence. The incidence of breast cancer varies greatly around the world, with breast cancer more prevalent in countries that have more sedentary societies. In addition, experiments on animals and humans have provided confirmation of lifestyle effects on breast cancer biology (Barnard et al., 2006). Of the studies that examined the role of exercise on reducing the risk of developing breast cancer (Campbell & McTiernan, 2007; Barnard et al., 2006), the majority have found that increasing exercise levels can reduce a woman's risk of developing breast cancer. On average, moderate exercise at a moderate to vigorous level can reduce a woman's breast cancer risk by 25–30 percent (Angeles-Llerenas et al., 2010; Friedenreich & Cust, 2008). Reductions in breast cancer risk applied to both premenopausal and postmenopausal women.

CONCLUSION

An understanding of the anatomy and physiology of the breasts can help women to recognize the changes that occur in their breasts throughout their lifetimes. Breast screening is an important component of maintaining breast health, because it can distinguish benign from potentially cancerous conditions. If a malignancy is found, early detection increases the odds that the treatment can be successful. Chapter 8 will address reproductive system conditions and cancers, including breast cancer.

WEBLINKS

Le Leche League
www.llli.org

American Academy of Pediatrics
**www.aap.org/healthtopics/
breastfeeding.cfm**

REVIEW QUESTIONS

1. Describe the anatomy of a mammary gland.

2. How do the breasts develop and change throughout a lifetime?

3. What are the advantages of breastfeeding? What are some potential obstacles to breast- feeding?

4. What is a fibroadenoma? Which age group is most susceptible to this type of tumor?

5. Describe the symptoms of breast cancer.

6. What screening or diagnostic tools would be used to diagnose breast cancer?

CRITICAL THINKING QUESTIONS

1. Why is breast cancer screening so important?

REFERENCES

Abbas, S., Linseisan, J., & Chang-Claude, J. (2007). Dietary vitamin D and calcium intake and premenopausal breast cancer risk in a German case-control study. *Nutrition and Cancer, 59*(1), 54–61.

American Academy of Family Physicians. (2001). *AAFP policy statement on breastfeeding.* Leawood, KS: American Academy of Family Physicians.

American Academy of Pediatrics. (2001). The transfer of drugs and other chemicals into human milk. *Pediatrics, 108*(3), September 2001.

American Cancer Society. Non-cancerous breast conditions. Retrieved June 16, 2010, from http://www.cancer.org/docroot/CRI/content/CRI_2_6X_Non_Cancerous_Breast_Conditions_59.asp.

American College of Obstetricians and Gynecologists. (2000). Breastfeeding: Maternal and infant aspects (ACOG Educational Bulletin No. 258). Washington, DC: American College of Obstetricians and Gynecologists.

Angeles-Llerenas, A., Ortega-Olvera, C., Perez-Rodriguez, E., Esparza-Cano, J. P., Lazcano-Ponce, E., Romieu, I,, & Torres-Mejfra, G. (2010). Moderate physical activity and breast cancer risk: The effect of menopausal status. *Cancer Causes & Control, 21*(4), 577–586.

Barnard, R. J., Gonzalez, J. H., Liva, M. E., & Ngo, T. H. (2006). Effects of a low-fat, high-fiber diet and exercise program on breast cancer risk factors in vivo and tumor cell growth and apoptosis in vitro. *Nutrition and Cancer, 55*(1), 28–34.

Brinton, L. A., & Brown, S. L. (1997). Breast implants and cancer. *Journal of the National Cancer Institute, 89*(18), 1341–1349.

Brook, M. A. (2006). Platinum in silicone breast implants. *Biomaterials, 27*(17), 3274–3286.

Byers, T., Graham, S. L., Rzepka, T., et al. (1985). Lactation and breast cancer: Evidence for a negative association in premenopausal women. *American Journal of Epidemiology, 121*(5), 664–674.

Campbell, K. L., & McTiernan, A. (2007). Exercise and biomarkers for cancer prevention studies. *Journal of Nutrition, 137*(1 Suppl), 161S–169S.

Chen, J., Power, K. A., Mann, J., Cheng, A., & Thompson, L. U. (2007). Flaxseed alone or in combination with tamoxifen inhibits MCF-7 breast tumor growth in ovariectomized athymic mice with high circulating levels of estrogen. *Experimental Biology and Medicine (Maywood), 232*(8), 1071–1080.

Dunn, R. A., Tan, A., & Samad, I. (2010). Does performance of breast self-exams increase the probability of using mammography: Evidence from Malaysia. *Asian Pacific Journal of Cancer Prevention, 11*(2), 417–421.

Dupont, W. D., & Page, D. L. (1985). Risk factors for breast cancer in women with proliferative breast disease. *New England Journal of Medicine, 312*(3), 146–151.

Early Breast Cancer Trialists' Collaborative Group. (1992). Systemic treatment of early breast cancer by hormonal, cytotoxic, or immune therapy. *Lancet, 339*(8784–8785), 1-15, 71–85.

Ekstrom, A., & Nissen, E. (2006). A mother's feeling for her infant are strengthened by excellent breastfeeding counseling and continuity of care. *Pediatrics, 118*(2), e309–314.

Evans, W. P., Lee, C. H., Monsees, B. S., Monticciolo, D. L., & Rebner, M. (2010). U.S. Preventive Services Task Force: the unbalanced view. *Radiology, 257*(1), 297–298.

Fifty Fourth World Health Assembly. *Global strategy for infant and young feeding: The optimal duration of exclusive breastfeeding.* Geneva, Switzerland: World Health Organization.

Fiorica, J. V. (1994). Fibrocystic changes. *Obstetrics & Gynecology Clinics of North America, 21*(3), 445–452.

Fleming, R. M. (2003). What effect, if any, does soy protein have on breast tissue? *Integrative Cancer Therapies, 2*(3), 225–228.

Friedenreich, C. M., & Cust, A. E. (2008). Physical activity and breast cancer risk: Impact of timing type and dose of activity and population subgroup effects. *British Journal of Sports Medicine, 42*(8), 636–647.

Gartner, L. M., Morton, J., Lawrence, R. A., Naylor, A. J., O'Hare, D., Schanler, R. J., Eidelman, A. I., & American Academy of Pediatrics Section on Breastfeeding. (2005). Breastfeeding and the use of human milk. *Pediatrics, 115*(2), 496–506.

Harbor, V., Harbor, A., Copptoiu, C., & Pantiru, A. (2010). Fibrocystic breast disease-breast cancer sequence. *Chirurgia (Bucur), 105*(2), 191–194.

Hedelin, M., Lof, M., Osson, M., Adlercreutz, H., Sandin, S., & Weiderpass, E. (2008). Dietary phytoestrogens are not associated with risk of overall breast cancer but diets rich in coumestrol are inversely associated with risk of estrogen receptor and progesterone receptor negative breast tumors in Swedish women. *Journal of Nutrition, 138*(5), 938–945.

Helewa, M., Levesque, P., Provencher, D., Lea, R. H., Rosolowich, V., Shapiro, H. M., & Breast Disease Committee and Executive Committee and Council, Society of Obstetricians and Gynaecologists of Canada. (2002). Breast cancer, pregnancy, and breastfeeding. *Journal of Obstetrics and Gynaecology Canada, 24*(2), 164-180, 181–184.

Holmes, M. D., Hunter, D. J., Colditz, G. A., et al. (1999). Association of dietary intake of fat and fatty acids with risk of breast cancer. *Journal of the American Medical Association, 281,* 914–920.

Howe, G. R., Hirhata, T., Hislop, G. T., et al. (1990). Dietary factors and the risk of breast cancer: Combined analysis of 12 case control studies. *Journal of the National Cancer Institute, 82*(7), 561–569.

Humphrey, L., Chan, B. K. S., Detlefsen, S., & Helfand, M. (2002). Screening for Breast Cancer [Internet]. Rockville, MD: Agency for Healthcare Research and Quality, US Preventive Services Task Force Evidence Synthesis, formerly Systematic Evidence Reviews.

Hurley, K. M., Black, M. M., Papas, M. A., & Quigg, A. M. (2008). Variation in breastfeeding behaviors, perceptions, and experiences by race/ethnicity among a low-income statewide sample of special supplemental nutrition programs for women, infants and children (WIC) participants in the United States. *Maternal & Child Nutrition, 4*(2), 95–105.

Hutchins, A. M., Martini, M. C., Olson, B. A., Thomas, W., & Slavin, J. L. (2001). Flaxseed consumption influences endogenous hormone concentrations in postmenopausal women. *Nutrition and Cancer, 39*(1), 58–65.

International Agency for Research on Cancer, World Health Organization. (2002). *IARC handbooks of cancer prevention: Weight control and physical activity* (Vol. 6). Lyon, France: Author.

Ip, S., Chung, M., Ramen, G., Chew, P., Magula, N., De Vine, D., Trikalinos, T., & Lau, J. (2007). Breastfeeding and maternal and infant health outcomes in developed countries. *Evidence Report/Technology Assessment* (No. 153).

James, D. C., Lessen, R., & American Dietetic Association. (2009). Position of the American Dietetic Association: Promoting and supporting breastfeeding. *Journal of the American Dietetic Association, 109*(11), 1926–1942.

Kopans, D. B. (2009). The 2009 US Preventative Services Task Force guidelines ignore important scientific evidence and should be revised or withdrawn. *Radiology. 256*(1), 15–20.

Kramer, M. S., & Kakuma, R. (2002). Optimal duration of exclusive breast feeding. *Cochrane Database Systematic Review,* (1), CD003517.

Krebs, N. F., Jacobson, M. S., & American Academy of Pediatrics Committee on Nutrition. (2003). Prevention of pediatric overweight and obesity. *Pediatrics, 112*(2), 424–430.

Lee, C. H., Dershaw, D. D., Kopans, D., Evans, P., Monsees, B., Monticciolo, D., Brenner, R. J., Bassett, L., Berg, W., Feig, S., Hendrick, E., Mendelson, E., D'Orsi, C., Sickles, E., & Burhenne, L, W. (2010). Breast cancer screening with imaging: Recommendations from the Society of Breast Imaging and the ACR on the use of mammography, breast MRI, breast ultrasound, and other technologies for the detection of clinically occult breast cancer. *Journal of the American College of Radiology, 7*(1), 18–27.

Lee, J. H., & Zuckerman, D. (2002). Silicon, silicone, and breast implants. *Pediatrics, 110*(5), 1030.

Leis, H. P., Cammarata, A., LaRaja, R., & Cruz, E. (1983). Fibrocystic breast disease. *Female Patient, 8,* 56–77.

Lin, J., Manson, J. E., Lee, I. M., Cook, N. R., Buring, J. E., & Zhang, S. M. (2007). Intakes of calcium and vitamin D and breast cancer risk in women. *Archives of Internal Medicine, 167*(10), 1050–1059.

London, R. S., Solomon, D. M., & London, E. D. (1978). Mammary dysplasia: Clinical response and urinary excretion of 11-deoxy-17-ketosteroids and pregnanediol following alphatocopherol therapy. *Breast, 4,* 19.

London, R. S., Sundaram, G. S., & Goldstein, P. J. (1982). Medical management of mammary dysplasia. *Obstetrics and Gynecology, 59*(4), 519–523.

London, R. S., Sundaram, G. S., Murphy, L., et al. (1985). The effect of vitamin E on mammary dysplasia: A double-blind study. *Obstetrics and Gynecology, 65*(1), 104–106.

London, S. J., Connolly, J. L., Schnitt, S. J., et al. (1992). A prospective study of benign breast disease and the risk of breast cancer. *Journal of the American Medical Association, 267*(7), 941–944.

Love, S. (1995). *Dr. Susan Love's breast book* (2nd ed.). Reading, MA: Addison-Wesley Longman.

Lykissa, E. D., & Maharaj, S. V. (2006). Total platinum concentration and platinum oxidation states in body fluids, tissues, and explants from women exposed to silicone and saline breast implants by IC-ICPMS. *Analytical Chemistry, 78*(9), 2925–2933.

Maharaj, S. V. (2007). Exposure dose and significance of platinum and platinum salts in breast implants. *Archives of Environmental and Occupational Health, 62*(3), 139–146.

Marcus, J. A. (2008, May/June). Pumping 9 to 5. *Mothering.* Retrieved March 31, 2009, from http://www.mothering.com/articles/new_baby/ breastfeeding/pumping-9-to-5.html.

Mardaleishvili, K. G., Nemsadze, G. G., Metreveli, D. S., & Roinishvili, T. L. (2006). About correlation of dysfunction of the thyroid gland with fibrocystic diseases in women. *Georgian Medical News,* (140), 30–32.

Margolies, L. (2010). Mammographic screening for breast cancer: 2010. *Mount Sinai Journal of Medicine, 77*(4), 398–404.

McCullough, M. L., Rodriguez, C., Diver, W. R., Feigelson, H. S., Stevens, V. L., Thun, M. J., & Calle, E. E. (2005). Dairy, calcium, and vitamin D intake and postmenopausal breast cancer risk in the Cancer Prevention Study II Nutrition Cohort. *Cancer Epidemiology, Biomarkers & Prevention, 14*(12), 2898–2904.

McLaughlan, P., & Coombs, R. R. (1983). Latent anaphylactic sensitivity of infants to cow's milk proteins. Histamine release from blood basophils. *Clinical & Experimental Allergy, 13*(1), 1–9.

McTiernan, A., & Thomas, D. B. (1986). Evidence for a protective effect of lactation on risk of breast cancer in young women. *American Journal of Epidemiology, 121*(3), 353–358.

Minton, J. P., Foecking, M. K., & Webster, D. J. (1979b). Response of fibrocystic disease to caffeine withdrawal and correlation of cyclic nucleotides with breast disease. *American Journal of Obstetrics and Gynecology, 135,* 147–149.

Minton, J. P., Foecking, M. K., Webster, D. J., et al. (1979a). Caffeine, cyclic nucleotides and breast disease. *Surgery, 86,* 105–109.

Mofenson, L. M. (2010). Prevention in neglected subpopulations: Prevention of mother-to-child transmission of HIV infection. *Clinical Infectious Diseases, 50* Suppl 3, S130–148.

Morrison, A. S. (1990). Is self-examination effective in screening for breast cancer? *Journal of the National Cancer Institute, 83*(4), 226–227.

Nelson, H. D., Tyne, K., Naik, A., Bougatsos, C., Chan, B., Nygren, P., & Humphrey, L. (2009). Screening for breast cancer: Systematic evidence review update for the US Preventive Services Task Force. Rockville, MD: Agency for Healthcare Research and Quality (US).

Newcomb, P. A., Weiss, N. S., Storer, B. E., et al. (1991). Breast self-examination in relation to the occurrence of advanced breast cancer. *Journal of the National Cancer Institute, 83*(4), 260–265.

Norlock, F. E. (2002). Benign breast pain in women: A practical approach to evaluation and treatment. *Journal of the American Medical Women's Association, 57*(2), 85–90.

Oezaras, G., Durualp, E., Civelek, F. E., Gul, B., & Uensal, M. (2010). Analysis of breast self-examination training efficiency in women between 20-60 years of age in Turkey. *Asian Pacific Journal of Cancer Prevention, 1*(3), 799–802.

Pan, I. J., Daniels, J. L., Herring, A. H., Rogan, W. J., Siega-Riz, A. M., Goldman, B. D., & Sjodin, A. (2010). Lactational exposure to polychlorinated biphenyls, dichlorodiphenyltrichloroethane and dichlorodiphenyltrichloroethylene and infant growth: An analysis of pregnancy, infection, and nutrition babies study. *Paediatric and Perinatal Epidemiology, 24*(3), 262–271.

Pearlstein, T. (2008). Perinatal depression: Treatment options and dilemmas. *Journal of Psychiatry & Neuroscience, 33*(4), 302–318.

Power, K. A., & Thompson, L. U. (2007). Can a combination of flaxseed and its lignans with soy and its isoflavones reduce the growth stimulatory effect of soy and its isoflavones on established

breast cancer? *Molecular Nutrition & Food Research, 51*(7), 845–856.

Ravert, P. K., & Huffaker, C. (2010). Breast cancer screening in women: An integrative literature review. *Journal of the American Academy of Nurse Practitioners, 22*(12), 668–673.

Reynolds, F. (2010). The effects of maternal labour analgesia on the fetus. *Best Practices & Research: Clinical Obstetrics & Gynaecology, 24*(3), 289–302.

Rosolowich, V., Saettler, E., Szuck, B., Lea, R. H., Levesque, P., Weisberg, F., Graham, J., McLeod, L., Rosolowich, V., & Society of Obstetricians and Gynecologists of Canada. (2006). Mastalgia. *Journal of Obstetrics and Gynaecology Canada, 28*(1), 49–71.

Saarinen, N. M., Power, K. A., Chen, J., & Thompson, L. U. (2006). Flaxseed attenuates the tumor growth stimulating effect of soy protein in ovariectomized athymic mice with MCF-7 human breast cancer xenographs. *International Journal of Cancer, 119*(4), 925–931.

Saarinen, N. M., Power, K. A., Chen, J., & Thompson, L. U. (2008). Lignans are accessible to human breast cancer xenographs in athymic mice. *Nutrition and Cancer, 60*(2), 245–250.

Sardanelli, F., Podo, F., Santoro, F., Manoukian, S., Bergonzi, S., Trecate, G., Vergnaghi, D., Federico, M., Cortesi, L., Corcione, S., Morassut, S., Di Maggio, C., Cilotti, A., Martincich, L., Calabrese, M., Zuiani, C., Preda, L., Bonanni, B., Carbonaro, L. A., Contegiacomo, A., Panizza, P., Di Cesare, E., Savarese, A., Crecco, M., Turchetti, D., Tonutti, M., Belli, P., & Maschio, A. D. (2010). Multicenter surveillance of women at high genetic breast cancer risk using mammography, ultrasonography, and contrast-enhanced magnetic resonance imaging (the High Breast Cancer Risk Italian 1 Study): Final results. *Investigative Radiology.*

Semple, J. L. (2007). Breast-feeding and silicone implants. *Plastic and Reconstructive Surgery, 120*(7 Suppl 1), 123S–128S.

Shirley, S. E. (1999). Beyond fibrocystic disease. The evolving concept of pre-malignant breast disease. *West Indian Medical Journal, 48*(4), 173–178.

Singhal, A., Kennedy, K., Lanigan, J., Clough, H., Jenkins, W., Elias-Jones, A., Stephenson, T.,

Dudek, P., Lucas, A., & Childhood Nutritional Research Center, Institute of Child Health. (2010). Dietary nucleotides and early growth in formula fed infants: A randomized controlled trial. *Pediatrics, 126*(4), e946–953.

Smith, D. (1999). Worldwide trends in DDT levels in human breast milk. *International Journal of Epidemiology, 28,* 179–188.

Smith, R. A., Cokkinides, V., Brooks, D., Daslow, D., & Brawley, O. W. (2010). Cancer screening in the United States, 2010: A review of current American Cancer Society guidelines and issues in cancer screening. *CA: A Cancer Journal for Clinicians, 60*(2), 99–119.

Stuebe, A. (2009). The risks of not breastfeeding for mothers and infants. *Reviews in Obstetrics and Gynecology, 2*(4), 222–231.

Suzuki, R., Rylander-Rudqvist, T., Ye, W., Saji, S., Adlercreutz, H., & Wolk, A. (2008). Dietary fiber intake and risk of postmenopausal breast cancer defined by estrogen and progesterone receptor status—A prospective cohort study among Swedish women. *International Journal of Cancer, 122*(2), 403–412.

Touillaud, M. S., Thiebaut, A. C., Fournier, A., Niravong, M., Boutron-Ruault, M. C., & Clavel-Chapelon, F. (2007). Dietary lignan intake and postmenopausal breast cancer risk by estrogen and progesterone receptor status. *Journal of the National Cancer Institute, 99*(6), 475–486.

United Nations Children's Fund. (1999). *Breastfeeding: Foundation for a healthy future.* New York, NY: Author.

Wolin, K. Y., & Colditz, G. A. (2008). Can weight loss prevent cancer? *British Journal of Cancer, 99*(7), 995–999.

World Health Organization. (2007). First food first. Retrieved from http://www.who.int/nutrition/topics/world_breastfeeding_week/en/index.html.

Zoccali, G., Lomartire, N., Mascaretti, G., & Giuliani, M. (2008). Silicone gel mammary prosthesis: Immune pathologies and breast feeding. *Clinical & Experimental Obstetrics & Gynecology, 35*(3), 187–189.

Zuckerman, D. (1999). No end to breast-implant controversy. *Network News, National Women's Health Network, 24*(2), 1–2.

chapter 8

CANCERS AND OTHER DISEASES OF THE REPRODUCTIVE SYSTEM

CHAPTER COMPETENCIES

Upon completion of this chapter, the reader will be able to:

- Identify the major gynecological pathologies that affect women
- Explain prevention methods for reproductive pathologies

- Explain treatment options for reproductive pathologies

KEY TERMS

carcinoma	fibroids	polycystic ovarian	prolapse
dysplasia	mastectomy	syndrome	vulvodynia
endometriosis	ovarian cyst	(PCOS)	

INTRODUCTION

That collection of illnesses that once fell under the euphemistic category of "female complaints" encompasses a range of conditions affecting the cervix, uterus, ovaries, and breasts. In the 1800s, diseases of the reproductive system were blamed on everything from poor diet to emotional stress. In turn, the uterus was considered the cause of hysteria and diseases of the nervous system (Hayes, 1869). The symptoms of some reproductive system pathologies are difficult to pinpoint, and, because there are often not obvious, external symptoms, it can be easy to deny anything is wrong (Figure 8-1). Structural abnormalities, endometriosis, and ovarian cysts often produce no symptoms or vague "discomfort" rather than a localized pain. Cancers affecting reproductive organs can go undiagnosed for years. Unfortunately, denial will not make these conditions go away. The National Cancer Institute predicts that in 2010, over 4000 American women will die from cervical cancer, 21,000 American women will be diagnosed with ovarian cancer, and over 40,000 American women will be diagnosed with uterine cancer (National Cancer Institute).

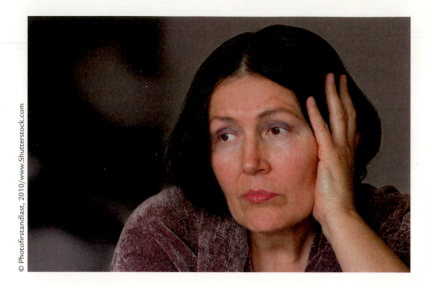

© Photofirstandlast, 2010/www.Shutterstock.com

FIGURE 8-1: Reproductive diseases can be difficult to visually assess and often have limited external symptoms. They often cause vague discomfort that women ignore or deny, leading to a more progressed disease when it is diagnosed.

Many factors can contribute to the development of reproductive system pathologies. Development may depend on an interplay between genes and steroid hormones. Mutations in two specific genes, BRCA1 and BRCA2, are implicated in both breast and ovarian cancer (NCI, 2010). Other genes are under investigation for their possible role in altering normal growth and function of the reproductive organs. Estrogen—either natural or synthetic—can encourage the growth of breast and endometrial cancer, particularly in association with the gene mutations (NCI, 2010). Environmental exposure to chemicals may also be a factor. Endocrine disruptors, chemicals that mimic naturally occurring steroids in the body, have been implicated in breast cancer (Bidgoli et al., 2010) and the growth of uterine fibroids (Gao et al., 2010). By identifying and minimizing her risk factors, recognizing symptoms, and getting regular testing, a woman can reduce her chances of developing reproductive system diseases.

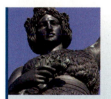

Historical Considerations
THE CAUSE OF FEMALE COMPLAINTS

Before the advent of modern diagnostic equipment, a variety of causes were blamed for diseases of the female reproductive system. The uterus was considered to be a highly "impressionable" organ, subject to damage from external events. Explanations for reproductive disorders ranged from warm weather, living in a large city, or eating a rich diet, to emotional conditions such as jealousy, an unhappy love life, and too much excitement. Singing, dancing, and carriage rides could cause the "womb to drop", a condition now called uterine prolapse. Even the "morbid emotions" caused by reading novels took some blame for uterine disorders. Many of the constraints put on young women during the eighteenth and nineteenth century were explained as an attempt to protect them from damaging their reproductive organs. Yet even by the mid-1800s, some physicians recognized the possibility of congenital causes as well as the impact of infection and frequent pregnancy or abortion rather than strong emotions as the cause of damage to the cervix or uterus and the surrounding tissue (Hayes, 1869). However, the unsubstantiated idea that the uterus was damaged by sports and emotion remained common into the 1970s and is still an explanation in some parts of the world.

IDENTIFICATION OF CERVICAL PATHOLOGIES

In its position at the base of the uterus, the cervix is in contact with the vaginal normal flora, as well as with potential pathogens. The condition of the cervix gives hints about the condition of the uterus and can indicate benign polyps, infections, or cancer. Identification of changes to the cervix is most commonly identified using a Pap smear, also called a Pap test.

The Pap Smear

In 1928, George Papanicolaou, first described the use of the vaginal smear for the diagnosis of early cervical cancer. His staining technique for cervical and vaginal cells forms the basis of the Pap smear, a test that is used to identify cervical cancer, inflammation, and infections. Use of the test has lead to a steady decrease in the number of deaths from cervical cancer through early diagnosis and identification of precancerous cells. A woman should discuss with her healthcare provider how frequently she needs a Pap smear. The current recommendations for most women are to test once every three years after becoming sexually active or starting at age 21 (NCI, 2010). Abnormal results may indicate a need for more frequent testing.

A woman should not have the sample taken during her period because the menstrual flow may interfere with the test results.

To perform the test, cells from the cervical canal are sampled using a small brush or swab (Figure 8-2). The swab may be smeared onto a glass slide. The smear is immediately "fixed" to prevent deterioration of the cells by spraying it with a commercial fixative or by dropping the slide into a solution of 95 percent ethyl alcohol. The cells are later stained and examined microscopically for malignant changes. Another technique involves adding the cells to a vial of fixative solution which is sent to the lab for analysis. Some labs use a computer-automated reader to initially screen samples. Abnormal slides are examined by a pathologist and any abnormal or precancerous cells, known as **dysplasia,** can be identified. The precancerous growths can then be removed before they progress to cancer.

An abnormal Pap test does not necessarily mean that a woman has cervical cancer, only that some of the cells are atypical and should be investigated further. The Pap test is the best kind of preventive medicine; if all women were screened, deaths from invasive cancer of the cervix could be prevented. However, only 82 percent of American women had a

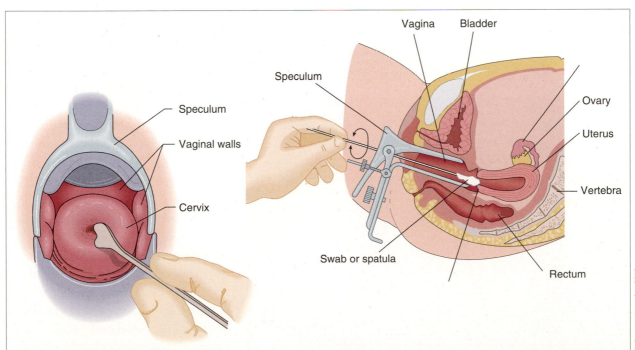

FIGURE 8-2: A pap smear for sampling cervical cells.

© Cengage Learning 2013

Pap smear in 2003 (Swan et al., 2003). In 2005, that number dropped to 78 percent (NCI, 2010), a trend in the wrong direction if cervical cancer deaths are to be reduced. Access to affordable healthcare could reverse this trend.

CERVICAL CANCER

Symptoms of cervical cancer include vaginal bleeding not associated with menstruation, pelvic pain, unusual vaginal discharge, and pain during intercourse. However, a lack of symptoms does not mean there is not a problem. Cervical cancer often has no symptoms, particularly in the early stages. A study of 9657 women who received screenings for cervical cancer between 2003 and 2005 found the greatest incidence of HPV infection was in women ages 14–19 (Datta et al., 2008).

Most cervical cancers begin in the transformation zone of the squamocolumnar junction, where the cells have the ability to differentiate into squamous or columnar cells. More than 90 percent of cervical cancer is squamous cell carcinoma on the outside of the cervix; the rest are malignancies of the glandular columnar cells of the endocervical canal.

Cervical intraepithelial neoplasia (CIN) is the first abnormality in the normal squamous epithelium of the vaginal cervix that may evolve into invasive cancer (Figure 8-3). It means that there are atypical cells, some with multiple nuclei. According to the numbers of atypical cells, CIN is characterized as very mild or mild (CIN-I or Grade 1) dysplasia, moderate

(CIN-II or Grade 2) dysplasia, and severe (CIN-III or Grade 3) dysplasia and carcinoma in situ, depending upon how much of the epithelium is involved in the proliferation of the abnormal cells. Cases of dysplasia may regress and return to normal epithelium, but the likelihood of regression is decreased as the number of atypical cells increases. **Carcinoma** in situ (CIS), literally "cancer in place", is the next stage in progression with the entire thickness of the epithelial cell layer involved. This stage is still a superficial condition, considered noninvasive because the abnormality has not broken through the epithelium into the connective tissue lying underneath. Dysplasia and carcinoma in situ are currently referred to as cervical intraepithelial neoplasia (CIN), with the implication that once CIN is diagnosed, there is the capability for progression to invasion if it is untreated. Long term studies show that 30–70 percent of untreated cases will progress to invasive cancer.

Cervical cancer is usually slow growing, and can take 10 or more years to develop. It first appears as a mild abnormality of atypical cells, which progresses through a series of intermediate stages, each more atypical than the last. Some of these early stages have the ability to return to normal or may remain stable without further progression toward cancer for an indefinite period. Even if left untreated, an area of abnormality does not inevitably become cancerous. The Pap test, however, detects abnormal cells when they are pre-invasive, and the possible evolution to cancer can be stopped.

Because there may be no visible difference between a normal cervix and one with CIN, the Schiller test can be utilized to aid in defining the suspicious area that should be biopsied after a positive Pap smear report. The Schiller test is based on the difference in color of normal cervical epithelium cells and cancerous cells when stained with a three percent potassium iodide solution. Abnormal cells metabolize differently and remain unstained, appearing white or yellow against the background of normal cells which stain dark brown. Once suspicious cells have been identified, a sample of tissue can be biopsied.

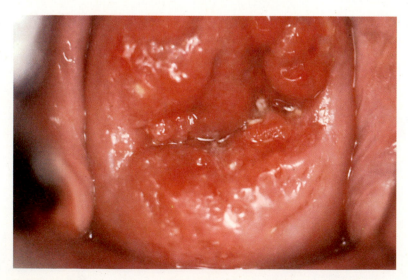

FIGURE 8-3: Early cervical cancer with a cervical erosion. *(Courtesy of CDC)*

The most common method of investigating an abnormal Pap smear is by conization, which removes a cone-shaped section of diseased tissue. The operation is associated with a number of postoperative complications, unless the cone is shallow. However, a shallow sample may not provide the pathologist with enough tissue to rule out invasive cancer. When the cone is deep and extends up into the endocervical canal, damage to the internal os and the canal itself is not uncommon. The subsequent scarring can threaten a woman's ability to conceive and deliver a child. Another procedure, LEEP (loop electrosurgical excision procedure) uses a thin wire and an electrical current to remove abnormal tissue. LEEP allows the abnormal tissue to be excised as a button-shaped specimen rather than to be vaporized by a laser beam. The intact tissue can serve as the biopsy specimen that can be sent to the laboratory for examination for invasive cancer. Like a cone biopsy, LEEP can prevent the development of invasive disease but may produce cervical scarring.

Invasive Cancer of the Cervix

If the abnormal cells have spread beyond the cervical epithelium, the cancer is considered invasive. The cancer is staged based on the TNM categories. The "T" refers to how far the tumor has spread and range from T0 with no invasion to T4 in which the tumor has spread far enough into the pelvic cavity to invade the bladder or colon. The "N" describes the lymph node involvement. N0 means no nodes in the area of the tumor are involved. N1 indicates the cancer cells have moved into the nearby nodes. The "M" designation refers to distant metastases, how far the cancer has spread. M0 indicates the tumor has not metastasized. M1 indicates it has spread beyond the reproductive system. The American Joint Committee on Cancer (AJCC) defines the stage of the cancer based on the TNM categories with Stage I designated as T1N0M0 (cancer is limited to the cervix and uterus) up to Stage IVB defined as any T, any N, M1 (cancer has metastasized) (AJCC, 2002).

Prevention of Cervical Cancer

The prevention of cervical cancer has become one of the success stories. The approval in 2007 of Gardasil, a vaccine which protects against four strains of HVP

Critical Thinking

Should Cervical Cancer Vaccines Be Required?

Most cases of cervical cancer are caused by the human papilloma virus (HPV), and there is now a vaccine that protects women from the virus. As a result, some states are considering laws that mandate cervical cancer vaccinations for all young girls as part of the regular vaccination schedule required for school. The vaccine is effective only before exposure to the virus. The intention is to vaccinate girls while they are still in elementary school, before they were likely to become sexually active, so that they will be protected from future infection with HPV. Some groups are concerned that vaccinating girls will require explaining about STIs and sex before the girls are old enough. They argue that it could encourage promiscuity and over stepped the boundary between State and parental rights. Should the cervical cancer vaccine be required? If so, at what age?

which are linked to 70 percent of all cervical cancers, should prevent vaccinated women from developing the disease. However, not all cases of cervical cancer are caused by the HPV virus. Pap smears combined with HPV testing can identify 90 percent of cervical cancers at the early, most treatable stages (NCI, 2010). Annual Pap smears are recommended for women who are at high risk for cervical cancer. Some of the risk factors for cervical cancer include cigarette smoking, having sexual partners, and having sexual intercourse before age 20. These factors are consistent with the epidemiological evidence associating cervical cancer with a sexually transmitted virus. Women who are celibate or in a mutually monogamous relationship, are nonsmokers, or have had a total hysterectomy for benign disease are at low risk for cervical cancer. A woman's decision on the frequency of her Pap smears should take into account her own risk status for cervical cancer.

The Hunt for the Cause of Cervical Cancer

Cervical cancer is found almost exclusively in women who have been sexually active, and the more partners a woman has had, the higher her risk of developing the disease. That pattern hinted that cervical cancer was associated with an infection. Various STIs were explored as possible causes. In 1981, Meisels et al. identified atypical, flat, genital warts on the cervix that were almost indistinguishable from very early carcinoma of the cervix. Another researcher Reid (1982) presented data for the association of genital warts caused by human papilloma virus and cervical cancer. Based on epidemiologic evidence in the early 1980s, however, that women with cervical cancer had higher serum levels of antibodies to genital herpes simplex virus (HSV), than did control women, it was theorized that HSV caused cervical cancer. However, additional epidemiological studies found no relationship between the presence of antibodies to HSV-2 and the development of cervical cancer (Vonka et al., 1984; Adam et al., 1985). With doubt cast on the connection between herpes and cervical cancer, interest in the human papilloma virus (HPV) as a causative agent in cervical cancer was renewed.

There are many different strains of HPV and not all are associated with cervical cancer. Identifying the virus strains associated with cervical cancer has allowed for the development of vaccines. The first vaccine was approved in 2007. Another, which targets only strains 16 and 18, is currently going through testing. In women with no prior viral exposure, both vaccines provided protection for up to five years in 90 percent of cases (Cutts et al., 2007). HPV Types 6, 11, 16, 18, 31, 33, 35, 40, and 58 have now been linked to cervical cancer (Ferreira, 2008), but are not included in any current vaccine.

Treatment of Cervical Cancer

Treatment options for cervical cancer involve surgery, radiation, and chemotherapy and depend on the stage of the cancer. Early in 1999, the National Cancer Institute released a clinical statement for physicians announcing that the results of five randomized Phase III trials indicated that concurrent chemotherapy along with radiation conferred an overall survival advantage in women with advanced cervical cancer. Analysis of the data from several studies has indicated that the combination of chemotherapy and radiation produced better survival rates than radiation alone, reducing deaths by up to 50 percent (Vale et al., 2008). The use of brachytherapy involves implanting small radioactive seeds directly into tumors. It is also successful for treating tumors that have invaded the uterus (Leung, 2008).

NON-CANCEROUS CERVICAL ABNORMALITIES

While cervical cancer is the most recognized abnormality of the cervix, several other conditions can also be detected during a gynecological exam. Inflammation, erosions, and polyps are the most common of these abnormalities.

Cervical Inflammation (Cervicitis)

Chronic cervicitis, which is an inflammation of the cervix, indicates the presence of a chronic, low-grade infection and is usually caused by *Candida,* STIs, or irritation from a contraceptive. Women with chronic cervicitis may complain of backache, feelings of urgency and frequent urination, and spotting or bleeding after intercourse. Acute cervicitis is a more defined infection, accompanied by vaginal inflammation and fever. The cervix becomes red and swollen. The swelling can obstruct the openings of some endocervical glands which produce mucus. The cervical mucus continues to accumulate but has no way of exiting the gland and forms small round bumps or nabothian cysts. The treatment of cervicitis is accomplished by treating the specific organism that is causing the infection.

Cervical Erosions

Cervical erosions are patches of the red columnar epithelium of the endocervical canal that have shifted

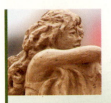

Economic Considerations
CANCER ON A BUDGET

Marie was 51 when she was diagnosed with stage II cervical cancer. A yoga instructor who followed a vegetarian diet and relied on homeopathic treatments for minor ailments, Marie had interpreted her symptoms merely as signs of menopause. Cancer wasn't on her mind, even though she had just devoted two months of the previous year to move home and provide daily end-of-life care for her father who died of cancer. But now she was back at home working on her Ph.D. again. Like many students, she relied on part-time work and student loans to support herself. She had never owned a home, and she always bought used cars, so she had no assets on which to draw. And like 24 percent of Americans aged 18–64, she had no health insurance (American Cancer Society, 2009). This diagnosis meant that she would become quickly familiar with California's medical safety net.

She initially went for a blood test in order to have work done on a tooth. But the test revealed more and after repeated examinations, blood tests, and a D and C, doctors were able to give her a diagnosis. Her cancer involved a tumor the size of a tennis ball and it would require chemotherapy in addition to 32 external and four internal radiation treatments. It was October 13. Still exhausted from the heavy bleeding and cramping she had thought were menopause symptoms, and now frightened by her diagnosis, she began the application process for CSMP, California State Medical Program. Proving that she was "indigent" was trickier than she imagined it would be. In addition to being a full-time student, she worked 25 hours a week doing clerical tasks for a local church, and that income just barely covered her monthly expenses for rent, food, and car insurance. But even that scant income put her over the guideline for assistance. How was she going to continue to pay the rent and keep the car running to get to treatment sessions across town AND qualify for medical help? She began to fill out the three-inch stack of application papers. She had been told that there would be no treatment until all of the papers cleared.

About 11,000 women are diagnosed with cervical cancer each year (American Cancer Society, 2009). And in the early 2000s when Marie was treated, direct medical costs to those with cancer similar to hers averaged $6,373 per month (Chang et al., 2004). Marie's prognosis for full recovery was good, but 40 very expensive chemotherapy and concurrent radiation treatments stood between her and restored health. It was a frightening time, and she was at a loss for strategies to negotiate the CSMP requirements. A sympathetic worker finally said, "If I had a friend in this situation, here's what I'd advise her to do…" Marie negotiated with her employer to reduce her wages and instead pay her rent directly to the landlord. She emailed friends and family asking them to cover added costs directly, paying for gasoline, food, and other necessities.

And then she waited for the papers to clear. Marie hadn't used traditional medicine for years, so this wait was even more stressful. She had always relied on homeopathic remedies, acupuncture, and the benefits of a fresh, vegetarian diet, exercise, and not smoking or drinking in order to stay healthy. And now she stood at the edge of the huge medical complex that would take on her cancer. She didn't yet know that, in addition to treatment costs, she would need several blood transfusions, intravenous iron and erythropoietin infusions for severe anemia, ambulance calls, and expensive shots to raise her white blood count…and on and on. The bill for the diagnostic hospital stay (one night) and D and C surgery had just arrived and it was already frighteningly large.

It was November 24 when the radiation treatments finally began, with chemotherapy starting a few days later. Through the next few months, Marie kept working, attended all of her classes, and drove

(continued)

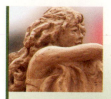

Economic Considerations (*continued*)
CANCER ON A BUDGET

herself to almost all of the treatments. A few weeks into the treatments, a classmate insisted on preparing meals for Marie and brought a week's supply of vegetarian fare each Sunday. What a gift! Friends near and far paid her acupuncturist to keep treating her for the side effects. And the holidays came and went.

In January, it was time for the four brachytherapy (internal radiation) treatments. These involved inserting a mesh of needles into her cervix, packing her vagina tightly, and immobilizing her entire body for the treatment, on four separate occasions. It was an intense time, and Marie was trying to keep up her strength to be able to work and continue classes. At one point, she passed out at home in her bathroom. When she regained consciousness, she crawled to the living room and called 911. The apartment, in the upstairs of a large house, was locked. The dispatcher asked if there were any windows that were accessible—the bathroom window wasn't latched. So the emergency workers climbed through the second floor bathroom window to find Marie on the floor a few feet from the phone. The bill for that rescue was even more shocking than the rescue itself. And during all of this time, the bills kept coming, with statements at the bottom of each bill saying, "If you fail to cooperate with the social service agency, you will be responsible for paying your bill in full", or even worse "We have no record of your medical application. Please contact this office immediately."

On January 18, the treatments were finally over and she had survived it all. It wasn't until February 20, her first follow-up visit, when Marie knew the treatments had been successful. Relief, gratitude! But the bills were still coming. A March 4th statement for a portion of January's treatments was $13,184.84. The CSMP workers kept saying it's okay, it's covered; just keep the statements for your records. And then came the letters from the collection agency—a glitch in the paperwork had sent her account there. The collection agency letter threatened to send a negative credit report to a credit agency if she didn't pay immediately. This particular notice was in error for Marie, but it points to a larger issue.

The cost of cancer treatment and the stress of covering that cost add to the already huge burden of cancer itself. A 2008 survey by Thomson Reuters revealed a "clear link between patients' annual income and their decisions to curb cancer treatment due to cost." Even late-stage cancer patients are passing up recommended treatment because it's too expensive. And nearly all cancer patients are distressed by the out-of-pocket costs of treatment (Thomson Reuters, 2008). The American Cancer Society estimates that Americans spent $93.2 billion in direct medical costs associated with cancer in 2008 (American Cancer Society, 2009, Costs of Cancer). But that figure only includes what was spent. Untreated cancer has a cost, too. Marie was fortunate enough to fall into California's medical safety net. What about all the others who also have cancer but who do not qualify?

position and extend out beyond their normal position to replace the paler squamous epithelium of the vaginal cervix. The patches, which have a velvety appearance, contain the same glands as the regular lining of the endocervical canal, and they produce the same clear mucus leading to abnormal levels of mucus secretion. Why the endocervical mucosa moves from its ordinary location is not understood. In adult women, cervical erosion has been linked to a previous inflammation of the cervix, oral contraceptives, and the hormonal influence of pregnancy. It can also result from childbirth.

Erosions commonly cause no symptoms, although in some women more than the usual amount of a clear vaginal discharge may be produced. Erosions may be associated with chronic cervicitis. Even without other symptoms, a high percentage of women with cervical erosions test positive for Chlamydia infections (Bułhak-Kozioł, 2007).

There are a variety of treatment options for cervical erosions. Some doctors regard any erosions with suspicion, believing that any change in the normal growth pattern of cells in the cervix can be a forerunner of cervical cancer. Electrocautery (burning) or cryosurgery (freezing) can be used to destroy the area of displaced tissue. After treatment, the epithelium regenerates and heals over, restoring the cervix to a more normal appearance. Since sensory nerve endings on the surface of the cervix are very sparse, electrocautery and cryosurgery cause little or no discomfort. Recent research has identified cryosurgery as the preferred option (Gay et al., 2006). There is evidence that the destruction of cellular overgrowth prevents the progression to cervical cancer. If a woman is not experiencing symptoms associated with the erosion, it may not be necessary to treat it because even minor surgical procedures on the cervix carry some risk of complication. However, the criteria of symptomatic or asymptomatic may not be enough to determine whether erosions should be treated or left alone. A Pap smear may be necessary to determine if the erosions contain precancerous cells.

Cervical Polyps

Cervical polyps are small extensions of the uterine endometrium or the endocervical canal that extend beyond the external os into the vagina. They may be single or multiple and are most common after age 40. If manipulated, the polyp may bleed easily. Polyps very rarely become cancerous, but they also are not likely to spontaneously disappear. Small polyps can sometimes be removed by twisting and then cauterization of the base to prevent bleeding. Larger polyps mimic cervical cancer, reaching several centimeters in size and may bleed after intercourse (Bucella, 2006). Larger polyps can also block the os and cause dysmenorrhea or even secondary amenorrhea. In some cases, the polyps may calcify. Larger polyps may require surgery to prevent bleeding and to unblock the os. Others which remain small do not require treatment, only monitoring, unless additional changes occur

VULVODYNIA

Vulvodynia also known as vulvar vestibulitis, or burning vulva syndrome, is characterized by chronic burning or painful itching of the vulva with none of the physical findings present in the usual forms of vaginal infection. It can be a frustrating condition because it is frequently misdiagnosed and the symptoms can be sporadic. Because physicians were unable to find any apparent cause for the complaint, they initially believed vulvodynia was a psychological problem. The condition affects 18 percent of women and is now classified as a chronic pain syndrome (Gumus et al., 2008).

There are no firmly established treatments for vulvodynia. The anxiety and depression that many women with vulvodynia have is the result and not the cause of the condition, but a number of women have responded to small doses of antidepressant medication. There is evidence that antidepressant medication may relieve pain, possibly by blocking neurotransmitter serotonin uptake by brain neurons. Psychotherapy (Mascherpa et al., 2007) and symptomatic treatments have proven effective in some women. Because there are probably multiple causes for the condition, treatments need to be tailored to the patient (Groysman, 2010).

UTERINE PATHOLOGIES

The endometrium of the uterus responds to changes in estrogen and progesterone levels, multiplying then shedding over the monthly cycles. Pathologies of the uterine tissues—endometriosis, fibroids, and endometrial cancer—rely heavily on those cyclical patterns. In addition, the physical changes produced by pregnancy can induce uterine prolapse, a shifting of the position of the uterus.

Endometriosis

In some women, cells from the basal layer of the endometrium establish themselves outside the uterus, a condition known as **endometriosis**. While the outside of the uterus, the intestines, and the fallopian tubes are the most common sites for the tissue to grow (Figure 8-4), endometrial

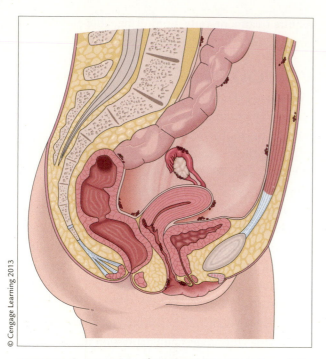

© Cengage Learning 2013

FIGURE 8-4: Common sites of misplaced tissue in endometriosis.

deposits can occur anywhere in the body. Up to 15 percent of premenopausal women have endometrial tissue outside of the uterus (Grow & Hsu, 2006). The cause of endometriosis remains unknown. Research has identified a collection of 76 genetic variations, most associated with chromosomes 7 and 10, which appear to be linked to the condition; however, no specific genes have been identified as the cause (Montgomery et al., 2008). Early menarche and very long or very short cycles are also risk factors. Whatever triggers the condition, with each menstrual cycle, the pain and damage caused by the tissue can accumulate. The endometrial tissue responds to the hormonal fluctuations just as it normally would inside the uterus—thickening in response to rising estrogen levels, and then shedding as estrogen and progesterone levels drop. The complications occur because the shed tissue has nowhere to go, and remains in the body, deteriorating, and eventually becoming scar tissue. The scarring can inhibit fertility, and the cyclic building of the tissue produces increasing pain.

The location of the endometrial tissue influences the symptoms that appear. Symptoms of endometriosis are often vague and fluctuate depending on the point in the menstrual cycle, peaking premenstrually and declining after menstruation. Backache, pelvic pain, bloating, and pain when urinating or defecating are common. As endometriosis progresses, infertility becomes a major concern. Up to 70 percent of infertile women suffer from endometriosis (Grow & Hsu, 2006). Treatment of endometriosis depends on the severity of the condition, the location of the growth, and plans for future fertility. Current treatment recommendations advise an initial six month suppression of ovarian function by altering reproductive hormone levels. Other options include surgical removal of the endometrial tissue, although adhesions and scar tissue formation are common complications of surgery (Kennedy et al., 2005). In cases where endometriosis has compromised the fallopian tubes but the woman still wishes to become pregnant, IVF is sometimes a viable option.

Uterine Fibroids

The most common gynecological tumors are benign masses of muscle and connective tissue in the uterus called **fibroids** or leiomyomas (from *leios*, smooth, and *myos*, muscle). Because small fibroids usually do not produce symptoms, their true incidence is unknown, but it is estimated that they occur in anywhere from 20–50 percent of women after the age of 35. Uterine fibroids are rare before menarche and after menopause, and estrogen appears to stimulate their growth. Both pregnancy and contraceptives containing estrogen may stimulate the growth of existing fibroids. Genetic factors, too, may play a role in their incidence. Fibroids are found somewhat more frequently in Jewish and African-American women, but can appear in women of any ethnic background. New research indicates that a chromosomal abnormality, a deletion of genes on chromosome 7, is implicated in 50 percent of fibroids (Okolo, 2008).

Fibroids may be single or multiple; they may be microscopic in size, or they may grow quite large. Although fibroids that have grown to 40–50 pounds are occasionally seen, earlier and better diagnosis has made large fibroids uncommon in the United States. Most fibroids average about 4–5 cm in diameter.

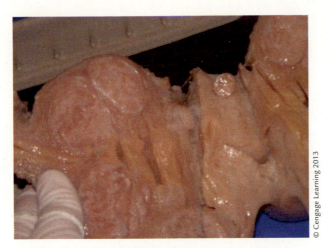

FIGURE 8-5: Fibroids in a human uterus.

© Cengage Learning 2013

They are round, smooth, quite firm in consistency, and when they are cut open, often display pinkish white whorls (Figure 8-5).

Depending on their location in the uterus, fibroids are classified as intramural, submucous, and subserous. The symptoms associated with fibroids also depend on their location in the uterus. Intramural are the most common and are found in the center of the myometrium. If they are small, they are frequently asymptomatic. Submucous fibroids grow between the endometrium and the myometrium. They may project into the uterine cavity and distort and stretch the endometrium. The subsequent increase in the surface of the endometrial lining may result in menorrhagia and dysmenorrhea, although small fibroids rarely produce discomfort. Submucosal fibroids may also be a cause of habitual miscarriage because they can interfere with the placenta. Subserous tumors develop between the perimetrium and the external peritoneal covering or serosa. Because they can grow into the abdominal cavity, these fibroids can become much larger than the uterus itself. They are often attached by a stalk to the uterus and are referred to as pedunculated. Occasionally, subserosal pedunculated fibroids can even become separated from the uterus. Fibroids can spontaneously deteriorate into calcified scar tissue. Large fibroids may encroach on the bladder or rectum and cause pressure symptoms, such as urinary frequency, constipation, or sensations of abdominal fullness. Fibroids have also been shown to increase uterine contractility, suggesting a reason for the menstrual pain and irregularity that some women experience with them.

The presence of fibroids, even if they produce no other symptoms, may be associated with infertility problems if they obstruct the opening of the fallopian tubes. If pregnancy does occur, small fibroids generally do not affect the pregnancy. If the fibroids are large, however, they may interfere with implantation and cause miscarriage or block the birth canal to prevent vaginal delivery.

The majority of small fibroids are symptomless, grow very slowly, and do not require immediate treatment. If they are not showing any evidence of rapid growth and are not causing any symptoms, they are usually left alone. If a woman is close to menopause and the symptoms are those she can live with, the discomfort should disappear with menopause as the fibroids stop growing and diminish in size with the natural drop in estrogen levels.

If the fibroids are large enough to cause symptoms, several treatment options exist. One technique involves placement of a progestin-releasing IUD to control menorrhagia (Sayed et al., 2010). Another treatment option is uterine artery embolisation (UAE) which blocks the blood supply to the fibroid, inhibiting its growth. The procedure is minimally invasive and has few reported complications. A myomectomy (surgical removal of the fibroid only) or hysterectomy are surgical options. In a study comparing UAE to hysterectomy for the treatment of fibroids, UAE was found to produce fewer complications, have greater patient satisfaction, and be more cost effective (Hirst et al., 2008). In some cases, a focused ultrasound beam can be used to treat fibroids (Stewart et al., 2003). Determining the course of treatment—hysterectomy, UAE, or a hands-off approach—needs to take into account the size of the fibroids, any complications, and the future plans for children. UAE does run the risk of reduced fertility, and a hysterectomy removes the option of pregnancy completely.

Uterine Prolapse

The uterus is held in position by a collection of ligaments. However, if those ligaments are overstretched or the pelvic floor muscles weakened, the uterus can **prolapse**, or drop out of position and protrude into

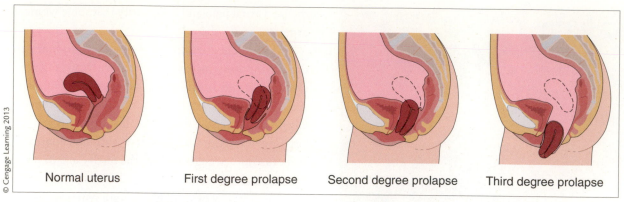

Normal uterus   First degree prolapse   Second degree prolapse   Third degree prolapse

FIGURE 8-6: Example of uterine prolapse.

the vagina (Figure 8-6). In extreme cases, the uterus may protrude outside the body. Prolapse is most often associated with difficult deliveries, delivery of very large babies, closely-spaced pregnancies, and early child bearing.

In some women, prolapse will spontaneously resolve, though this is usually only in mild cases. Weight loss can help by relieving some of the pressure on the displaced uterus. A devise called a pessary can be placed inside the vagina to hold the uterus in position, but this is usually only effective with mild cases. Pessaries may irritate the vaginal tissues, harbor microbes, and interfere with sexual intercourse. In more severe cases of uterine prolapse, a surgical procedure may be used to tighten the ligaments, reposition the uterus, and tighten the pelvic floor. When this condition does not respond to any treatments or the uterus is damaged, a hysterectomy is usually required.

Cancer of the Uterus

Endometrial cancer is one of the most common gynecological cancers in women. It is most common in postmenopausal women and in women who have used a form of hormone therapy called ERT that uses estrogen unopposed by progesterone for more than five years (NCI, 2010). In addition to age and estrogen exposure, other risk factors for endometrial cancer include a family history of cancer (uterine, colon, or ovarian), a history of fertility problems, a weight of more than 200 pounds, and use of Tamoxifen (CDC, 2008). Tamoxifen, used as an anti-estrogen in the treatment of breast cancer, can paradoxically behave as an estrogen in some women, increasing the thick-

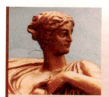

Cultural Considerations
PROLAPSE IN NEPAL

In a study of women's reproductive health in eastern Nepal, 98 percent of the women who sought medical attention (345 out of 351 respondents) reported suffering symptoms of uterine prolapse. Despite reporting symptoms of vaginal bleeding, incontinence, backache and pain during intercourse, many women (56 percent) did not seek treatment. In the sample of women surveyed, most did not have access to money of their own and relied on their husbands or mothers-in-law for financial support. This limited their access to healthcare. Twenty percent of the women placed a ball in the vagina to serve as a pessary or took medications to treat the condition. Thirty-six percent of the women dealt with the prolapse symptoms for more than two years before getting medical help (Basnet, 2005).

ness of the endometrium and stimulating cancerous cells (Lindahl et al., 2008). Women on Tamoxifen must be carefully monitored for endometrial changes during treatment. The use of combination oral contraceptives (estrogen with progesterone) has been shown to reduce the risk of developing endometrial cancer (NCI, 2010).

The most common initial symptom of endometrial cancer is abnormal and painless vaginal bleeding, especially in postmenopausal women.

Case Study

Post-menopausal Uterine Bleeding

Elena, a very active and vigorous woman in her late 50s, is looking forward to her granddaughter's quinciñera. She was finally through menopause. It had been a very difficult transition for her between hot flashes, insomnia, and night sweats, and she resorted to hormone therapy for relief, but she doesn't remember what kind it was. It has now been years since her last period. Now as she is preparing for the party, she realizes that she seems to be having a period—bright red vaginal bleeding. She wants to ignore it because she is feeling fine. But when she asks her daughter, a nurse, for a pad, the daughter insists she make an appointment immediately to see a doctor. Upon reviewing her medical records, the doctor finds she was on unopposed estrogen replacement for six years. The doctor orders an endometrial biopsy which finds endometrial cancer.

1. Why was her daughter so concerned about the post-menopausal bleeding?

2. Why is the type of hormone replacement she took important?

3. What are her treatment options?

While abnormal uterine bleeding is very rarely the result of uterine malignancy in a young woman, in postmenopausal women, it should be regarded with suspicion.

Pap smears are unreliable for detecting endometrial cancer, and diagnosis is made by biopsy of the lining of the uterus. The sample can be taken with a local anesthesia to the cervix. In microcurettage, a small strip of endometrium is scraped away with a sharp spoon-shaped instrument called a curette. In suction biopsy, the curette tip is incorporated into a hollow tube inserted into the uterine cavity. When light suction is applied, the tissue sample is drawn out through the tube. A positive diagnosis through endometrial biopsy is conclusive evidence of cancer, but a negative finding does not necessarily exclude it. The carcinoma may have been missed in an area of the endometrium that was not sampled. The most definitive diagnosis is made by a D and C (dilation and curettage), a procedure in which the cervix is dilated and the entire endometrium removed.

Early endometrial cancer is usually treated by a hysterectomy plus removal of the fallopian tubes and the ovaries. More extensive carcinoma is generally considered an indication for preoperative radiation treatment followed by surgery. Chemotherapy and anti-estrogen hormone therapy are also effective. When metastases have spread to the vagina, pelvis, and lungs, chemotherapy in the form of massive doses of progestins has produced remissions. As in all cancers, the most successful treatment depends on early diagnosis.

OVARIAN PATHOLOGIES

The ovaries are highly active organs, producing a constantly changing collection of hormones and maturing eggs each month during a woman's reproductive years. Ovarian pathologies often produce symptoms which include irregular cycles, pain (often mistaken for appendicitis), and infertility issues. Unfortunately, ovarian cancer produces few symptoms until it has progressed quite far.

Ovarian Cysts

Functional follicular and corpus luteum cysts occur frequently, and women are probably seldom aware of their existence because most experience no symptoms. Commonly, and probably due to some alteration in the usual hypothalamic-pituitary-ovarian hormonal axis, a follicle does not ovulate normally but continues to grow, accumulate fluid, and produce

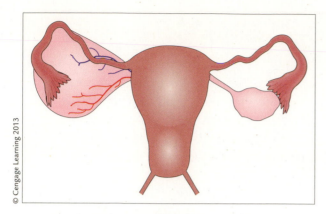

© Cengage Learning 2013

FIGURE 8-7: An ovarian cyst causes distention of the ovary.

estrogen, becoming an **ovarian cyst**. These cysts can become quite large (Figure 8-7). More rarely, the corpus luteum may not regress normally but continues to grow and produce progesterone. These cysts are called functional follicular or corpus luteum cysts. The hormones secreted by such a functional follicular cyst may produce disruptions of the menstrual cycle. There may be some abdominal pain as a result of pressure from the cyst on the ovarian connective tissue capsule. These cysts may spontaneously disappear by fluid absorption or rupture within a month or two, and do not have to be treated by surgery or any other method, unless there is some complication.

Large cysts may cause an ovary to shift position, twisting the ligaments that hold it in place and possibly cutting off the blood supply to the ovary. In these cases, the damaged ovary may need to be removed. Occasionally, a cyst will rupture through a small blood vessel on the surface of the ovary, producing

intraperitoneal bleeding. If the bleeding is scant and spontaneously stops, there may be few symptoms. If the bleeding is extensive, the source can be diagnosed by laparoscopy (the examination of the pelvic cavity by an instrument inserted through a small incision in the abdominal wall). Surgery may then be necessary to control the bleeding and repair the ovary.

Polycystic Ovarian Syndrome

Polycystic ovarian syndrome (PCOS) is an endocrinological disorder also known as a type of Stein-Leventhal disease. Symptoms include a failure to ovulate, large numbers of follicular cysts, enlarged ovaries with thickened capsules, excessive androgen production, and amenorrhea. The excess androgen production may alter blood sugar levels, increase acne, and increase facial hair. Menstrual irregularities and infertility are common symptoms. PCOS is also associated with metabolic syndrome including type 2 diabetes, hypertension, high triglyceride levels, and high LDL cholesterol levels (Beckman et al., 2010).

Treatment of PCOS involves relieving symptoms and reducing the metabolic changes associated with the disease. Oral contraceptives can readjust the menstrual cycle. PCOS also appears to respond well to dietary therapy (Moran et al., 2008) and exercise that leads to weight loss.

Ovarian Cancer

Ovarian cancers are classified according to their cellular origin. There are more than 60 kinds of ovarian tumors, but the most common are ovarian epithelial carcinomas and ovarian germ cell tumors. Ovarian cancers can be deadly, primarily because as they develop they usually remain silent and symptomless until they have progressed beyond the point where treatments are effective. Nearly 50 percent of cases are diagnosed in women between the ages of 45 and 65 (Altekruse et al., 2010). Risk factors for ovarian cancer include a family history of ovarian cancer, having another reproductive cancer, having never given birth, and endometriosis. Women with two or more first-degree

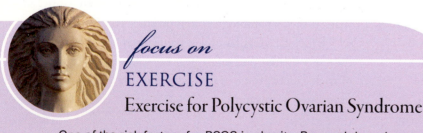

focus on

EXERCISE

Exercise for Polycystic Ovarian Syndrome

One of the risk factors for PCOS is obesity. Research has shown that increased exercise can be effective as a therapy for PCOS (Hoeger, 2008). Exercise, combined with controlled calorie intake and reduced weight, has helped stabilize blood sugar levels. Moderate exercise produced the same beneficial effects as vigorous exercise. The combination of exercise with dietary changes produced positive effects in the management of PCOS.

relatives (mother, sister, or daughter) who had ovarian cancer are at high risk. Ovarian cancer is also associated with the BRCA 1 and BRCA 2 gene mutations (NCI, 2010), which are also associated with an increased risk of developing breast cancer. A review of 45 epidemiological studies found that oral contraceptive use lowered the risk of ovarian cancer, creating a protective effect that strengthens with the length of time a woman uses the contraceptive and continues providing protection long after the medication is stopped (Collaborative Group on Epidemiological Studies of Ovarian Cancer et al., 2008). While this provides one protective mechanism, a great deal of research is still needed.

Ovarian cancer produces few obvious symptoms, although there are some changes that are cause for concern—back pain or lower abdominal pain, abnormal vaginal bleeding, unusual vaginal discharge, changes in bowel or bladder habits, digestive upset and bloating. Unfortunately, these symptoms often develop slowly and are not recognized as something to be concerned about. Gilda Radner, the comedian who died in 1988 at the age of 42, was unaware of her family history. She had two, and possibly three, blood relatives who had died of ovarian cancer. In her book, *It's Always Something,* she described how she was sick for nine months with bloating and abdominal cramps, going from doctor to doctor, before she was finally diagnosed with cancer that had already spread.

Several screening techniques for early detection of ovarian cancer have been developed, but as yet none has proven effective (NCI, 2010). CA-125, for example, is an antigen found in blood serum that becomes elevated in women with ovarian cancer. This antigen is not exclusive to ovarian cancer, however, and is increased in other cancers as well as in a number of benign conditions, including endometriosis and early pregnancy. A large pilot study in Great Britain by Ian Jacobs and colleagues (1999) found that when detection of elevated CA-125 is combined with vaginal ultrasound to measure for increased ovarian volume and followed up with continued surveillance, this kind of screening can save lives by detecting cancer

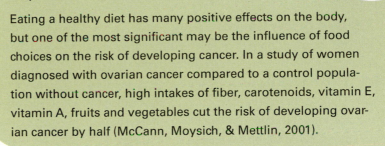

focus on

NUTRITION
Phytochemicals and Ovarian Cancer

Eating a healthy diet has many positive effects on the body, but one of the most significant may be the influence of food choices on the risk of developing cancer. In a study of women diagnosed with ovarian cancer compared to a control population without cancer, high intakes of fiber, carotenoids, vitamin E, vitamin A, fruits and vegetables cut the risk of developing ovarian cancer by half (McCann, Moysich, & Mettlin, 2001).

early when it is symptomless and confined to the ovaries. Unfortunately, this protocol does not work for all ovarian tumor types. Work by Kurman et al., (2008) found that ovarian cancers can be grouped into two categories—type I tumors that grow slowly and undergo a series of diverse mutations and type II tumors that contain a mutation in the P53 gene, which controls apoptosis, a self-induced cell death. The type II tumors are highly aggressive and account for the majority of ovarian tumors. Because they are so aggressive, type II tumor cells can rapidly metastasize and move beyond the ovary to invade other tissues.

Ovarian cancer is most effectively treated with surgery supplemented by radiation and chemotherapy. For women who are treated while the tumor is still localized in the ovary, the five-year survival rate is 93.5 percent. Unfortunately, the majority of ovarian cancers (62 percent) are not diagnosed until they have metastasized. In those cases, the five-year survival rate drops to just under 27 percent (Altekruse et al., 2010).

BREAST CANCER

It has been suggested that the increasing incidence of breast cancer should be considered within the context of the accelerating rise in reproductive system cancers. Inheriting the BRCA1 and BRCA2 gene mutations increases the risk of developing both breast cancer and ovarian cancer. According to the National Cancer Institute (Altekruse et al., 2010), one of every eight women in the United States will develop breast cancer during her lifetime. It is estimated that 207,000 new cases of breast cancer will be diagnosed in women this year, as well as approximately 2000 cases in men (NCI, 2010). Breast cancer is the most common cancer in women and is second only to lung cancer in terms of how many women die from it each year. Breast cancer rates are increasing world-wide, including in developing nations.

Types of Breast Cancer

The breasts are composed of several different types of tissues and may develop several different types of cancer. Ductal cancer is the most common and develops from the cells lining the milk ducts. Ductal cancers account for approximately 88 percent of breast cancer cases. Less common are lobular cancers which develop in the mammary glands themselves. Lobular cancer makes up only five percent of the breast cancer cases. Other types include inflammatory breast cancer and Paget's disease of the nipple (National Breast Cancer Foundation, 2010). All types of breast cancer have the ability to metastasize to other parts of the body if not identified and treated early.

RISK FACTORS FOR BREAST CANCER

The most important risk factor for breast cancer is being a woman. Although breast cancer occurs in men, it occurs 100 times more frequently in women. The second most important risk factor is age. Breast cancer is rarely found in girls younger than 15, and only two percent of all mammary cancers occur in women between 20 and 34. At 45, the incidence of the disease increases and continues to rise rapidly with age. Forty-seven percent of breast cancers are diagnosed in women between 45 and 64. However, by the time a woman reaches her 80s, her risk has declined to less than six percent (Altekruse et al., 2010). Other risk factors include genetics, chemical exposures, and lifestyle choices such as smoking, alcohol consumption, diet, and physical activity level. Individual risk factors for breast cancer do not necessarily cause breast cancer; instead they may provide a circumstance where breast cancer is more likely to develop. Having one or several of the risk factors is associated with increased frequency of breast cancer. Women diagnosed with atypical hyperplasia are four times more likely to develop breast cancer. A diagnosis of **hyperplasia** means that abnormal

cells have been detected, but they are not currently cancerous. Some risk factors such as age, sex, and family history of breast cancer cannot be changed. Other risk factors such as diet, smoking, and activity level are under an individual's control and can be influenced by personal lifestyle decisions.

Genetic Factors

About five to ten percent of breast cancer cases have the mutations that are associated with specific inherited genes, most commonly BRCA1 and BRCA2. These genes are believed to be tumor-suppresser genes, and when they function normally, tumor development is inhibited. When BRCA-1 is mutated, there is interference with DNA repair in other genes, and unchecked cell growth can occur (Gowen et al., 1998; Lancaster, Carney, & Furtreal, 1997). Female carriers of BRCA1 and BRCA2 mutations have a marked predisposition to develop breast and ovarian cancer, and male carriers have a small increase in risk of developing prostate or colon cancer (Gallagher et al., 2010). Even with a mutation, however, there is no certainty when and whether a cancer will occur. Some women who carry the BRCA gene mutations opt for a preventative mastectomy, having both breasts removed to reduce their risk of developing breast cancer. Other genes contribute to the risk of developing breast cancer, but the majority of mutations that lead to breast cancer are not inherited. Instead, they are acquired during a person's lifetime. These mutations can develop through exposure to radiation, and through exposure to chemicals and hormones.

Risk Factors Associated with Endogenous Hormones

Endogenous hormones are hormones that are made by a woman's own body. For example, women produce progesterone, testosterone, and three different forms of estrogen, all in different proportions depending on the stages of the menstrual cycle, pregnancy, and menopausal status. Research indicates that the pattern of long term exposure of a woman to her own hormones, especially some forms of estrogen, throughout her reproductive life, can have an impact on her chances of developing breast cancer. The period of time between the onset of menarche and the completion of menopause is sometimes referred to as the estrogen window.

Both early menarche and late menopause increase the estrogen window and can contribute to an increased risk of breast cancer. The hormonal changes that accompany pregnancy are protective, but the evidence currently available suggests that the degree of protection is associated with the age of the woman at the time of the first full-term delivery. Having a child within five years of menarche appears to lower a woman's risk for breast cancer. However, having a first child after age 40 increases the risk. Prolonged breast-feeding also appears to have a protective effect against the subsequent development of breast cancer (Byers et al., 1985; McTiernan and Thomas, 1986. Collaborative Group on Hormonal Factors in Breast Cancer, 2002).

Excess estrogen stimulation in the absence of cyclic progesterone has been suggested as a risk factor, and several studies have shown an increased incidence of breast cancer in women with anovulatory cycles (Cowan et al., 1981; Gonzalez, 1983). During their reproductive lives, women produce three types of estrogen: estradiol, estrone, and estriol. All of these are carcinogenic when administered to laboratory animals. Estradiol is the strongest of the estrogens in biological activity, but it has less carcinogenic potential in animals than estrone. Estriol is the weakest estrogen and has very little or no carcinogenic activity in mice. On this basis, some investigators have credited an increased risk of breast cancer to estradiol and estrone and a protective effect to estriol. During pregnancy, the production of all three estrogens is greatly increased, but estradiol and estrone increase over prepregnancy levels by a hundredfold while estriol increases a thousand fold. This has led to speculation that the higher levels of estriol during pregnancy, acting on the breast, provide protection against cancer.

Risk Factors Associated with Exogenous Hormones

Exogenous hormones are hormones that come from outside the body, either intentionally by taking a medication such as birth control or hormone replacement therapy, or unintentionally by exposure to endocrine disruptors from the environment. Hormonal forms of birth control, hormone replacement therapies, and other medications contain either purified natural hormones or synthetic versions of hormones normally found in the body. It should be noted that synthetic hormones are not always identical to natural hormones. For example, the hormone progesterone is difficult to administer as a pill or by a transdermal patch, so a synthetic version of the hormone, progestin, is usually used. Progestin is not identical to progesterone in its properties or its effects on the body. In fact, in some of the ways that natural progesterone is protective or beneficial to the body, synthetic progestins may have negative effects. Researchers (Béguelin et al., 2010) have identified a specific progesterone-binding receptor which stimulates the growth of some breast cancers.

There is conflicting evidence about how hormonal birth control methods such as oral contraceptives, the patch, the vaginal ring, and depo provera influence a woman's risk of developing breast cancer. The changes associated with combination oral contraceptives are thought to cause a slight increase in breast cancer rates (Garcia y Narvaiza et al., 2008). For many years, progestin used in contraceptives and HRT was thought to have no impact on breast cancer rates. However, new research is now calling that assumption into question (Geirsig, 2008).

Researchers have pointed out the link between hormone replacement therapy (HRT) and the development of breast cancer, highlighting the role that endogenous estrogens can play in the development of this disease. As the number of women using HRT has declined, there has been a steep drop in the number of cases of breast cancer in postmenopausal women (Key et al., 2002; Surhke et al., 2009; Missmer et al., 2004).

Endocrine disruptors frequently have estrogenic properties. In some cases, chemicals that are not estrogenic by themselves can act in combination with other chemicals to have an effect. This opens the possibility that endocrine disruptors, present in the environment, may play a role in the dramatic increases in breast cancer rates over the past decades. These chemicals, which have already been detected in human tissues, can act in combination to influence the physiology of estrogen within the body (Kortenkamp, 2006). Exposure is through food or water, contamination from plastics, or absorption through the skin from cosmetics and personal care or household products. However, a recent review of the literature found no direct links between personal care products, breast cancer, and endocrine disruptors (Witorsch & Thomas, 2010).

Other Risk Factors for Developing Breast Cancer

Women who have received radiation treatments as a child or as a young adult are more likely to develop breast cancer later in life. If the exposure occurred during puberty when the breasts were developing, the risk is greater. There is some controversy currently about the effect of the small amount of radiation associated with mammography on the development of breast cancer. Both smoking and exposure to second-hand smoke increase a woman's risk for developing breast cancer (Reynolds et al., 2009; Sadri & Mahjub, 2007). Studies examining the effect of alcohol consumption on breast cancer risk have yielded mixed results. There is increasing evidence that alcohol affects recurrent breast cancer (Knight et al., 2009). Heavy drinking has also been associated with an increased risk of breast cancer, but low and moderate alcohol, particularly wine, does not appear to increase the risk (Bessaoud & Daurès, 2008).

Obesity is also a risk factor for breast cancer, but the relationship between excess weight and cancer is complex. The risk is greatest if excess weight is gained after menopause, but gaining excess weight as an adolescent also increases risk. Estrogens are produced by conversion from a precursor called androstenedione in adipose tissue, and more estrogen is produced in obese women. Premenopausal obese women also have higher blood levels of estrogen and frequently have irregular menstrual periods and anovulatory cycles. Other data imply that a relationship between increased weight and increased risk may have to do with where on the body the excess weight is distributed. Schapira et al. (1990) compared the body measurements of 432 healthy women to 216 women of the same age with breast cancer. The women who were "apple-shaped", that is, with excess weight around the middle and a waist-to-hip ratio greater than 0.8, were five times more likely to develop breast cancer than "pear-shaped" women who have more fat on their hips or thighs. The waist-to-hip ratio is computed by dividing the waist measurement by the measurement of the hips taken at the widest point between the hips and the buttocks.

A recent large prospective study has not found a link between dietary fat intake and breast cancer risk (Michels & Willett, 2009). However, increased dietary fat intake is often associated with obesity, and obesity does contribute to the risk of developing breast cancer. It will likely take further study to fully understand the role of dietary fat intake in the development of breast cancer.

A further link between diet and estrogen metabolism is suggested by studies that compare vegetarian women with non-vegetarian women. For example, Goldin and associates (1982) found that vegetarian women have decreased levels of estrogen in the blood. The amount of fat and fiber eaten could be a factor explaining the high risk of breast cancer in Western countries where a diet high in fat and animal protein is consumed and the much lower risk of breast cancer in Third World countries where women eat vegetarian or semi-vegetarian low-protein, high-fiber diets.

There is also evidence from animal and human studies linking specific vegetables to a beneficial effect. The risk of breast cancer, as well as other cancers, may be reduced when foods rich in selenium, vitamin C, and the cruciferous vegetables (brussels sprouts, cabbage, turnips, broccoli, and cauliflower) are part of the diet. While the lower fat content of a vegetarian diet is believed to be a factor, a further explanation for the protective effect is the presence of carcinogenic inhibitors in the food. The inhibitors are indoles, or plant growth factors, which have been found to prevent tumors in various animals. Michnovicz and Bradlow (1990) provided evidence that the role of indoles in estrogen metabolism may enable them to reduce estrogen-responsive tumors such as breast cancer in humans. The workers extracted indole from cruciferous vegetables and administered it to a small group of men (to avoid any influence of fluctuating hormone levels and because previous research had indicated that estrogen metabolism is independent of gender). The result was a significant increase in the metabolic conversion of strong estradiol to weak estrogens with little carcinogenic activity.

LIFESTYLE FACTORS TO REDUCE THE RISK OF BREAST CANCER

There are many steps that individual women can take to reduce their risk of developing breast cancer. Many of the steps that can help prevent breast cancer can also reduce a woman's risk of developing cardiovascular disease, diabetes, dementia, and many other cancers.

They are part of maintaining a healthy lifestyle. The following is a list of steps that can be taken to minimize the risk of developing breast cancer:

- Maintain a healthy weight
- Maintain a healthy level of daily physical activity
- Avoid smoking and limit exposure to secondhand smoke
- Limit alcohol consumption
- Eat foods high in fiber and monounsaturated oils
- Avoid exposure to endocrine disruptors
- Avoid long term hormone therapy

While these changes are no guarantee that breast cancer will not develop, research supports the idea that these changes can significantly reduce a woman's risk.

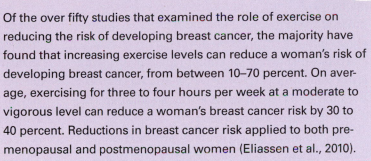
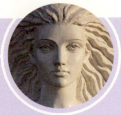

focus on

EXERCISE
Exercise and Breast Cancer Risk

Of the over fifty studies that examined the role of exercise on reducing the risk of developing breast cancer, the majority have found that increasing exercise levels can reduce a woman's risk of developing breast cancer, from between 10–70 percent. On average, exercising for three to four hours per week at a moderate to vigorous level can reduce a woman's breast cancer risk by 30 to 40 percent. Reductions in breast cancer risk applied to both pre-menopausal and postmenopausal women (Eliassen et al., 2010).

SCREENING AND DIAGNOSIS OF BREAST CANCER

With one in eight women developing breast cancer in their lifetime, it is important to take the threat of this deadly disease seriously. The most effective way to survive breast cancer is to detect it and treat it as early as possible. Therefore, it is important to recognize the symptoms of breast cancer. However, breast tumors are usually painless and the disease often does not present noticeable symptoms during the early stages. This is why regular screening is important for detecting breast cancer in its earliest stages, while treatments are most likely to be successful. The most common types of screening for breast cancer include breast self examination, clinical breast exam, and mammogram. Recently, MRI and ultrasound have been added to the screening tools. Breast screening is discussed in detail in Chapter 7.

STAGING BREAST CANCER

Diagnostic and screening tests for breast cancer are used to determine the size and location of a tumor. They are also used to determine how advanced the cancer is and whether or not it has metastasized. Staging the cancer is an important component of determining the best plan for treatment. Breast cancer is classified as stages 0–4, in an increasing order of seriousness. Stage 0 cancers are also called in situ, which means in one place. Ductal cancer in situ (DCIS) and lobular cancer in situ (LCIS) are noninvasive. The majority of breast cancers are identified at this stage, and the five-year survival rate with treatment is 98 percent (Altekure et al., 2010). Stage 1 cancers are small (2 cm or less) and cancerous cells can be detected in the lymph nodes. Tumors in nodes that are small and have not moved beyond the breast lymph nodes (NCI, 2010) are classified as stage 1. The five-year survival rate at this stage drops slightly, down to 83 percent (Altekure et al., 2010), but the prognosis for most patients is still very good. Stage 2 cancers are larger (up to 5 cm) and have invaded the axillary lymph nodes. Stage 3 cancers have metastasized to the chest wall and the skin of the breast producing the peau d'orange (orange peel) changes in the skin of the breast characteristic of inflammatory breast cancer (NCI, 2010). Survival rates on stage 2 and 3 drop to 23 percent (Altekure et al., 2010). The most severe form is stage 4 by which time the cancer has metastasized to other locations in the body, especially the bone, liver, lungs, and brain (NCI, 2010). Survival rates at this stage are poor.

TREATMENTS FOR BREAST CANCER

Breast cancer is treated with surgery and another adjuvant or additional types of treatment such as radiation, chemotherapy, and hormone therapy. Recent advances in treatment include the use of monoclonal antibodies and treatments based on genetic testing results.

Surgical Treatments

In the past, the most common treatment for breast cancer was radical **mastectomy** which involved the removal of a breast plus removal of the pectoral and axial lymph nodes, and part of the underlying pectoral muscle. Because so much tissue was removed, this procedure lead to several long term problems, including problems of edema from disrupted lymph flow and difficulty moving the arm. A radical mastectomy is not commonly performed today. Instead, less invasive procedures are available. Figure 8-8 illustrates the different types of mastectomies.

In a modified radical mastectomy, the entire breast is removed, plus some axillary lymph nodes, but the chest muscles are left intact. Leaving the chest muscles intact reduces future complications for the woman and makes breast reconstruction easier, if it is desired. With a simple mastectomy the entire breast is removed. Follow-up tests after the surgery will determine if radiation, chemotherapy or hormone therapy is needed.

In the case of a lumpectomy, only the tumor and some of the surrounding tissue is removed, thus preserving as much of the breast as possible. This surgery can be used when the cancer is small, localized, and close to the skin surface. If the tumor is located deep in the breast, or if there is more than one tumor dispersed over a larger area, a lumpectomy is not an option. In some cases, if a woman has a large tumor but still wants to have a lumpectomy rather than a mastectomy, chemotherapy will be used to shrink the tumor prior to surgery.

Adjuvant Treatments for Breast Cancer

There are four major forms of adjuvant therapies that can be used to treat breast cancer: radiation therapy, chemotherapy, hormonal therapies, and biological therapies.

Radiation treatment can be administered through several different methods ranging from X-rays to implanted radioactive pellets. Radiation is used in many circumstances including, following both lumpectomy and mastectomy especially when cancer has invaded the chest wall or invaded multiple sentinel lymph nodes. When it is used as an adjunct to conservative surgery in early breast cancer, radiotherapy is given postoperatively to destroy any cancer cells that may have been left in the breast or the lymph nodes after surgery. Radiation therapy can cause tiredness, damage to the heart, lungs, or nerves, and edema.

Chemotherapy functions at the cellular level to destroy or inhibit the growth of cancer cells. The compounds that are used for chemotherapy do not selectively seek out the cancer cells. Generally, these drugs affect all rapidly dividing cells, normal as well as malignant. Chemotherapy can damage the cells of the skin, the hair follicles, the mouth, the gastrointestinal tract, and the bone marrow. Side effects of chemotherapy include loss of hair, skin changes, sores in the mouth, nausea, and vomiting. Tiredness and lowered resistance to infection may occur as bone marrow suppression results in fewer red and white blood cells. Sometimes chemotherapy can damage the heart, nerves, kidneys, and other organs, and because it

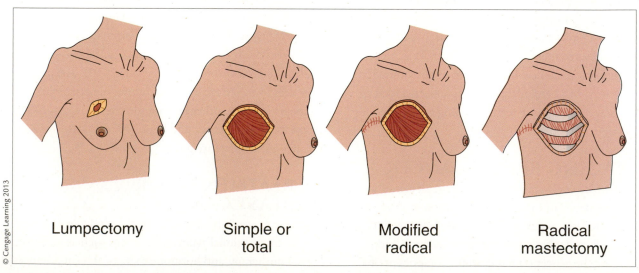

Lumpectomy   Simple or total   Modified radical   Radical mastectomy

© Cengage Learning 2013

FIGURE 8-8: The types of mastectomy.

damages white blood cells, it can reduce the effectiveness of a woman's immune system while she is receiving treatments. Chemotherapy can even lead to myeloid leukemia, which is cancer of the white blood cells. This effect is a rare effect, however. Other possible side effects of chemotherapy are premature menopause and infertility. Memory and concentration problems can also occur while undergoing chemotherapy.

Usually a tumor is analyzed when it is removed to determine if it is positive for estrogen receptors (ER). If it is, there is a very good chance that the woman will respond to hormonal therapy to treat the cancer. It should be noted that hormone therapy in the context of breast cancer treatment is not the same as hormone replacement therapy (HRT) sometimes prescribed for women going through menopause. In fact, hormone therapy in this context could probably

be better called hormone blocking therapy because it blocks estrogen receptors on the cancer cells and slows their growth. There is a correlation between ER status and a woman's prognosis for surviving breast cancer. Women diagnosed with ER-positive tumors usually survive longer and have longer disease-free intervals than women who have ER-negative tumors, regardless of the size of the tumor or the presence or absence of cancer in the axillary nodes.

Like chemotherapy, hormone therapy can be used to decrease the chance of cancer returning, or it can be used to shrink tumors and control metastasized cancer. There are two types of hormone therapy: selective estrogen receptor modulators (SERMS) and aromatase inhibitors. The drug tamoxifen is an example of a SERM. Tamoxifen is a nonsteroid antiestrogen that competes with estrogen binding at the

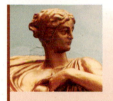

Cultural Considerations
BREAST CANCER IN WOMEN OF AFRICAN DESCENT

African American women are 50 percent more likely to get breast cancer in their 20s, 30s, or 40s, than are women of European descent, who usually develop breast cancer at an older age. They are also twice as likely to be diagnosed with ER-negative tumors which are more likely to spread aggressively. Many of the new anti-cancer drugs are not effective against these ER-negative cancer cells.

A Chicago physician, Funmi Olopade noticed these trends with her African American patients in the South Side of Chicago. On a trip to a niece's wedding in her native Nigeria, she discovered that the same patterns that she observed in the breast cancers of African American patients were also present in the young women of Nigeria. Convinced that there were important unaddressed differences in the cancers of women of African and women of European descent, she decided to study breast cancer in both North America and Africa.

She began with a small pilot study in 2000, and then designed a much larger study through the Center for Interdisciplinary Health Disparities

Research in 2003. Both the National Institute of Health and the John D and Catherine T McArthur Foundation have provided funding for her to conduct her research. As part of this work, Olopade is collaborating with physicians and researchers in Nigeria to conduct clinical trials of two anti-cancer drugs in Africa. These clinical trials have also received support from the Breast Cancer Research Foundation. In Chicago, Olopade is investigating how breast cancer tumors differ between African American women and women of other groups. Her project is also addressing questions about how pre-scribed screening protocols and treatments must be re-evaluated. For example, in high risk populations, screening for ER-negative breast cancer may need to begin earlier and occur more often. At present, most insurance policies only pay for mammograms after age 40, and the ER-negative tumors of concern in women of African descent can develop at a much younger age. Her study is also addressing issues of unequal access and utilization of preventative screening and medical services (Burton, 2005).

estrogen receptor sites. This drug is prescribed as an adjuvant treatment for women with estrogen receptor positive breast cancer, and as a treatment for women with metastatic breast cancer. It is also sometimes prescribed as a preventative to women who are at high risk of developing breast cancer.

Tamoxifen has minimal side effects compared with chemotherapy or radiation and does not cause nausea, vomiting, or hair loss, although it is not without adverse effects. Many premenopausal women experience menopausal symptoms such as hot flashes. Tamoxifen has been shown to increase the risk of uterine endometrial cancer, deep vein thrombosis (a blood clot in a major vein), and pulmonary embolism, which can occur when a blood clot travels in the circulation to the lung. Other risks that may be more common in women on tamoxifen include visual difficulties, such as an increased incidence of cataracts and macular degeneration (Colleoni & Giobbie-Hurder, 2010).

While tamoxifen is an anti-estrogen in tumors, it mimics the effects of estrogen in other parts of the body. It may decrease osteoporosis and may reduce the risk of heart disease because it decreases the levels of LDL cholesterol. There also is evidence, first reported a number of years ago, that tamoxifen reduces the level of certain stimulatory growth factors in the blood (Pollak et al., 1990) and promotes the production of cellular inhibitory growth factors, therefore acting as an inhibitor of tumor growth (Jordon, 1988). There also are numerous reports of the beneficial therapeutic effect of tamoxifen in patients with a wide range of malignancies other than breast cancer (Jordon, 1988).

Aromatase inhibitors prevent the production of estrogen in cells other than the ovaries, such as adipose cells and cells of the adrenal glands. Recent evidence has indicated that arormatase inhibitors may be more effective at preventing breast cancer than tamoxifen, and with fewer side effects (Colleoni & Giobbie-Hurder, 2010). These medications are less likely to cause blood clots or endometrial cancer. The major drawback, however, is an increased risk of osteoporosis.

Biological therapies target the specific biological properties that distinguish cancer cells from other body cells. This approach to treating cancer is relatively new compared to radiation, chemotherapy, and hormone therapy. Three biological therapies are now available and they each target cancer cells in a different way. Trastuzumab (Herceptin) uses

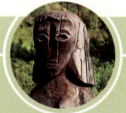

focus on NUTRITION

Lignans are chemical components of some plants that can act as weak estrogens in the human body. Because they are derived from plants, lignans are classified as a type of phytoestrogen. There are many other phytoestrogens found in plants including soy isoflavonoids and coumestrol.

Animal studies have demonstrated that lignans can interact with cancer tumors (Saarinen et al., 2008; Touillaud et al., 2007), and it is hypothesized that they have the ability to block some types of estrogen receptors, thus depriving tumors of the stimulation for further growth. Lignans are also found in typical high fiber foods, and the fiber itself may aid in removal of metabolized estrogens out of the body and the prevention of their reabsorption back into the bloodstream from the gut (Suzuki et al., 2008).

Lignans can be found in flaxseeds, which are sometimes called linseeds (Chen et al., 2007; Saarinen et al., 2006). Oils made from flaxseed do not contain significant amounts of lignans, but they do contain a compound called alpha lipoic acid, which has also been found to have cancer fighting properties. These compounds can also influence hormone metabolism and estrogen levels, and cancer risk (Hutchins et al., 2001). Flaxseeds must be ground up in order to be easily digested, and in the ground form can be sprinkled on foods or mixed into beverages. It is recommended that between 1–2 tablespoons of flaxseed per day will have a protective effect. Flaxseeds and sesame seeds have the highest concentrations of lignans, but other sources include pumpkin seeds, whole grains, cranberries, and black or green tea.

monoclonal antibody technology to target and attack a specific protein that is commonly found on the cell surface of breast cancer cells. This reaction mimics that action of the body's own immune response to invading viruses or bacteria. By attacking the protein on the surface of the cancer cell, the medication is able to destroy that cell. Another biological therapy prevents new blood vessels from growing, thereby depriving the cancer cells of the blood supply they need to divide and grow. A third biological treatment attacks proteins inside the cancer cells.

CONCLUSION

Cancers and other pathologies that affect the organs of the reproductive system and the breasts often present with few symptoms until the conditions are advanced. Many of these diseases share common risk factors including genetic mutations and hormone sensitivity. Lifestyle changes can mitigate the symptoms of some conditions or reduce the risk of developing others. In the case of cancers, screening and preventative measures can reduce the risk of developing metastatic disease.

REVIEW QUESTIONS

1. What are the symptoms of ovarian cancer?

2. What are the symptoms of uterine cancer?

3. Why is a virgin less likely to develop cervical cancer than a sexually active woman?

4. What happens when endometrial tissue is located outside the uterus?

5. Why is early diagnosis of reproductive issues important?

CRITICAL THINKING QUESTIONS

1. Thinking about the hormone interactions, why does polycystic ovarian disease produce problems throughout the body?

2. Breast cancer and reproductive system cancers are often linked. What are some of the possible reasons?

WEBLINKS

Centers for Disease Control
www.cdc.gov
National Cancer Institute
www.cancer.gov

WOREC
www.worecnepal.org

REFERENCES

Adam E., Kaufman R. H., & Adler-Storthz K., et al. (1985). A prospective study of association of herpes simplex virus and human papillomavirus with cervical neoplasia in women exposed to diethylstilbesterol in utero. *International Journal of Cancer, 35,* 19–27.

Altekruse, S. F., Kosary, C. L., Krapcho, M., Neyman, N., Aminou, R., Waldron, W., Ruhl, J., Howlader, N., Tatalovich, Z., Cho, H., Mariotto, A., Eisner, M. P., Lewis, D. R., Cronin, K., Chen, H. S., Feuer, E. J., Stinchcomb, D. G., & Edwards, B. K. (Eds). (2010). *SEER Cancer Statistics Review, 1975–2007,* National Cancer Institute. Bethesda, MD, http://seer.cancer.gov/csr/1975_2007/, based on November 2009 SEER data submission, posted to the SEER web site.

American Cancer Society. (2009). *Cancer facts & figures 2009*. Retrieved from http://www.cancer.org/Research/CancerFactsFigures/cancer-facts-figures-2009.

American Joint Committee on Cancer. (2002). *AJCC cancer staging manual* (6th ed.). New York, NY: Springer.

Basnet, M. (2005). Women's Reproductive Health Situation in Eastern-Terai, Nepal.

Beckman, C. R., Ling, F. W., & Barzansky, B. M. (2010). *Obstetrics and gynecology* (6th ed.). Philadelphia, PA: Wolters Kluwer/Lippincott Williams and Wilkens.

Béguelin, W., Díaz Flaqué, M. C., Proietti, C. J., Cayrol, F., Rivas, M. A., Tkach, M., Rosemblit, C., Tocci, J. M., Charreau, E. H., Schillaci, R., & Elizalde, P. V. (2010). Progesterone receptor induces ErbB-2 nuclear translocation to promote breast cancer growth via a novel transcriptional effect: ErbB-2 function as a coactivator of Stat3. *Molecular and Cellular Biology, 30*(23), 5456–5472.

Ben-Baruch, G., Rothenberg, O., Modan, M., & Menczer, J. (1991). Abnormal cervical cytologic, colposcopic and histologic findings in exposed DES young Israeli Jewish women. *Clinical and Experimental Obstetrics and Gynecology, 18*(2), 71–74.

Bessaoud, F., & Daurès, J. P. (2008). Patterns of alcohol (especially wine) consumption and breast cancer risk: A case-control study among a population in Southern France. *Annals of Epidemiology, 18*(6), 467–475.

Bidgoli, S. A., Ahmadi, R., & Zavarhei, M. D. (2010). Role of hormonal and environmental factors on early incidence of breast cancer in Iran. *Science of the Total Environment, 408*(19), 4056–4061.

Bucella, D., Frédéric, B., & Noël, J. C. (2008). Giant cervical polyp: A case report and review of a rare entity. *Archives of Gynecology and Obstetrics, 278*(3), 295–298.

Bułhak-Kozioł, V., Zdrodowska-Stefanow, B., Ostaszewska-Puchalska, I., Maćkowiak-Matejczyk, B., Pietrewicz, T. M., & Wilkowska-Trojniel, M. (2007). Prevalence of *Chlamydia trachomatis* infection in women with cervical lesions. *Advances in Medical Science, 52*, 179–181.

Burton, K. (2005). The face of breast cancer. Retrieved from http://www.uchospitals.edu/pdf/uch_009154.pdf.

Byers, T., Graham, S., Rzepka, T., & Marshall, J. (1985). Lactation and breast cancer. Evidence for a negative association in premenopausal women. *American Journal of Epidemiology, 121*(5), 664–674.

Chang, S., Long, S. R., Kutikova, L., Bowman, L., Finley, D., Crown, W. H., & Bennett, C. L. (2004). Estimating the cost of cancer: Results on the basis of claims data analyses for cancer patients diagnosed with seven types of cancer during 1999 to 2000. *Journal of Clinical Oncology, 22*(17), 3524–3530.

Chen, J., Power, K. A., Mann, J., Cheng, A., & Thompson, L. U. (2007). Flaxseed alone or in combination with tamoxifen inhibits MCF-7 breast tumor growth in ovariectomized athymic mice with high circulating levels of estrogen. *Experimental Biology and Medicine* (Maywood), *232*(8), 1071–1080.

Collaborative Group on Epidemiological Studies of Ovarian Cancer. Beral, V., Doll, R., Hermon, C., Peto, R., & Reeves, G. (2008). Ovarian cancer and oral contraceptives: collaborative reanalysis of data from 45 epidemiological studies including 23 257 women with ovarian cancer and 87 303 controls. *Lancet, 371*(9609), 303–314. doi:10.1016/S0140-6736(08)60167-1.

Collaborative Group on Hormonal Factors in Breast Cancer. (2002). Breast cancer and breastfeeding: Collaborative reanalysis of individual data from 47 epidemiological studies in 30 countries, including 50 302 women with breast cancer and 96 973 women without the disease. *Lancet, 360*(9328), 187–195. doi:10.1016/S0140-6736(02)09454-0.

Colleoni, M., & Giobbie-Hurder, A. (2010). Benefits and adverse effects of endocrine therapy. *Annals of Oncology, 21* Suppl 7, vii107–vii111.

Cowan, L. D., Gordis, L., Tonascia, J. A., & Jones, G. S. (1981). Breast cancer incidence in women with a history of progesterone deficiency. *American Journal of Epidemiology, 114*(2), 209–217.

Cutts, F. T., Franceschi, S., Goldie, S., Castellsague, X., de Sanjose, S., Garnett, G., Edmunds, W. J.,

Claeys, P., Goldenthal, K. L., Harper, D. M., & Markowitz, L. (2007). Human papillomavirus and HPV vaccines: A review. *Bulletin of the World Health Organization, 85*(9), 719–726.

Datta, S. D., Koutsky, L. A., Ratelle, S., Unger, E. R., Shlay, J., McClain, T., Weaver, B., Kerndt, P., Zenilman, J., Hagensee, M., Suhr, C. J., & Weinstock, H. (2008). Human papillomavirus infection and cervical cytology in women screened for cervical cancer in the United States, 2003–2005. *Annals of Internal Medicine, 148*(7), 493–500.

Dunn, R. A., Tan, A., & Samad, I. (2010). Does performance of breast self-exams increase the probability of using mammography: Evidence from Malaysia. *Asian Pacific Journal of Cancer Prevention, 11*(2): 417–421.

Eliassen, A. H., Hankinson, S. E., Rosner, B., Holmes, M. D., & Willett, W. C. (2010). Physical activity and risk of breast cancer among postmenopausal women. *Archives of Internal Medicine, 170*(19), 1758–1764.

Ferreira, M., Crespo, M., Martins, L., & Félix, A. (2008). HPV DNA detection and genotyping in 21 cases of primary invasive squamous cell carcinoma of the vagina. *Modern Pathology, 21,* 968–972.

Gallagher, D. J., Gaudet, M. M., Pal, P., Kirchhoff, T., Balistreri, L., Vora, K., Bhatia, J., Stadler, Z., Fine, S. W., Reuter, V., Zelefsky, M., Morris, M. J., Scher, H. I., Klein, R. J., Norton, L., Eastham, J. A., Scardino, P. T., Robson, M. E., & Offit, K. (2010). Germline BRCA mutations denote a clinicopathologic subset of prostate cancer. *Clinical Cancer Research, 16*(7), 2115–2121. doi:10.1158/1078-0432.

Gao, X., Yu, L., Castro, L., Moore, A. B., Hermon, T., Bortner, C., Sifre, M., & Dixon, D. (2010). An endocrine-disrupting chemical, fenvalerate, induces cell cycle progression and collagen type I expression in human uterine leiomyoma and myometrial cells. *Toxicology Letters, 196*(3), 133–141.

Garcia y Narvaiza, D., Navarrete, M. A., Falzoni, R., Maier, C. M., & Nazário, A. C. (2008). Effect of combined oral contraceptives on breast epithelial proliferation in young women. *Breast Journal, 14*(5), 450–455.

Gardner, H. L., & Dukes, C. D. (1955). *Hemophilus vaginalis* vaginitis. *American Journal of Obstetrics and Gynecology, 69*(5), 962–975.

Gay, C., Riehl, C., Ramanah, R., Desmoulin, G., & Violaine, B. (2006). Cryotherapy in the management of symptomatic cervical ectopy. *Gynécologie Obstétrique & Fertilité, 34*(3), 214–223.

Giersig, C. (2008). Progestin and breast cancer. The missing pieces of a puzzle. *Bundesgesundheitsblatt Gesundheitsforschung Gesundheitsschutz, 51*(7), 782–786.

Goldin, B. R., Adlercreutz, H., Gorbach, S. L., Warram, J. H., Dwyer, J. T., Swenson, L., & Woods, M. N. (1982). Estrogen excretion patterns and plasma levels in vegetarian and omnivorous women. *New England Journal of Medicine, 307*(25), 1542–1547.

González, E. R. (1983). Chronic anovulation may increase postmenopausal breast cancer risk. *Journal of the American Medical Association, 249*(4), 445–446.

Gowen, L. C., Avrutskaya, A. V., Latour, A. M., Koller, B. H., & Leadon, S. A. (1998). BRCA1 required for transcription-coupled repair of oxidative DNA damage. *Science, 281*(5379), 1009–1012.

Grow, D. R. & Hsu, A. L. (2006). Endometriosis, part 1: Clinical diagnosis and analgesia. *Female Patient, 31*(11).

Groysman, V. (2010). Vulvodynia: New concepts and review of the literature. *Dermatology Clinics, 28*(4), 681–696.

Gumus, I. I., Sarifakioglu, E., Uslu, H., & Turhan, N. O. (2008). Vulvodynia: case report and review of literature. *Gynecologic and Obstetric Investigation, 65*(3), 155–161.

Hayes, A. H. (1869). *Sexual physiology of woman, and her diseases.* Boston, MA: Peabody Medical Institute.

Herbst, A. L., Anderson, S., & Hubby, M. M., et al. (1986). Risk factors for the development of diethylstilbestrol associated clear cell adenocarcinoma. *American Journal of Obstetrics and Gynecology, 154,* 814–820.

Herbst, A. L., Senekjian, E. K., & Frey, K. W. (1989). Abortion and pregnancy loss among diethylstilbestrol-exposed women. *Seminars in Reproductive Endocrinology, 7,* 124–129.

Hirst, A., Dutton, S., Wu, O., Briggs, A., Edwards, C., Waldenmaier, L., Maresh, M., Nicholson, A., & McPherson, K. (2008). A multi-centre retrospective cohort study comparing the efficacy, safety and cost-effectiveness of hysterectomy and uterine artery embolisation for the treatment of symptomatic uterine fibroids. The HOPEFUL study. *Health Technology Assessment, 12*(5), 1–248.

Hoeger, K. M. (2008). Exercise therapy in polycystic ovary syndrome. *Seminars in Reproductive Medicine, 26*(1), 93–100.

Hutchins, A. M., Martini, M. C., Olson, B. A., Thomas, W., & Slavin, J. L. (2001). Flaxseed consumption influences endogenous hormone concentrations in postmenopausal women. *Nutrition and Cancer, 39*(1), 58–65.

Jordan, V. C. (1988). Chemosuppression of breast cancer with tamoxifen: Laboratory evidence and future clinical investigations. *Cancer Investigation, 6,* 589–595.

Kennedy, S., Bergqvist, A., Chapron, C., D'Hooghe, T., Dunselman, G., Greb, R., Hummelshoj, L., Prentice, A., & Saridogan, E., and on behalf of the ESHRE Special Interest Group for Endometriosis and Endometrium Guideline Development Group. (2005). ESHRE guideline for the diagnosis and treatment of endometriosis. *Human Reproduction, 20*(10), 2698–2704. doi:10.1093/humrep/dei135.

Key, T., Appleby, P., Barnes, I., & Reeves, G., and Endogenous Hormones and Breast Cancer Collaborative Group. (2002). Endogenous sex hormones and breast cancer in postmenopausal women: Reanalysis of nine prospective studies. *Journal of the National Cancer Institute,94*(8), 606–616.

Knight, J. A., Bernstein, L., Largent, J., Capanu, M., Begg, C. B., Mellemkjaer, L., Lynch, C. F., Malone, K. E., Reiner, A. S., Liang, X., Haile, R. W., & Boice, J. D., Jr., WECARE Study Collaborative Group, & Bernstein, J. L. (2009). Alcohol intake and cigarette smoking and risk of a contralateral breast cancer: The Women's Environmental Cancer and Radiation Epidemiology Study. *American Journal of Epidemiology, 169*(8), 962–968.

Kortenkamp, A. (2006). Breast cancer, oestrogens and environmental pollutants: A re-evaluation from a mixture perspective. *International Journal of Andrology, 29*(1), 193–198.

Kurman, R. J., Visvanathan, K., Roden, R., Wu, T. C., & Shih, I.M. (2008). Early detection and treatment of ovarian cancer: shifting from early stage to minimal volume of disease based on a new model of carcinogenesis. *American Journal of Obstetrics and Gynecology, 198*(4), 351–356.

Lancaster, J. M., Carney, M. E., & Futreal, P. A. (1997). BRCA 1 and 2—A genetic link to familial breast and ovarian cancer. *Medscape Women's Health, 2*(2), 7.

Leung, F., Terzibachian, J. J., Aouar, Z., Govyadovskiy, A., & Lassabe, C. (2008). Uterine sarcomas: Clinical and histopathological aspects. Report on 15 cases. *Gynécologie Obstétrique & Fertilité, 36*(6), 628–635.

Lindahl, B., Andolf, E., Ingvar, C., Ranstam, J., & Willén, R. (2008). Adjuvant tamoxifen in breast cancer patients affects the endometrium by time, an effect remaining years after end of treatment and results in an increased frequency of endometrial carcinoma. *Anticancer Research, 28*(2B), 1259–1262.

Mascherpa, F., Bogliatto, F., Lynch, P. J., Micheletti, L., & Benedetto, C. (2007). Vulvodynia as a possible somatization disorder. More than just an opinion. *Journal of Reproductive Medicine, 52*(2), 107–110.

McCann, S. E., Moysich, K. B., & Mettlin, C. (2001). Intakes of selected nutrients and food groups and risk of ovarian cancer. *Nutrition and Cancer, 39*(1), 19–28.

McKay, M., Frankman, O., & Horowitz, B. J., et al. (1991). Vulvar vestibulitis and vestibular papillomatosis. Report of the ISSVD committee on vulvodynia. *Journal of Reproductive Medicine, 36*(6), 413–415.

McTiernan, A., & Thomas, D. B. (1986). Evidence for a protective effect of lactation on risk of breast cancer in young women. Results from a case-control study. *American Journal of Epidemiology,124*(3), 353–358.

Meisels, A., Roy, M., & Fortier, M., et al. (1981). Human papillomavirus virus infection of the cervix: The atypical condyloma. *Acta Cytologica, 25*(1), 7–16.

Michels, K. B., & Willett, W. C. (2009). The Women's Health Initiative randomized controlled dietary modification trial: A post-mortem. *Breast Cancer Research and Treatment, 114*(1), 1–6.

Michnovicz, J. J., & Bradlow, H. L. (1990). Induction of estradiol metabolism by dietary indole-3-carbinol in humans. *Journal of the National Cancer Institute, 82*(11), 947–949.

Missmer, S. A., Eliassen, A. H., Barbieri, R. L., & Hankinson, S. E. (2004). Endogenous estrogen, androgen, and progesterone concentrations and breast cancer risk among postmenopausal women. *Journal of the National Cancer Institute, 96*(24), 1856–1865.

Montgomery, G. W., Nyholt, D. R, Zhao, Z. Z., Treloar, S. A., Painter, J. N., Missmer, S. A., Kennedy, S. H., & Zondervan, K. T. (2008). The search for genes contributing to endometriosis risk. *Human Reproduction Update, 14*(5), 447–457.

Moran, L. J., Brinkworth, G. D., & Norman, R. J. (2008). Dietary therapy in polycystic ovary syndrome. *Seminars in Reproductive Medicine, 26*(1), 85–92.

National Breast Cancer Foundation. (2010). Retrieved from http://www.nationalbreastcancer.org/About-Breast-Cancer/Types.aspx.

National Cancer Institute. (2010). Retrieved from www.cancer.gov.

Okolo, S. (2008). Incidence, aetiology and epidemiology of uterine fibroids. *Best Practices & Research Clinical Obstetrics & Gynaecology, 22*(4), 571–588.

Pollak, M., Costantino, J., Polychronakos, C., Blauer, S. A., Guyda, H., Redmond, C., Fisher, B., & Margolese, R. (1990). Effect of tamoxifen on serum insulinlike growth factor I levels in stage I breast cancer patients. *Journal of the National Cancer Institute, 82*(21), 1693–1697.

Reid, R., Stanhope, R., & Herschman, B. R., et al. (1982). Genital warts and cervical cancer. *Cancer, 50,* 377–383.

Reynolds, P., Goldberg, D., Hurley, S., Nelson, D. O., Largent, J., Henderson, K. D., & Bernstein, L. (2009). Passive smoking and risk of breast cancer in the California teachers study. *Cancer Epidemiology, Biomarkers & Prevention, 18*(12), 3389–3398.

Saarinen, N. M., Power, K. A., Chen, J., & Thompson, L. U. (2006). Flaxseed attenuates the tumor growth stimulating effect of soy protein in ovariectomized athymic mice with MCF-7 human breast cancer xenographs. *International Journal of Cancer, 119*(4), 925–931.

Saarinen, N. M., Power, K. A., Chen, J., & Thompson, L. U. (2008). Lignans are accessible to human breast cancer xenographs in athymic mice. *Nutrition and Cancer, 60*(2), 245–250.

Sadri, G., & Mahjub, H. (2007). Passive or active smoking, which is more relevant to breast cancer. *Saudi Medical Journal, 28*(2), 254–258.

Sardanelli, F., Podo, F., Santoro, F., Manoukian, S., Bergonzi, S., Trecate, G., Vergnaghi, D., Federico, M., Cortesi, L., Corcione, S., Morassut, S., Di Maggio, C., Cilotti, A., Martincich, L., Calabrese, M., Zuiani, C., Preda, L., Bonanni, B., Carbonaro, L. A., Contegiacomo, A., Panizza, P., Di Cesare, E., Savarese, A., Crecco, M., Turchetti, D., Tonutti, M., Belli, P., & Maschio, A. D. (2010). Multicenter surveillance of women at high genetic breast cancer risk using mammography, ultrasonography, and contrast-enhanced magnetic resonance imaging (the High Breast Cancer Risk Italian 1 Study): Final results. *Investigative Radiology, 46*(2), 94–105.

Sayed, G. H., Zakherah, M. S., El-Nashar, S. A., & Shabaan, M. M. (2010). A randomized clinical trial of a levonorgestrel-releasing intrauterine system and a low-dose combined oral contraceptive for fibroid-related menorrhagia. *International Journal of Gynaecology and Obstetrics, 112*(2), 122–130.

Schapira, D. V., Kumar, N. B., Lyman, G. H., & Cox, C. E. (1990). Abdominal obesity and breast cancer risk. *Annals of Internal Medicine, 112*(3), 182–186.

Schmidt, G., & Fowler, W. D. (1982b). Ovarian cystadenofibromas in three women with antenatal exposure to diethylstilbestrol. *Gynecologic Oncology, 14*(2), 175–184.

Senekjian, E. K., Frey, K. W., Stone, C., & Herbst, A. L. (1988). An evaluation of stage II vaginal clear cell adenocarcinoma according to substages. *Gynecologic Oncology, 31*(1), 56–64.

Senekjian, E. K., Potkul, R. K., Frey, K. W., & Herbst, A. L. (1988). Infertility among daughters either exposed or not exposed to diethylstilbestrol. *American Journal of Obstetrics and Gynecology, 158*(3 Pt. 1), 493–498.

Stewart, E. A., Gedroyc, W. M., Tempany, C. M., Quade, B. J., Inbar, Y., Ehrenstein, T., Shushan, A., Hindley, J. T., Goldin, R. D., David, M., Sklair, M., & Rabinovici, J. (2003). Focused ultrasound treatment of uterine fibroid tumors: Safety and feasibility of a noninvasive thermoablative technique. *American Journal of Obstetrics and Gynecology, 189*(1), 48–54.

Suhrke, P., Zahl, P. H., & Maehlen, J. (2009). Declining breast cancer incidence and decreased HRT use. *Lancet, 373*(9662), 460–461.

Suzuki, R., Rylander-Rudqvist, T., Ye, W., Saji, S., Adlercreutz, H., & Wolk, A. (2008). Dietary fiber intake and risk of postmenopausal breast cancer defined by estrogen and progesterone receptor status—a prospective cohort study among Swedish women. *International Journal of Cancer, 122*(2), 403–412.

Swan, J., Breen, N., Coates, R. J., Rimer, B. K., & Lee, N. C. (2003). Progress in cancer screening practices in the United States: Results from the 2000 National Health Interview Survey. *Cancer, 97*(6), 1528–1540.

Thompson Reuters. (2008, October 13). Thomson Reuters survey finds cancer patients forgoing treatment because of cost. Retrieved from http://thomsonreuters.com/content/press_room/healthcare/TR_Survey_Finds_Cancer_Patients.

Touillaud, M. S., Thiebaut, A. C., Fournier, A., Niravong, M., Boutron-Ruault, M. C., & Clavel-Chapelon, F. (2007). Dietary lignan intake and postmenopausal breast cancer risk by estrogen and progesterone receptor status. *Journal of the National Cancer Institute, 99*(6), 475–486.

U.S. Cancer Statistics Working Group. (2007). *United States cancer statistics: 2004 incidence and mortality.* Atlanta, GA: Department of Health and Human Services, Centers for Disease Control and Prevention, and National Cancer Institute.

Vale, C., Tierney, J. F., Stewart, L. A., Brady, M., Dinshaw, K., Jakobsen, A., Parmar, M. K., Thomas, G., Trimble, T., Alberts, D. S., Chen, H., Cikaric, S., Eifel, P. J., Garipagaoglu, M., Keys, H., Kantardzic, N., Lal, P., Lanciano, R., Leborgne, F., Lorvidhaya, V., Onishi, H., Pearcey, R. G., Pras, E., Roberts, K., Rose, P. G., Thomas, G., & Whitney, C. W. (2008). Reducing uncertainties about the effects of chemoradiotherapy for cervical cancer: A systematic review and meta-analysis of individual patient data from 18 randomized trials. *Journal of Clinical Oncology, 26*(35), 5802–5812.

Vonka, V., Kanka, J., & Hirsch, I., et al. (1984). A prospective study of the relationship between cervical neoplasia and herpes simplex type-2 virus. *International Journal of Cancer, 33,* 61–70.

Witorsch, R. J., & Thomas, J. A. (2010). Personal care products and endocrine disruption: A critical review of the literature. *Critical Reviews in Toxicology, 40* Suppl 3, 1–30.

chapter 9

FEMALE SEXUALITY

CHAPTER COMPETENCIES

Upon completion of this chapter, the reader will be able to:

- Outline and describe the physiological components of the female sexual response and orgasm
- Outline the health benefits of sexual activity
- Describe and understand the potential health risks of sexual activity, as well as ways to reduce the risks

- Describe and understand the nature and treatment of sexual dysfunction in women
- Discuss the current medical opinion regarding sexual activity during pregnancy and in regard to other medical conditions
- Identify and describe the impact of a variety of drugs and substances on female sexual response

KEY TERMS

anorgasmia	dyspareunia	orgasm	vasocongestion
coitus	myotonia	orgasmic platform	

INTRODUCTION

For most animal species **coitus**, or sexual intercourse, is linked directly to reproduction. Sexual activity is likely to take place only during particular seasons of the year, in order to time the arrival of offspring to coincide with the richest availability of food or other resources that are needed to raise the young. During the breeding season, females of a species will often signal their receptivity to mating, either through temporary changes in appearance or through the release of pheromones, which serve to attract males to them. Humans are relatively unique in that sexual activity is neither confined to a breeding season nor limited only to reproduction. Some other species of primates share this characteristic with humans, with bonobo chimpanzees probably being the best known example. Bonobo chimpanzees engage in a wide range of sexual activity throughout the year, and in fact use sexual contact to maintain social cohesion within the troop, and to reduce stress (Figure 9-1).

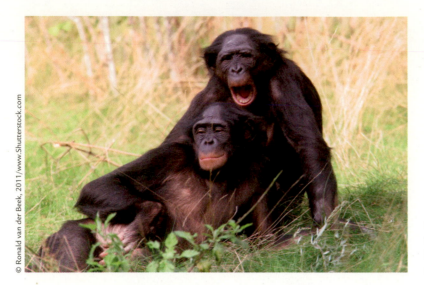

© Ronald van der Beek, 2011//www.Shutterstock.com

FIGURE 9-1: Bonobo chimpanzees are among the only mammals besides humans to engage in sexual contact for reasons other than reproduction.

PHYSIOLOGY OF THE FEMALE SEXUAL RESPONSE

It is important to remember that the physiology of the female sexual response is the same no matter how it is initiated. As a result of their groundbreaking research on human sexuality, Masters and Johnson divided the female and male sexual response cycle into four phases: excitement, plateau, orgasm, and resolution. These stages were considered successive; each phase following the other along a continuum, and this progression was considered to be the same in both sexes. Masters and Johnson identified the sequence as excitement, plateau, and orgasm, followed by resolution. During the four phases, there are two basic kinds of physiological mechanisms that cause the sexual response. One is congestion or an increased flow of blood into the organs so that the tissues become engorged (swollen) and usually undergo a color change. This increase in blood flow and concentration is called **vasocongestion**. The other main physiological phenomenon is **myotonia**, the increased muscular tension that occurs both in voluntary (skeletal) muscles and in involuntary smooth muscles. Vasocongestion and myotonia result in the physical manifestations that are visible in the genitalia and also appear as body responses such as changes in heart rate, breathing rate, blood pressure, and perspiration. More recent analysis of female sexuality suggests that the four stage progression is not universal to all women or for all sexual encounters.

The Excitement Phase of the Sexual Cycle

Sexual stimulation causes sensory nerve impulses primarily from the clitoris but also from the vulva to travel to the spinal cord and then to the brain. Reflexes in the spinal cord result in parasympathetic nerve impulses that cause arteries to dilate in the tissues of the genitals, and the subsequent vasocongestion that sets the stage for orgasm. The first sign of physiological response occurs in the vagina within 10–30 seconds of the initiation of sexual stimulation. The "sweating" of the vaginal walls as a result of the vasocongestion of the vaginal blood vessels results in the lubrication of the entire vagina. Almost simultaneously with lubrication, and as a result of vasocongestion, the entire vagina dilates. The increased flow of blood also produces a color change in the vaginal wall, turning it deeper shades of purple.

As the uterus becomes engorged with blood, it moves up and out of its regular position, rising slightly in the pelvic cavity. The shifting position, along with the expansion of the vaginal walls, produces a tenting or ballooning out of the inner two-thirds of the interior of the vagina (Figure 9–2). This happens only if the uterus is in the typical ante-verted position; it does not occur in a retroverted uterus. Vasocongestion causes changes in the clitoris as well, and the constriction of the ischiocavernosus and bulbocavernosus muscles contribute to clitoral enlargement. In approximately 50 percent of the women observed by Masters and Johnson, the glans

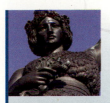

Historical Considerations
THE HISTORY OF HUMAN SEX RESEARCH

The nature of the female sexual response or any kind of sex research at all was largely a taboo subject in science until a zoologist at Indiana University, Alfred C. Kinsey, started to teach a marriage course in 1937. Dr. Kinsey was an entomologist, a specialist on insects, when he took over the marriage course. Kinsey quickly discovered that there was very little scientific perspective about human sexual behavior. In order to provide his students with facts, he decided he would have to gather data about human sexuality himself. He approached his task with the same meticulous precision with which he studied insects. With the publication of his observations in 1948 and 1953, popularly known as The Kinsey Report, he opened up the field of sex research as a valid scientific discipline. Kinsey's work foreshadowed the laboratory studies of human sexual responses observed by gynecologist William Masters and his associate, Virginia Johnson, at Washington University in St. Louis that took place 20 years later. Masters and Johnson were interested in studying the physiological changes that take place during sexual intercourse. Under controlled laboratory conditions, they reported on the physiological responses of 382 women and 312 men between the ages of 18 and 89 during more than 10,000 sexual response cycles. They made observations during manual masturbation, during masturbation with a vibrator, during intercourse in several positions, while the breasts alone were stimulated without genital contact, and also during "artificial coitus" with a plastic penis containing a movie camera to record internal changes.

Masters and Johnson received criticism for focusing on the anatomical and physiological aspects of sexual activity at the expense of emotional aspects. However, until their research findings were published, little was known about the mechanics of the female sexual response. Important physiological events of the female sexual response, such as vaginal lubrication, the distension of the inner two-thirds of the vagina, the gaping of the cervical os, and the elevation of the uterus, had not been previous observed. In addition to expanding understanding about the physiology of sex, these observations have had clinical value in understanding infertility problems and contraceptive research.

---

of the clitoris doubled in diameter; in the other half of the subjects, however, there was no visible difference in the size of the glans, although swelling could be seen if the glans were observed through endoscopy. The blood that flows into the corpora cavernosa of the shaft of the clitoris causes the shaft to increase in diameter, but only in about 10 percent of the women does the clitoral shaft visibly elongate. Since recent studies have found that the clitoris is much larger than previously understood and wraps around the vaginal vault. The enlargement of the clitoris is likely to affect sensation in the vagina itself. Additional studies found swelling in the erectile tissue near the opening of the urethra in eighty percent of women.

As vasocongestion increases, the labia minora swell, and their color darkens. The labia majora also undergo congestive changes, but the extent can depend on whether the woman has delivered children or not. Pregnancy results in a general increase in pelvic blood flow, and this may account for the differences. Usually, in a nonexcited state, the major lips meet in the midline of the vaginal orifice. During the excitement phase in women who have not had children, the labia majora thin out and flatten themselves against the perineum, elevated away from and opening up the entrance to the vagina. In a woman who has had children, the major lips often do not flatten but become swollen and distended. Very late in the excitement phase, the Bartholin's glands may secrete

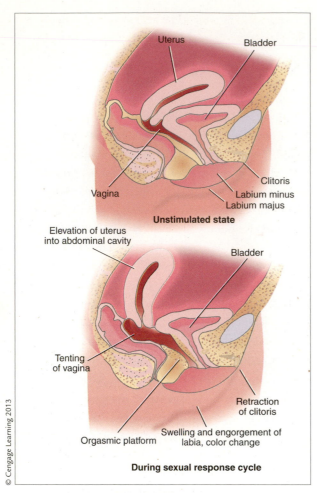

Uterus

Bladder

Vagina

Clitoris

Labium minus

Labium majus

Unstimulated state

Elevation of uterus
into abdominal cavity

Bladder

Tenting
of vagina

Retraction
of clitoris

Orgasmic platform

Swelling and engorgement of
labia, color change

During sexual response cycle

© Cengage Learning 2013

FIGURE 9-2: Changes that occur in the pelvic area during the excitement and the orgasmic phases of the sexual response cycle.

a trace amount of fluid, but this is after the vagina is well lubricated. These glands, therefore, play only a small role in vaginal lubrication.

Nipple erection occurs in many women early in the excitement phase. Sometimes one nipple becomes erect before the other. There may be an increase in nipple length of 0.5–1.5 cm and in diameter of the nipple base of 0.25–1.0 cm. The areola enlarges and swells later in the excitement phase. By the end of this phase, the breasts have increased in size by 20–25 percent, more noticeably in women who have not breastfed a child. The veins of the breasts may become more apparent because of engorgement with blood.

Another vascular change that occurred in the laboratory in approximately 75 percent of the women and 25 percent of the men during the sexual cycle was the "sex flush." Beginning on the upper part of the abdomen and spreading up to the chest, throat, and

neck, a pink mottling appears on the skin. It is especially obvious in fair-skinned people. As the excitement phase progresses, there is increased tension in the voluntary muscles of the arms and legs, the rectal muscles, some of the abdominal muscles, and the intercostal muscles of the ribs. In addition, heart rate and blood pressure increase, although there is usually no observable change in respiration or perspiration at this point.

Plateau Phase of the Sexual Cycle

During the plateau stage, the bulbocavernosus muscles contract and compress the veins in the bulbs of the vestibule, the highly vascular tissue that is equivalent to the corpus spongiosum in males. The bulbs become turgid and swollen, producing a vulvar erection that reduces the diameter of the outer third of the vaginal barrel by approximately 50 percent. This is what Masters and Johnson called the orgasmic platform. The elevation of the uterus and the vasocongestion produce an increasing sensitivity in the smooth muscle of the uterus. This sensitivity can trigger uterine contractions late in the plateau phase.

The clitoris also elevates in the plateau phase from its normal position of overhanging the lower border of the pubic bone. In this stage of the cycle, the body and glans of the clitoris retract from their non-stimulated overhanging position and withdraw deep under the prepuce, carrying the labia minora and the suspensory ligament along toward the pubic symphysis. The clitoris is no longer externally visible after this elevation, but it still responds to stimulation by pressure on the mons pubis over the pubic bone and/or by the thrusting that pulls on the labia minora, producing traction on the prepuce. A finger, a vibrator, or other kind of tactile friction will have the same effect. For 25 percent of women, pulling on the labia minora during vaginal intercourse is sufficient to stimulate the clitoris and trigger an orgasm. For most women, however, more direct stimulation of the clitoris is required.

The labia majora continues to show more of the changes that started during the excitement phase. In women who have not had children, the labia majora flatten out even more; in women who have had children, they become more swollen and engorged. Late in the plateau phase, the labia minora experience more of a vivid color change, and orgasm will usually occur within a few minutes if clitoral stimulation is continued. More turgidity of the nipples occurs, and there is further swelling of the areola and entire breasts. If a sex flush has occurred, it spreads over the shoulders, down the inner surface of the arms, and perhaps onto the abdomen, thighs, buttocks, and back. There is a further increase in the tightening of both voluntary and involuntary muscles and intercostals of the ribs. There may also be voluntary tightening of the rectal sphincter and the buttock and thigh muscles. The heart rate increases from a normal 70 beats per minute to 100–175 beats per minute and there is an elevation in blood pressure. Late in the plateau phase, there is also an increase in respiratory rate.

The Orgasm Phase of the Sexual Cycle

During an orgasm the **orgasmic platform**, the muscles that make up the outer third of the vaginal wall and those surrounding the turgid tissues of the vulva, undergoes rhythmic contractions that occur at roughly 0.8 second intervals. In a mild **orgasm**, there may be three to five such contractions; a more intense orgasm results in more contractions. The onset of rhythmic muscle contractions around and in the vagina causes most of the blood and fluid to then empty from the pelvis. Both the clitoris and the vagina form an integral part of the orgasmic reaction. Along with the throbbing sensation in the vagina, the uterus undergoes contractions; each begins at the top (fundus) of the uterus and works its way toward the cervix. If sex flush is present, it reaches a peak of intensity with the onset of orgasm.

The entire body is so involved in the experience of orgasm that some voluntary muscular control is lost as the involuntary contraction of many muscle groups takes place. The spontaneous involuntary contractions of the muscles of the pelvic floor cause the throbbing of the orgasmic platform and may result in the same 0.8-second contractions of the external rectal sphincter. If they occur, the anal contractions do not last as long and usually involve only a few spasms. Both superficial and deep muscles of the arms, legs, neck, abdomen, and buttocks also contract. The hands and feet are extended while the fingers and toes curl under. This spastic posture is called carpopedal spasm. The amount of muscle contraction that occurs with orgasm is an individual response. It may be so mild as to barely be visible, or it may be uncontrollably convulsive.

Resolution Stage of the Sexual Cycle

Within a few seconds of orgasm, the two physiological mechanisms that created the sexual responses, vasocongestion and contractions, are rapidly dissipated. The blood rapidly drains out of the engorged tissues, and the orgasmic platform relaxes. The anterior wall of the vagina returns to meet the posterior wall, and the deep color fades, although the complete return to normal coloring may take as long as 10–15 minutes. The elevated uterus returns to its normal unstimulated position. The cervix returns to its relaxed position in the posterior fornix, the location where semen pools if the woman has been lying on her back during intercourse. The external os of the cervix remains slightly dilated for approximately 20–30 minutes. If orgasm does not occur after a progression through the plateau phase, the vasocongestion that produced the enlargement of the uterus takes much longer to resolve, and engorgement may persist for as long as an hour, or even longer in women who have had children.

Ten seconds after the last vaginal contraction, the external portion of the clitoris returns to its normal position overhanging the pubic symphysis, but the engorgement with blood that produced the size increase takes longer to dissipate. The glans remains very sensitive for several minutes; in some women it is actually painful to the touch. The labia minora return to their original color and size within 10–15 seconds. The labia majora return to the normal midline position and size more quickly in nulliparous women. In a woman who has had several children, the labia majora may retain their engorgement for several hours.

All body responses, including muscle tension, heart rate, blood pressure, and respiratory rate rapidly return to preorgasmic levels unless there is further sexual stimulation. The sex flush disappears in reverse order of its appearance, and in approximately one-third of the women subjects there is the appearance of a widespread film of perspiration over the chest, back, and thighs. Heavier sweating occurs on the forehead, upper lip, and under the arms. The swelling of the areolae of the breasts promptly disappears.

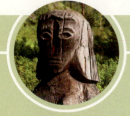

focus on

NUTRITION

Nutritional Supplements: Effects on Female Desire

The physiology and mechanics of genital arousal are similar for males and females. Dilating blood vessels allow increased blood flow to the genitals, which causes them to swell. In men, this causes the penis to become erect. In women, this increased blood flow causes swelling in the clitoral and vaginal tissues and makes them more sensitive and responsive to sexual stimulation. This in turn increases feelings of arousal and increases the possibility of reaching orgasm. Blood flow in the body, including blood flow related to sexual arousal is mediated by a chemical called nitric oxide (NO). Therefore, NO is important to normal sexual function in both men and women. An amino acid, L-arginine, is a chemical precursor of nitric oxide (NO) and without it, NO cannot be manufactured. Fortunately, L-arginine is a non-essential amino acid, which means that it is manufactured by the human body, and does not have to be obtained from the diet. However, studies have shown that for women, supplementation with L-arginine can heighten sexual response and may be helpful in maintaining female sexual function. Some foods high in L-arginine include peanuts, walnuts, brazil nuts, coconut, meat, and dairy products.

In one study involving 77 women, 73.5 percent of the women who took a supplement including L-arginine experienced greater sexual satisfaction, including heightened desire and clitoral sensation, frequency of intercourse and orgasm, and less vaginal dryness (Ito et al., 2001). Sexual arousal was measured by measuring vaginal pulse amplitude, a measure of blood flow to the genitals. However, despite these physical changes, the subjective evaluation of their arousal by the women who took the supplement was not different from that of the women who took a placebo; more evidence that female sexual response is complex (Meston & Worcel, 2002).

The nipple erection usually remains longer than the areolar swelling.

In males, the resolution phase after orgasm and ejaculation is followed by a refractory period during which the man cannot respond to sexual stimulation by another sexual cycle. The duration of the period is generally directly related to the age of the male; the younger he is, the sooner he is able to have another erection, ejaculation, and orgasm. In women, there is no such refractory period, and they are said to be multiorgasmic, having the physiological capacity to reach repeated orgasms.

VARIABILITY IN WOMEN'S EXPERIENCE OF ORGASM

When women between the ages of 14 and 92 were surveyed by the National Survey of Sexual Health and Behavior, 64 percent reported that they had an orgasm during their last sexual encounter (Herbenick et al., 2010). According to the survey, women who engaged in a variety of sexual activities, including oral sex and vaginal intercourse, were more likely to report having an orgasm. It is estimated that 75 percent of women require more direct clitoral stimulation than vaginal intercourse alone provides to orgasm. About 10–16 percent of women never experience orgasm (Hooper, 2005). This variability in female orgasm has been the focus of research and some debate.

Natural variability in the anatomy of women's genitals is likely to contribute to the diversity of women's orgasmic experiences. Some have suggested that the distance between the clitoris and the vagina (Davidson, 2010), the presence or absence of glandular tissue (G-spot) located in the anterior wall of the vagina (Battaglia et al., 2010; Jannini et al., 2010, Foldes & Buisson, 2009; Thabert, 2009), and genetics (Hooper, 2005) may play a role in whether a woman experiences orgasm from vaginal intercourse alone, or through more direct stimulation of her clitoris. Others point out that psychosocial and emotional factors can have profound effects on women's sexual experiences.

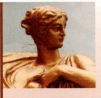

Cultural Considerations
A New Classification for Labia Elongation

Starting at puberty, young women in Rwanda apply medicinal herbs to their labia minora and pull on their labia minora to elongate them. This practice is continued into adulthood. The elongation of the labia is said to enhance sexual pleasure for the woman and her partner and to facilitate both female ejaculation and orgasm. Until recently the World Health Organization classified elongation of the labia as female genital mutilation (FMG), a term that describes the harmful traditional practice of altering female genitals for cultural or religious reasons. In most cases, alterations to a woman's genitals classified as female genital mutilation have the effect of reducing a woman's desire or sexual pleasure, and can have many other negative effects on her health (Fahmy et al., 2010; Al Sibiani & Rouzi, 2010). In contrast, the women of Rwanda view their practice of labial elongation as a positive modification of the genitals that enhances their sexual pleasure. In response, the World Health Organization has released an amendment that distinguishes between labial elongation and female genital mutilation (Koster & Price, 2008).

Physiologically, orgasm is a relatively simple reflex: tactile stimulation causes sensory impulses to travel to a center in the spinal cord and results in a motor response, the contraction of muscles. However, the orgasm reflex can be influenced, either positively or negatively, by thought processes in the brain. The entire life experience of a woman is involved in her sexual response. If the brain says "go," then the appropriate responses are initiated from the spinal cord, and the sensory nerves transmit impulses back to the brain, which perceives the pleasure of orgasm. However, psychological inhibition can block the experience of orgasm, even in the presence of adequate stimulation. By measuring physiological signs of arousal, Chivers et al. (2010) was able to show that women's conscious perception of their arousal state does not always match their physical arousal, underlining the role that thoughts or emotions can have on women's experience. Scans taken of women's brains while they were experiencing an orgasm have found that neural activity increases in the parts of the brain that process sensations, and decrease in the portions of the brain that control alertness and anxiety (LePage, 2005). Hebenich (2010) found that women who feel relaxed with themselves and who were not burdened with feelings of shame or self consciousness with their bodies were more likely to orgasm.

HEALTH BENEFITS OF SEXUAL ACTIVITY

Regular sexual activity has several documented health benefits. For example, sexual activity is good exercise and burns about 170 calories or more an hour. The hormones released during orgasm—oxytocin and DHEA—protect against cancer and heart disease (Komisarukl et al., 2006). Frequent sexual intercourse has been linked with reduced blood pressure and improves cardiovascular health. Although this has not been studied specifically yet in women, it has been found that men who have sex twice or more per week reduced their risk of dying from a heart attack by half. The hormone oxytocin, which is released during orgasm, helps to improve intimacy, and helps to build trust between sexual partners. In addition to these emotional benefits, the surge of oxytocin and endorphins that can accompany sex can also decrease pain. Oxytocin can help to improve sleep, and improved sleep helps to strengthen the immune system and lower blood pressure. Having sexual intercourse once or twice per week strengthens the immune system by increasing the body's production of the antibodies (Charnetski & Brennan, 2004). Interestingly, having sex either less frequently or more than two times per week resulted in lower antibody production.

Finally, many women report that headache, arthritis, and PMS symptoms are reduced after sexual activity.

HEALTH RISKS OF SEXUAL ACTIVITY

The two primary health risks of sexual activity are the contraction of a sexually transmitted infection (STI) or the initiation of an unwanted pregnancy. While there is no way to completely eliminate all of the potential risks associated with sexual activity, steps can be taken to make sexual activity safer. Chapter 6, Reproductive Tract Infections, provides information about sexually transmitted infections and their prevention. Chapter 13, Birth Control, provides comprehensive information about preventing pregnancy.

Safer Sex

It is important to remember that many STIs, including the most deadly ones such as HIV and Hepatitis B, can be present in an individual without any visible symptoms. Until both partners are tested for STIs, it is important to take precautions against infection, and if either partner engages in unprotected sex or other risky behavior, there can be danger of infection. In terms of the chances of acquiring an STI, unprotected sexual behaviors can be categorized as high risk, lower risk, and no risk. Table 9-1 lists sexual behaviors and their risks, and was compiled by Planned Parenthood.

SEXUAL PREFERENCE

The National Survey of Sexual Health and Behavior interviewed nearly 6,000 people in the United States and found that seven percent of women identified themselves as lesbian or bisexual and eight percent of men identified themselves as gay or bisexual. (Figure 9-3) (Zhao et al., 2010).

There is a growing body of research exploring the biological basis for sexual orientation. Same sex sexual behavior is widespread in the natural world, with a broad range of species engaging in a wide range of sexual behaviors (Bailey & Zuk, 2009). In humans, much of the scientific research to date has focused on homosexuality in men. There is evidence that many factors, including genetics, hormonal influences while in the womb, and psychosocial factors appear to contribute to the development of sexual orientation (Jannini et al., 2010; Langstom et al., 2010). For example, studies of identical twins have revealed a genetic component in the development of sexual preference. Langstom et al. (2010) found that genetics accounted for 35 percent of the variation of sexual preference in men, while the rest was influenced by individual-specific environmental factors such as hormonal influences during fetal development. For women, genetics accounted for 18 percent of variation in sexual preference, with 64 percent of variation influenced by individual-specific environmental factors,

Table 9-1 Planned Parenthood: Ranking of Risks for Sexual Behaviors.		
High Risk	**Lower Risk**	**No Risk**
Anal Sex - Putting the penis inside the anus	Oral Sex with a dental dam or a condom	Masturbation—Touching your own body in an erotic manner, without the exchange of body fluids
Vaginal Sex - Putting the penis inside the vagina	Vaginal Sex with a male or female condom	Mutual masturbation—Each partner touching his/her own body
Oral Sex - Putting the mouth on the penis, vagina, or anus	Anal Sex with a male or female condom	Body rubbing—Also known as outercourse; involves pressing and rubbing against your partner's body while your clothes are on
		Erotic massage—Caressing your partner's neck, back, belly, thighs, etc.
		Kissing—"Locking Lips," with or without tongue

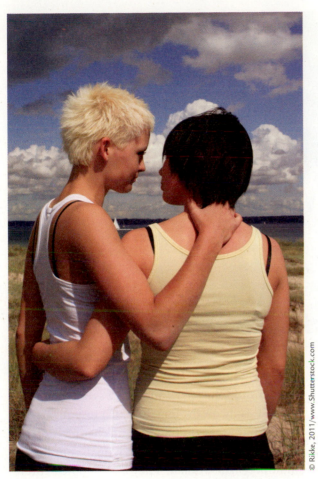

FIGURE 9-3: Components that make up a person's sexual orientation include: sexual identity, attraction or fantasy, and behavior.

© Rikke, 2011/www.Shutterstock.com

and 16 percent by shared environmental factors such as family environment. Differences in brain structure and physiology of homosexuals and heterosexuals have been demonstrated. These differences may be the result of genetics, hormonal, or other influences while in the womb (Garcia-Falgueras & Swaab, 2010; Rahman & Koerting, 2008; Blanchard, 2008). Falgueras and Swaab (2010) suggest that the timing of hormonal influences during pregnancy can have a profound effect on sexual orientation. The presence or absence of testosterone facilitates two important changes during fetal development. During the first two months of pregnancy the level of testosterone present facilitates the development of either male or female genitals, with high levels resulting in male anatomy and low levels resulting in female anatomy. During the second half of pregnancy, the levels of testosterone present shape brain development toward either male or female characteristics, that is, to identify

as either male or female. In this way, sexual orientation is programmed into the developing brain while the fetus is still developing in the womb. Because of this months-long time lag between the differentiation of the genitals and the brain, these two developmental processes can be influenced independently, resulting in same-sex sexual preference. When asked how large of a role choice played in the development of their sexual preference, 95 percent of gay men and 84 percent of gay women reported that they had little or no choice about their sexual orientation (Herek et al., 2010).

There are wide disparities in the cultural acceptance of lesbians, homosexuals, and bisexual (LGB) individuals around the world, with some cultures demonstrating openness and others demonstrating more bigoted or homophobic attitudes. In light of this, lesbian, gay and bisexual individuals often face added challenges. For example LGB youth are more likely to be targeted for bullying while in school (Berlan et al., 2010; Kosciw et al., 2009; Almeida et al., 2009) and LGB individuals are more likely to suffer physical and sexual assault and develop post-traumatic stress disorder (Roberts et al., 2010). In spite of these challenges, recent studies have shown that children in lesbian households are doing well (Gartrell & Bos, 2010; Bos et al., 2008; Lev, 2010). There is evidence that lesbian, gay and bisexual young people in the United States are self-identifying and disclosing their sexual orientation at an earlier age now than in the past (Herek et al., 2010).

Teen and Adolescent Sexuality

The average age at which adolescents or teenagers first engage in sexual activities varies across cultures. The recent National Survey of Sexual Health and Behavior found that in the United States, adolescents between the ages of 14 to 17 engaged in a wide range of sexual activities, with solo masturbation being the most prevalent. Partnered sexual activity, primarily oral sex and vaginal intercourse, became more prevalent in the older age levels surveyed (Fortenberry et al., 2010; Song, 2010). The Kinsey Institute reports that by age seventeen, about half of United States teenagers have had sexual intercourse, and this statistic moves to 70 percent by age 18. Of particular concern for girls having sexual experiences during their teenage years is the potential for

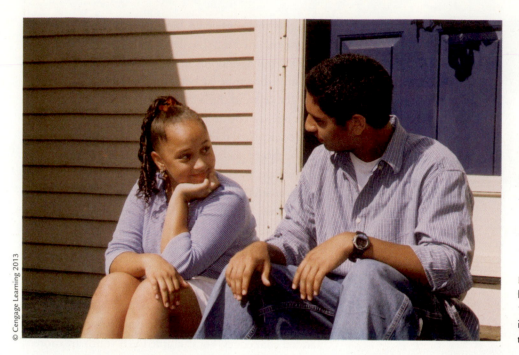

© Cengage Learning 2013

FIGURE 9-4: Adolescents between the ages of 15-19 have the highest infection rate for sexually transmitted infections.

unplanned pregnancies or the acquisition of sexually transmitted infections. Adolescents between the ages of 15-19 have the highest infection rate for sexually transmitted infections, including infections that can potentially diminish future fertility (Figure 9-4). Recent research has found that girls are more likely to have an unprotected first sexual encounter than boys are (Arizona State University, 2010), putting them at greater risk.

Several factors contribute to a teenager's likelihood to engage in more risky sexual behavior, such as having sexual intercourse without a condom. Borowsky (2009) found that teens (both male and female), who are not able to envision a hopeful future for themselves are more likely to participate in risky sexual behaviors. In addition, teens who work part-time jobs in adult environments with inadequate supervision are more likely to become involved with older partners and engage in risky behaviors (Bauermeister et al., 2009). Drug and alcohol use by teens have also been shown to correlate with higher risk sexual behavior (Santelli et al., 2008; Kilgree et al., 2000). In contrast, teens who plan to attend college immediately following high school are less likely to engage in casual sex or high risk sex (Bailey, 2008). Reducing exposure to alcohol and other drugs, plus having positive goals and a strong self esteem can allow girls to make more empowered choices about sex.

Sexuality During Pregnancy

Masters and Johnson conducted a small but detailed study on the female sexual response throughout pregnancy and found that physiology of the sexual response did not change from that of a non-pregnant woman. They later supplemented their direct observation of a small sample of six women with the subjective responses of a larger sample of 111 women who regularly reported their sexual feelings, behavior, and responses as their pregnancies progressed. Other investigators (Solberg, Butler, & Wagner, 1973; Kenny, 1973; Tolor & DiGrazia, 1976; Reamy, White, Daniell, & LeVine, 1982) used a similar technique of regular oral interviews or used a retrospective questionnaire to determine sexual attitudes of women during and after pregnancy. In general, the conclusions drawn from these studies indicate that the usual wide range of individual response exists but that sexual interests, frequency, and the enjoyment derived from activity was essentially the same as it is in non-pregnant women until the last trimester of pregnancy, when a progressive decline in desire and frequency occurred (Figure 9-5).

Medical opinions vary about the risks and benefits of sexual activity during pregnancy, although the risks during the first two trimesters appear to

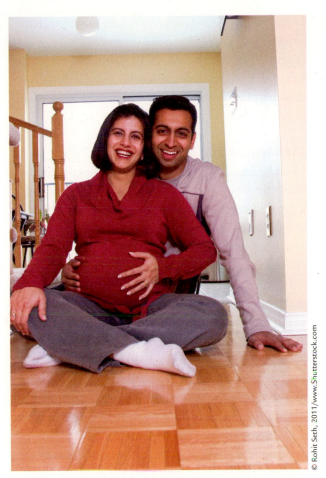

FIGURE 9-5: In general, sexual interest, frequency and enjoyment during the first and second trimesters of pregnancy tends to be similar to non-pregnant women, until the last trimester when there is typically a progressive decline in desire and frequency.

be minimal. For a small group of women who have already miscarried several times and who are having difficulty in maintaining a pregnancy, it may be prudent to avoid all sexual activity, including masturbation, because the uterine contractions could cause a miscarriage. There is very little evidence, however, that intercourse or orgasm can cause miscarriage in the majority of pregnancies. Women in the first trimester do have an increased pelvic awareness that accompanies the uterine changes; if they are concerned that intercourse may be damaging to the fetus, it will tend to decrease the satisfaction derived from stimulation, and orgasm may not be as frequent (Malarewicz et al., 2006). The sensations during intercourse may be different from those usually experienced, but they are not believed to be harmful.

By the second and third trimester, a woman has usually adjusted to the changes that she is experiencing in the pelvic area. Masters and Johnson reported an increase in sexual functioning at this time. However, other researchers have not confirmed heightened arousal, and instead report the same desire for and frequency of sexual activity as before. There is some concern that the uterine contractions during orgasm can trigger the onset of pre-term labor or that there is more possibility of infection during the last four to six weeks of pregnancy. However, at present, research does not support this concern for most women (Tan et al., 2007). Sometimes, the glans of the penis hitting the cervix may result in a little spotting; this need not discourage sexual relations if they are desired.

In their survey of women's sexual experiences during pregnancy, Malarewicz et al. (2006) found that sexual satisfaction during pregnancy contributed to their self-esteem, and helped to strengthen their bond with their partner. It is common for sexual desire to return between two weeks and three months after the delivery of a baby. Desire often reappears earlier in women who are breast-feeding. However, the significant drop in estrogen and progesterone levels after delivery may cause a temporary vaginal dryness and decrease in lubrication during intercourse. If a woman has undergone medical procedures during the delivery, such as episiotomy or a cesarean section, more time may be needed for incisions to have healed sufficiently to make resumption of sexual relations comfortable.

Disease, Disability, and Sexuality

Approximately one out of 10 adults have a permanent physical impairment that was either present at birth, developed later as a result of an illness, or was suddenly acquired through accident or injury. Almost everyone will experience some form of temporary disability during periods of their life when they are ill or injured. The sexuality of the physically ill or disabled is a reality that has been largely ignored by the medical profession as well as by the general public. The effects of illness or disability can be wide ranging but generally fall into several broad categories. Some of the difficulties may be in the realm of the psychological and social aspects of sexual relationships, in which the increased stress or depression resulting from the illness reduces the sexual drive. Other problems are physical or physiological

© Rohit Seth, 2011/www.Shutterstock.com

and involve concerns about physical comfort and safety during the sexual activity or the loss of sexual capability as a result of paralysis or lack of sensation. For example, for women who have suffered from a spinal cord injury, the physiological manifestations of the sexual response cycle usually differ little from women who are not injured. The vasocongestion responses are consistently present, but muscle responses in the genitals may be absent. The clitoris and labia become engorged with blood and swell, but the uterine and vaginal responses that contribute to the orgasmic platform may be missing. Usually, extragenital responses such as increased heart rate, respiration, pulse, blood pressure, and skin flush are still present. Women with spinal cord injuries have reported that, given the opportunity, they can experience full sexual pleasure and satisfaction psychologically even if a physical sensation is lacking. For some, the areas of the body that are still innervated become new erogenous zones to compensate for those parts that no longer respond to touch, and many individuals have the ability to produce sexual satisfaction by concentrating on the sensations received from those areas.

Some of the diseases a woman may experience during her lifetime that can have an impact on her sexuality include heart disease, cancer, and diabetes. For example, it is common for sexual activity to decline for months or years after a woman experiences a heart attack because of fear of triggering another heart attack, even though the likelihood of dying of a heart attack during sexual activity is very small (American Heart Association, 2010; Swedish Research Council, 2009). The American Heart Association recommends that sexual activity is safe as soon as a woman is comfortable resuming moderate exercise. Cancer can also have a wide range of impacts on a woman's sexuality, depending on the type of cancer and the kinds of treatments that she undergoes. Women going through chemotherapy or radiation therapy often experience a loss of libido. Decreases in estrogen or testosterone production during treatments can contribute to a decrease in vaginal lubrication, resulting in pain during intercourse. Many women who undergo a hysterectomy as part of their cancer treatment experience similar problems (Zippe et al., 2006). Sexual problems in women with diabetes have not been as well studied as in men (Brown &

Lowry, 2008). Some researchers have reported that women with diabetes experience more sexual dysfunction (Zied-Rad et al., 2010; Esposito et al., 2010) but others suggest that depression associated with diabetes may be more closely correlated with sexual problems than diabetes itself (Wallner et al., 2010).

Menopause and Sexuality

Given reasonably good health, sexual function continues for women well past menopause. In fact, in the United States the National Survey of Sexual Health and Behavior found that between 20 and 30 percent of women remain sexually active into their 80s (Schick et al., 2010). Masters and Johnson, who studied women aged 40–73 and men aged 51–89, found that while there are sometimes decreases in the intensity of the physical responses in the sexual cycle with increasing age, all of the physiological changes that occur in younger women during the excitement, plateau, orgasm, and resolution stages also take place in older women. They found this to be especially true for women who had remained sexually active throughout their lives. The first Hite Report (Hite, 1976) quotes some older women who felt that sex was not that important to them anymore, but the majority indicated that their sexual pleasure had actually increased with age and that they were now enjoying more new and gratifying experiences. In a survey of the sexual experiences of Swedish women in their 70s, Beckman (2008) found a similar result. Postmenopausal women, perhaps free for the first time in their lives from the fear of any unwanted pregnancy and with fewer family responsibilities, may experience an increase in their desire for sexual activity. In another study, McCall (2007) found that physiologically, postmenopausal women are equally responsive to sexual desire cues as premenopausal women (Figure 9-6).

The cumulative effects of aging along with changes in hormone levels that accompany menopause do have potential impacts on the neural, muscular and vascular responses that contribute to the physiology of the female sexual response (Nappi, 2007). For half a century, a large body of research has focused on how these hormonal changes, particularly in estrogen and testosterone levels, reduce sexual function in postmenopausal women. These studies have contributed to a widespread perception that sexual

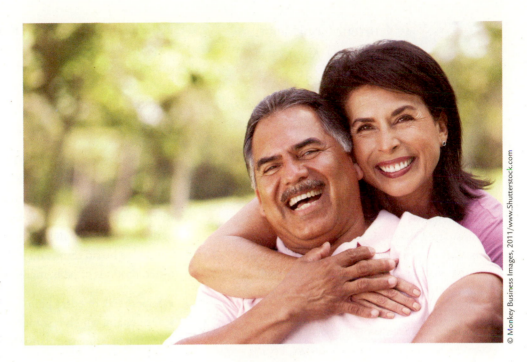

FIGURE 9-6: Menopause does not mean an end to sexual pleasure. For many postmenopausal women, there may be an increase in sexual desire and enjoyment.

response diminishes drastically in all women after they experience menopause. For many years, the prescribed remedy for this decline was hormone replacement therapy, until the significant risks associated with these medications were revealed. Currently, vaginal estrogen creams and testosterone transdermal patches are often prescribed to address physical changes brought on by hormone level changes (Kingsberg, 2007). Recently, there has been increasing attention focused on additional factors that either hinder or promote sexual function in postmenopausal women. For example, Hincliff et al. (2010) found that social and psychological factors, such as the demands of providing care to relatives, their partner's low sex drive, and the quality of their relationship play as large a role influencing women's sexual behavior during menopause as do biological changes that result from declining hormone levels. Likewise, Hartmann et al. (2004) found that a broad range of issues, including current stress levels, past sexuality, self esteem and mental health problems have more impact on postmenopausal women's sexual function than does menopause itself. It is important to take these studies into consideration as much of the current research is focused on finding medications to treat declines in female sexual function such as low sex drive, lack of orgasm, and pain during intercourse after menopause (Goldstein, 2007; Walsh & Berman, 2004).

Regular sexual activity itself, either alone or with a partner, is important to help women remain sexually active. After menopause, there can be vaginal changes that result from the decrease in estrogen levels. These changes may decrease the ability of the vagina to undergo adequate lubrication in preparation for intercourse, a circumstance that can lead to pain during intercourse. Women who maintain regular intercourse or masturbation throughout their lives have much less difficulty with vaginal lubrication and expansion of the vagina than do women who are not sexually active (Figure 9-7). They also experience

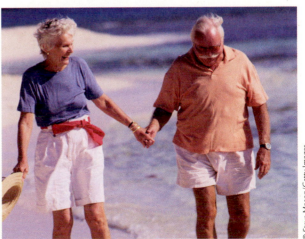

FIGURE 9-7: Sexual function continues for women well past menopause.

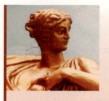

Current Considerations
OLDER WOMEN ARE VULNERABLE TO SEXUALLY TRANSMITTED INFECTIONS

Many women find new partners after divorce or the death of a spouse. While an unplanned pregnancy may not be of concern after menopause, there is still a risk of contracting sexually transmitted infections from unprotected sex. In their survey of Americans between the ages of 50-92, the National Survey of Sexual Health and Behavior (NSSHB) found that adults over age fifty are the least likely of all age groups surveyed to use condoms to protect themselves from STIs. According to the responses gathered, approximately two-thirds of men and women in this age group did not use a condom during their last sexual encounter, even if that encounter was not with a committed partner (Schick et al., 2010).

less thinning of the vaginal lining and inflammation caused by irritation. The mechanism by which sexual activity helps to prevent vaginal changes secondary to estrogen decline is unknown. It may be that the principle of disuse atrophy, more commonly known as "use it or lose it," is playing a role. The National Survey of Sexual Health and Behavior (NSSHB) found that vaginal lubrication and orgasm were the components of the sexual response that declined the most with age (Schick et al., 2010).

FEMALE SEXUAL DYSFUNCTION

Female sexual dysfunction refers to persistent or recurring problems that occur in one or more of the stages of sexual response. According to the medical definition, problems experienced at any of the stages is only considered sexual dysfunction if it is causing distress to the woman who is experiencing it, or if it negatively affects their relationship with their partner. The most common problems that occur are dyspareunia, or pain during intercourse; anorgasmia, or lack of orgasm; and low sex drive. According to a study published in 1999 in the Journal of the American Medical Association, 43 percent of women in the United States experience some form of sexual dysfunction during their lifetime. These problems can occur at any time during a woman's life. Although sexual problems can be complex, in general they are treatable.

Dyspareunia: Pain During Intercourse

Dyspareunia refers to genital pain that is experienced just before, during or after intercourse. It is estimates that up to 60 percent of women experience episodes of dyspareunia at some point in their lifetime. Dyspareunia is a broad term, and it refers to a variety of different kinds of pain, including:

- Superficial, or entry pain
- Deep pain, which is sometimes described as a feeling of "something inside being bumped"
- Burning pain
- Aching pain

Dyspareunia can begin unexpectedly, after previously pain-free intercourse. Each of the different types of pain can be caused by different problems or circumstances. For example, inadequate lubrication can cause pain during intercourse. There are many circumstances that can result in inadequate lubrication, such as not enough foreplay or drops in estrogen levels that occur after menopause, immediately after childbirth or while a woman is breastfeeding. Many common medications can also decrease lubrication, including many antidepressant medications, antihistamines, blood pressure medications and even some birth control pills.

Irritation due to inflammation or infection can also cause dyspareunia. This could be caused by either a vaginal or a urinary tract infection. If a woman has eczema or other skin disorders in her genital area, there can be irritation and pain. Allergic reactions to some birth control products can also cause pain. Some women are allergic to latex, so using a latex condom, dental dam, diaphragm, or cervical cap can cause inflammation. An ill-fitting cervical cap or diaphragm can also cause irritation and pain. It is possible to have an allergic reaction to spermicides. Injury of the genitals or vagina can also cause pain during intercourse. If a woman has had an episiotomy during childbirth the scar tissue can result in long term pain. Pelvic surgeries, injuries, and female circumcision can also lead to dyspareunia.

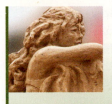

Economic Considerations

FEMALE SEXUAL DYSFUNCTION: DISEASE OR DISEASE MONGERING?

There has been a recent increase in research into female sexual dysfunction. Increased attention and research is good news for women who are distressed by problems with their sexual experience. However, there is also concern that some of this interest is motivated by previous successes diagnosing and treating male sexual dysfunction. Financial incentives can lead to a phenomenon called "disease mongering," when relatively common conditions are re-branded as potentially dangerous medical conditions. Some of the characteristics of disease mongering include (Payer, 1992 page 292):

- Taking a normal function and implying that there's something wrong with it and it should be treated
- Imputing suffering that isn't necessarily present
- Defining the largest proportion of the population possible as suffering from the "disease"
- Defining a condition as a deficiency disease or a disease of hormonal imbalance
- Taking a common symptom that could mean anything and making it sound as if it is a sign of a serious disease

Two medical conditions, vaginismus and vestibulitis can also make intercourse painful. With vaginismus, the muscles of the vaginal walls spasm involuntarily, making penetration difficult and painful. With vestibulitis, a woman experiences an unexplained stinging or burning sensation in the vagina. The pelvic floor muscles are sensitive to stress, and for this reason, emotional factors can also play a role in dyspareunia. In addition, experiencing pain during intercourse can cause additional anxiety and stress, which can lead to more pain. For that reason, it is important to seek treatment. The view that dyspareunia is primarily a psychological problem is outdated, and it is important to identify the cause or causes of the pain.

Deeper pain can be caused by a variety of conditions, including many illnesses. Endometriosis, pelvic inflammatory disease, uterine prolapse, ovarian cysts and uterine fibroids can all contribute to feelings of deep pain during intercourse. Nonreproductive problems such as cystitis, irritable bowel syndrome and hemorrhoids can also cause problems. Many women experience painful intercourse following hysterectomy because of scarring left over from the surgery. Chemotherapy and radiation therapy can also contribute to dyspareunia.

There are many potential treatments for dyspareunia, and the treatment prescribed will depend, in many cases, to the underlying cause of the pain. Sometimes a change as simple as avoiding scented bath products which can cause irritation or switching sex positions can alleviate the problem. If an infection or a medical condition is causing the problem, then it is important to get treatment for that condition. It may be necessary to switch medications if possible if side effects of a medication are interfering with lubrication. Pain medications, either to be taken orally or as an injection may be prescribed to treat the pain. In the past, HRT was prescribed to menopausal and postmenopausal women to treat vaginal dryness. Current recommendations are to avoid or minimize exposure to HRT in order to reduce the many health risks associated with therapy. If estrogen is prescribed for vaginal dryness, it can be prescribed as a vaginal cream or vaginal ring, which minimizes the negative impacts of the hormone on other parts of the body. Counseling and sex therapy can also be helpful to treat the stress and negative feeling that may be associated with the experience of dyspareunia.

Anorgasmia

Anorgasmia is the medical term for difficulty achieving orgasm either through vaginal intercourse or by direct stimulation to the clitoris. This condition can be caused by a variety of physical, psychological or relationship issues. Anorgasmia affects approximately 15 percent of women. It should be noted that even women who have orgasms regularly usually climax only about 50–70 percent of the time. Counseling, couples counseling, or sex therapy may be helpful for addressing the underlying problems that are contributing to anorgasmia. Medical conditions that cause dyspareunia can also contribute to anorgasmia, including hysterectomy and cancer surgeries and treatment. In addition, diseases such as multiple sclerosis and diabetes can interfere with nerve transmission and the orgasmic response. The effects of aging and reduction of estrogen after menopause can also result in changes to the nervous system and the circulatory systems that can make orgasm more difficult to achieve. Medications used to treat depression can also reduce a woman's ability to have an orgasm.

The vasocongestion and muscle responses that facilitate orgasm are under the control of the parasympathetic and sympathetic divisions of the autonomic nervous system. Anything that interferes with parasympathetic and sympathetic impulses can inhibit orgasm. For example, anticholinergic drugs block parasympathetic nerve impulses and are frequently used in the treatment of gastrointestinal disturbances because they decrease muscle spasm of the digestive tract and inhibit acid secretion in the stomach. It is possible that high doses of anticholinergics may result in erection difficulties in the male and, by extrapolation to the female, swelling and lubrication difficulties. Drugs that inhibit the sympathetic nerve impulses are often used to lower high blood pressure. These drugs have been reported to cause difficulty with ejaculation and decreased libido in men, and may have similar effects in women.

Hypoactive Sexual Desire Disorder: Low Sex Drive

Hypoactive sexual desire disorder is the medical terminology for a persistent and recurrent lack of interest in sex that causes personal distress. This disorder is also called low sex drive. It is estimated to affect 40 percent of women at some point in their lives. It is natural for interest in sex to fluctuate over time and to depend on circumstances. In addition, everyone has their own view about the frequency of sex that seems optimal to them. The key to determining if a woman has this disorder is if the lack of desire for sex is causing personal distress.

Dyspareunia and anorgasmia can both contribute to low sex drive, as can many diseases, including: cancer, diabetes, arthritis, heart disease and many neurological diseases. In addition, many of the medications used to treat diseases can also have a negative impact on libido. Antidepressants, blood pressure medications, chemotherapy, and even antihistamines can reduce sex drive. For some couples, it has been found that infertility and the stress of infertility treatments can also play a role. Consuming

---

Case Study

Hysterectomy and Sexual Dysfunction

Jennifer, a 50-year-old woman, had a total hysterectomy a year ago. Her recovery has gone very well. She's back to walking two miles a day, gardening, and returned back to work. The only thing she is concerned about is that even though she and her husband had a very intimate and satisfying relationship before the surgery, she is now having problems with arousal. She is feeling emotionally very romantic, but the physical response is just not there any longer. The few times they have been intimate since the surgery, vaginal dryness has made it uncomfortable and she has been unable to have an orgasm. She is wondering if these changes in her sexuality are due to her age or if they are linked to the hysterectomy.

1. What factors might be contributing to this disruption in Jennifer's sex life?

2. How could a hysterectomy influence the sexual response?

too much alcohol and the use of other recreational drugs can also disrupt libido. In some cases, women have reported a lessening of desire for sexual activity while on oral contraceptives, while others have claimed an increased interest in sex occurs while on the pill. There have been indications from both men and women that tranquilizers and other kinds of anti-anxiety, antidepressant drugs result in decreases in sexual interest, and some men have reported potency difficulties while on thiazide diuretics. Although effects of drugs on sexual function can occur at any age, they are more frequent and troublesome after age 50.

In addition, changes throughout the lifetime influence libido. The hormonal changes associated with pregnancy, breastfeeding or menopause can alter a woman's sex drive. In the case of pregnancy and breastfeeding, fatigue may also play a role along with hormonal changes. During menopause, both estrogen and testosterone levels drop, and this can, in some cases reduce sex drive for some women. Finally, the same psychological and relationship issues that may contribute to anorgasmia are likely to contribute to low sex drive.

A trained sex therapist can suggest behavioral options for improving sex drive. Medical treatments can help if behavioral changes are not effective. Usually, any underlying medical condition that is interfering with sex drive will be addressed. Medications that may be interfering with sex drive may need to be adjusted. In some cases, hormones may be prescribed, but it is always important to consider the long term risks and benefits of hormone therapies before they are prescribed. Estrogen, alone or with progesterone, might be prescribed as a pill, patch, or gel. Estrogen, in the form of a vaginal cream or as a vaginal ring that distributes hormones slowly over time, can increase blood flow

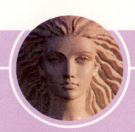

focus on

EXERCISE
Exercise and Libido

Exercise can have a dramatic effect on a women's sex drive. Vigorous exercise stimulates the sympathetic nervous system which causes an increase in blood flow to the genitals, and promotes other indicators of arousal (Hamilton et al., 2008). This effect continues even after an exercise session has ended. In addition, exercise causes the release of endorphins, which increase a women's perception of pleasure. For some women, testosterone levels also rise as a result of exercise, and testosterone is an important hormone for moderating sexual desire in both men and women. In addition, women who exercise tend to report feelings of having more energy, and improved self esteem, both of which contribute in a positive way to libido.

Yoga in particular has positive effects on women's sex drives and experiences. Paying attention to breath and postures creates body awareness, which can heighten pleasure. Yoga also increases flexibility and strengthens pelvic floor muscles, which can contribute to stronger orgasms. Finally, many of the postures direct blood flow to the genitals, which can help to improve the vasocongestion that accompanies arousal (Dhikav et al., 2010).

to the vagina and increase libido. Testosterone has an important influence on the sex drives of both men and women. Testosterone therapy seems to be more effective for women who have unusually low testosterone levels to begin with. Treatment with testosterone can also lead to side effects such as increasing acne, increasing body hair and personality or mood changes.

RAPE, SEXUAL ASSAULT AND DATE RAPE DRUGS

Rape and sexual assault include any sexual activities that take place against an individual's will. Rape and sexual assault are both violent crimes that can result in long term physical and psychological impacts on their victims. In the United States, it is estimated that about one in five women experience sexual assault during their lifetime. College age women are approximately four times more likely to be sexually assaulted than other age groups. Although rape can happen at any age, about half of all rape victims are teens or adolescents under the age of 18. It is common for the victim of rape or sexual assault to know her assailant.

Women should be aware that alcohol plays a role in half of all violent crimes, including rape and sexual assault. In addition, drugs, commonly called "date-rape drugs" can be added to food or drinks that render a woman unconscious and vulnerable to sexual assault. Some drugs that are used include gamma-hydroxybutric acid (GHB) and benzo-diazepines such as rohypholor "roofies." Police suggest that women can safeguard themselves from these drugs by ordering bottled drinks with caps or closed cans, and not accepting drinks from strangers.

Women who have been sexually assaulted are at risk of pregnancy and sexually transmitted infection. It is important to seek medical help, immediately if possible, as steps can be taken to prevent a pregnancy and to mitigate the effects of some types of infections. In addition, evidence can be collected. In most places, emotional and psychological support is available for survivors of rape and sexual assault, and these can be an important component of healing from this traumatic experience.

CONCLUSION

With its associated risks and benefits, sexuality is an important component of women's lives. Sexual experience is highly variable between women and even throughout an individual woman's lifetime. This is not surprising considering the interactions between psychosocial expectations and anatomical and physiological differences that influence and orchestrate the female sexual response. Increasing attention has been focused in recent years on female sexual function and on the maintenance of sexual health throughout the lifespan. While this added attention can have positive effects for women, there is some concern about the potential for increased medicalization of female sexuality. A woman's own experience of what is pleasurable and desirable for her is important for distinguishing between natural variability or changes, and signs of a disorder that she would like to address.

REVIEW QUESTIONS

1. List some of the health benefits of sexual activity.

2. What are some of the potential health risks of sexual activity?

3. Describe the four stages of the female sexual response, as described by Masters and Johnson?

4. What is meant by dyspareunia?

5. How does anorgasmia differ from hypoactive sex drive?

6. Which types of medications can impair sexual function in women?

7. What are date rape drugs? How can a woman avoid falling victim to sexual predators using date rape drugs?

CRITICAL THINKING QUESTION

1. If orgasm is a physiological reflex, why is there so much variability in women's experience of orgasm?

WEBLINKS

National Survey of Sexual Health and Behavior
   www.nationalsexstudy.indiana.edu
The Kinsey Institute
   www.kinseyinstitute.org

Planned Parenthood
   www.plannedparenthood.org
The National Center for Victims of Crime
   www.ncvc.org

REFERENCES

Abel, E. L. (1985). *Psychoactive drugs and sex.* New York, NY: Plenum Press.

Almeida, J., Johnson, R. M., Corliss, H. L., Molnar, B. E., & Azael, D. (2009). Emotional distress among LGBT youth: The influence of perceived discrimination based on sexual orientation. *Journal of Youth and Adolescence, 38*(7), 1001–1014.

Alsibisani, S. A., & Rouzi, A. A. (2010). Sexual function in women with female genital mutilation. *Fertility and Sterility, 93*(3), 722–724.

American Heart Association. (2010, May 21). Sexual activity declines after heart attack. Patients not getting doctor's advice, study finds. *Science Daily.* Retrieved November 20, 2010, from http://www.sciencedaily.com/releases/2010/05/100521092424.htm.

Arizona State University. (2010, November 8). Research into adolescent sexual habits reveals surprising findings. *Science Daily*. Retrieved November 20, 2010, from http://www.sciencedaily.com/release/2010/11/101108190135.htm.

Bailey, J. A., Fleming, C. B., Henson, J. N., Catalano, R. F., & Haggerty, K. P. (2008). Sexual risk behavior 6 months post-high school: associations with college attendance, living with a parent, and prior risk behavior. *Journal of Adolescent Health, 42*(6), 573–579.

Bailey, N. W., & Zuk, M. (2009). Same-sex sexual behavior and evolution. *Trends in Ecology and Evolution, 24*(8), 439–446.

Battaglia, C., Nappi, R. E., Mancini, F., Alvisi, S., Del Forno, S., Battaglia, B., & Venturoli, S. (2010). 3-D volumetric and vascular analysis of the urethrovaginal space in young women with or without vaginal orgasm. *Journal of Sexual Medicine, 7*(4 Pt 1), 1445–1453.

Bauermeister, J. A., Zimmerman, M. A., Caldwell, C. H., Xue, Y., & Gee, G. C. (2010). What predicts sex partners' age differences among African American youth? A longitudinal study from adolescence to young adulthood. *Journal of Sexual Research, 47*(4), 330–344.

Beckman, N., Waern, M., Gustafson, D., & Skoog, I. (2008). Secular trends in self reported sexual activity and satisfaction in Swedish 70 year olds: Cross sectional survey of four populations, 1971–2001. *BMJ, 337,* a279. doi:10.1136/bmj.a279.

Berlan, E. D., Corliss, H. L., Field, A. E., Goodman, E., & Austin, S. B. (2010). Sexual orientation and bullying among adolescents in the growing up today study. *Journal of Adolescent Health, 46*(4), 366–371.

Blanchard, R. (2008). Review and theory of handedness, birth order, and homosexuality in men. *Laterality, 13*(1), 51–70.

Borowsky, I. W., Ireland, M., & Resnick, M. D. (2009). Health status and behavioral outcomes for youth who anticipate a high likelihood of early death. *Pediatrics, 124*(1), e81–88.

Bos, H. M., Gartrell, N. K., van Balen, F., Peyser, H., & Sandfort, T. G. (2008). Children in planned lesbian families: A cross-cultural comparison between the United States and the Netherlands. *American Journal of Orthopsychiatry, 78*(2), 211–219.

Brotto, L. A., Klein, C., & Gorzalka, B. (2008). Laboratory-induced hyperventilation differentiates female sexual arousal disorder. *Archives of Sexual Behavior, 38*(4), 463–475.

Brown, A. J., & Lowry, K. P. (2008). Sexual dysfunction in women with type 2 diabetes. In *Type 2 Diabetes Mellitus. Contemporary Endocrinology, 2008*, 399–402. doi: 10.1007/978-1-60327-043-4_25.

Buisson, O., Foldes, P., Jannini, E., & Mimoun, S. (2010). Coitus as revealed by ultrasound in one volunteer couple. *Journal of Sexual Medicine, 7*(8), 2750–2754. doi: 10.1111/j.1743-6109.2010.01892.x.

Charnetski, C. J., & Brennan, F. X. (2004). Sexual frequency and salivary immunoglobulin A (IgA). *Psychological Reports, 94*(3 Pt 1), 839–844.

Chivers, M. L., Seto, M. C., Lalumiere, M. L., Laan, E., & Grimbos, T. (2010). Agreement of self-reported and genital measures of sexual arousal in men and women: A meta-analysis. *Archives of Sexual Behavior, 39*(1), 5–56.

Cole, T. M. (1975). Sexuality and physical disabilities. *Archives of Sexual Behavior, 4*(4), 389–403.

Davidson, J. (2010, January 28). Women's orgasmic capability [Web log post]. Retrieved from http://www.sexualhealth.com/article/read/women-sexual-health/pleasure/561/

Dhikav, V., Karmarkar, G., Gupta, R., Verma, M., Gupta, R., Gupta, S., & Anand, K. S. (2010). Yoga in female sexual functions. *Journal of Sexual Medicine, 7*(2 Pt 2), 964–70.

Duke, N. N., Borowsky, I. W., Pettingell, S. L., & McMorris, B. J. (2009). Examining youth hopelessness as an independent risk correlate for adolescent delinquency and violence. *Maternal and Child Health Journal, 15*(1), 87–97.

Esposito, K., Maiorino, M. I., Bellastella, G., Giugliano, F., Romano, M., & Giugliano, D.(2010). Determinants of female sexual dysfunction in type 2 diabetes. *International Journal of Impotence Research, 22*(3),179–184.

Fahmy, A., El-Mouelhy, M. T., & Rwgab, A. R. (2010). Female genital mutilation/cutting and issues of sexuality in Egypt. *Reproductive Health Matters, 18*(36), 181–190.

Foldes, P., & Buisson, O. (2009). The clitoral complex: A dynamic sonographic study. *Journal of Sexual Medicine, 6*(5), 1223–1231.

Fortenberry, J. D., Schick, V., Herbenick, D., Sanders, S. A., Dodge, B., & Reece, M. (2010). Sexual behaviors and condom use at last vaginal intercourse: A national sample of adolescents ages 14 to 17 years. *Journal of Sexual Medicine, 7*(Supplement 5), 305–314.

Freud, S. (1905). *Three essays on the theory of sexuality.* New York, NY: Avon Books.

Garcia-Falgueras, A., & Swaab, D. F. (2010). Sexual hormones and the brain: An essential alliance for sexual identity and sexual orientation. *Endocrine Development, 17*, 22–35.

Gartrell, N., & Bos, H. (2010). US National Longitudinal Lesbian Family Study: Psychological adjustment of 17-year-old adolescents. *Pediatrics 126*(1), 28–36.

Goldstein, I. (2007). Current management strategies of the postmenopausal patient with sexual health problems. *Journal of Sexual Medicine, 4*(Supplement 3), 235–253.

Hamilton, L. D., Fogle, E.A., & Meston, C. A. (2008). The roles of testosterone and alpha-amylase in exercise-induced sexual arousal in women. *Journal of Sexual Medicine, 5*(4), 845–853.

Hartmann, U., Philippsohn, S., Heiser, K., & Ruffer-Hesse, C. (2004). Low sexual desire in midlife and older women: Personality factors, psychosocial development, present sexuality. *Menopause, 11*(6 Pt 2), 726–740.

Herbenick, D. L. (2009). The development and validation of a scale to measure attitudes towards women's genitals. *International Journal of Sexual Health, 21*(3), 153.

Herbenick, D. L., Reece, M., Schick, V., Sanders, S., Dodge, B., & Fortenberry, J. D. (2010). An event-level analysis of the sexual characteristics and composition among adults ages 18 to 59: Results from a national probability sample in the United States. *Journal of Sexual Medicine, 7*(Supplement 5), 346–361.

Herek, G. M., Norton, A. T., Allen, T. J., & Sims, C. L. (2010). Demographic, psychological and social characteristics of self-identified lesbian, gay and bisexual adults in a US probability sample. *Sexuality Research and Social Policy, 7*(3), 176–200. doi:10.1007/s13178-010-0017-y.

Hinchcliff, S., Gott, M., & Ingleton, C. (2010). Sex, menopause and social context: A qualitative study with heterosexual women. *Journal of Health Psychology, 15*(5), 724.

Hite, S. (1976). *The Hite report.* New York, NY: Macmillan.

Hooper, R. (2005). Genes blamed for fickle female orgasm. *Biology Letters.* doi: 10.1098/rsbl.2005.0308.

Ito, T. Y., Trant, A. S., & Polan, M. L. (2001). A double-blind placebo-controlled study of ArginMax, a nutritional supplement for enhancement of female sexual function. *Journal of Sex & Marital Therapy, 27*(5), 541–549.

Jannini, E. A., Blanchard, R., Camperio-Ciani, A., & Bancroft, J. (2010). Male homosexuality: Nature or culture? *Journal of Sexual Medicine, 7*(10), 3245–3253.

Jannini, E. A., Fisher, W. A., Bitzer, J., & McMahon, C. G. (2009). Is sex just fun? How sexual activity improves health. *Journal of Sexual Medicine, 6*(10), 2640–2648.

Jannini, E. A., Whipple, B., Kingsberg, S. A., Buisson, O., Foldes, P., & Vardi, Y. (2010). Who's afraid of the G-spot? *Journal of Sexual Medicine, 7*(1 Pt 1), 25–34.

Kaplan, H. S. (1983). *The evolution of sexual disorders: Psychological and medical aspects.* New York, NY: Bunner/Mazel.

Kaplan, S. A., Reis, R. B., Kohn, I. J., et al. (1999). Safety and efficacy of sildenafil in postmenopausal women with sexual dysfunction. *Urology, 53*(3), 481–486.

Kenny, J. A. (1973). Sexuality of pregnant and breast-feeding women. *Archives of Sexual Behavior, 2*(3), 201–203.

Kingree, J. B., Braithwaite, R., & Woodring, T. (2000). Unprotected sex as a function of alcohol and marijuana use among adolescent detainees. *Journal of Adolescent Health, 27*(3),179–185.

Kingsberg, S. (2007). Testosterone treatment for hypoactive sexual desire disorder in postmenopausal women. *Journal of Sexual Medicine, 4*(Supplement 3), 227–234.

Kinsey, A., Pomeroy, W. B., Martin, C. E., & Gebhard, P. H. (1953). *Sexual behavior in the human female.* New York, NY: Saunders.

Kim, N. N., Christianson, D. W., & Traish, A. M. (2004). Role of arinase in the male and female sexual arousal response. *Journal of Nutrition, 134,* 2873S–2879S.

Kohler, P. K., Manhart, L. E., & Lafferty, W. E. (2008). Abstinence-only and comprehensive sex education and the initiation of sexual activity and teen pregnancy. *Journal of Adolescent Health, 42*(4), 344–351.

Komisaruk, B. R., Beyer-Flores, C., & Whipple, B. (2006). *The science of orgasm.* Baltimore, MD: Johns Hopkins University Press.

Kosciw, J. G., Greytak, E. A., & Diaz, E. M. (2009). Who, what, where, when and why: Demographic and ecological factors contributing to hostile school climate for lesbian, gay, bisexual, and transgender youth. *Journal of Youth and Adolescence, 38*(7), 976–988.

Koster, M., & Price, L. L. (2008). Rwandan female genital modification: Elongation of the labia minora and the use of local botanical species. *Culture, Health & Sexuality, 10*(2), 191–204.

Laumann, E. O., Paik, A., & Rosen, R. C. (1999). Sexual dysfunction in the United States: Prevalence and predictors. *Journal of the American Medical Association, 281,* 537–544.

LePage, M. (2005, June 25). Women's orgasms are a turn-off for the brain. *New Scientist,17*(54), 14.

Lev, A. I. (2010, September). How queer!—The development of gender identity and sexual orientation in LGBTQ-headed families. *Family Process, 49,* 268–290. doi:10.1111/j.1545-5300.2010.01323.x.

Malarewicz, A., Szymkiewicz, J., & Rogala, J. (2006). Sexuality in pregnant women. *Ginekologia Polska, 77*(9), 733–739.

Masters, W. H., & Johnson, V. E. (1966). *Human sexual response.* Boston: Little, Brown.

McCall, K., & Meston, C. (2007). Differences between pre- and postmenopausal women in cues for sexual desire. *Journal of Sexual Medicine,4*(2), 364–371.

Meston, C. M., & Gorzalka B. B. (1996). Differential effects of sympathetic activation on sexual arousal in sexually dysfunctional and functional women. *Journal of Abnormal Psychology, 105*(4), 582–591.

Meston, C. M., & Worcel, M. (2002). The effects of yohimbine plus L-arginine glutamate on sexual arousal in postmenopausal women with sexual arousal disorder. *Archives of Sexual Behavior, 31*(4), 323–332.

Muller, J. E., Mittleman, A., Maclure, M., et al. (1996). Triggering myocardial infarction by sexual activity. Low absolute risk and prevention by regular physical exertion. *Journal of the American Medical Association, 275*(18), 1405–1409.

Nappi, R. E. (2007). New attitudes to sexuality in the menopause: Clinical evaluation and diagnosis. *Climacteric, 10*(Supplement 2), 105–108.

Naylor, J., & Cohen, J. S. (1999, March 17). Elixir becomes date-rape killer. *Detroit News,* p. A1.

Payer, L. (1992). *Disease-mongers: How doctors, drug companies, and insurers are making you feel sick.* New York, NY: Wiley & Son.

Rahman, Q., & Koerting, J. (2008). Sexual orientation-related differences in allocentric spatial memory tasks. *Hippocampus 18*(1), 55–63.

Reamy, K., White, S., Daniell, W. C., & LeVine, E. (1982). Sexuality and pregnancy. *Journal of Reproductive Medicine, 27*(6), 321–327.

Reamy, K. J. (1991). A management guide to postpartum problems. *Medical Aspects of Human Sexuality,* 20–25.

Roberts, A. L., Austin, A. B., Corliss, H. L., Vandermorris, A. K., & Koenen, K. C. (2010). Pervasive trauma exposure among US sexual orientation minority adults and risk posttraumatic stress disorder. *American Journal of Public Health, 100*(12), 2433–2441.doi:10.2105/AJPH.2009.168971.

Rosen, R. C. (1998). Medical advance or media event. *Lancet, 353,* 1599–1600.

Safer Sex, How Can I Lower My Risk Using Safer Sex? Retrieved November 20, 2010 from http://www.plannedparenthood.org/health-topics/stds-hiv-safer-sex/safer-sex-4263.htm.

Santelli, J., Carter, M., Orr, M., & Dittus, P. (2009). Trends in sexual risk behaviors, by nonsexual risk behavior involvement, U.S. high school students, 1991-2007. *Journal of Adolescent Health, 44*(4), 372–379.

Schick, V., Herbenick, D., Reece, M., Sanders, S., Dodge, B., Middlestadt, S. E., & Fortenberry, J. D. (2010). Sexual behaviors, condom use, and sexual

health of Americans over 50: Implications for sexual health promotion for older adults. *Journal of Sexual Medicine, 7*(Supplement 5), 315–329.

Solarz, A. (1999, October/November). Lesbian healthcare issues. Exploring options for expanding research and delivering care. *AWHONN Lifelines, 3*(5), 13–14.

Solberg, D. A., Butler, J., & Wagner, N. N. (1973). Sexual behavior in pregnancy. *New England Journal of Medicine, 288,* 1098–1103.

Song, A. V., & Halpern-Felsher, B. L. (2010). Predictive relationship between adolescent oral and vaginal sex: Results from a perspective, longitudinal study. *Archives of Pediatrics and Adolescent Medicine, 165.* doi:10.1001/archpediatrics.2010.214

Steinke, E., & Patterson-Midgley, P. (1996). Sexual counseling following acute myocardial infarction. *Clinical Nursing Research, 5*(4), 462–472.

Swedish Research Council. (2009, July 3). Healthy sex life after a cardiac event. *Science Daily,* Retrieved November 20, 2010, from http://www.science-daily.com/releases/2009/07/090703065458.htm

Tan, P. C., Yow, C. M., & Omar, S. Z. (2007). Effect of coital activity on onset of labor in women scheduled for labor induction: A randomized controlled trial. *Obstetrics & Gynecology, 110*(4), 820–826.

Thabet, S. M. (2009). Reality of the G-spot and its relation to female circumcision and vaginal surgery. *Journal of Obstetrics and Gynaecology Research, 35*(5), 967–973.

Tolor, A., & DiGrazia, P. V. (1976). Sexual attitudes and behavior patterns during and following pregnancy. *Archives of Sexual Behavior, 5*(6), 539–551.

Vance, E. B., & Wagner, N. N. (1976). Written descriptions of orgasm: A study of sex differences. *Archives of Sexual Behavior, 5*(1), 87–98.

Wallner, L. P., Sarma, A. V., & Kin, C. (2010). Sexual functioning among women with and without diabetes in the Boston Area Community Health Study. *Journal of Sexual Medicine, 7*(2Pt 2), 881–887.

Walsh, J. J. (1976). The spinal cord disabled. *Nursing Mirror, 142*(5), 53–54.

Walsh, K. E., & Berman, J. R. (2004). Sexual dysfunction in the older woman: An overview of the current understanding and management. *Drugs and Aging, 21*(10), 655–675.

Wiegel, M., Meston, C., & Rosen, R. (2005). The Female Sexual Function Index (FSFI): Cross-validation and development of clinical cutoff scores. *Journal of Sexual & Marital Therapy, 31*(1), 1–20.

Zhao, Y., Montoro, R., Igartua, K., & Thrombs, B. D. (2010). Suicidal ideation and attempt among adolescents reporting "unsure" sexual identity or heterosexual identity plus same-sex attraction or behavior: Forgotten groups. *Child & Adolescent Psychiatry, 49*(2), 104–113.

Ziaei-Rad, M., Vahdaniania, M., & Montazeri, A. (2010). Sexual dysfunctions in patients with diabetes: A study from Iran. *Reproductive Biology and Endocrinology, 18*(8), 50.

Zippe, C., Nandipati, K., Agarwal, A., & Raina, R. (2006). Sexual dysfunction after pelvic surgery. *International Journal of Impotence Research, 18*(1), 1–18.

chapter 10

GENETICS AND FETAL DEVELOPMENT

CHAPTER COMPETENCIES

Upon completion of this chapter, the reader will be able to:

- Differentiate between mitosis and meiosis
- Describe the development of the embryo
- Identify what each germ layer becomes

- Describe the role of the placenta
- Explain the importance of genetics and genetic testing

KEY TERMS

blastocyst

chorionic thyrotropin

chromosomes

deoxyribonucleic
  acid (DNA)

diploid

ectoderm

embryo

endoderm

fetus

gastrulation

genome

haploid

human chorionic
  gonadotropin (hCG)

Human Genome Project

karyotype

meiosis

mesoderm

mitosis

morula

neural tube
  defects

placenta

placental growth
  hormone

placental lactogen

single nucleotide
  polymorphisms
  (SNPs)

teratogens

zygote

INTRODUCTION

In sexually reproducing species such as humans, a potential pregnancy begins with fertilization, the fusion of a sperm and an egg. Each of these cells contains one-half of the genetic instructions to form the structures, tissues and organs of a new body, and these instructions—the genes—are coded for by molecules of **DNA (deoxyribonucleic acid)**. When a sperm fertilizes an egg, the genes combine and a potential new individual is formed. Fertilization is the first embryonic event in a series that culminates in the birth of a baby (Figure 10-1). In order to understand the developmental processes that take place during the 38 weeks between fertilization and birth, a basic understanding of genetics and the physiology of cells is required.

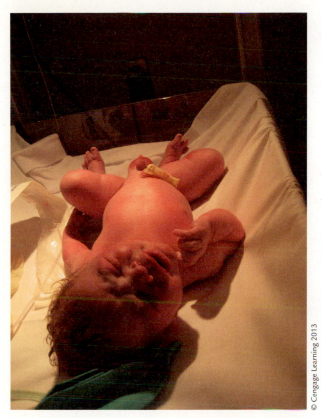

© Cengage Learning 2013

FIGURE 10-1: The birth of a baby is the end of a journey that begins when a single sperm fertilizes a single egg.

CELLS

Cells are the basic units of life. In the case of single celled organisms such as bacteria, each individual cell is relatively self sufficient, able to obtain nutrients, produce energy, eliminate waste products, and reproduce independently. Cells in multicellular organisms like plants or animals perform these same functions, but the cells are differentiated, or specialized, and are dependent on the cooperation of other cells making up the organism to survive. Figure 10-2 shows a basic human cell without differentiation. All cells contain genes that allow them to accomplish their physiological tasks, and they are able to pass these genes on to descendent cells when they divide. In the case of most multicellular organisms, the genes are stored in a structure called a nucleus within the cell.

The metabolic activities of the cell are performed under the control of the nucleus. Whatever a cell does at any time in its life—muscle cells contracting, nerve cells conducting an impulse, stomach cells secreting digestive enzymes, etc.—is directed by the genetic instructions from its nucleus. Even natural cell death is programmed by its nucleus. When cells deteriorate or become damaged, they are usually replaced by division of other cells. In some cases, the cells that divide to replace other cells are called stem cells. Cell division is also controlled by the nucleus.

DNA Structure and the Genetic Code

The DNA molecule (Figure 10-3) is shaped like a ladder that is twisted into a spiral staircase, a shape often called the double helix. The side pieces of the ladder, or its backbone, are made of a sugar called deoxyribose and phosphate, occurring in alternating groups. The cross connections, or rungs of the ladder, are attached to the deoxyribose and are composed of compounds called nitrogenous bases which bond together to form base pairs. DNA contains two different sets of nitrogenous bases—guanine (G) which pairs with cytosine (C) and thymine (T) which pairs with adenine (A). The sequence of the bases forms the instructions for the cell. All of the bases that code for a single trait comprise a gene. Thousands of genes can be stored on a single DNA strand. It is estimated that human DNA contains more than 3.4 billion base pairs arranged into 25000 genes (Canadian Museum of Nature, 2008).

Chromosomes

In a cell, DNA molecules wrap around proteins called histones to form a structure called a **chromosome**. Each chromosome contains thousands of genes that direct the functions of the body. The chromosomes are usually stored in the nucleus of the cell. While in the nucleus, the chromosomes are dispersed and are not visible under the microscope. In this state the chromosomes are called chromatin. During the brief period when the cell divides, the chromosomes become more tightly packed around the histone proteins, a process call condensation. Once the chromosomes condense, they become visible under the microscope. The number of chromosomes varies in different species. Human cells have 46 chromosomes, with the exception of the eggs and sperm. This complete set is called a **karyotype**. Instead of 46 chromosomes, the egg and sperm cells

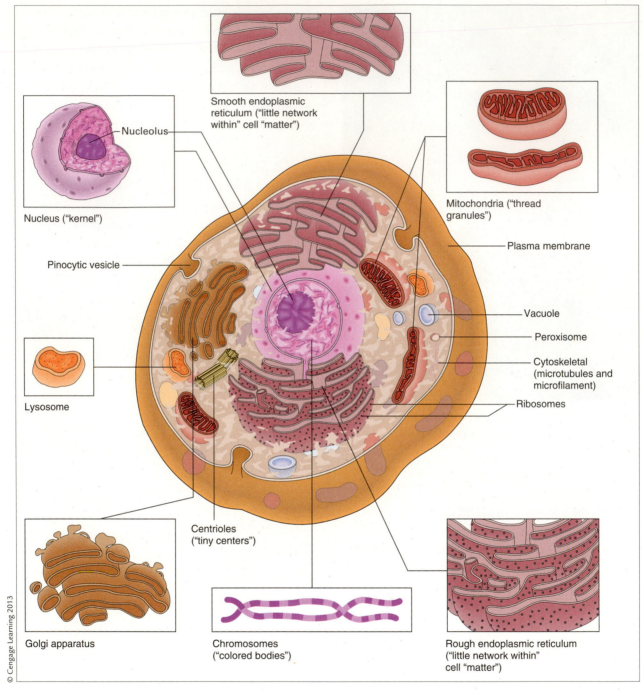

Smooth endoplasmic reticulum ("little network within" cell "matter")

Nucleolus

Nucleus ("kernel")

Pinocytic vesicle

Lysosome

Golgi apparatus

Centrioles ("tiny centers")

Chromosomes ("colored bodies")

Mitochondria ("thread granules")

Plasma membrane

Vacuole

Peroxisome

Cytoskeletal (microtubules and microfilament)

Ribosomes

Rough endoplasmic reticulum ("little network within" cell "matter")

FIGURE 10-2: The basic human cell.

each have only 23 chromosomes. Cells with two sets of chromosomes—one from each parent—are referred to as **diploid**. Eggs and sperm, with only one set, are referred to as **haploid**. The 46 chromosomes of a typical body cell are made up of 23 pairs of matching chromosomes, with one chromosome from each pair inherited from the individual's mother and the other chromosome in the pair inherited from the father. These matching pairs of chromosomes are called homologous pairs (Figure 10-4). The exceptions are the X and Y chromosomes which determine the genetic sex of the individual. The X and Y chromosomes are called the sex chromosomes. The other 22 pairs are referred to as autosomes.

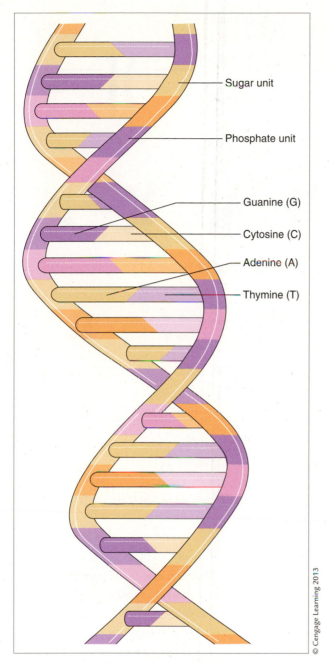

FIGURE 10-3: The structure of the basic DNA molecule.

Sugar unit

Phosphate unit

Guanine (G)

Cytosine (C)

Adenine (A)

Thymine (T)

© Cengage Learning 2013

Reading the Code

Although all of the cells contain copies of the same set of chromosomes and therefore, the same genes, different genes are utilized in different cells. Some genes are active in nearly all cells, while other genes are active in only a few cells. For example, follicle-stimulating hormone (FSH) is synthesized in the cells of the anterior pituitary gland but not in other cells of the body, even though all of the other cells of the body contain the genes that code for this hormone. The kinds of genes that code for the synthesis of a specific protein that is concerned with the specific functions of a cell, like growth or secretion, are called structural genes. Regulator genes switch structural genes on and off, so that appropriate traits are expressed at the proper time. These regulator genes dictate which genes in the particular cell are functional and which remain inactive. Identifying regulator genes and understanding their complex interactions are the major focus of molecular genetics research. A relatively new field of study, called epigenetics, explores how environmental factors such as diet and lifestyle influence gene regulation and gene expression.

The genes on homologous chromosomes also exist in pairs called alleles. Each chromosome of a pair carries a copy of a gene that governs a particular trait, and the homologous chromosome carries the same gene's partner at the same location. While both genes code for the same trait, their arrangement of nitrogenous bases may not be exactly the same, in which case the individual is said to be heterozygous for that particular trait. For example, a person who inherits a gene for brown eyes from one parent and a gene for blue eyes from the other is heterozygous for that trait. In some cases, one of these alleles is dominant over the other allele, and it will be expressed in the appearance or the physiology of the individual. The allele that is not expressed is said to be recessive. If the sequence of nitrogenous bases is exactly the same for both of the alleles, the individual is said to be homozygous for that trait.

If the arrangement of nitrogenous bases in a gene is altered by mutation, an abnormality may result. These mutations can be beneficial, neutral, or detrimental. Mutations in the DNA will be transmitted to future generations. Tay-Sachs disease, cystic fibrosis, and sickle cell anemia are examples of hereditary diseases caused by genetic mutations. Genetic mutations may result from environmental factors such as x-rays, chemicals, and infections, as well as a spontaneous mismatching of the base pairs, the equivalent of a genetic typo.

The Human Genome Project and Gene Mapping

The base pairs coding for the genes embedded in the DNA of the human chromosomes provide a blue

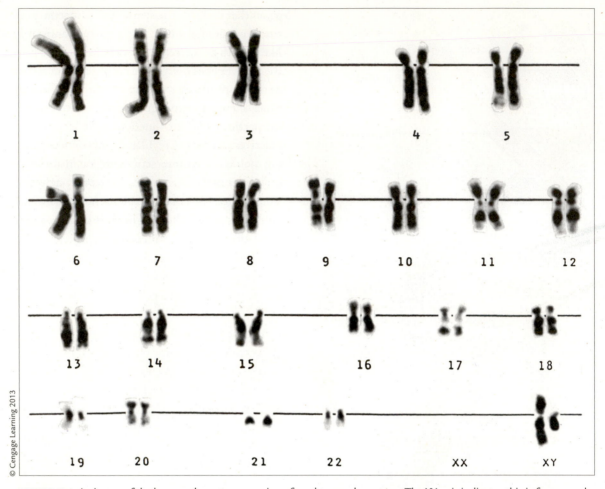

FIGURE 10-4: An image of the human chromosome pairs referred to as a karyotype. The XY pair indicates this is from a male.

print for the human body. The **genome** is the term for the entire DNA in an organism. The **Human Genome Project**, coordinated by the National Institutes of Health (NIH) and the Department of Energy (DOE), was started in 1990 as a 15-year project with the ambitious goal of mapping the entire human genome. In 2000, a first draft of the human genome was released and, with the combined efforts of labs across the world, a completed map was released in 2003. Additional projects have mapped the genomes of rice, sheep, several bacteria, dogs, and several other species. These projects identify the nucleotide sequences along the chromosomes, and the information can then be used in a variety of applications, including evolutionary and medical research.

Single nucleotide polymorphisms (SNPs) are minute changes in the nucleotide sequence, normally only a single base pair, that represent mutations in the DNA. These slight variations are part of what makes each person unique. In most cases, these mutations are of no major consequence, but in others, the change in DNA is sufficient to produce a different trait. Perhaps it is resistance to a specific disease or a unique metabolic property. Disease conditions, or at least a predisposition to a condition, can be identified. SNPs have been linked to Alzheimer's disease (Bekris et al., 2008), cholesterol levels (Klos et al., 2008), osteoporosis (Mullin et al., 2008), and diabetes (Bronstein et al., 2008). The Online Mendelian Inheritance in Man (OMIM) database provides information on thousands of SNPs and their relation to traits. The database is accessible online. Genome maps are also used for tracking human migrations across the world and have forced a rethinking of the accepted history of how early humans moved across the globe (Hellenthal et al., 2008).

Critical Thinking

Designer Babies

The 1997 movie GATTACA presented a future in which the world is divided into two groups – the genetically enhanced and selected, upper class and the unenhanced, lower class individuals. Genetic engineering has moved this possibility from the realm of science fiction closer to the realm of the possible. Gene recombination in bacteria and plants is now a common procedure. The Human Genome Project has identified thousands of genes linked to different traits. Should people be able to create "designer babies"? Who should determine which traits are desirable? What are the potential advantages and disadvantages of engineered traits? Should there be limits placed on the technology?

Pre-implantation Genetic Diagnosis (PGD)

For women undergoing infertility treatments such as in vitro fertilization (IVF) procedures (Chapter 14), pre-implantation genetic diagnosis offers an opportunity to identify genetic problems in an embryo. During the first week of development, a cell or two can be removed for testing and screened for genetic disorders. In a study of 20,000 IVF cases, the use of PGD produced a higher rate of successful pregnancies than procedures that did not use the screening (Kuliev & Verlinsky, 2008). One advantage to this procedure is the ability to implant fewer embryos, and, in some cases, only one. This reduces the risk of multiple pregnancies and also lowers the risk of miscarriage (McArthur et al., 2005).

GENETIC ETHICS

Genetic testing has raised a number of ethical questions (Bredenwood et al., 2008). DNA analysis is still in its infancy, and new genes are identified daily. However, genetic testing and reproductive technologies have outpaced the scientific understanding of many people. A wide range of legal questions about genetically engineered organisms remain unresolved and are currently being debated. Should stem cell research be allowed? Should human cloning be allowed? Can a company own a gene? Who decides which alleles are desirable and which should be rejected? Can an insurance company refuse to cover someone because they carry a specific gene? These issues are beginning to appear in the mainstream media. On May 21, 2008, the Genetic Information Nondiscrimination Act (GINA) was signed into law. GINA does not address every issue, but does begin to address some of the legal issues surrounding the genes and genetic engineering. The law is designed to protect Americans from discrimination based on genetics, and contains the following provisions:

- Forbids discrimination by insurance companies via reduced coverage or increased pricing based on genetic testing.
- Prevents employers from making adverse employment decisions based on genetics.
- Neither employers nor insurers can demand genetic testing.

CELL DIVISION BY MITOSIS

Most cells must undergo cell division to facilitate growth, repair and maintenance. Some cells divide less frequently than others. Nerve cells, for example, have a limited ability to divide and usually must last a lifetime. On the other hand, every second, millions of blood cells die and must be replaced from a dividing stem cell. The most common form of cell division is called **mitosis**, which results in an orderly splitting of a cell into two new daughter cells (Figure 10-5). In humans, each new daughter cell contains 46 chromosomes and is genetically identical to the original cell that formed it. The majority of cell divisions that occur through embryonic development and throughout a lifetime are by mitosis.

Meiosis

While the majority of the cells in the body have 46 chromosomes, eggs and sperm have only half that many, or 23 chromosomes. When eggs and sperm are formed, a reduction division takes place that ensures that each gamete contains only half of the usual number of chromosomes. This reduction division is called **meiosis**. The reduction in chromosome number found in eggs and sperm is essential because these gametes combine to form a new individual

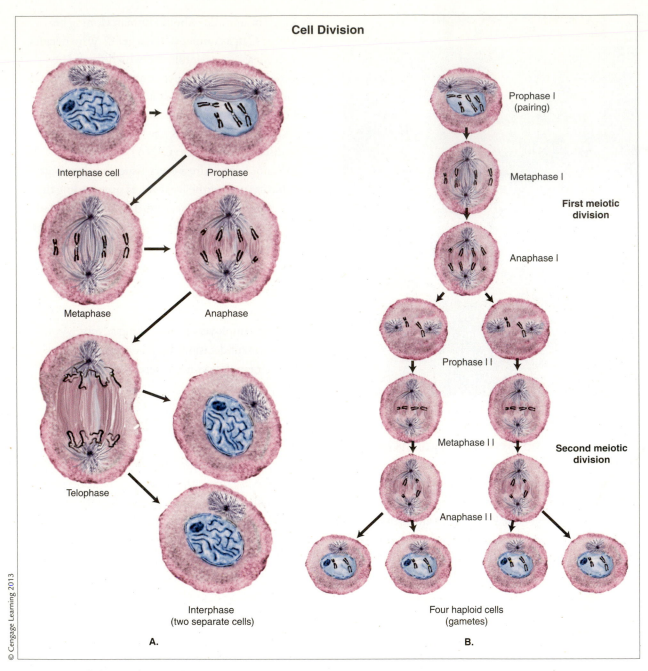

Cell Division

A.

Interphase cell → Prophase → Metaphase → Anaphase → Telophase → Interphase (two separate cells)

B.

Prophase I (pairing) → Metaphase I → Anaphase I — First meiotic division

Prophase II → Metaphase II → Anaphase II — Second meiotic division

Four haploid cells (gametes)

FIGURE 10-5: Cell division: (A) mitosis (B) meiosis.

with 46 chromosomes. During meiosis, progenitor cells with 46 chromosomes undergo two cell divisions that result in four new cells (Figure 10-5). In males, all of these cells become sperm. In females, only one of the resulting four cells becomes a viable egg. The other three become polar bodies and fail to develop. Because progenitor cells in females carry two X chromosomes, the eggs that they produce will contain only an X sex chromosome. By contrast, progenitor cells in males contain both an X and

a Y chromosome. As a result, half of the resulting sperm contain an X chromosome and half contain a Y chromosome.

FERTILIZATION AND EARLY EMBRYONIC DEVELOPMENT

As the unfertilized egg travels through the fallopian tube toward the uterus, it is surrounded by a protective coating of cells called the zona pellucida. If the egg and the sperm fuse, changes occur in the outer layers of the egg, forming an impermeable fertilization membrane which prevents additional sperm from fusing with the egg. The resulting fertilized egg is called a **zygote**. The initial cell divisions that take place after fertilization are called cleavages. The first cleavage occurs about 20 hours after fertilization (Figure 10-6). These early cell divisions take place while the zygote is slowly being transported through the fallopian tubes toward the uterus. With each cleavage, the number of cells in the zygote increases, but the size of the new daughter cells decreases, resulting in little net change in the size of the zygote. These cell divisions take place within the fertilization membrane. After four cleavage divisions, the resulting 16 cells appear as a solid ball or **morula**, meaning "little mulberry" (Figure 10-7). The morula reaches the uterine cavity 72–80 hours after fertilization.

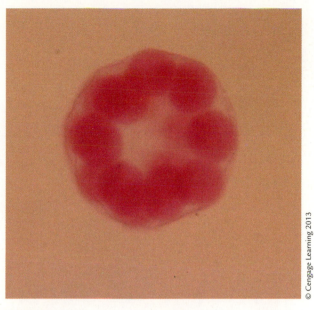

FIGURE 10-8: Blastocyst.

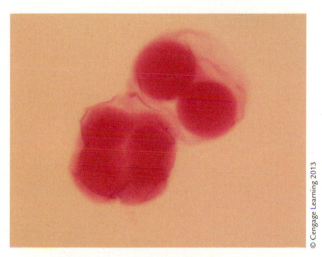

FIGURE 10-6: Early cleavages.

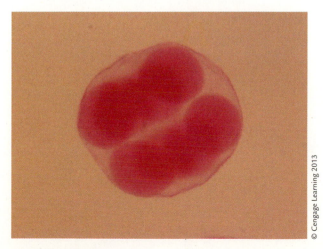

FIGURE 10-7: Morula.

Within the morula, a fluid-filled space appears, transforming it into a hollow ball of cells called a **blastocyst** (Figure 10-8). The clump of cells on the inner surface of the blastocyst is called the inner cell mass, and it is destined to become the embryo. The outer wall of the blastocyst becomes the trophoblast and contains the cells responsible for forming the placenta.

By the sixth day after ovulation, the blastocyst is ready to implant in the endometrium of the uterus. The events from fertilization to implantation are summarized in Figure 10-9.

DEVELOPMENT OF THE PLACENTA

Prior to implantation, the zygote has been nourished by the secretions from the fallopian tube and the uterus, but further growth requires more nutrients and oxygen which must be provided by the mother's blood. The blastocyst accesses the maternal blood supply by burrowing into the uterine lining. The trophoblast secretes enzymes that dissolve some of the cells of the endometrium. The trophoblast cells then proliferate to form small, finger-like projections called the chorionic villi of the placenta. The chorionic villi facilitate the transfer of nutrients and wastes between the maternal and fetal circulation

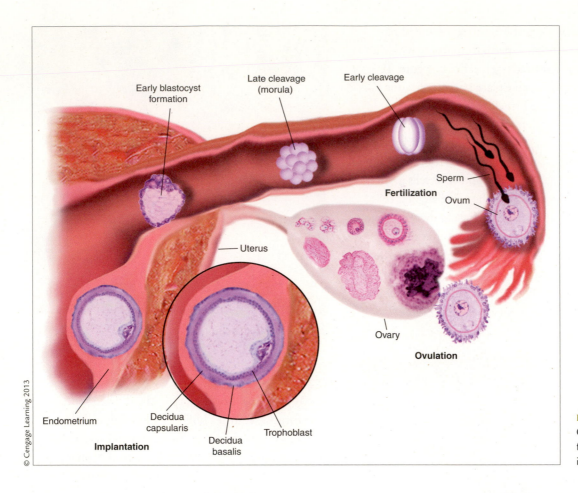

Early blastocyst formation

Late cleavage (morula)

Early cleavage

Sperm

Fertilization

Ovum

Uterus

Ovary

Ovulation

Endometrium

Decidua capsularis

Decidua basalis

Trophoblast

Implantation

© Cengage Learning 2013

FIGURE 10-9: Ovulation, fertilization, and implantation.

while keeping the maternal and fetal blood seperated. The thick endometrium is called the decidua, meaning "to shed." The portion of the endometrium under the blastocyst is the decidua basalis (Figure 10-10). The process of attachment and placental formation is called implantation. From a medical perspective, a pregnancy has not occurred until successful implantation has taken place.

Originally, the chorionic villi are present over the entire surface of the blastocyst, but as the embryo enlarges, the surface that is not in contact with the endometrium and projects into the uterine cavity loses its villi and becomes smooth. Two layers of fetal membranes form around the developing embryo—the inner amnion, which secretes the amniotic fluid, and the outer chorion. As placental development continues, a complicated network of blood vessels develops in which the fetal chorionic villi are surrounded by and bathed in the maternal blood sinuses of the decidua basalis. Later, the fetal blood vessels, two umbilical arteries, and one umbilical vein will form the umbilical cord,

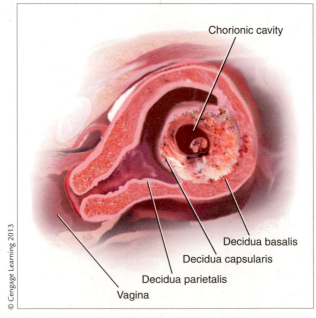

Chorionic cavity

Decidua basalis

Decidua capsularis

Decidua parietalis

Vagina

© Cengage Learning 2013

FIGURE 10-10: Implantation, and the formation of the placenta.

which connects the embryo to the placenta. These blood vessels continue into the chorionic villi (Figure 10-11).

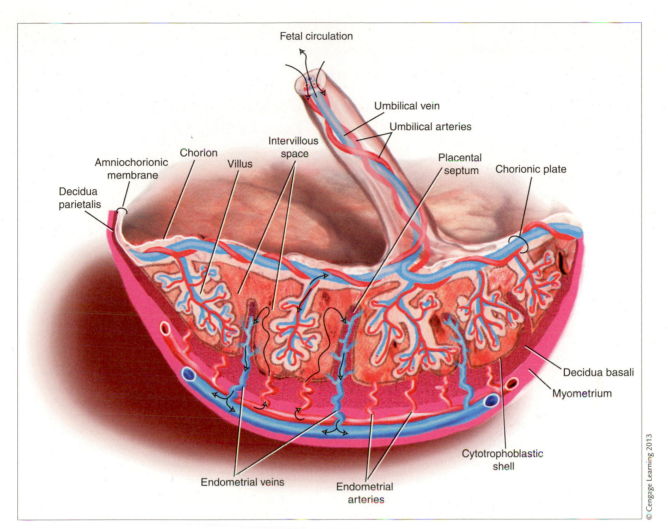

FIGURE 10-11: Placental circulation.

The **placenta** is an organ that serves to prevent the direct exchange between the blood of the fetus and the blood of the mother. Layers of placental tissue separate the maternal and the fetal blood, forming the placental barrier. The nutrients and oxygen delivered by the maternal vessels diffuse across the placental barrier into the bloodstream of the fetus. In turn, the waste products from the fetus travel in the opposite direction and diffuse into the mother's blood. Many substances are prevented from crossing the placental barrier including many microbes and some medications. However, the placental barrier does not stop all transfers. Microbes such as hepatitis B and *Treponema pallidum* and chemicals such as alcohol, retinol, and tetracycline can pass from mother to fetus.

The placenta is not only a transfer organ but a factory as well. It is capable of synthesizing enzymes

and proteins, and it manufactures fats and carbohydrates that serve as a source of stored energy. The placenta also functions as an endocrine gland, manufacturing and secreting hormones. Maternal hormones set the stage for ovulation, conception, and implantation, but very early in pregnancy, the placenta begins to synthesize its own collection of hormones that play a vital role in maintaining the pregnancy. Placental **human chorionic gonadotropin (hCG)** is a hormone secreted very early by the cells of the trophoblast. The biological effect of hCG is similar to luteinizing hormone. Its function is to preserve the corpus luteum and progesterone production so that the endometrial lining of the uterus is not shed and the pregnancy is maintained. While the production of hCG begins soon after implantation, it rises to a peak production between the eighth and twelfth weeks of pregnancy, and then falls to a much lower level for the remainder of gestation. Pregnancy tests are designed to detect levels of hCG.

After the eighth week, the placenta becomes a major source of progesterone, which it produces in large quantities to maintain the pregnancy. The placenta also forms estrogen from androgen precursors, many of which are provided by the developing fetal endocrine glands. **Placental lactogen**, also known as human somatomammotropin, increases maternal blood sugar levels by breaking down fat and decreasing glucose uptake by the maternal cells. This means that high levels of glucose are present in the mother's bloodstream to diffuse across the placenta and provide energy to the rapidly growing embryo. In addition, placental lactogen increases urine output in the mother, facilitating the removal of increased wastes from the mother's system. Another placental hormone, **chorionic thyrotropin,** mimics thyroid stimulating hormone, causing an increase in the production of thyroid hormone in the mother's body. Placental growth hormone secretion usually surpasses the levels of maternal growth hormone by four months into the pregnancy. Research indicates that **placental growth hormone** may be one factor in regulating maternal insulin resistance (McIntyre, Zeck, & Russell, 2009) and may play a role in the development of gestational diabetes. The influence of the placenta extends even after birth. A review by Thornburg et al. (2010) found that the quality of placental development predicted risks for the development of heart disease, hypertension, and cancer for the offspring later in life.

EMBRYONIC GERM LAYERS

As the trophoblast develops into the placenta, the cells of the inner mass of the blastocyst continue to divide and differentiate. During a process called **gastrulation**, three layers of embryonic cells form, and the blastocyst becomes a gastrula. As the divisions continue, the cells begin to differentiate,

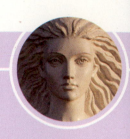

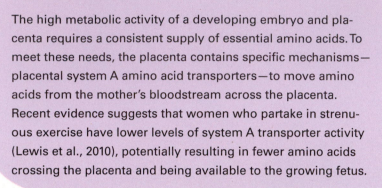

focus on

EXERCISE
Maternal Exercise and the Placental Transfer of Essential Amino Acids

The high metabolic activity of a developing embryo and placenta requires a consistent supply of essential amino acids. To meet these needs, the placenta contains specific mechanisms—placental system A amino acid transporters—to move amino acids from the mother's bloodstream across the placenta. Recent evidence suggests that women who partake in strenuous exercise have lower levels of system A transporter activity (Lewis et al., 2010), potentially resulting in fewer amino acids crossing the placenta and being available to the growing fetus.

and from then on, will no longer be identical to each other. Some will become brain cells, some bone cells, some will be the eye, heart, or kidney cells, and some will become segregated from the other cells at an early stage to become future egg or sperm cells.

The outermost layer of the gastrula is called the **ectoderm**, the innermost is called the **endoderm**, and sandwiched between them is the layer called the **mesoderm**. The cells of the ectoderm will give rise to such structures as the nervous system, the skin, and some of the endocrine glands. The endoderm differentiates into the digestive and respiratory systems and parts of the reproductive system. The mesoderm will differentiate into the skeletal, muscular, urinary, circulatory, and reproductive systems. Details about the structure derived from each of the germ layers are shown in Table 10-1. While most of the embryonic cells are taking on specific forms and functions, some cells remain at least partially undifferentiated. These will remain as stem cells which retain the ability to become many different types of cells in the body. After gastrulation and differentiation of the germ layers (14 days after ovulation), the blastocyst becomes an **embryo**.

Neural Tube Formation
Two of the first structures to take shape in the embryo are the brain and the spinal cord. Starting

Table 10-1 Embryonic Germ Layers.		
Ectoderm Will Form:	**Mesoderm Will Form:**	**Endoderm Will Form:**
Skin, hair, nails, lens of the eye, lining of the internal and external ear, nose sinuses, mouth, anus, tooth enamel, pituitary gland, mammary glands, and all parts of the nervous system	Muscles, bones, lymphatic tissue, spleen, blood cells, heart, lungs, and reproductive and excretory systems	Lining of the lungs, tongue, tonsils, urethra, associated glands, bladder, and digestive tract

© Cengage Learning 2013

at one end of the ectodermal surface and extending along the length of the embryo, two folds of tissue begin to bulge upward and form a structure called the neural tube. The neural tube will become the brain and spinal cord. The area of the initial tube formation becomes the brain. From this point onward, development progresses from this area, which becomes the head, downward toward the feet. Small blocks of mesodermal tissue called somites orient along each side of the neural tube.

As development continues, cells from the somites migrate to other sections of the embryo to become the axial skeleton, the skeletal muscles, and the dermis layer of the skin.

By the third week after fertilization, a primitive heart begins to form and pumps blood throughout the embryo. At this point in development, the embryo has a distinct tail and limb buds. The tail is eventually reabsorbed and only the remnant tailbone remains. By the sixth week, the trachea and the lungs are beginning to form. The hands have also formed, but webbing remains between the fingers. At nine weeks, the foundation of each of the organ systems has developed, though none of the systems are fully functional. From this point to the end of the pregnancy, the embryo is called a **fetus**. Although the fetus' organ systems have formed, it will be several more months before the fetus is capable of surviving on its own. Around week 17, the fetal nervous system has matured enough to coordinate larger scale muscle movements which the mother can often feel. By the 20th week, the fetal heart beat can be heard using a stethoscope. By seven months, the fetus has developed enough to reliably survive if born prematurely. Table 10-2 illustrates the stages of fetal development from implantation to delivery and identifies major events in the development.

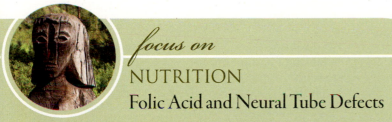

focus on

NUTRITION
Folic Acid and Neural Tube Defects

Sometimes during embryonic development, the neural tube that becomes the brain and spinal cord does not close, producing a **neural tube defect**. Neural tube defects include conditions such as spina bifida (failure of the vertebrae to close, leaving the spinal cord exposed) and anencephaly (failure of the brain to develop). Normally, the neural tube forms and seals in the first two weeks following conception, a time when many women do not even know they are pregnant. Consuming adequate amounts of folic acid before becoming pregnant and continuing throughout the pregnancy dramatically reduces the risk of a child developing a neural tube defect. Women are encouraged to eat foods high in folic acid (fresh dark greens and fortified cereals) if there is any possibility of becoming pregnant. The recommendation from the CDC is 400 micrograms of folic acid per day.

Table 10-2 Stages of Fetal Development.

	Stage	Fetal Development
	Embryonic or Germinal Stage Weeks 1 and 2	Rapid cell division and differentiation. Germinal layers form.
	Embryonic Stage Week 3*	Primitive nervous system, eyes, ears, and RBCs present. Heart begins to beat on day 21.
4 weeks	Week 4* Wt 0.4 g L 4–6 mm (crown–rump, C–R)	Half the size of a pea. Brain differentiates. GI tract begins to form. Limb buds appear.
	Week 5* L 6–8 mm (C–R)	Cranial nerves present. Muscles innervated.
	Week 6* L 10–14 mm (C–R)	Fetal circulation established. Liver produces RBCs. Central autonomic nervous system forms. Primitive kidneys form. Lung buds present. Cartilage forms. Primitive skeleton forms. Muscles differentiate.
	Week 7* L 22–28 mm (C–R)	Eyelids form. Palate and tongue form. Stomach formed. Diaphragm formed. Arms and legs move.
8 weeks	Week 8* Wt 2 g L 3 cm (1.5 in) (C–R)	Resembles human being. Eyes moved to face front. Heart development complete. Hands and feet well formed. Bone cells begin replacing cartilage. All body organs have begun forming.
	Fetal Stage Week 9	Finger and toenails form. Eyelids fuse shut.
	Week 10 Wt 14 g (1/2 oz) L 5–6 cm (2 in) crown–heel (C–H)	Head growth slows. Islets of Langerhans differentiated. Bone marrow forms, RBCs produced. Bladder sac forms. Kidneys make urine.

(*continued*)

Table 10-2   Stages of Fetal Development.

	Stage	Fetal Development
	Week 11	Tooth buds appear. Liver secretes bile. Urinary system functions. Insulin forms in pancreas.
 12 weeks	Week 12 Wt 45 g (1.5 oz) L 9 cm (3.5 in) (C–R) 11.5 cm (4.5 in) (C–H)	Lungs take shape. Palate fuses. Heart beat heard with Doppler ultrasound. Ossification established. Swallowing reflex present. External genitalia. Male or female distinguished.
 16 weeks	Second Trimester Week 16 Wt 200 g (7 oz) L 13.5 cm (5.5 in) (C–R) 15 cm (6 in) (C–H)	Meconium forms in bowels. Scalp hair appears. Frequent fetal movement. Skin thin, pink. Sensitive to light. 200 mL amniotic fluid. (Amniocentesis possible.)
 20 weeks	Week 20 Wt 435 g (15 oz) L 19 cm (7.5 in) (C–R) 25 cm (10 in) (C–H)	Myelination of spinal cord begins. Peristalsis begins. Lanugo covers body. Vernix caseosa covers body. Brown fat deposits begun. Sucks and swallows amniotic fluid. Heartbeat heard with fetoscope. Hands can grasp. Regular schedule of sucking, kicking, and sleeping.
 24 weeks	Week 24 Wt 780 g (1 lb, 12 oz) L 23 cm (9 in) (C–R) 28 cm (11 in) (C–H)	Alveoli present in lungs, begin producing surfactant. Eyes completely formed. Eyelashes and eyebrows appear. Many reflexes appear. Chance of survival if born now.

(continued)

Table 10-2   Stages of Fetal Development.

	Stage	Fetal Development
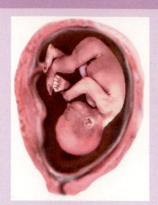 28 weeks	**Third Trimester** Week 28 Wt 1200 g (2 lb. 10 oz) L 28 cm (11 in) (C–R) 35 cm (14 in) (C–H)	Subcutaneous fat deposits begun. Lanugo begins to disappear. Nails appear. Eyelids open and close. Testes begin to descend.
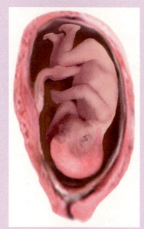 32 weeks	Week 32 Wt 2,000 g (4 lb, 6.5 oz) L 31 cm (12 in) (C–R) 41 cm (16 in) (C–H)	More reflexes present. CNS directs rhythmic breathing movements. CNS partially controls body temperature. Begins storing iron, calcium, phosphorus. Ratio of the lung surfactants lecithin and sphingomyelin (L/S) is 1.2:2.
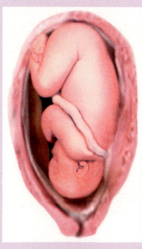 36 weeks	Week 36 Wt 2,500–2.750 g (5 lb, 8 oz) L 35 cm (14 in) (C–R) 48 cm (19 in) (C–H)	A few creases on soles of feet. Skin less wrinkled. Fingernails reach fingertips. Sleep-wake cycle fairly definite. Transfer of maternal antibodies.
	Week 38	L/S ratio 2:1

(continued)

Table 10-2	Stages of Fetal Development.	
	Stage	**Fetal Development**

40 weeks | Week 40
Wt 3,000–3,600 g
  (6 lb, 10 oz–7 lb, 15 oz)
L 50 cm (20 in) (C–H) | Lanugo only on shoulders and upper back.
Creases cover sole.
Vernix mainly in folds of skin.
Ear cartilage firm.
Less active, limited space.

Ready to be born. |

*Vulnerable to teratogenic effects.
Courtesy of Littleton, L.Y. & Engebretson, J.C. (2002) *Maternal, Neonatal, and Women's Health Nursing.* Clifton Park, NY: Cengage Learning.

SEX DETERMINATION

While females can produce only eggs with an X chromosome, males can produce two kinds of sperm—those carrying an X and those carrying a Y. If a sperm bearing an X chromosome fertilizes an egg, the resulting XX zygote will be genetically female. If a Y-carrying sperm fertilizes an egg, the XY zygote will be genetically male. Because half the sperm will carry an X and the other half will carry a Y, the chances of a male or a female being conceived are, theoretically, 50–50. In actuality, the birth sex ratio favors male embryos. World wide, for every 100 females born, 107 males are born. The ratio varies from country to country, ranging from 100 females per 102 males in Kenya to 100 females per 112 males in India (CIA, 2010).

For many years, the sex ratio imbalance was explained as the result of smaller and faster Y-bearing sperm reaching and fertilizing the egg before the slightly heavier and slower X-bearing sperm. However, new research has discredited this theory by showing that the speed that an individual sperm can swim is unrelated to whether it carries an X or a Y (Yan et al., 2006). Furthermore, in an *in vitro* study in which sperm were mixed with eggs, 20 male zygotes were conceived compared to only eight females despite the fact that equal numbers of X- and Y-bearing sperm were introduced simultaneously and neither had to swim any appreciable distance to fertilize an egg. Bowmen et al., proposed that eggs bind preferentially to Y-bearing sperm, resulting in the skewed ratio (2004). Another factor that can influence the sex ratio is smoking. Men who smoke heavily are more likely to father female children than male children. Smoking did not impact the sex ratio in women, however (Viloria et al., 2005). In cultures that favor male children, genetic testing and selection of male embryo and selective abortion of female fetuses can also shift the sex ratio in favor of males.

Development of the Reproductive System

While most organ systems of both male and female embryos develop nearly identically, there are differences in the development of their reproductive

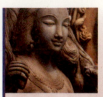

Social Considerations
SEX-SELECTION ABORTIONS

One factor which shifts the sex ratio in favor of male babies is selective abortion. Families in cultures that place high value on males compared to females are more likely to use sex-selective abortions to prevent the birth of daughters even when laws are in place to prevent them. Nepal, India, Bangladesh, and China have the highest reported rates of sex-selective abortions (Abrejo et al., 2009). Unfortunately, the practice is not limited to Asia. Thiele and Leier (2010) report that the practice is becoming more common in North America as well. In response to the increased number of sex-selective abortions, the Society of Obstetricians and Gynaecologists of Canada has adopted a policy against sex-selective abortions for non-medical reasons.

systems. The genetic sex of each individual is established by the X and Y chromosomes at fertilization, but the early embryo is anatomically neither male nor female. It has the potential to become either. The gonads and two sets of ducts—Wolffian ducts and Müllerian ducts—as well as the external structures remain undifferentiated for the first few weeks of embryonic development. During the fourth week after fertilization, a small swelling called the genital tubercle forms in the approximate position of the future external genitalia. Below it, the outer labioscrotal swellings and the inner urogenital folds form on either side of the common exit of the developing urinary, digestive, and reproductive systems. By the seventh week of embryonic life, each gonad consists of an outer zone called the cortex and an inner area called the medulla, which contain masses of cells which form the primary sex cords. The primary sex cords contain the primordial germ cells which can later develop into eggs or sperm.

Female Differentiation

In a female embryo, several gene sequences, specifically the ROBO and SLIT genes, trigger the formation of follicles in the developing ovary. However, the exact mechanisms though which an undifferentiated gonad becomes an ovary have not yet been fully identified (Dickinson et al., 2010). It does not appear that hormones are involved in the development of the female reproductive tract and external genitalia. The upper portions of the paired Müllerian ducts become the fallopian tubes, while the lower portions fuse to form the uterus and the upper portion of the vagina. The Wolffian ducts spontaneously regress without the presence of testosterone, a hormone not present in high levels in a female embryo.

Male Differentiation

In the male embryo, differentiation of the gonads into the testes takes place earlier than ovarian differentiation. The Y chromosome contains a gene called SRY, which is responsible for transforming each undifferentiated gonad into a testes (Sinclair et al., 1990). Under the influence of SRY, the testes will secrete hormones, including testosterone and Müllerian inhibiting factor, which will direct further differentiation of the male reproductive tract and male genitalia. The primary sex cords become the seminiferous tubules of the testes, and the cells that lie between the seminiferous tubules increase in size and number to become the interstitial cells. These interstitial cells secrete testosterone. Testosterone and its derivatives are responsible for the stabilization of the Wolffian ducts and cause the masculinization of the external genitalia. The Wolffian ducts are incorporated into the male reproductive system as the epididymis, the vas deferens, and the ejaculatory duct, and give rise to the seminal vesicle. The fetal testes also secrete a Müllerian duct inhibiting factor (MIF) that causes the regression of the Müllerian ducts as the embryo becomes anatomically male.

Differentiation of the External Genitalia

In both males and females, the genital tubercle elongates rapidly at first. In a female embryo, its growth gradually slows and it becomes the clitoris. The urogenital folds become the labia minora, and the urogenital sinus outlet that they originally enclosed becomes the vestibule. The labioscrotal swellings become the labia majora, fusing anteriorly to form the mons pubis.

In a male embryo, testosterone causes the genital tubercle to elongate further to form the penis. As it elongates, the penis pulls the urogenital folds forward to form the lateral walls of a urethral groove. The urogenital folds close over the urethral groove along the undersurface of the penis to form the penile urethra, and the external urethral opening moves from its original location at the root of the penis to its ultimate opening at the tip of the penis. The labioscrotal swellings develop and merge with each other in the midline to form the scrotum. Later in fetal life, the testes will descend from the body cavity to lie within the two scrotal sacs. Figure 10-12 shows the development of the external genitalia. Sexual differentiation is essentially completed by the twelfth week after fertilization.

In female embryos, the developing ovaries produce estradiol which may play a role in differentiating the ovarian tissue, but the hormone is not essential to female development. Mammalian embryos seem to be innately programmed to become female and only differentiate into males under the influence of the SRY gene and testosterone. In test mammals, if the embryonic gonads are removed before differentiation occurs, the embryo develops the reproductive tract of a female,

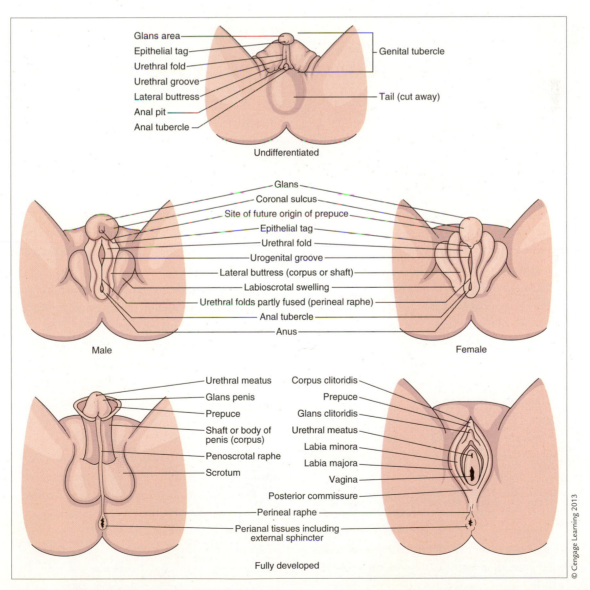

Glans area
Epithelial tag
Urethral fold
Urethral groove
Lateral buttress
Anal pit
Anal tubercle
Genital tubercle
Tail (cut away)
Undifferentiated

Glans
Coronal sulcus
Site of future origin of prepuce
Epithelial tag
Urethral fold
Urogenital groove
Lateral buttress (corpus or shaft)
Labioscrotal swelling
Urethral folds partly fused (perineal raphe)
Anal tubercle
Anus
Male   Female

Urethral meatus
Glans penis
Prepuce
Shaft or body of penis (corpus)
Penoscrotal raphe
Scrotum

Corpus clitoridis
Prepuce
Glans clitoridis
Urethral meatus
Labia minora
Labia majora
Vagina
Posterior commissure
Perineal raphe
Perianal tissues including external sphincter
Fully developed

FIGURE 10-12: Development of the external genitalia.

although it lacks ovaries. Embryos of both sexes are exposed to high levels of estrogen and progesterone produced by the mother and the placenta. Sufficient quantities of testosterone must be secreted by the male embryo's testes to overcome not only the innate predisposition toward femaleness, but also the high circulating levels of maternal hormones. As a result, mammalian males, even after sexual differentiation is complete, continue to show high resistance to experimentally injected estrogens and require large doses before any feminization appears. Mammalian females are, in contrast, easily masculinized and respond to even minute quantities of testosterone. The presence of endogenous (from the mother) or exogenous (administered) testosterone during the critical differentiation period in a female fetus can interfere with normal female development of both her internal reproductive organs and her external genitalia. For the female pattern of anatomical development to be shifted toward male, the Y chromosome must be present and the SRY gene must trigger the testes to secrete testosterone and MIF. The MIF inhibits the development of the fallopian tubes and uterus.

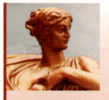

Cultural Considerations
THE GODDESS AND FEMALE EMBRYO

According to many of the world's religions, in the beginning there was the Creatrix, the Great Cosmic Mother, who was known by many names. She is Ilmatar, the Finnish birthing goddess. In Venezuela, she is Kuma, from whom everything sprang. In the Acoma Pueblo, they call her Thinking Woman who fed the sisters who then gave life to all. In the Truk Islands, she is Ligoubufanu, the mother of people, animals, grain, and coconuts who made the coconut in the image of her first child's face. In West Africa, the Fon people call her Mawu. The ancient Koreans honored her as Mago, the triune deity who birthed her daughters parthenogenetically—without male fertilization. The Greek Gaia, herself born from Chaos, also gave birth without a male god's participation (Leeming & Leeming, 1995; Hwang, 2007; Leadbetter, 1997).

As far back as 25,000 B.C.E., clay and bone and stone sculptures of women, many pregnant, were plentiful throughout what is now Spain, France, Germany, Austria, Czechoslovakia and Russia (Stone, 1976). In the more recent Neolithic period, European sites have yielded twenty times more female figurines than male (Dexter, 1990). Analyses of Neolithic creation myths suggest that the role of the male in procreation was unclear or unknown.

So it is natural that the mother and her reproductive capacity were the preeminent life-giving symbols (Biaggi, 2000). These matrifocal Neolithic societies appear to have also been socially egalitarian, matrilineal, and peaceful (Biaggi, 2000). Present-day goddess scholars suggest that these social results are linked to these societies' religious systems where the goddess embodied the entire life process: birth, life, and death (Dexter, 1990).

From a scientific perspective, it would be centuries before reproduction theory would evolve to suggest that sperm played a role in life-giving. Dutch biologist Jan Swammerdam observed frogs reproducing in the fourteenth century and speculated that the male frog's semen fertilized the female's eggs. Charles Darwin theorized that in the beginning, primordial life gestated within the ocean and reproduced parthenogenetically. In 1914, Emil Witschi discovered that all mammalian embryos are undifferentiated during the early stages of fetal life. The default body plan is female, and fetuses only become male if sufficient testosterone is present during development (Segal, 2007). This intrinsic developmental program of spontaneous female development in embryos is common scientific knowledge today (LeVay & Baldwin, 2009).

CHROMOSOMAL DISORDERS

The mechanisms underlying cell division are complex and chromosomal abnormalities can occur during the early stages of meiosis, as eggs and sperm are forming. In addition, failure of the chromosomes to divide properly during mitosis can create abnormal numbers of chromosomes in the daughter cells. When cells arise with an incorrect number of chromosomes, the condition is called aneuploidy. Because there are usually two homologous chromosomes, the presence of an extra chromosome results in what is called a trisomy. The absence of a chromosome results in a monosomy. In some cases, a piece of a chromosome breaks off, producing a deletion. Deleted fragments can combine with other chromosomes, rearranging the sequence of base pairs and altering the genes. When broken segments are exchanged between two chromosomes, it is called a translocation. These chromosomal abnormalities result in damage to the developing embryo and may trigger an early miscarriage. The exact number of embryos with chromosomal abnormalities is unknown, but there is evidence that zygotes with severe abnormalities frequently do not survive long enough to implant.

A Sample of Aneuploidies

Trisomies, which result in a total of 47 chromosomes instead of the usual 46, cause severe mental and physical abnormalities. Most occur during meiosis when one homologous pair of chromosomes which would normally separate remains together, creating an abnormal gamete with an extra chromosome. When this occurs, it is called a nondisjunction. Factors which influence the rate of nondisjunction include increased age, smoking, and other environmental factors. Cells in an arrested state of meiotic division are particularly susceptible to environmental influences—viruses, x-rays, toxic chemicals—that can interfere with normal cell division. The older a woman is, the longer her oocytes have been exposed to these damaging agents. Age does not have as strong of an effect on sperm, although the incidence of aneuploidies is also higher in older men.

The most frequent trisomy found in live births, affecting one in 800 children, is trisomy 21, or Down syndrome, in which there are three copies of chromosome 21. Trisomy 21 is almost always due to an egg with the extra chromosome that is fertilized by a normal sperm. Despite the maternal age effect, two-thirds of the children with Down syndrome are born to mothers younger than 35, in part because there are so many more children born to women in the younger age group. Down syndrome cases due to nondisjunction are not hereditary.

There are several other kinds of autosomal abnormalities that can result in multiple congenital birth defects. Most aneuploidies result in physical, developmental, and metabolic abnormalities. Trisomy 18, formerly called Edwards' syndrome, has an incidence of one in 6500 live births but usually causes the death of the child within the first year. Lejeune syndrome, the "cri-du-chat" or "cat-cry" syndrome is a very rare condition caused by a deletion of the shorter arm on chromosome 5. Affected babies have physical deformities, are developmentally disabled, and, as a result of a defect in the larynx, have a characteristic high-pitched cry that sounds like the meowing of a kitten. Another aneuploidy, monosomy 15, is associated with Angelman syndrome which affects nearly every cell in the body producing developmental delays, seizures, a failure to speak, and difficulties with balance (Pujana et al., 2002).

Sex Chromosome Abnormalities

The random accidents during meiotic development of the gametes that cause autosomal abnormalities can also produce aneuploidies of the sex chromosomes. Sometimes these result in abnormal development of the gonads and impaired fertility, but frequently, the change in chromosome number has no visible effects. The body's ability to tolerate variations in the number of sex chromosomes can result in a wide range of sex chromosome arrangements. These include Turner's syndrome with only a single X and no Y, Klinefelter's syndrome (XXY), trisomy X (XXX), double Y syndrome (XYY) and several other variations. Embryos with a Y chromosome usually develop male reproductive anatomy, even when extra X chromosomes are present. A zygote, however, must have at least one X to survive. Embryos with combinations such as YO or YY have never been observed, and it is assumed that zygotes with these combinations die very early in development.

Generally, any physical or mental abnormalities produced by sex chromosome anomalies are mild compared with those produced by autosomal trisomies and monosomies. There does seem to be a tendency for some developmental disability to be associated with extra X chromosomes, but the impairment is usually minimal. Surveys of patients in schools, hospitals, and institutions for the mentally disabled indicate there is a higher incidence of XXX females and Klinefelter's males than in the general population. Studies have shown XYY males score slightly lower on IQ tests than XY males and are slightly taller than normal, but show no other changes (Witkin et al., 1976; Owen 1979; Aksglaede et al., 2008).

TERATOGENS AND CONGENITAL ABNORMALITIES

Teratogens are agents that can induce damage to the developing embryo and cause birth defects or congenital abnormalities. They are another factor women must be concerned about during and even before pregnancy. Microbes, medications, and many common chemicals have the potential to cause birth defects. The type of damage caused by specific teratogens depends on a variety of factors including the level of exposure, the stage of pregnancy when the exposure occurred, and several other, less understood factors. Research by Włoch et al. (2009) found that the metabolic activity of both the placenta and the fetus influences the teratogenic effects of some drugs. The nutritional condition of the mother also appears to have an effect, with good nutrition offering some protection from the effects of some teratogens.

The most critical period in the development of an embryo is from approximately day 15 to day 56, the time period when the organ systems are forming. Each of the organs has its own particularly sensitive period, and influence of a teratogen at that time can result in malformations. Because the development of many organ systems overlaps, the outcome of teratogen exposure can include clusters of abnormalities. The effect of rubella virus, for example, is known to be most harmful if the disease occurs within the four or five weeks after fertilization when the brain, heart, eyes, and ears are undergoing rapid development. Although the risk to the child is greatest during the

first trimester, susceptibility to environmental influences can continue throughout the pregnancy. Brain development, for example, takes place throughout gestation and even extends into the postnatal period. Babies born to mothers who used cocaine or methamphetamine, even late in pregnancy, showed neurological damage (Lester & Lagasse, 2009).

When a child is born with a developmental defect, parents often look for something to blame. While a woman should be concerned about what she exposes herself and her child to during pregnancy, she cannot avoid every potential threat. Nor is everything a teratogen. For many years caffeine was considered a teratogen, and pregnant women were warned about the dangers of even a single cup of tea or coffee. However, a review of 25 scientific studies on the teratogenic effects of caffeine found no evidence of damage to the fetus from a moderate caffeine intake (Browne et al., 2006). Other substances, such as alcohol, cause well-documented damage to the fetus.

Medications as Teratogens

Data bases such as the Teratogen Exposure Registry and Surveillance (TERAS) and the FDA track potential and known teratogens. The FDA places drugs into specific pregnancy risk categories: A, B, C, D, and X. Drugs in category A have been tested in large, well controlled studies and have shown no teratogenic effects. Category X drugs are proven teratogens in which the risk outweighs the benefits of taking the drug. The other categories represent levels between these two extremes (Sachdeva et al., 2009).

Thirty years ago, researchers who investigated women's medication use during pregnancy discovered that 65–95 percent of women use over-the-counter (OTC) medications during pregnancy (Nelson and Fortar, 1973; Hill, Craig, and Chaney, 1977; McManus et al., 1982). However, as women become more aware of the potential teratogenic effects of medications, there is more concern about potential negative impact. A recent study of 180 women who either were pregnant at the time of the study or had recently given birth found that the women commonly overestimated the potential risks of both prescription and OTC medications (Nordeng et al., 2010), raising the possibility that women may forego necessary medication in an attempt to protect the fetus. While many medications carry risks, pregnant women should discuss medically-necessary drugs and their effects on the fetus with their healthcare provider. Many common prescription medications—ACE inhibitors, warfarin, tetracycline, methotrexate, retinol—are recognized teratogens. However, in some cases, the risk of untreated maternal illness may be greater for the woman and her fetus than the possible harmful effect of a drug.

Microbes as Teratogens

Several microbes have the ability to cross the placenta and damage the fetus. For example, the virus rubella was once a common cause of congenital deafness and visual problems. The wide spread use of the rubella vaccine has dramatically reduced the incidence of these birth defects. Cytomegalovirus (CMV) also attacks the fetal nervous system, but there is no vaccine for CMV. *Toxoplasma* is a protozoan, or single-celled animal, that is commonly associated with cat feces. Pregnant women are advised to avoid contact with cat litter boxes to reduce the risk of exposure. Like CMV, *Toxoplasma* targets the nervous system of the fetus. *Listeria* is a bacteria found in contaminanted dairy products and foods containing dairy by-products such as processed lunch meats. If a pregnant woman is infected, it produces minor, flu-like symptoms. However, during the first trimester, *Listeria* can cause severe deformities and miscarriage. The STI *Treponema pallidum*, which causes syphilis, can cross the placenta and cause a number of structural birth defects including skull malformation and heart damage. It can also cause stillbirth.

Alcohol

The teratogenic effects of alcohol consumption have been recognized since 1973, when fetal alcohol syndrome (FAS) was first described. Now called fetal alcohol spectrum disorder (FASD), the condition includes a pattern of structural, behavioral, and neurocognitive disabilities that include low birth weight and fetal growth retardation, microcephaly, underdeveloped jaws, nonparallel low-set ears, and a variety of cardiac, urogenital, cutaneous, and musculoskeletal defects. A Finnish study which followed a group of FASD children from birth through adolescence found that 70 percent had growth deficiencies,

55 percent had deformed fingers (camptodactyly), 38 percent had crossed eyes (strabismus), 43 percent had tooth abnormalities, 22 percent had urogenital abnormalities, and 18 percent had congenital heart defects. These conditions occurred at much higher rates in FASD children than in the general population (Autti-Rämö et al., 2006). One analysis of the effects of moderate drinking (three drinks per week) during pregnancy found a decline in the children's IQ scores, as well as learning problems at age 7.5 years (Streissguth et al., 1990). Even light drinking, defined as having a drink once a week, has been linked to an increased risk of miscarriage and low birth weight. Avoiding alcohol during pregnancy prevents FASD.

Tobacco

Tobacco smoke is another potential teratogen. Reduced birth weight with maternal smoking has been shown to be independent of all the other factors that can influence the size of a baby. Although it is possible that heavy smokers have lower maternal weight gain, which could concurrently slow fetal growth, the cause of the decrease in fetal weight (an average of 6 oz or 170 g) may also be related to the

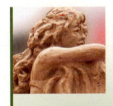

Economic Considerations

A SMALL INVESTMENT RETURNS BIG REWARDS

Teratogens are widespread. During pregnancy, a woman is likely to be exposed to some chemicals that have the potential to harm her developing fetus. While concerns have been raised about the potential damage caused by severe nutritional deficiencies, slight declines in the nutritional status of the mother can have negative effects, as well. Research shows that a suboptimal level of minerals increases the damage caused by fetal alcohol exposure (Keen et al., 2010). The implication is that the fetal damage caused by teratogens could be partially mitigated by inexpensive prenatal vitamin and mineral supplementation.

presence of excess carbon monoxide in the mother's blood. Studies have found up to 10 times the level of carbon monoxide in the blood of infants born to smoking mothers compared to infants born to nonsmoking mothers. Hemoglobin preferentially binds to carbon monoxide instead of oxygen. This results in hypoxia (low blood oxygen) which deprives the embryonic cells of oxygen needed for growth and metabolism. Kink and Fabro's review (1982) of the effects of cigarette smoking on pregnancy documents an increased frequency of miscarriage and a greater incidence of pregnancy complications such as bleeding in women who smoked. A study in Israel that examined the smoking habits of more than 16,000 mothers found that infants delivered by women aged 35 years and older who smoked had an increased rate of major malformations such as cleft palate, heart defects, and central nervous system anomalies and a significantly higher risk for minor malformations (Seidman et al., 1990). Karatza, et al., (2009) found that the number of cigarettes a woman smoked while pregnant had a direct effect on congenital heart defect rates. Smoking more than 10 cigarettes per day poses the greatest risk. The long-term growth and development of the children born to smoking mothers is also affected.

Endocrine disruptors

In recent years, the problem of endocrine disruptors and their impact on cancer and fertility in adults has captured media attention. Research has now turned to the impact of these compounds on the developing fetus, particularly the effects on the development of the reproductive system. Two chemicals of particular, recent interest are the plasticizers BPA and phthalates. Phthalates have been shown to reduce the number of germ cells in the fetal testes (Habert et al., 2009). BPA has been shown to disrupt meiosis of the fetal oocytes, leading to nondisjunctions and the lack of polar body formation (Lenie et al., 2008). Both of these effects can contribute to infertility.

Endocrine disruptors have additional effects on the body. BPA is shown to alter the function of thyroid hormone in the developing fetus (Heimeier & Shi, 2010), interfering with the signaling pathways for the hormone. Since thyroid hormone influences the metabolic rate of cells, BPA has implications beyond reproductive system damage.

CONCLUSION

The events that take place during development between fertilization and birth have impacts that will continue throughout the life of an individual. Understanding the sequence of events during development, the influence of teratogens, and the roles that genes play in development can help a woman make informed choices and provide the best possible outcome if she decides to have children.

REVIEW QUESTIONS

1. Why is the first trimester the most sensitive for terotagens?

2. What is the Human Genome Project?

3. What does each embryonic germ layer develop into?

4. What happens during neural tube development?

5. What role does the placenta play during pregnancy?

CRITICAL THINKING QUESTIONS

1. How can knowing your family history help predict the health of your children?

2. What criteria should be used to determine the "best" genetic traits?

3. Why are researchers working on stem cell research?

WEBLINKS

Centers for Disease Control
     www.cdc.gov
March of Dimes
     www.marchofdimes.com

Online Mendelian Inheritance in Man
     www.ncbi.nlm.nih.gov/sites/entrez?db=omim

REFERENCES

Abrejo, F. G., Shaikh, B. T., & Rizvi, N. (2009). 'And they kill me, only because I am a girl' . . . A review of sex-selective abortions in South Asia. *European Journal of Contraception and Reproductive Healthcare, 14*(1),10–16.

Aksglaede, L., Skakkebaek, N. E., & Juul, A. (2008). Abnormal sex chromosome constitution and longitudinal growth: Serum levels of insulin-like growth factor (IGF)-I, IGF binding protein-3, luteinizing hormone, and testosterone in 109 males with 47,XXY, 47,XYY, or sex-determining region of the Y chromosome (SRY)-positive 46,XX karyotypes. *Journal of Clinical Endocrinology & Metabolism, 93*(1), 169–176.

Autti-Rämö, I., Fagerlund, A., Ervalahti, N., Loimu, L., Korkman, M., & Hoyme, H. E. (2006). Fetal alcohol spectrum disorders in Finland: Clinical delineation of 77 older children and adolescents. *American Journal of Medical Genetics Part A,140*(2), 137–143.

Bekris, L. M., Millard, S. P., Galloway, N. M., Vuletic, S., Albers, J. J., Li, G., Galasko, D. R., Decarli, C., Farlow, M. R., Clark, C. M., Quinn, J. F., Kaye, J. A., Schellenberg, G. D., Tsuang, D., Peskind, E. R., & Yu, C.E. (2008). Multiple SNPs within and surrounding the apolipoprotein E gene influence cerebrospinal fluid apolipoprotein E protein levels. *Journal of Alzheimer's Disease, 13*(3), 255–266.

Biaggi, C. (Ed.). (2000). *In the footsteps of the Goddess: Personal stories.* Manchester, CT: Knowledge, Ideas & Trends, Inc.

Bowman, M., de Boer, K., Cullinan, R., Catt, J., & Jansen, R. (1998). Do alterations in the sex ratio occur at fertilization? A case report using fluorescent in situ hybridization. *Journal of Assisted Reproduction and Genetics, 15*(5), 320–322.

Bredenoord, A. L., Pennings, G., Smeets, H. J., & de Wert, G. (2008). Dealing with uncertainties: Ethics of prenatal diagnosis and preimplantation genetic diagnosis to prevent mitochondrial disorders. *Human Reproduction Update, 14*(1), 83–94.

Bronstein, M., Pisanté, A., Yakir, B., & Darvasi, A. (2008). Type 2 diabetes susceptibility loci in the Ashkenazi Jewish population. *Human Genetics, 124*(1), 101–104.

Browne, M. L. (2006). Maternal exposure to caffeine and risk of congenital anomalies: A systematic review. *Epidemiology, 17*(3), 324–331.

Canadian Museum of Nature. (2008). Retrieved April 24, 2010 from http://nature.ca/ genome/03/a/03a_11a_e.cfm.

Centers for Disease Control. (2010). Folic acid. Retrieved April 24, 2010 from http://www.cdc. gov/ncbddd/folicacid/index.html.

Central Intelligence Agency. (2010). *The world factbook.* Washington, DC: Retrieved April 24, 2010 from https://www.cia.gov/library/publications/ the-world-factbook/index.html.

Collins, T. (1986). Mythic reflections: Thoughts on myth, spirit, and our times, an interview with Joseph Campbell. *In Context: A Quarterly Of Humane Sustainable Culture, 12.* Retrieved March 11, 2009 from http://www.context.org/ ICLIB/IC12/Campbell.htm.

Dexter, M. R. (1990). *Whence the goddesses: A source book.* Elmsford, NY: Pergamon Press.

Diav-Citrin, O., Shechtman, S., Bar-Oz, B., Cantrell, D., Arnon, J., & Ornoy, A. (2008). Pregnancy outcome after in utero exposure to valproate: Evidence of dose relationship in teratogenic effect. *CNS Drugs, 22*(4), 325–334.

Dickinson, R. E., Hryhorskyj, L., Tremewan, H., Hogg, K., Thomson, A. A., McNeilly, A. S., & Duncan, W. C. (2010). Involvement of the SLIT/ROBO pathway in follicle development in the fetal ovary. *Reproduction, 139*(2), 395–407.

GINA becomes law 2008, May 21. Retrieved May 25, 2008 from http://www.ornl.gov/sci/techresources/Human_Genome/home.shtml.

Habert, R., Muczynski, V., Lehraiki, A., Lambrot, R., Lécureuil, C., Levacher, C., Coffigny, H., Pairault, C., Moison, D., Frydman, R., & Rouiller-Fabre, V. (2009). Adverse effects of endocrine disruptors on the fetal testis development: Focus on the phthalates. *Folia Histochemica et Cytobiologica, 47*(5), S67–74.

Heimeier, R. A., & Shi, Y. B. (2010). Amphibian metamorphosis as a model for studying endocrine disruption on vertebrate development: Effect of bisphenol A on thyroid hormone action. *General and Comparative Endocrinology, 168*(2), 181–189.

Hellenthal, G., Auton, A., & Falush, D. (2008). Inferring human colonization history using a copying model. *PLoS Genetics, 4*(5), e1000078. doi:10.1371/journal.pgen.1000078

Hesselgrave, D. (2002). Enculturation and acculturation: A reading for cultural anthropology. Retrieved from http://home.snu.edu/-hculbert/encultur.htm

Hill, R. M., Craig, J. P., Chaney, M. D., Tennyson, L. M., & McCulley, L. B. (1977). Utilization of over-the-counter drugs during pregnancy. *Clinical Obstetrics and Gynecology, 20*(2), 381–394.

Hruby, E., Sassi, L., Görbe, E., Hupuczi, P., & Papp, Z. (2007). The maternal and fetal outcome of 122 triplet pregnancies. *Orv Hetil, 148*(49), 2315–2328.

Kaplowitz, P. B., Drug and Therapeutics and Executive Committees of the Lawson Wilkins Pediatric Endocrine Society & Oberfield, S. E.

(1999). Reexamination of the age limit for defining when puberty is precocious in girls in the United States: Implications for evaluation and treatment. *Pediatrics, 104*(4 Pt. 1), 936–941.

Karatza, A. A., Giannakopoulos, I., Dassios, T. G., Belavgenis, G., Mantagos, S. P., & Varvarigou, A. A. (2009). Periconceptional tobacco smoking and X isolated congenital heart defects in the neonatal period. *International Journal of Cardiology, 148*(3), 295–299.

Keen, C. L., Uriu-Adams, J. Y., Skalny, A., Grabeklis, A., Grabeklis, S., Green, K., Yevtushok, L., Wertelecki, W. W., & Chambers, C. D. (2010). The plausibility of maternal nutritional status being a contributing factor to the risk for fetal alcohol spectrum disorders: the potential influence of zinc status as an example. *Biofactors, 36*(2), 125–135.

Kink, J. C., & Fabro, S. (1983). Alcohol consumption and cigarette smoking: Effect on pregnancy. *Clinical Obstetrics and Gynecology, 26*(2), 437–448.

Klos, K., Shimmin, L., Ballantyne, C., Boerwinkle, E., Clark, A., Coresh, J., Hanis, C., Liu, K., Sayre, S., & Hixson, J. (2008). APOE/C1/C4/C2 hepatic control region polymorphism influences plasma apoE and LDL cholesterol levels. *Human Molecular Genetics, 17*(13), 2039–2046.

Kuliev, A., & Verlinsky, Y. (2008). Impact of preimplantation genetic diagnosis for chromosomal disorders on reproductive outcome. *Reproductive BioMedicine Online, 16*(1), 9–10.

Leadbetter, Ron. (1997). Gaia. Retrieved March 12, 2009 from http://www.pantheon.org/articles/g/gaia.html.

Leeming, D., & Leeming, M. (1995). *A cictionary of creation myths.* New York, NY: Oxford University Press.

Lenie, S., Cortvrindt, R., Eichenlaub-Ritter, U. & Smitz, J. (2008). Continuous exposure to bisphenol A during in vitro follicular development induces meiotic abnormalities. *Mutation Research, 651*(1–2), 71–81.

Lester, B. M., & Lagasse, L. L. (2010). Children of addicted women. *Journal of Addictive Diseases, 29*(2), 259–276.

LeVay, S., and Baldwin, J. (2009). *Human sexuality.* Sunderland, MA: Sinauer Associates, Inc.

Lewis, R. M., Greenwood, S. L., Cleal, J. K., Crozier, S. R., Verrall, L., Inskip, H. M., Cameron, I. T., Cooper, C., Sibley, C. P., Hanson, M. A., & Godfrey, K. M. (2010). Maternal muscle mass may influence system A activity in human placenta. *Placenta, 31*(5), 418–422.

McArthur, S. J., Leigh, D., Marshall, J. T., de Boer, K. A., & Jansen, R. P. S. (2005). Pregnancies and live births after trophectoderm biopsy and preimplantation genetic testing of human blastocysts. *Fertility and Sterility, 84*:1628–1636.

McManus, K. A., Brackbill, Y., Woodward, L., Doering, P., & Robinson, D. (1982). Consumer information about prenatal and obstetric drugs. *Women & Health, 7*(1), 15–29.

McIntyre, H. D., Zeck, W., & Russell, A. (2009). Placental growth hormone, fetal growth and the IGF axis in normal and diabetic pregnancy. *Current Diabetes Reviews, 5*(3), 185–189.

Mullin, B. H., Prince, R. L., Dick, I. M., Hart, D. J., Spector, T. D., Dudbridge, F., & Wilson, S. G. (2008). Identification of a role for the ARHGEF3 gene in postmenopausal osteoporosis. *American Journal of Human Genetics, 82*(6), 1262–1269.

Nelson, M. M., & Fortar, J. O. (1971). Association between drugs administered during pregnancy and congenital abnormalities of the fetus. *British Medical Journal, 1,* 523–527.

Nordeng, H., Ystrøm, E., & Einarson, A. (2010). Perception of risk regarding the use of medications and other exposures during pregnancy. *European Journal of Clinical Pharmacology, 66*(2), 207–214.

Owen, D. R. (1979). Psychological studies in XYY males. In H. L. Vallet & I. H. Porter (Eds.), *Genetic mechanisms of sexual development* (pp. 465–471). New York, NY: Academic Press.

Prescott, J., & Doerr, E. (1989). Fetal personhood: Is an Acorn an oak tree? *Truth Seeker.* Vol. 1 (2) May/June. 21–28.

Pujana, M. A., Nadal, M., Guitart, M., Armengol, L., Gratacòs, M., & Estivill, X. (2002). Human chromosome 15q11-q14 regions of rearrangements contain clusters of LCR15 duplicons. *European Journal of Human Genetics, 10*(1), 26–35.

Randall, T. (1991). Pregnancy hormone levels signal trisomy 21, improved screening, lower costs possible. *Journal of the American Medical Association, 265*(14), 1797–1798.

Sachdeva, P., Patel, B. G., & Patel, B. K. (2009). Drug use in pregnancy; a point to ponder! *Indian Journal of Pharmaceutical Sciences, 71*(1), 1–7.

Schlaepfer, T. E., Harris, G. J., & Tien, A. Y., et al. (1995). Structural differences in the cerebral cortex of healthy female and male subjects: A magnetic resonance imaging study. *Psychiatry Research, 61*(3), 129–135.

Segal, S. (2007). Life of Emil Witschi. Retrieved March 12, 2009 from http://daisyfield.com/ew/segal.htm.

Seidman, D. S., Ever-Hadani, P., & Gale, R. (1990). Effect of maternal smoking and age on congenital anomalies. *Obstetrics & Gynecology, 76*(6), 1046–1050.

Sinclair, A. H., Berta, P., & Palmer, M. S. (1990). A gene from the human sex-determining region encodes a protein with homology to a conserved DNA-binding motif. *Nature, 346,* 240–245.

Stone, M. (1978). *When God was a woman.* New York, NY: Mariner Books.

Streissguth, A. P., Barr, H. M., & Sampson, P. D. (1990). Moderate prenatal alcohol exposure: effects on child IQ and learning problems at age 7 1/2 years. *Alcoholism: Clinical and Experimental Research, 14*(5), 662–669.

Thiele, A. T., & Leier, B. (2010). Towards an ethical policy for the prevention of fetal sex selection in Canada. *Journal of Obstetrics and Gynaecology Canada, 32*(1), 54–57.

Thornburg, K. L., O'Tierney, P. F., & Louey, S. (2010). Review: The placenta is a programming agent for cardiovascular disease. *Placenta, 31* Suppl, S54–59.

Verkerk, A. J., Pieretti, M., Sutcliffe, J. S. (1991). Identification of a gene (FMR-1) containing a CGG repeat coincident with a breakpoint cluster region exhibiting length variation in fragile X syndrome. *Cell, 65,* 905–914.

Viloria, T., Rubio, M. C., Rodrigo, L., Calderon, G., Mercader, A., Mateu, E., Meseguer, M., Remohi, J., & Pellicer, A. (2005). Smoking habits of parents and male: Female ratio in spermatozoa and preimplantation embryos. *Human Reproduction, 20*(9), 2517–2522.

Witkin, H. A., Mednick, S. A., & Schulsinger, F. (1976). Criminality in XYY and XXY men. *Science, 193,* 547–555.

Włoch, S., Pałasz, A., & Kamiński, M. (2009). Active and passive transport of drugs in the human placenta. *Ginekologia Polska, 80*(10), 772–777.

Yan, J., Feng, H. L., Chen, Z. J., Hu, J., Gao, X., & Qin, Y. (2006). Influence of swim-up time on the ratio of X- and Y-bearing spermatozoa. *European Journal of Obstetrics & Gynecology and Reproductive Biology, 129*(2), 150–154.

chapter 11

PREGNANCY, LABOR, AND DELIVERY

CHAPTER COMPETENCIES

Upon completion of this chapter, the reader will be able to:

- Describe the physiological events that lead to the establishment of a pregnancy
- Identify and describe the changes that take place to a woman's body during pregnancy
- Identify practices that contribute to a healthy pregnancy
- Describe the physiological process of labor and delivery
- Identify issues that are important to the immediate after care of the mother and infant following delivery

KEY TERMS

apgar score	gestational period	malaria	parturition

INTRODUCTION

Pregnancy is a normal physiological process. Chapter 10 focused on the process of development and pregnancy from the fetal perspective. This chapter examines pregnancy, labor, and delivery primarily as it is experienced by the mother during a typical pregnancy. Potential complications of pregnancy and medical interventions are discussed in Chapter 12.

DETERMINATION OF PREGNANCY

Individual women vary in terms of the degree to which they experience the preliminary signs of pregnancy. Before the advent of modern pregnancy tests, a combination of signs were used to establish if a woman was pregnant, with some signs carrying an increased probability of accuracy. Usually one of the first signs noticed is the absence of menstruation. Of course, just being late or even skipping a period is not a reliable sign of pregnancy, but when the cessation of menstruation is accompanied by other pregnancy signs such as morning nausea, fatigue, breast tenderness, and an increased frequency of urination, pregnancy is likely. A sustained elevation of the basal body temperature (BBT) is another indication of pregnancy. A woman who keeps a record of her BBT should suspect she is pregnant if her temperature remains at 37°C–38°C (98.8°F–99.8°F) for three weeks after ovulation and stays elevated.

Pregnancy tests use an immunoassay to detect hCG levels which indicate that implantation has taken place. Immunoassay tests are capable of detecting very low levels of hCG in the blood serum or urine even before the first missed period. These tests can be taken at home, using an over-the-counter pregnancy test, which measures hCG in a woman's urine or as a blood or urine test in a healthcare setting. In the absence of a pregnancy test, changes that take place in the mother's body after implantation can also be interpreted as signs of pregnancy.

Some signs of pregnancy appear upon physical examination by a healthcare professional. Changes in the size, shape, and consistency of the uterus can be observed. Piskack's sign appears after implantation of the fertilized egg as a soft bulge at the implantation site. Skilled hands can detect this softening of the uterus on one side while the other side remains firm. Goodell's sign, a softening of the cervix, also appears early in pregnancy. Hegar's sign refers to the softening of the neck or isthmus of the uterus, the narrow part between the body and the cervix. First detectable at about six weeks, Hegar's sign disappears later when the entire cervix and the uterus have become soft and spongy in consistency. Another sign of pregnancy visible during a pelvic exam is Chadwick's sign, in which the walls of the vagina change from the usual pink to a dusky bluish color due to the increased blood supply and venous congestion. Such a color change can also be present, however, with heart disease or with a pelvic tumor.

Additional signs of pregnancy can be detected when the fetus starts growing larger in the uterus.

Around 16–18 weeks, a woman will begin to feel a fluttering sensation known as quickening, or "feeling life." This sensation can be mistaken for intestinal gas in a first pregnancy. For the doctor or midwife, fetal heart sounds, a fetal electrocardiogram, or an ultrasound image of the fetus are all signs that confirm a diagnosis of pregnancy (Figure 11-1). By 14 weeks, a procedure called internal ballottement can be performed gently during a vaginal examination (Figure 11-2). With the finger up against the cervix, the cervix is gently tapped. The fetus within the amniotic sac bounces up against the top of the uterus, and as it sinks back down, the rebound is felt against the finger. By 24 weeks, external ballottement can be performed. In this case, a push on one side of the abdomen with one hand will cause the fetus to move to the other side and can be felt by a hand that is placed there.

The Gestation Period

The **gestational period** is the time that the developing fetus spends in the uterus before being born. This is the length of time that it takes for all of the organ systems to become mature enough to function outside of the mother's body. The World Health Organization (WHO) defines "full term" for delivery as 37 to 42 weeks gestation. Infants delivered before 37 weeks gestation are considered preterm. Medical intervention is often required with preterm or premature infants (Rimawi, 2006). Gestations longer than 42 weeks are considered post term, and these pregnancies can also be prone to complications for both the mother and the fetus (The American College of

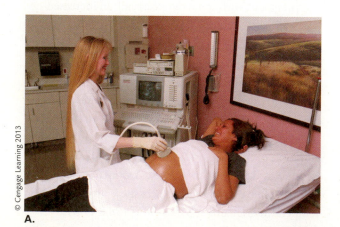

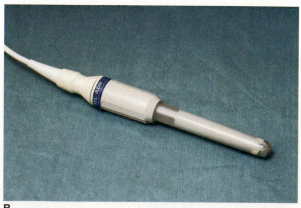

© Cengage Learning 2013

FIGURE 11-1: A. Abdominal ultrasound. B. Transducer for transvaginal ultrasound.

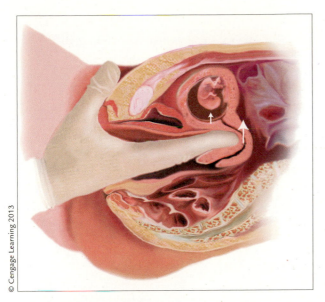

FIGURE 11-2: Ballottement.

Obstetricians and Gynecologists, 2006). If a woman knows the date of conception, she can, based on statistical averages, expect to deliver a baby 266 days, or 38 weeks, later. Because the precise time of fertilization is rarely known, the usual method to predict a due date is to determine the first day of the last menstrual period and add 280 days, or 40 weeks. It should be noted, however, that actual delivery dates can vary up to two weeks on either side of an estimated due date. In fact, less than five percent of births occur on a calculated due date, 50 percent are within one week of the calculated due date, and 90 percent are within two weeks (ACOG, 2006).

The gestational period is divided into three trimesters, each consisting of three calendar months. By week 10 of the first trimester, the embryo becomes a fetus. The first trimester is a critical period of development because of the great sensitivity of the embryo and fetus to teratogens, which are agents that can cause malformations and birth defects. By the end of the first trimester, all of the major organ systems are formed but not fully developed, even though the fetus is only about 6 cm long and weighs only 14 grams. The rest of the fetal period is a time for further growth and differentiation of the organs. Figure 11-3 illustrates fetal size by gestational age.

There is concern that recent increases in spontaneous preterm deliveries and medical decisions to schedule induction of labor or cesarean section have shifted the average gestation in the United States from 40 weeks to 39 weeks. Davidoff et al. (2006) reported that between 1992 and 2002, the most common gestational age at birth for single babies was 39 weeks. The consequences of preterm deliveries will be addressed in Chapter 12. In 2005, 52 percent of childbirths were the result of induced labor or cesarean section before the onset of labor. Prenatal techniques for estimating gestational age have a margin of error of up to two weeks, so elective deliveries may result in infants that are younger gestationally than expected (Sakela, 2006a). There is strong evidence that suggests that fetal development, especially of the brain and lungs, is still occurring after 37 weeks gestation (Kinney, 2006; Zanardo, 2004). Recent research has found that brain volume increases dramatically during the last weeks of gestation and continues to the 41st week. The development of white matter in the brain, which facilitates the interconnections within the brain, is especially pronounced between weeks 34-41 gestation (Kinney, 2006). It is not known whether there are differences between continued brain and lung development outside verses inside the womb (Sakela & Corry, 2008).

Multiple Pregnancy

The human uterus is shaped to accommodate one fetus at a time, although it can accommodate more. When one fetus develops in the uterus, it is called a singleton pregnancy. When more than one fetus develops, it is termed a multiple pregnancy or a multiple gestation. The most common type of multiple pregnancy occurs when two eggs are simultaneously ovulated from two separate follicles and are then fertilized by two different sperm. The two zygotes implant in separate areas in the uterus to produce dizygotic or fraternal twins. These twins may be the same or opposite sexes, and they resemble each other as much as any other siblings would. Monozygotic twins originate from one fertilized egg that splits into two zygotes early in development. Such twins are the same sex, and begin their lives genetically identical. They are born identical in physical appearance unless there has been some environmental factor during fetal life to cause a difference between them. Conjoined twins, often referred to as Siamese twins, develop when monozygotic twins fail to separate completely. Figure 11-4 illustrates the formation of both fraternal and identical twins.

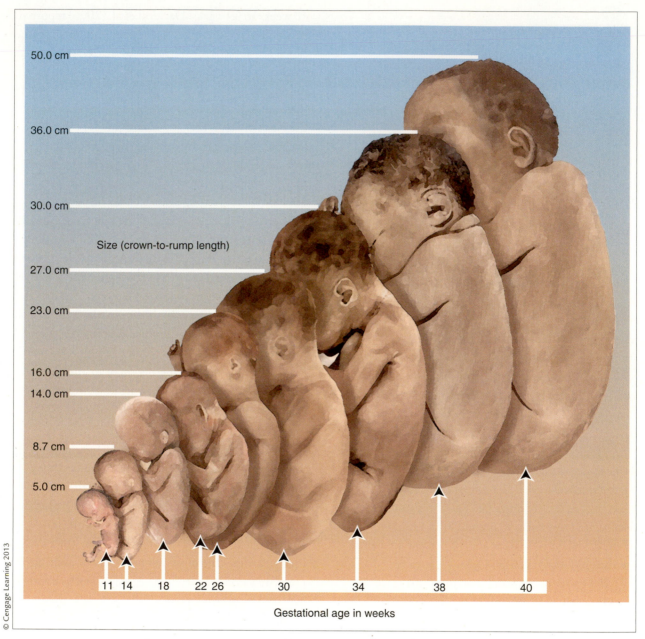

Size (crown-to-rump length)

50.0 cm
36.0 cm
30.0 cm
27.0 cm
23.0 cm
16.0 cm
14.0 cm
8.7 cm
5.0 cm

11 14   18   22 26   30   34   38   40

Gestational age in weeks

© Cengage Learning 2013

FIGURE 11-3: Fetal size by gestational age.

Twins occur in approximately one in 90 pregnancies in the United States, and the prevalence of twins varies across the globe. There have not been specific risk factors identified that increase a woman's chances of becoming pregnant with identical twins, but the American Society for Reproductive Medicine (2004) has identified the following characteristics that increase the incidence of conceiving fraternal twins:

- Age and Reproductive History of the Mother—The likelihood of twins increases with the age of the mother, and once a woman has given birth to twins, a multiple birth is about five times more likely to occur the next time. In addition, women between the ages of 35–40 who have had four or more children are three times more likely to have twins than are younger women without children.

- Heredity—Women who are fraternal twins or who have a family history of fraternal twins are more likely to conceive twins themselves. This trend does not appear to be true for male twins as fathers.

- Ethnic Background—Women of African descent are more likely to have twins than are women of European descent. Women of Asian descent are the least likely to have twins.

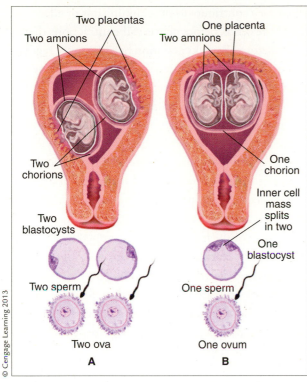

FIGURE 11-4: Formation of twins: A. Fraternal (nonidentical); B. Identical.

- Maternal Height and Weight—Larger and taller women are more likely to have twins than are smaller women.
- Infertility Treatments—Women who have undergone infertility treatments, including assisted reproductive technology (ART) are more likely to have twins.

Multiple births other than twins can be of the identical type, the fraternal type, or combinations of the two. Triplets occur once in 7000 births and quadruplets once in 660,000 births. In recent years, the use of fertility drugs to induce ovulation as well as other fertility treatments has resulted in a greater frequency of quadruplets, quintuplets, sextuplets, and even octuplets. However, the number of these extreme multiple pregnancies has been decreasing in recent years due to new guidelines for Assisted Reproductive Technology advocated by the American Society for Reproductive Medicine (ASRM) in 2009. The placentas of multiple pregnancies have to compete for physical space and nutrients in the uterus, resulting in babies born at a lower birth weight than are singleton babies. There is also an increased risk of miscarriage and premature

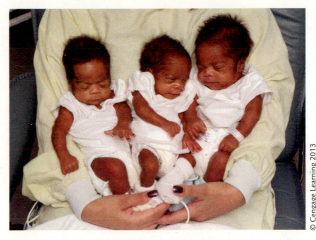

FIGURE 11-5: These male triplets were delivered before 37 weeks gestation; now, at 6 weeks of age, they are each showing different rates of growth and weight gain.

labor and delivery. In the United States, the average gestation period for twins is about 35 weeks, a full five weeks shorter than the normal gestation of 40 weeks. Triplets, on average are delivered after 33 weeks, (Figure 11-5) and quadruplets after only 29 weeks gestation. Babies are considered premature if they are delivered before 37 weeks gestation, thus the chance of being born premature is about 50 percent for twins, 90 percent for triplets, and virtually 100 percent for quadruplets and higher multiples. Premature infants face increased risks of death or serious complications as newborns that can lead to lifelong disabilities. These risks will be discussed in more detail in Chapter 12. Mothers also face additional risks when they are pregnant with multiples. They are more likely to develop serious conditions during their pregnancies such as gestational hypertension, preeclampsia, gestational diabetes, and excessive bleeding associated with delivery (ASRM, 2008). The risks, both to the mother and to the developing fetuses, increase with the number developing in the uterus at the same time. For example, twins are seven times more likely than singletons to die during their first month, while triplets are 20 times more likely to die during the same time period (ASRM, 2004).

MATERNAL CHANGES DURING PREGNANCY

In spite of how it is often portrayed by popular media, it is important to remember that pregnancy is a normal physiological condition and not an illness.

Many women experience relatively trouble free pregnancies and few discomforts. A woman's body will experience both physical and physiological changes during her pregnancy. Denying that pregnancy can be anything but a healthy, happy, productive, problem-free period is unrealistic, but so is the other extreme in which pregnancy is treated as a serious illness. Sometimes all the emphasis on the "naturalness" of pregnancy can produce unrealistic expectations about how a woman "should" feel and behave. How a woman experiences these changes has a lot to do with her personality, life situation, relationship with her partner and the rest of her family, and her feelings about having a baby.

It is also important to consider that no two pregnancies are identical, even for the same woman. Some pregnancies bring few difficulties. Others bring nausea, backaches, swelling, hemorrhoids, stretch marks, or varicose veins. The physical aspects of pregnancy are frequently unpredictable and sometimes uncomfortable, but an understanding of what is taking place and why, and an appreciation that other women have similar experiences, can provide a woman with the knowledge to work with her body and not against it.

Changes in the Reproductive System During Pregnancy

During pregnancy, all of the components of the reproductive system undergo dramatic changes. In response to hormonal secretion and the growth of the zygote to a full term fetus, organs both shift position and change shape.

Uterus

At full term, a pregnant uterus weighs around one kilogram and is about five to six times larger than a nonpregnant uterus. This enormous enlargement of the pregnant uterus is accomplished by the growth of the individual smooth muscle cells, which become wider and longer. Blood vessels elongate, dilate, and form new branches to support and nourish the growing muscle tissue, leading to a dramatic increase in uterine blood flow. The contractility of the smooth muscle that makes up the walls of the uterus is also enhanced. Spontaneous, irregular contractions, called Braxton Hicks contractions, begin in the first trimester. They continue throughout pregnancy, becoming especially noticeable during the last month

when they contribute to the thinning out or effacing of the cervix before delivery. If contractions that occur before 37 weeks gestation become more regular and occur less than 10 minutes apart, steps may need to be taken to prevent preterm delivery.

The entire uterus remains in the pelvic cavity for the first three months, after which the fundus portion of the uterus expands, pushing into the abdominal cavity. As the uterus grows, it presses on the urinary bladder and causes the increased frequency of urination noticed in early pregnancy. By about 20 weeks it is at the level of the mother's umbilicus. Thereafter, the growth of the fetus can be determined by measuring the distance from the pubic symphysis to the top of the uterine fundus. The expanding uterus usually becomes obvious around the fourth to fifth month, although the waistline tends to thicken earlier in each subsequent pregnancy. Figure 11-6 shows the change in abdominal shape during pregnancy.

Cervix

Softening of the cervix by the sixth week (Goodell's sign) has been mentioned earlier in the chapter as a sign of pregnancy. Along with the softening, which is the result of vasocongestion, the endocervical glands increase in size and number and produce more cervical mucus. Under the influence of progesterone, a thick mucus plug forms which blocks the cervical

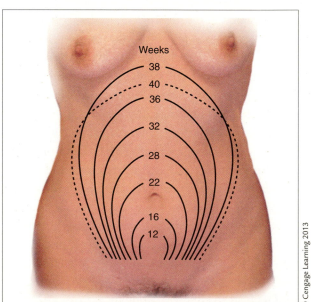

FIGURE 11-6: Approximate height of the fundus as the uterus enlarges.

© Cengage Learning 2013

os and reduces the risk of microbes from the vagina entering into the uterus. The increase in cervical secretions results in leukorrhea, or increased vaginal secretion. The secretion is markedly acidic, which also helps to prevent bacterial infection. Under a slow steady pull of the muscles of the uterus, the cervix stretches but has very little rebound and can, therefore, progressively dilate. This dilation of the cervix will eventually allow the baby to pass through during delivery.

Ovaries and Fallopian Tubes

The increased blood supply to the ovaries and fallopian tubes causes some enlargement during pregnancy. This is also responsible for the enlargement of the ovary containing the corpus luteum as it continues to secrete progesterone during the first trimester. After the placenta takes over the major production of progesterone, the corpus luteum of pregnancy regresses. The anterior pituitary gland is inhibited by the large amounts of circulating progesterone, which prevents additional follicles in the ovaries from maturing during pregnancy.

Vagina

Ordinarily a highly distensible organ, the vagina prepares for even greater distensibility during delivery by a thickening of the vaginal lining, a reduction in the density of the connective tissue in the walls of the vagina, and an increased growth of the muscle tissue. The increased blood supply results in the color change from pink to dusky blue, previously described as Chadwick's sign. After giving birth, folds in the walls of the vagina become smoothed out, and the firmness of the walls may diminish for women who have given birth to many children.

Breasts

Many women experience a tenderness and enlargement of the breasts during the progestational phase of each menstrual cycle. This sensitivity remains and intensifies in early pregnancy. Tingling and soreness are common in the first two months. Thereafter, the breasts become enlarged, more tender, and nodular. The primary areolae become wider and deepen in color, and Montgomery's glands are more prominent, as the nipples enlarge (Figure 11-7). Under the influence of hormones from the corpus luteum and the placenta, the ducts, lobules, and alveolae of the mammary glands multiply in preparation for lactation. By the 10th week of gestation, colostrum can be expressed from the nipples, but actual milk synthesis is inhibited by the high sex hormone levels circulating in the blood.

Changes to the Digestive System

A variety of changes take place in the digestive system during pregnancy. One symptom of early pregnancy, experienced by about 80 percent of pregnant women, is the nausea and vomiting familiarly known as "morning sickness." While it occurs most often in the morning, the nausea can be present any time of day, and some women have it all day. For most women, morning sickness subsides after week 16 of their pregnancy, although for about 20 percent, the condition can last throughout pregnancy (Gill & Einarson, 2007). About one percent experience an extreme and persistent form of morning sickness called hyperememsis gravidarum, which will be addressed in more detail in Chapter 12. Women who are pregnant for the first time or who are carrying multiples are more prone to morning sickness. There is some evidence that the chances of experiencing morning sickness increases with each successive pregnancy (Einarson et al., 2007).

The nausea that is experienced with morning sickness can be precipitated by odors from cooking, paint, cigarettes, or other strong odors. For each particular woman, a period of trial and error may be necessary to find something that alleviates her nausea. Avoiding an empty stomach can help to alleviate morning sickness. Some strategies might include having a small snack before sleeping, and eating something sweet immediately upon waking. Some women find that drinking a sweet beverage upon waking can prevent nausea and vomiting. Eating several small meals throughout the day rather than three large ones may also help prevent these symptoms. There is evidence that women in populations who eat a diet high in sugars, meat, or alcohol are more likely to experience morning sickness than do women in other populations. Avoiding these types of foods in the diet may help (Pepper & Roberts, 2006). There is also evidence that getting adequate vitamin B6, either through the diet or from supplements, can help prevent morning sickness. Several explanations for the physiological basis of morning

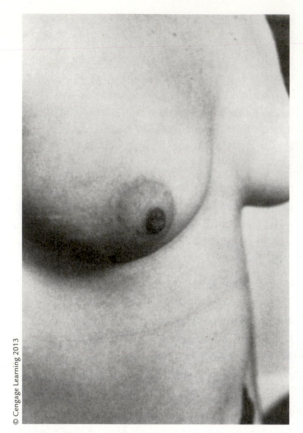 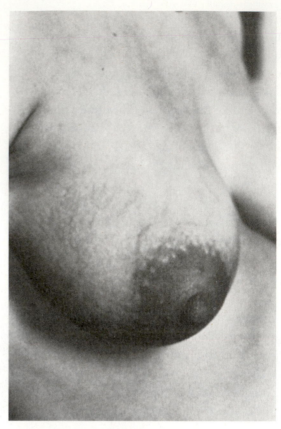

© Cengage Learning 2013

FIGURE 11-7: Comparison of the breasts of a nonpregnant woman (left) with the breast of a woman who is 7 months pregnant (right). Note the size, the deeply pigmented areola, signs of increased vascularity, and prominent Montgomery's gland elevations in the breast during pregnancy. The second areola, a further pigmented mottling effect surrounding the primary areola, is evident.

sickness have been proposed, and it is likely that multiple factors contribute to this condition. It has been proposed that high levels of human chorionic gonadotropin and high levels of circulating estrogens reduce stomach acidity, and lower the tone and motility of the digestive tract. The principal nutrient utilized by the fetus is glucose, and it derives its supply from the mother's blood. As a result of the placental transfer of glucose, the pregnant woman's fasting blood sugar level is about 10 percent lower than normal. This, and other changes in maternal carbohydrate metabolism, may play a role in morning sickness.

It is interesting to note that women who experience nausea and vomiting during their pregnancies are less likely to experience miscarriage (Weigel & Weigel, 1989). This observation has led to the proposal that the nausea and vomiting of morning sickness might be a protective mechanism that causes pregnant women to physically expel or avoid foods containing substances that could harm the developing embryo. The usual timing of morning sickness supports this proposal, since women normally experience nausea and vomiting during the first trimester, during which the embryo is forming its organ systems and is the most vulnerable to teratogens (Flaxman & Sherman, 2008). In an earlier study, Flaxman and Sherman (2000) also found that the incidence of morning sickness varies considerably between populations that consume different types of foods. Populations that consume more animal products, especially meats, poultry, and fish, are more likely to experience morning sickness. Before the advent of refrigeration, and throughout most of human evolution, these foods were more likely to carry parasites or pathogens than available plant-based foods.

Other digestive tract complaints may include excessive salivation, which occasionally occurs and then spontaneously disappears by the middle of the second trimester. Heartburn is often experienced, especially during the last three months of pregnancy.

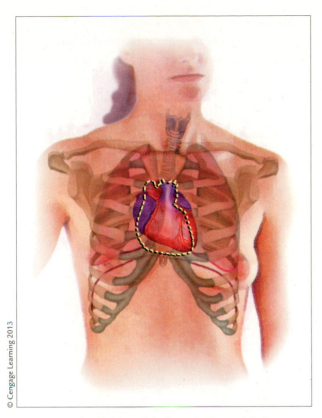

© Cengage Learning 2013

FIGURE 11-8: The position of the heart is changed during pregnancy. The dotted lines represent the nonpregnant position of the heart. The point of maximal impulse (PMI) is altered and heart sounds may be louder.

It is caused by regurgitation of the stomach contents into the upper esophagus and may be associated with the general relaxed muscle tone of the entire gastro-intestinal tract during pregnancy and the increased intra-abdominal pressure caused by the enlarging uterus. Sleeping on several pillows so that the head and the esophagus are elevated can help prevent heartburn at night. Decreased muscle tone in the large intestine results in decreased motility and increased water absorption leads to other common complaints: constipation and flatulence, or gas. Adequate fiber in the diet and exercise will usually minimize the problem.

The effect of hormones on the gums in the mouth may cause gingivitis, resulting in swollen, spongy gums that bleed easily. Improved diet may help, especially foods rich in vitamin C. There is no truth to the folk belief that pregnancy results in tooth decay because the fetus needs the calcium from its mother's teeth. Calcium in the teeth is fixed and is not withdrawn. Instead, tooth loss is associated with lower levels of vitamin C and a reduction in tooth

ligament repair. Dental work can be done at any stage, but because of exposure to the anesthetic, pregnancy is not the best time to have oral surgery.

Changes to the Cardiovascular System

Cardiovascular alterations occur early in pregnancy to meet the demands of the enlarging uterus and the placenta for more blood and more oxygen. The heart works harder and pumps more blood per minute (Figure 11-8). By the end of the first trimester, cardiac output has increased by 25–50 percent, and there is an accompanying increase in blood volume. By the end of the pregnancy, blood volume will increase 45–50 percent, depending on the size of the mother and the size of the fetus. The number of red blood cells also increases, but there is a greater rise in the plasma volume as a result of hormonal factors and sodium and water retention. Combined with added demand for red blood cells to carry oxygen to the placenta and fetus, it is no wonder that pregnant women are at an increased risk for anemia. As the hemoglobin concentration falls, the heart rate increases rising to a maximum of 15 beats above the nonpregnant state. Arterial blood pressure usually drops, and reaches its low point at about 22 weeks of gestation, and thereafter slowly rises to pre-pregnancy levels until delivery (Figure 11-9). The ability of the blood to clot also increases significantly.

With pregnancy, blood flow to the extremities is increased. Women who have always had cold hands

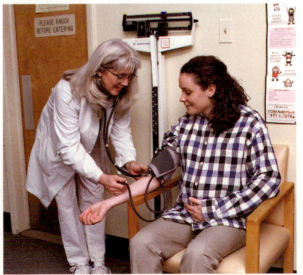

© Cengage Learning 2013

FIGURE 11-9: Blood pressure drops during pregnancy, reaches a low point at 22 weeks gestation, then slowly rises until delivery.

and feet will find them uncharacteristically warm and even clammy during pregnancy. This change is associated with changes in thyroid hormone levels that result from the secretion of the hormone chorionic thyrotropin from the placenta.

Varicose veins in the legs and the vulva are common during pregnancy. There may be a genetic predisposition to weakened venous walls and supporting tissues; women whose mothers or other family members have varicosities are more likely to have them. The developing uterus presses on the large veins that return blood from the legs to the heart and impedes the flow of venous blood (Figure 11-10). This slowing of circulation, coupled with the engorgement of the pelvic veins, causes the blood to back up in the veins of the legs and exert increasing pressure on their walls.

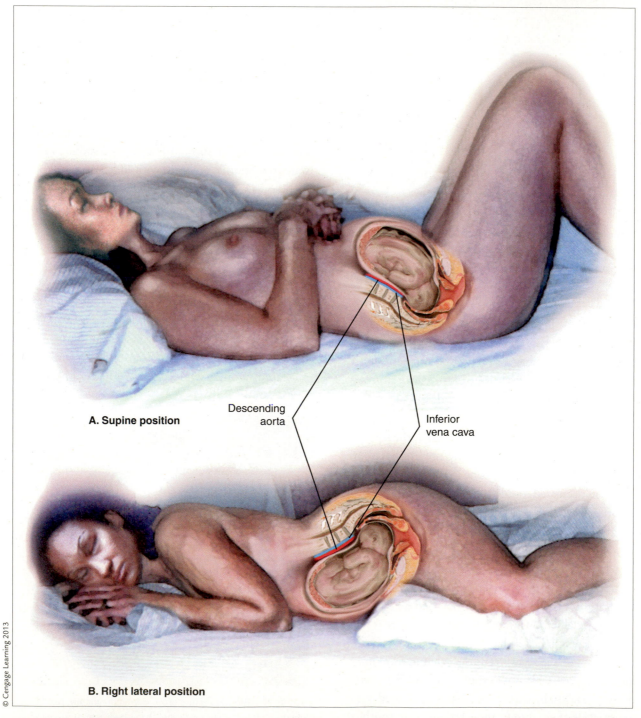

A. Supine position

Descending aorta

Inferior vena cava

B. Right lateral position

FIGURE 11-10: A. Lying on the back in a supine position can allow the weight of the uterus to press on the large blood vessels in the abdomen. B. Lying on the side relieves the pressure on the large blood vessels.

If the venous walls are not strong enough to withstand this increased pressure, they stretch and thin to become the large, tortuous varicose veins. They may not produce any symptoms, but some women experience varying amounts of discomfort ranging from mild burning and itching to aching pain. Relief can be obtained by avoiding standing for long periods, elevating the legs whenever possible, and wearing support hose. In addition, the elevated levels of progesterone during pregnancy may lead to increased flexibility of the connective tissue surrounding the vessels, allowing them to stretch farther than usual. Hemorrhoids are varicosities of the rectal veins and can be an annoying condition during pregnancy. Constipation aggravates hemorrhoids, and straining during defecation may cause bleeding when hemorrhoids are present. Eating a high fiber diet can help to relieve constipation. Finally, some women are more likely to experience mild nosebleeds during pregnancy. This may be related to increased blood volume and resultant capillary pressure. Nosebleeds can usually be controlled by remaining upright, bending the head forward, and pinching the bridge of the nose.

This increase in blood volume during pregnancy may lead to a generalized edema. Swollen ankles and fingers occur in many women (Figure 11-11). While some edema is normal, a rapid increase in weight of more than a kilogram (2.2 pounds) in a week, an increase in blood pressure, or protein appearing in the urine, may signal the beginnings of preeclampsia. There should be no attempts to reduce the edema with diuretics. In a large Danish study, researchers found that treatment with diuretics during the third trimester of pregnancy significantly increased the risk of the child developing schizophrenia later in life (Sorenson et al., 2003). A healthy diet, plenty of fluids, and moderate exercise will usually help with edema. Any changes in the circulatory system should be discussed with a woman's healthcare provider.

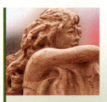

Economic Considerations

RACE AND INEQUALITY: THE CASE OF MATERNAL MORTALITY IN THE UNITED STATES

In a 2007 global survey of 171 countries sponsored by the World Health Organization, the United Nations Population Fund, the U.N. Children's Fund, the U.N. Population Division, and the World Bank, the United States ranked a dismal 41st in maternal mortality (Gosick, 2008). At that time, the United States was tied with the eastern European country of Belarus and just above Serbia and Montenegro, ranking far behind countries like Ireland, Italy, Greece, Austria, Germany, and Sweden.

As the United States Centers for Disease Control and Prevention has acknowledged, "It is a problem of racial disparity." In Chapter 2, the special risks that women of color encounter when it comes to heart disease, as well as the underlying triggers of obesity, hypertension, and diabetes were discussed. These underlying health conditions also make pregnancy less safe for women of color and make them more susceptible to complications. The Centers for Disease Control and Prevention have found that regardless of income, four times more black women die from pregnancy, deliver prematurely, or produce more low-weight babies than white women in the United States. Better access to family planning tools, reproductive health services, and good healthcare are the best ways to reduce maternal mortality in the United States.

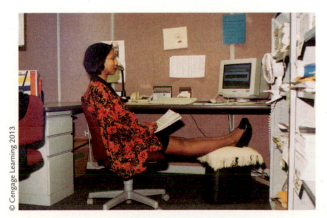

© Cengage Learning 2013

FIGURE 11-11: Elevating the feet while seated can help relieve edema of the ankles and feet.

Changes to the Respiratory System

Early in pregnancy, there is an increase in the minute respiratory volume—the total amount of air moved into and out of the lungs each minute. The number of breaths per minute does not increase, but the amount of air breathed in with each breath does. Later in gestation, there are anatomical changes that affect breathing as well. Even though the uterus in the abdominal cavity pushes up on the diaphragm and elevates it, the entire thoracic cavity compensates by an increase in its dimensions so that more air can be inspired. Shortness of breath, or dyspnea, develops in slightly more than half of women during the last month of pregnancy. Since breathing capacity is not limited, the mechanism for this is not understood and may be related to pressure on the diaphragm and lungs. Dyspnea usually subsides when the fetal head shifts into the true pelvis, a process called "lightening," when the uterus drops slightly, reducing the pressure on the diaphragm (Figure 11-12). Lightening is experienced several weeks before labor begins with a first baby, but usually takes place during labor in a woman who has already borne a child.

Changes to the Urinary System

Urinary frequency increases during pregnancy as a result of pressure from the enlarging uterus on the bladder and hormonal shifts (Figure 11-13). The hormone placental lactogen triggers an increase in the production of urine by the kidneys. Probably as a result of hormonal influences, the ureters leading from the kidneys to the bladder become dilated by the 10th week of pregnancy. The right side is generally more enlarged than the left side. This enlargement may predispose some women to kidney infections.

Musculoskeletal Changes During Pregnancy

By the 10th to 12th week of pregnancy, the hormones estrogen, progesterone, and relaxin cause the ligaments that hold the sacroiliac joints and the pubic symphysis in place to begin to soften and stretch, in preparation to make delivery easier. The relaxation of the joints is progressive and becomes maximal by the beginning of the third trimester. The shifting of the joints accompanied by the shift in a woman's center

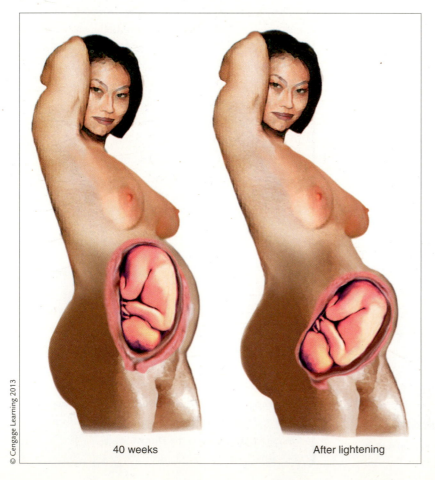

40 weeks   After lightening

© Cengage Learning 2013

FIGURE 11-12: The shift in the fetus's position after lightening relieves pressure on the diaphragm.

Many women experience leg cramps during the last few months of pregnancy. A painful spasm of the calf muscles is most likely to occur when lying down. Immediate relief of the cramp can be obtained by flexing the foot upward so that the toes point toward the face while simultaneously pushing down on the knee to straighten the leg. It is thought that high dietary phosphorus or insufficient calcium provokes leg cramps, but attempts to prevent them by adding calcium or restricting dietary phosphorus are not always successful. Some women notice occasional sensations in their hands, ranging from tingling to actual pain. The symptoms are similar to those in carpal tunnel syndrome and result from compression of the hand's median nerve. Incidence of carpal tunnel-like symptoms in pregnancy has been reported in up to 50 percent of women. Although some have related the condition to the hormone relaxin, fluid retention in pregnant women is more likely responsible for the symptoms.

Changes to the Integumentary System

Many pregnant women are concerned about the development of stretch marks, skin problems, and changes to the hair. Unfortunately, little is known about how to avoid them. Striae gravidarum, or stretch marks, are irregular reddish streaks that appear on the abdomen, breasts and buttocks in about half of pregnant women after the fifth month. After delivery, the red discoloration disappears but the striae persist indefinitely as whitish lines (Figure 11-14). The striae are the result of changes in the collagen and elastic fibers in the dermis of the skin and result from the relatively rapid weight gain of pregnancy.

Complexion changes during pregnancy are not unusual. Some women develop irregular patches of freckles on the forehead and cheeks that form the mask of pregnancy, or chloasma. Chloasma gradually disappears after delivery of the baby. The increased pigmentation that occurs on the breasts and genitals may develop in other areas as well. Dark haired women may notice a brownish-black line (linea nigra) appearing down the middle of the abdomen (Figure 11-15). Another skin manifestation believed to be secondary to the high estrogen concentrations, is the appearance of vascular "spider veins" or bright red

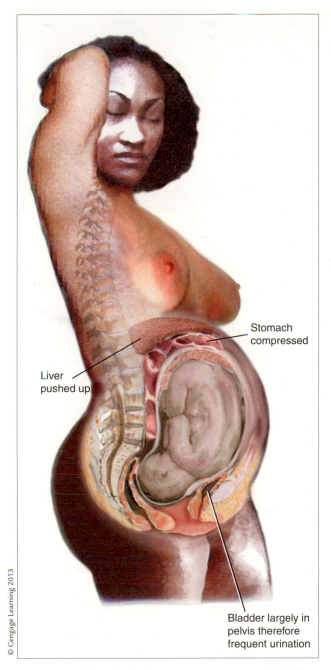

Liver pushed up

Stomach compressed

Bladder largely in pelvis therefore frequent urination

© Cengage Learning 2013

FIGURE 11-13: The enlarging uterus puts pressure on the bladder leading to frequent urination.

of gravity caused by the growing fetus may alter balance and affect a women's walk, producing the classic waddle so frequent in late pregnancy. The postural changes of pregnancy, which include an increased swayback and an upper spine extension to compensate for the enlarging abdomen, coupled with the loosening of the sacroiliac joints may also result in lower back pain. Backaches can be relieved by heat, rest, sleeping on a firmer mattress, and by exercises that strengthen abdominal and back muscles.

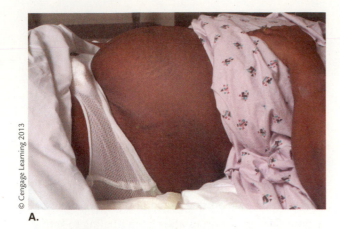

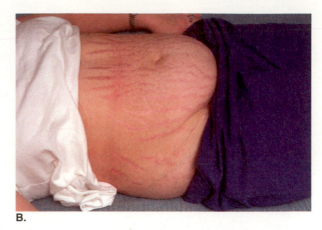

A.

B.

FIGURE 11-14: A. Postpartum striae, or stretch marks of a dark-skinned woman. B. Stretch marks of a light-skinned woman.

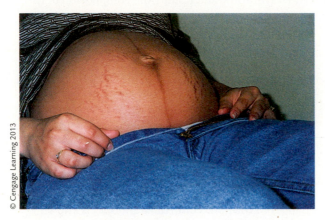

FIGURE 11-15: Dark line of pigmentation, called linea nigra, may appear in the midline of the abdomen.

circular areas of branching and dilated capillaries. These occur on the face, neck, thorax, and arms and are especially obvious in women with pale complexions, but disappear after childbirth.

Some women notice acceleration in fingernail and hair growth during pregnancy as a result of increased metabolism due to the hormone thyrotropin. The hair follicles on the scalp and on the rest of the body normally undergo a growing and a resting phase. The resting phase is followed by a loss of hairs, which are then replaced by new ones. During pregnancy, fewer hair follicles go into the resting phase, and after delivery, there is a catching-up period of greater hair loss until the follicles return to their normal cycle.

WEIGHT GAIN DURING PREGNANCY

There is no one-size-fits-all rule about how much weight should be gained during pregnancy. Several recent studies have demonstrated that overweight

and obese women experience more potentially serious complications such as miscarriage, gestational hypertension, preeclampsia, and gestational diabetes during pregnancy (Hincz et al., 2009; Eerdekens et al., 2009; Satpathy et al., 2008; ACOG, 2005). However, it is not a good idea to try to lose weight during pregnancy, as this can deprive the fetus of the nutrients that it needs to develop fully. Dieting that results in a metabolic condition called ketosis can release potentially harmful levels of ketones into the bloodstream, and these can cross the placenta to damage the fetus. While dieting without supervision by a healthcare professional is not advisable, there is evidence that moderate exercise during pregnancy is beneficial to both the mother and the developing fetus.

Some women undergo bariatric surgery to reduce their weight prior to becoming pregnant. Pregnancies following bariatric surgery are considered high risk and can result in a variety of serious complications for both the mother and the infant, many of them related to deficiencies of vitamin K, which plays an important role in blood clotting (Guelinckx et al., 2009; Eerdenkens et al., 2009). These pregnancies require close supervision by a doctor before, during, and after delivery.

In general, the amount of weight that a woman should gain depends on her weight and body size before pregnancy, and on the number of fetuses that she is carrying. This added weight is important to supporting the growth and health of the baby and contributes to its birth weight (Dietz et al., 2009; Jaruratanasirikul et al., 2009). Low birth weight babies, who are born at term weighing 2,500 g (5.5 lb) or less, have an increased susceptibility to illness and an increased rate of mortality compared with normal weight babies. A woman who has limited or inadequate weight gain during pregnancy has a substantially increased risk of delivering a baby of low birth weight. Animal studies have shown that maternal malnutrition decreases the ability of the placenta to transfer nutrients from the blood of the mother to the blood of the fetus. Prenatal malnutrition has also been shown to cause a reduction in the cell size and number in fetal tissues, with disproportionate effects occurring in the brain (Schieve, Cogswell, & Scanlon, 1998; Grantham, McGregor, & Fernald, 1997). Gaining too much weight during pregnancy, on the other hand, can also lead to problems including macrosomia (Viswanayhan et al., 2008), which is babies weighing 4,000 g (8.8 lbs) or more, and is linked to an increased need for a cesarean section (Vetr, 2005) as well as other complications.

If the total weight gained has not exceeded 11–14 Kg (24–30 lb), a woman can expect to lose 8–9 Kg (18–20 lb) within a week after delivery. The rest of the weight will likely be gone by three months after delivery, especially if a woman is breast-feeding, which increases calorie demands by the body. If she

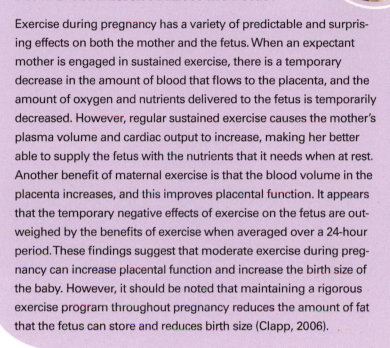

focus on
EXERCISE
How Does Exercise Affect the Fetus?

Exercise during pregnancy has a variety of predictable and surprising effects on both the mother and the fetus. When an expectant mother is engaged in sustained exercise, there is a temporary decrease in the amount of blood that flows to the placenta, and the amount of oxygen and nutrients delivered to the fetus is temporarily decreased. However, regular sustained exercise causes the mother's plasma volume and cardiac output to increase, making her better able to supply the fetus with the nutrients that it needs when at rest. Another benefit of maternal exercise is that the blood volume in the placenta increases, and this improves placental function. It appears that the temporary negative effects of exercise on the fetus are outweighed by the benefits of exercise when averaged over a 24-hour period. These findings suggest that moderate exercise during pregnancy can increase placental function and increase the birth size of the baby. However, it should be noted that maintaining a rigorous exercise program throughout pregnancy reduces the amount of fat that the fetus can store and reduces birth size (Clapp, 2006).

is not lactating, she can increase her activity level to speed up the weight loss.

Nutrition During Pregnancy

A woman's daily requirement for certain nutrients does increase during pregnancy. Table 11-1 outlines the nutrients that are especially important to

Table 11-1 Daily Guide to Essential Foods.		
	Servings Each Day	
To Be Consumed	Pregnant	Breast-feeding
Milk and milk products	4	4–5
Protein source (meat, fish, poultry, eggs, cheese, and at least one vegetable protein)	4	4–5
Leafy green vegetables	1–2	1–2
Source of vitamin C	1	1
Other fruits and vegetables	1	1
Whole grain breads and cereals	3	3–4
Water and other liquids (milk may be included in total)	6	6

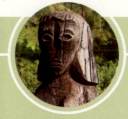

focus on

NUTRITION

Effect of Diet on Maternal and Fetal Weight Gain

What a woman eats while she is pregnant can influence her chances of developing insulin resistance and gestational diabetes and also can influence the future health of her infant. Recent studies have shown that women who eat primarily low glycemic index carbohydrates, also known as complex carbohydrates, are less likely to develop insulin resistance and gestational diabetes during the last trimester of pregnancy (Monroy et al., 2008).

When carbohydrates are consumed, the pancreas releases insulin to signal the cells of the body to absorb the glucose out of the bloodstream. When the body is exposed to too much high glycemic index carbohydrates, also known as simple sugars, the receptors for insulin stop working as efficiently and consequently, the cells stop absorbing the excess glucose. This results in elevated blood glucose and can develop into gestational diabetes, if it becomes chronic. The elevated blood sugar of gestational diabetes can lead to severe complications, and in some cases, miscarriage or stillbirth of the fetus.

High glucose levels in the mother's blood also cross the placenta to the fetus and can cause the fetus to grow larger than normal, leading to complications during delivery. There is increasing evidence that excessively high birth weights can lead to the development of diabetes and weight problems in children. On the other hand, too low a birth weight has been associated with reduced IQ, so when it comes to fetal birth weight it seems prudent to aim for the middle percentile. Eating primarily low glycemic index carbohydrates, combined with moderate exercise, results in healthy mothers and infants within the normal birth weight range (Allen et al., 2007).

nant, get sufficient folic acid in their diet to prevent these birth defects (Wilson et al., 2007).

Vitamin B12 and iron demand increases during pregnancy to meet the demands of manufacturing new red blood cells. Women who are prone to anemia or who eat a low iron diet, may become anemic during pregnancy. Iron rich foods or prenatal supplements can help prevent anemia.

Preventing Birth Defects

Birth defects can be caused by genetic abnormalities, by the absence of essential nutrients during development, or by exposure to harmful agents during gestation (Figure 11-16). Birth defects are discussed in Chapter 10. While birth defects cannot always be prevented, pregnant women can exercise common sense to minimize the risk. Some simple guidelines follow:

- Be sure to get adequate levels of nutrients, especially folic acid and B vitamins.
- Avoid alcohol and drugs that are not prescribed by a medical professional.
- Avoid smoking and exposure to secondhand smoke.
- Avoid excessive caffeine consumption.
- Obtain genetic counseling and birth defect screening.

maintaining a healthy pregnancy. One nutrient of particular interest is folic acid. The vitamin folic acid has been shown to play an important role in preventing a class of birth defects called neural tube disorders, in which the brain and spinal cord of the developing embryo do not form properly. Formation of these structures occurs very early in development, usually before a woman is even aware that she might be pregnant. For this reason, it is important that women who are pregnant, or who may become preg-

THE PHYSIOLOGY OF LABOR AND DELIVERY

Pregnancy culminates in childbirth, or **parturition**. Exactly what happens during labor is well known; what triggers it to begin is still somewhat of a mystery. Proposed theories to explain the onset of labor range from the rather unscientific—"the baby outgrows the uterus," to a group of theories that explain

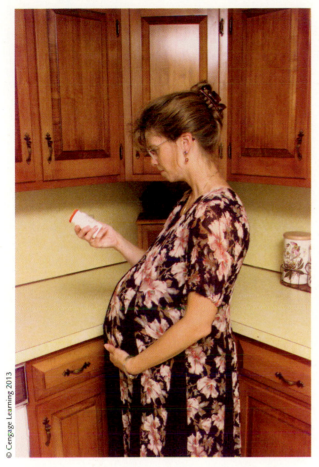

FIGURE 11-16: Avoiding exposure to harmful agents such as unnecessary and unprescribed drugs, including over-the-counter medications, can help prevent birth defects.

the chemical control of parturition including the withdrawal of systemic progesterone, the oxytocin effect, changes in the progesterone/estrogen ratio, the secretion of the fetal hormones, and the role of prostaglandins. Current theories assume that many, perhaps all, of these factors are implicated in causing labor, and that labor is initiated by a sequence of interacting endocrine events involving chemical and physical signals from both the fetus and the mother's body.

Pre-Labor Events

In the days or weeks before parturition, important changes take place in both the expectant mother and in the fetus. These changes, which include shifts in the baby's position in the uterus, are in preparation for labor and delivery of the baby. The timing of these changes is variable between pregnancies, but they do follow a fairly predictable pattern.

Fetal Positions

As the end of gestation approaches, the fetus will usually shift its position within the uterus in preparation for its decent through the birth canal. This shifting of position is called lightening. Figure 11-17 shows a fetus in the occipital anterior position, which is the most common position for the fetus to begin the birth process. This position is also the most favorable for labor and delivery because the smallest part of the baby's head will lead the way through the birth canal. In this position, the posterior portion of the baby's head can exert pressure on the cervix. This pressure helps to dilate the cervix and helps to shorten the time that the mother will be in labor to deliver the baby. In the occipital posterior position, the baby is presenting head first, but the occiput, or the back of the baby's head, is facing the mother's spine. This position does not allow close contact between the baby's head and the cervix and can lead to prolonged labor. A breech presentation means that the buttocks or feet of the baby present first, and this occurs about once in every 40 deliveries. Occasionally, the baby will lie in a transverse position, and the shoulder presents first, although this position is rare. The breech and transverse positions during labor are more likely to lead to delivery by Cesarean section, unless the baby can be repositioned into a more favorable position.

Changes in the Uterus Prior to Parturition

Several changes take place in the uterus before the start of true labor. In most women who are having their first baby, lightening usually occurs a few weeks before delivery. Sometimes a first baby does not drop until labor begins, which is the usual situation in

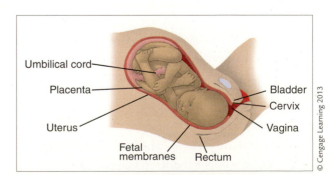

FIGURE 11-17: The most common position for the fetus to take to begin the birth process referred to as cephalic presentation.

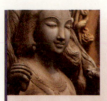

Social Considerations
MOSQUITO NETS TO PREVENT MALARIA IN PREGNANT WOMEN

April 25th is World Malaria Day. **Malaria** is a disease caused by a parasite carried by certain mosquitos. People with malaria often experience fever, chills, and flu-like symptoms, which can last for several days. Left untreated, they may develop severe complications and many die needlessly, particularly within the developing world. Each year, some 350–500 million people are infected with malaria, and over one million people die because of the disease, most of them young children in sub-Saharan Africa, the region of the world hardest hit by malaria (CDC, 2007).

Pregnant women also suffer unique problems because of malarial disease. Malaria during pregnancy can have adverse effects on both the mother and the fetus, including fetal loss (stillbirth), maternal anemia, premature delivery, and delivery of low birth weight babies. Low weight at birth is a major contributor to infant mortality. According to the Centers for Disease Control and Prevention, malaria infection is estimated to cause 400,000 cases of severe maternal anemia and from 75,000-200,000 infant deaths annually (CDC, 2004). In addition, maternal anemia contributes significantly to maternal mortality and causes an estimated 10,000 deaths per year. There is also increasing evidence that where they occur together, malaria and HIV infections interact. The World Health Organization notes that malaria worsens HIV by increasing viral load in adults and pregnant women. This means that malaria could accelerate the progression of AIDS. In addition, malaria infection appears to contribute to increasing the risk of HIV transmission between adults, as well as between a mother and her child.

In places where malaria is common, such as sub-Saharan Africa, insecticide-treated mosquito nets are used to prevent the transmission of the disease. Such prevention strategies are particularly important for pregnant women, so that they can ensure a healthy pregnancy. Insecticide-treated nets have consistently been shown to decrease both the number of malaria cases and malaria death rates in pregnant women and their children. An insecticide-treated net is a regular mosquito net that deters, immobilizes, or kills mosquitoes on contact through the use of an insecticide. Insecticide-treated nets have been proven to reduce disease and deaths due to malaria in regions which are particularly plagued by the disease. Untreated mosquito nets do form a protective barrier around persons using them. While they are better than no protection at all, mosquitoes are stubborn and persistent creatures. They can feed on people through the nets, and nets with even a few small holes provide little, if any, protection from the incessant, hungry mosquito.

In community trials across Africa, insecticide-treated mosquito nets have been shown to reduce mortality rates by about 20 percent (Hoebil, 2006). Where most community members have access to insecticide-treated mosquito nets, both the numbers and the longevity of mosquitoes are lessened, which adds another layer of protection for the community at large. One study in an area of high malaria transmission in Kenya showed that women protected by insecticide-treated mosquito nets every night during their first four months of pregnancy have 25 percent fewer underweight or premature babies (WHO, 2009). Insecticide-treated mosquito nets should be provided to pregnant women as early in their pregnancy as possible, and their use should be encouraged for women throughout their pregnancy and during the immediate postpartum period.

women who have previously borne children. After lightening, the upper abdomen becomes flatter and the lower abdomen becomes more prominent. Women notice they are able to breathe more easily

again, but the urge to urinate frequently returns because of the increased pressure on the bladder. Pressure on the rectum and sacrum may also result in diarrhea and backache.

Changes to the Cervix prior to Parturition

During the last few weeks of pregnancy, Braxton-Hicks contractions become more frequent. Each contraction shortens the muscle fibers in the cervix, thinning the cervix in a process called effacement. Further contractions of the uterus will bring about progressive cervical dilation, or enlargement, of the external os. With a first baby, complete cervical effacement usually occurs before there is any cervical dilatation. In women who have previously delivered a baby, dilation usually takes place when effacement is still incomplete, or concurrently with effacement (Figure 11-18). Cervical effacement is measured by percentage. A cervix one-half of its normal length is 50 percent effaced.

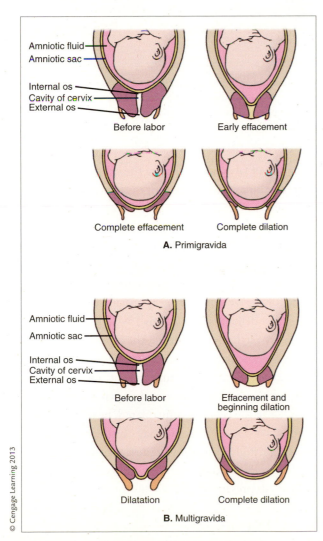

© Cengage Learning 2013

Amniotic fluid
Amniotic sac

Internal os
Cavity of cervix
External os

Before labor   Early effacement

Complete effacement   Complete dilation

A. Primigravida

Amniotic fluid
Amniotic sac

Internal os
Cavity of cervix
External os

Before labor   Effacement and beginning dilation

Dilatation   Complete dilation

B. Multigravida

FIGURE 11-18: A. Effacement and dilation in first delivery (primigravida); B. Previous deliveries (multigravida).

Loss of the Mucous Plug

The effacement and dilation of the cervix cause the fetal membranes that are attached to the uterine wall at the region of the internal os to become loosened. As they pull away from the uterine wall, the mucous plug is released (Figure 11-19). Loss of the plug is painless, but some blood often escapes with it, producing what is termed a "bloody show." Increased vaginal discharge during the period of cervical effacement is not unusual, but when pink-tinged or blood-streaked mucus is expelled from the vagina, it is a sign that active labor has started or is imminent.

The Three Stages of True Labor

Labor takes place in three stages, and each stage can last a variable amount of time. The labor process is a series of rhythmic and involuntary uterine muscle contractions that continues the effacement and dilatation of the cervix, and brings about a bursting of the fetal membranes. Then, accompanied by contractions of the abdominal muscles, the uterine contractions result in the expulsion of the baby through the birth canal. Labor depends on a positive feedback mechanism. Oxytocin, secreted from both the mother's pituitary gland and the fetus, triggers uterine contractions. These contractions cause the uterus to release prostaglandins, which help to trigger an increase in oxytocin secretion. Contractions build until the baby is delivered and the positive feedback cycle is broken.

The first stage of labor begins with the first true labor contractions and ends with the complete dilatation of the cervix, large enough to permit the passage of the infant. The second stage of labor ends with the delivery of the baby. The third stage is the period from the birth of the baby through delivery of the placenta. The timeline of labor and delivery varies dramatically and can range from an hour of active labor to a few days.

First Stage of Labor

The criteria used to differentiate true labor contractions from the Braxton Hicks prelabor contractions are regularity and discomfort. When the contractions become painful, less than 10 minutes apart, last 30–90 seconds, and are regular in frequency, labor has begun. For a woman having her first baby, the average duration of the first stage of labor is about

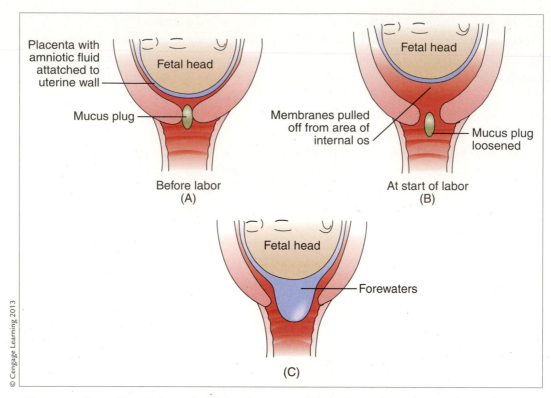

© Cengage Learning 2013

FIGURE 11-19: Illustration of "bloody show". *A.* Before onset of labor, the membranes are attached to the uterine wall. A mucous plug blocks the endocervical canal. B. With effacement and dilation of the cervix, the fetal membranes are pulled away from the internal os, and the mucous plug is set free along with a little bleeding. C. After the plug is lost, the forewaters bulge in front of the fetal head.

12 hours, but there are wide variations. The length may be as short as one hour if contractions are strong and frequent.

The fetal membranes, or amniotic sac, usually ruptures during the first stage of labor. However, they may burst earlier if the baby's head engages early with the cervix, or may even remain intact until delivery. The part of the membrane that ruptures is only a portion of the amniotic and chorionic sac, a little pocket of fluid called the forewaters that lies in front of the fetal head. The successive uterine contractions keep compressing the forewaters and eventually it breaks, permitting a little gush of amniotic fluid to exit. The rest of the fluid remains behind the baby's head as the hindwaters.

When the cervix is dilated to 10 cm in diameter, it is large enough to permit the passage of the fetal head, and the first stage of labor is over. Cervical dilatation is gauged subjectively by vaginal examination and is expressed in centimeters or finger widths. Depending on the birthing practices employed, there may be regular vaginal examinations throughout the first stage of labor to determine the degree of dilatation. The index and second finger are inserted into the vagina to feel the extent of the cervical rim that remains.

The end of the first stage of labor, when the cervix is open to complete dilation, is called transition. It is the most difficult and, fortunately, the shortest phase for the woman, lasting approximately one hour in the first delivery and perhaps 15–30 minutes in successive births. At transition, the contractions are stronger, more painful, somewhat erratic, and last longer. Pressure on the rectum is great, and there is a strong desire to contract the abdominal muscles and push. Until the cervix is fully dilated, however, bearing down is not helpful, and may cause cervical lacerations. Controlled breathing and relaxation techniques can help with the transition period as can supportive individuals present to help the mother through labor.

Second Stage of Labor

With each succeeding uterine contraction, the infant is pushed lower through the birth canal, and

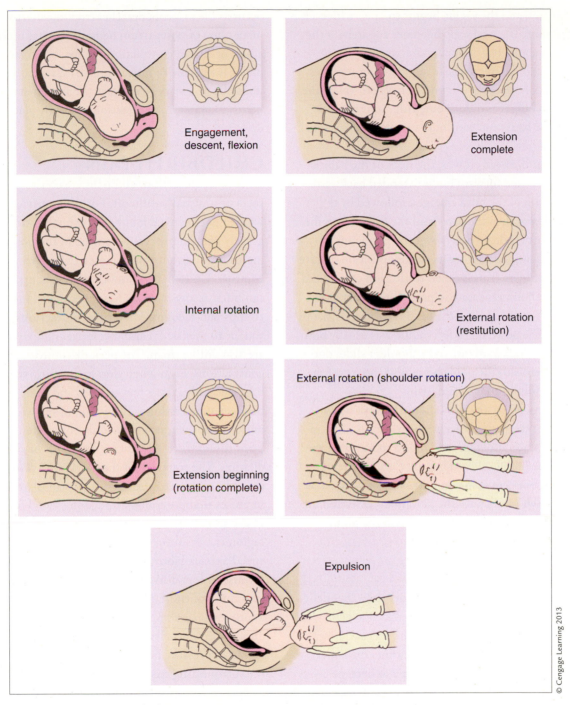

Engagement, descent, flexion

Extension complete

Internal rotation

External rotation (restitution)

Extension beginning (rotation complete)

External rotation (shoulder rotation)

Expulsion

© Cengage Learning 2013

FIGURE 11-20: Mechanisms of Labor.

its position alters as it accommodates itself to passage through the pelvis (Figure 11-20). At this stage of labor, the mother will experience a strong desire to contract her abdominal muscles and push. This pushing reflex is called the Ferguson Reflex, and it helps to propel the infant through the birth canal. At the beginning of the second stage of labor, the birth canal through which the baby descends is formed by the completely dilated cervix, the distended vagina, and the stretched and distended muscles of the pelvic floor. When the fetal head meets the resistance of the pelvic floor, it rotates 45° from its former position. The face is now directed posteriorly, facing the mother's sacrum. As further descent continues, the anus dilates, and the vagina begins to open with each contraction. The fetal scalp becomes apparent at the vaginal opening but disappears between contractions. When the top of the head no longer regresses between contractions, it is said to have crowned. The perineum bulges and thins out with each contraction as the fetal head continues to enlarge the vaginal opening.

When the head crowns, the neck of the baby is no longer flexed forward but is extended backward. First the top of the head emerges, followed by the forehead, and then the brow and the face. When the head is born, it drops down over the perineum and rotates sideways to restore its natural position relative to the shoulders. This is called restitution of the head. Then the shoulders rotate to present their narrowest diameter for passage and the head is turned farther to the side. The posterior or left shoulder is usually born first. It falls backward, the right shoulder slides out from underneath the pubic bone, and the rest of the body can follow quickly and easily.

After delivery, the baby should be kept below the level of the uterus for a minute or so to allow an adequate amount of placental blood to transfuse the infant. The umbilical cord may be clamped and then cut about one-half inch from the baby's abdomen or it may be left intact until the placenta is delivered. At this stage, the baby can be placed with the mother and may even begin to suckle.

Third Stage of Labor

Uterine contractions slow for a short time after delivery, but begin again to deliver the placenta, which has become partially separated from the uterus during expulsion of the baby. At the same time, the upper segment of the uterus changes shape to become smaller, firmer, and rounder. There is a small gush of blood from the vagina, and the umbilical cord appears to lengthen as the placenta is forced downward. Continued uterine contractions usually cause the placenta to be expelled within 5–30 minutes. Nursing the baby immediately after delivery will trigger the release of the hormone oxytocin from the brain, which will promote the continuation of uterine contractions to expel the placenta. These contractions also promote the constriction of the uterine blood vessels and diminish any bleeding that may occur as the placenta detaches from the uterus. The main cause of postpartum hemorrhaging is uterine atony, or lack of contractions. If, for some reason, the infant is not able to nurse immediately after delivery, it may be necessary to massage the abdomen and the uterus to maintain contractions until the placenta is delivered.

CHILDBIRTH PAIN

Only 8–10 percent of all births are considered dystocia or unusually difficult. For the vast majority of women with typical labor, giving birth is not the acutely painful process portrayed in the popular media, but neither is it completely free from discomfort. Undeniably, smooth muscle contractions can hurt, as anyone who has experienced menstrual cramps will recognize. Uterine contractions are similar to menstrual and intestinal cramps, but they are also unlike them. The peak discomfort of labor contractions, even when they are coming very close together, only lasts a few seconds and disappears between contractions. The action of the uterine muscle, however, is not the only component of labor discomfort. Another is the result of cervical dilation. The traction on the cervix that results in the enlargement of the cervical os stimulates nerve impulses that are transmitted along sacral nerves to the spinal cord. Those sensations in the sacral region can result in the intense backache experienced as back labor by some women. A third reason for discomfort during labor and delivery is the stretching of the vagina and the perineum. When a full-term baby's head, usually 10 cm at its widest dimension, starts its descent into the birth canal, it creates pressure on the bladder, rectum, and all the surrounding tissues. This pressure may be interpreted as pain. A wide variety of techniques can be used to modify or alleviate the pain associated with labor and delivery. These interventions will be addressed in Chapter 12.

Apgar Score

In 1960, American anesthesiologist Virginia Apgar introduced a method of assessing the well-being of newborns at one minute and five minutes after delivery. This rating system is called the **Apgar score** and is used to evaluate the central nervous system. The baby is scored at zero, one, or two in each of five categories: heart rate (absent, slow, or fast); respiratory effort (absent, weak cry, or good strong yell); muscle tone (limp, lively or active); response to irritating stimulus; and skin color. A score of 7–10 means the baby is in the best possible condition, while three–six means moderately depressed; a score below two indicates problems. Babies born to mothers who have been heavily drugged for pain relief, generally score around five or six.

The ability to predict developmental outcome and infant mortality on a long-term basis by use of the Apgar method is limited. Even very low scores at one and five minutes do not necessarily mean subsequent neurological dysfunction, illness, or mortality, particularly in low birth weight or premature infants. Similarly, high scores cannot guarantee that neurological development will be normal. Another problem with the Apgar system is its lack of objectivity. Assessment of the score is necessarily subjective, and Apgar believed that the emotional involvement of the delivery personnel could affect it. The general consensus is that the method can be used effectively if the limitations are understood and if an independent observer, and not the obstetrician or midwife, does the scoring.

After Care for Mother and Baby

Birth settings vary tremendously in terms of the routines or procedures that are likely to take place following the birth of a baby. In a home setting and in some hospitals and birthing centers, it is likely that there will be close contact between the mother and infant, as well as other family members in the moments immediately following the infant's birth. Breast-feeding may be initiated soon after birth.

In some hospital settings, post delivery procedures may keep the mother and baby separated for significant periods of time. Recovery on the part of the mother or the baby from the effects of pain medications or emergency procedures can also delay contact and the opportunity to initiate breast-feeding. The importance of the immediate period after birth for cementing the relationship between parent and child has been recognized (Figure 11-21). In a number of studies, Marshall Klaus (1972, 1976) and his colleagues emphasized the importance of contact,

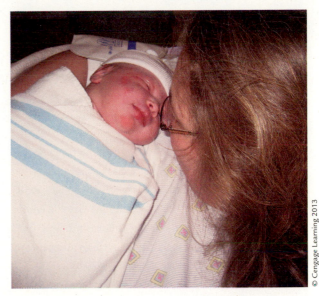

© Cengage Learning 2013

FIGURE 11-21: Bonding between mother and infant in the time immediately following delivery has been shown to be important for both the mother and baby.

both visual and tactile, between mother and baby in the first minutes, hours, and days after birth. Bonds of affection can be particularly strengthened if eye-to-eye and skin-to-skin contact take place. Klaus and Kennell (1986) advocate the value of mother, father, and infant togetherness for the first hour after birth in the delivery or recovery room. De Chateau (1980) reported that when mothers were given their naked babies for one hour within the first three hours after birth, such extra contact resulted in differences in maternal attachment behavior—smelling, kissing, close body contact—one month, one year, and even two years after delivery.

Hospital Stays After Delivery

Postpartum hospital stays lasting a week or 10 days were not uncommon during the 1950s and 1960s in the United States. But with an increased sensitivity toward what women wanted—less medicalized birth and more natural childbirth—the American College of Obstetricians and Gynecologists recommended shorter postpartum hospitalization with the intent of providing "a more family-centered birth experience." By 1970, four days in the hospital after delivery was average; by 1980, the average stay was 3.2 days.

As health insurance companies and managed care providers became more concerned about

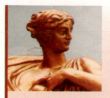

Cultural Considerations

SIMPLE WAYS TO MAKE PREGNANCY SAFER FOR WOMEN WORLDWIDE

Each year, around 210 million women become pregnant around the world. Yet every day, 1,500 women die due to complications during pregnancy or childbirth (WHO, 2009). That represents two women, every single minute of every single day. Add to this the fact that 10,000 babies per day die within the first month of life, with an equal number of stillbirths per day. Much can be done to avert these tragedies, and to ensure that almost every mother has a healthy pregnancy, and is able to deliver a healthy child into the world.

One of the most important things that can be done is to improve the quality of care available to women during their pregnancies. Skilled care, particularly around the time of birth, would greatly reduce the number of these needless deaths. Furthermore, gender equality and women's empowerment serve to enhance women's access to and control over resources, which are themselves linked to better health outcomes for women, including improving maternal and newborn health.

According to the World Health Organization, a majority of maternal and newborn deaths and illnesses can be prevented by access to quality skilled care during pregnancy, childbirth and in the postpartum period; timely access to emergency obstetric and newborn care; and access to family planning services to prevent unwanted pregnancy. On the first point, having a skilled birth attendant is crucial to reducing maternal mortality rates worldwide. The World Health Organization has defined a skilled attendant as a person with midwifery skills who:

- is able to give the necessary supervision, care, and advice to women during pregnancy, labor, and the postpartum period;
- is able to conduct deliveries on her/his own responsibility and to care for the mother and newborn; this care includes preventive measures and the detection and appropriate referral of abnormal conditions in the mother and newborn;
- is able to provide emergency measures as needed, for instance post-abortion care;
- is able to provide health counseling and education for the woman, her family, and community;
- may practice in hospitals, clinics, health units, domiciliary conditions or in any other service setting; has acquired the requisite qualifications to be registered and/or legally licensed to practice. (WHO, Regional Office for South-East Asia, 2004)

Ways to save the lives of mothers and of newborns are known, but the challenge remains to deliver these services and increase rates of access, particularly for the poorest, most marginalized, and often most difficult to reach women.

costs, the length of hospital stays for new mothers was shortened further. By the mid-1990s, many insurance companies would pay for only 24-hour hospital stays, and there was a public outcry over "drive-by deliveries." A number of states passed legislation mandating insurance coverage for a minimum stay, and in 1996, federal legislation, the Newborns and Mothers Health Protection Act, was passed and took effect in 1998. The law prohibits insurance companies from restricting post delivery hospital stays after a vaginal birth to fewer than 48 hours. According to a study released by the Centers for Disease Control and Prevention, 2.1 days was the average hospital stay by 1997 even before the federal law went into effect. For healthy women with uncomplicated deliveries having their second or third baby, even 24-hour stays may be all they need or want. First-time mothers, however, with a longer labor and more questions concerning baby care and breast-feeding, may want or need more care.

CONCLUSION

Pregnancy, labor, and delivery are normal physiological processes that more often than not take place without complications, or the need for medical interventions. Women have been giving birth for millennia under a wide variety of circumstances. Problems can develop however, and have been a cause of mortality for both women and their infants. Complications and the medical interventions that are sometimes used to treat or prevent them will be addressed in Chapter 12.

REVIEW QUESTIONS

1. What are the signs and physiological changes that are used to determine pregnancy?

2. What is a gestation period? How long is the human gestation period?

3. Choose one body system and describe the changes that take place to that body system during pregnancy.

4. What steps can a pregnant woman take to reduce the chances of birth defects?

5. What changes take place in a woman's body during the days prior to the onset of labor?

6. Describe the events that take place during the first stage of labor.

7. Describe the events that take place during the second stage of labor.

8. Describe the events that take place during the third stage of labor.

9. What is the Ferguson reflex?

10. What is the APGAR score and why is it used?

CRITICAL THINKING QUESTION

1. The Newborns and Mothers Health Protection Act prohibits insurance companies from restricting post delivery hospital stays after a vaginal birth to fewer than 48 hours. What factors must be considered when determining appropriate hospital stays? What are the advantages and disadvantages of shorter or longer stays for both the mother and the baby?

WEBLINKS

Childbirth Connection:
www.childbirthconnection.org

REFERENCES

Allen, V. M., Armson, B. A., Wilson, R. D., Allen, V. M., Blight, C., Gagnon, A., Johnson, J. A., Langlois, S., Summers, A., Wyatt, P., Farine, D., Armson, B. A., Crane, J., Delisle, M. F., Keenan-Lindsay, L., Morin, V., Schneider, C. E., Van Aerde, J., & Society of Obstetricians and Gynecologists of Canada. (2007). Teratogenicity associated with pre-existing and gestational diabetes. *Journal of Obstetrics and Gynaecology Canada, 29*(11), 927–944.

American Congress of Obstetricians and Gynecologists, Committee on Obstetric Practice. (2005, September). *Obesity in pregnancy* (Committee Opinion No. 315). *Obstetrics & Gynecology, 106*(3), 671–675.

American Congress of Obstetricians and Gynecologists. (2007, January). *Screening for fetal chromosomal abnormalities* (Bulletin No. 77). *Obstetrics & Gynecology, 109*(1), 217–228.

American Congress of Obstetricians and Gynecologists. (2006, July 13). ACOG statement in support of IOM report, "Preterm birth: Causes, consequences, and prevention." Washington, DC: ACOG Office of Communications. Retrieved from http://www.acog.org/from_home/publications/press_releases/nr07-13-06.cfm.

American Society for Reproductive Medicine, Patient Education Committee and Publications Committee. (2004). *Multiple pregnancy and birth: Twins, triplets, and higher order multiples. A guide for patients.* Birmingham, AL.

American Society for Reproductive Medicine. (2008). Complications and problems associated with multiple births. Patient fact sheet. Retrieved from http://www.asrm.org/uploadedFiles/ASRM_Content/Resources/Patient_Resources/Fact_Sheets_and_Info_Booklets/complications_multiplebirths.pdf.

American Society for Reproductive Medicine. (2009). New SART data posted; Triplet and higher order multiples from ART are below two percent. *ASRM Bulletin, 11*(11).

Badell, M. L., Ramin, S. M., & Smith, J. A. (2006). Treatment options for nausea and vomiting during pregnancy. *Pharmacotherapy, 26*(9), 1273–1287.

Centers for Disease Control and Prevention. (2004). Malaria during Pregnancy. Retrieved June 1, 2009 from http://www.cdc.gov/mmwr/preview/mmwrhtml/ss5504a2.

Centers for Disease Control and Prevention. (2007). Malaria facts. Retrieved June 1, 2009 from http://www.cdc.gov/malaria/about/facts.html.

Clapp, J. F. (2006). Effects of diet and exercise on insulin resistance during pregnancy. *Metabolic Syndrome and Related Disorders, 4*(2), 84–90.

Clapp, J. F. (2006). Influence of endurance exercise and diet on human placental development and fetal growth. *Placenta, 27*(6–7), 527–534.

Davidoff, M. J., Dias, T., Damus, K., Russell, R., Bettegowda, V. R., Dolan, S., Schwarz, R. H., Green, N. S., & Petrini, J. (2006). Changes in the gestational age distribution among U.S. singleton births: Impact on rates of late preterm birth, 1992 to 2002. *Seminars in Perinatology, 30*(1), 8–15.

De Chateau, P. (1980). Parent–neonate interaction and its long-term effects. In E. G. Simmel (Ed.), *Early experience and early behavior.* New York, NY: Academic Press.

Dietz, P. M., Callaghan, W. M., & Sharma, A. J. (2009). High pregnancy weight gain and risk of excessive fetal growth. *American Journal of Obstetrics and Gynecology, 201*(1), 51, e1-6.

Dunnihoo, D. R. (1990). *Fundamentals of gynecology and obstetrics,* (p. 445). Philadelphia, PA: J. B. Lippincott.

Eerdekens, A., Debeer, A., Van Hoey, G., DeBorger, C., Sachar, V., Gudlinckx, I., Devlieger, R., Hanssens, M., & Vanhole, C. (2009). Maternal bariatric surgery: Adverse outcomes in neonates. *European Journal of Pediatrics, 169*(2), 191–196.

Einarson, T. R., Navioz, Y., Maltepe, C., Einarson, A., & Koren, G. (2007). Existence and severity of nausea and vomiting in pregnancy (NVP) with different partners. *American Journal of Obstetrics & Gynecology, 27*(4), 360–362.

Eskanazi, B., & Bracken, M. B. (1982). Bendectin (Debendox) as a risk factor for pyloric stenosis. *American Journal of Obstetrics and Gynecology, 144*(8), 919–924.

Fabro, S., & Sieber, S. M. (1969). Caffeine and nicotine penetrate the pre-implantation blastocyst. *Nature, 223*(204), 410–411.

Flaxman, S. M., & Sherman, P. W. (2008). Morning sickness: Adaptive cause or nonadaptive consequence of embryo viability? *American Naturalist, 172*(1), 54–62.

Flaxman, S. M., & Sherman, P. W. (2000). Morning sickness: A mechanism for protecting mother and embryo. *Quarterly Review of Biology, 75*(2), 113–148.

Forfar, J., & Nelson, M. M. (1973). Epidemiology of drugs taken by pregnant women: Drugs that may affect the fetus adversely. *Clinical Pharmacologies and Therapeutics, 14,* 632.

Gill, S. K., & Einarson, A. (2007). The safety of drugs for the treatment of nausea and vomiting in pregnancy. *Expert Opinion on Drug Safety, 6*(6), 685–694.

Golding, J., Vivian, S., & Baldwin, J. A. (1983). Maternal antinauseants and clefts of lip and palate. *Human Toxicology, 2,* 63–73.

Gosik, A. (2007, October 12). U.S. ranks 41st in maternal mortality: New report will be discussed at London meeting. Cox News Service. Retrieved from http://www.seattlepi.com/default/article/U-S-ranks-41st-in-maternal-mortality-1252472.php.

Grantham-McGregor, S. M., & Fernald, L. C. (1997). Nutritional deficiencies and subsequent effects on mental and behavioral development in children. *Southeast Asian Journal of Tropical Medicine and Public Health, 28* (Suppl. 2), 50–68.

Guelinckx, I., Devlieger, R., & Vansant, G. (2009). Reproductive outcomes after bariatric surgery: A critical review. *Human Reproductive Update, 15*(2), 189–201.

Hamilton, B. E., Martin, J. A., & Ventura, S. J. (2007). Births: Preliminary data for 2006. *National Vital Statistics Reports, 56*(7). Hyattsville, MD: National Center for Health Statistics.

Hincz, P., Borowski, D., Krekora, M., Podciechowski, L., Horzelski, W., & Wilczynski, J. (2009). Maternal obesity as a perinatal risk factor. *Ginekologia Polska, 80*(5), 334–337.

Jaruratanasirikul, S., Sangsupawanich, P., Koranantakul, O., Chanvitan, P., Sriplung, H., & Patanasin, T. (2009). Influence of maternal nutrient intake and weight gain on neonatal birth weight: A prospective cohort study in southern Thailand. *Journal of Maternal-Fetal and Neonatal Medicine, 16,* 1–6.

King, J. C., & Fabro, S. (1982). Alcohol consumption and cigarette smoking: Effect on pregnancy. *Clinical Obstetrics and Gynecology, 26*(2), 437–448.

Kinney, H. C. (2006). The near-term human brain and risk for periventricular leukomalacia: A review. *Seminars in Perinatology 30*(2), 81–88.

Klaus, M., Jerauld, R., & Kreger, N. (1972). Maternal attachment. *New England Journal of Medicine, 286*(9), 460–463.

Klaus, M., & Kennell, J. H. (1976). *Maternal-infant bonding.* St. Louis, MO: C. V. Mosby.

Klaus, M., & Kennell, J. (1983). Parent to infant bonding: Setting the record straight. *Journal of Pediatrics, 102*(4), 575–576.

Martin, J. A., Hamilton, B. E., Sutton, P. D., Ventura, S. J., Meacker, F., & Kirmeyer, S. (2006). Births: Final data for 2004. *National Vital Statistics Reports, 55*(1). Hyattsville, MD: National Center for Health Statistics.

Martin, J. A., Hamilton, B. E., Sutton, P. D., Ventura, S. J., Meacker, F., Kirmeyer, S., & Munson, M. L. (2007). Births: Final data for 2005. *National Vital Statistics Reports, 56*(6). Hyattsville, MD: National Center for Health Statistics.

Martin, J. A., et al. (2009). Births: Final data for 2006. *National Vital Statistics Reports, 57*(7). Hyattsville, MD: National Center for Health Statistics.

Monroy, T. R., Reeves, A. C. C., Naves Sanchez, J., & Macias, A. E. (2008). Influence of an individualized diet on control of gestational diabetes mellitus. *Ginecología y obstetricia de México, 76*(12), 722–729.

Page, E. W., Villee, C. A., & Villee, D. B. (1976). *Human reproduction* (2nd ed.). Philadelphia, PA: W. B. Saunders.

Pepper, G. V., & Roberts, S. C. (2006). Rates of nausea and vomiting in pregnancy and dietary characteristics across populations. *Proceedings: Biological Sciences, 273*(1601), 2675–2679.

Rimawi, L. (2006, September 22). Premature infant. In *Disease and conditions encyclopedia.* Discovery Communications, LLC. Retrieved January 16, 2008, from http://health.discovery.com/encyclopedias/illnesses.html?article=2728

Roll Back Malaria. Malaria in pregnancy. Retrieved June 1, 2009, from http://www.rbm.who.int/cmc_upload/0/000/015/369/RBMInfosheet_4.htm

Rycel, M., Wilczynski, J., Sobala, W., & Nowakowska, D. (2009). Analysis of teenage pregnancy outcomes and delivery between 2000 and 2006. *Ginekologia Polska, 79*(12), 867–870.

Sakela, C. (2006a). Carol Sakela's letter from North America: An uncontrolled experiment: Elective delivery predominates in the United States. *Birth, 33*(4), 332–335.

Sakela, C., & Corry, M. P. (2008). Achieving the Institute of Medicine's six aims for improvement of maternity care. *Women's Health Issues, 18*(2), 75–78.

Satpathy, H. K., Fleming, A., Frey, D., Barsoom, M., Satpathy, C., & Khandalavala, J. (2008). Maternal obesity and pregnancy. *Postgraduate Medicine,* 120(3), E01-9.

Schieve, L. A., Coqswell, M. E., & Scanlon, K. S. (1998). Trends in pregnancy weight gain within and outside ranges recommended by the Institute of Medicine in a WIC population. *Maternal and Child Health Journal, 2*(2), 111–116.

Vetr, M. (2005). Risk l factors associated with high birth weight deliveries. *Ceská Gynekologie, 70*(5), 347–354.

Weigel, M. M., & Weigel, R. M. (1989). Nausea and vomiting of early pregnancy and pregnancy outcome. An epidemiological study. *British Journal of Obstetrics and Gynecology, 96,* 1304–1311.

Wilson, R. D., Johnson, J. A., Allen, V., Gagnon, A., Langlois, S., Blight, C., Audibert, F., Desilets, V., Brock, J. A., Koren, G., Goh, I., Nyuyen, P., Kapur, B., & Genetics Committee of the Society of Obstetricians and Gynaecologists of Canada and the Mother Risk Program. (2007). Re-conceptional vitamin/folic acid supplementation 2007: The use of folic acid in combination with a multivitamin supplement for the prevention of neural tube defects and other congenital abnormalities. *Journal of Obstetrics and Gynaecology Canada, 29*(12), 1003–1026.

World Health Organization. (2005). *The World Health Report 2005: Make every mother and child count.* Geneva, Switzerland.

World Health Organization. (2008). *Maternal mental health and child health and development in low and middle income countries. Report to WHO meeting.* Geneva, Switzerland: Author.

World Health Organization Global Malaria Programme. Insecticide treated mosquito nets: A WHO position statement. Retrieved June 1, 2009 from http://apps.who.int/malaria/docs/itn/ITNspospaperfinal.pdf.

World Health Organization, Regional Office for South-East Asia. (2004). Introduction to the 'Making Pregnancy Safer' Initiative. Retrieved June 1, 2009, from http://www.searo.who.int/EN/Section13/Section36/Section129/Section396_1450.htm

Zanardo, V., Simibi, K. A., Vedovato, S., & Trevisanuto, D. (2004). The influence of elective cesarean section on neonatal resuscitation risk. *Pediatric Critical Care Medicine, 5*(6), 566–570.

chapter 12

COMPLICATIONS AND MEDICAL INTERVENTIONS DURING PREGNANCY

CHAPTER COMPETENCIES

Upon completion of this chapter the reader will be able to:

- Identify and describe the complications that can arise during pregnancy
- Identify the techniques used to monitor fetal health during pregnancy

- Describe medical procedures that are used during childbirth and the complications that can arise from them
- Identify methods that can be used to reduce the pain associated with childbirth

KEY TERMS

assisted vaginal birth
cesarean section
contraction stress
   test (cst)

eclampsia
ectopic pregnancy
epidural anesthesia
episiotomy

hyperemesis
  gravidarum
miscarriage
placenta previa

placental abruption
preeclampsia

PREGNANCY COMPLICATIONS

Complications during pregnancy can be a risk to the life of both the mother and her fetus. Although some pregnancies are considered more high risk than others, complications can arise in any pregnancy. Healthy women, over age 17 and under age 34, with no serious physical illnesses, who are well nourished, but not over- or underweight are considered low-risk pregnancy prospects. For younger or older women, women with health issues, or for women who are over- or underweight, prenatal visits are especially important to prevent or manage potential complications (Jahromi & Husseini, 2008). Regular prenatal visits provide an important step toward detecting problems and treating them before they become serious or potentially life-threatening (Figure 12-1). Evaluation of simple factors such as blood pressure, glucose or protein levels in the urine, and weight gain between visits can be important in early detection of potential complications. Women's access to prenatal care is widely variable around the world. Even in countries where prenatal care is available, many women are unable or unwilling to access services.

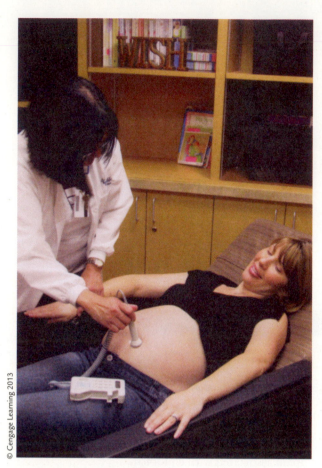

© Cengage Learning 2013

FIGURE 12-1: Prenatal visits are an important step towards detecting and treating pregnancy complications.

Complications with Implantation

Complications can occur when a fertilized egg implants somewhere other than the uterus, as in the case of ectopic pregnancies. In some cases, a placenta fails to develop and the result is a miscarriage. Complications can also occur when the placenta develops too close to the cervix causing placental bleeding during the pregnancy. This condition is called **placenta previa**.

Ectopic Pregnancy

After a fertilized egg arrives in the uterus, it normally implants in the upper part of the uterine cavity. Complications arise when implantation occurs in another location causing an **ectopic pregnancy** (Figure 12-2). In most of these ectopic pregnancies, the embryo implants in the fallopian tubes, and these are often called tubal pregnancies. Rarely, the fertilized egg may implant on the ovary, the cervix, or even the wall of the abdominal cavity. Ectopic pregnancies can be fatal. It is estimated that one out of 50 pregnancies is ectopic, however, the exact number is unknown. It is possible that many tubal pregnancies, like many uterine pregnancies, spontaneously regress or abort at a very early stage,

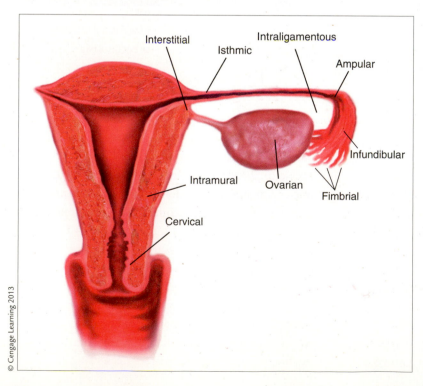

© Cengage Learning 2013

FIGURE 12-2: Implantation sites for ectopic pregnancies.

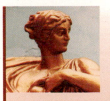

Cultural Considerations
EARLY MARRIAGE AND ADOLESCENT PREGNANCY

Child marriage has been classified as a harmful traditional practice that weds young people at an early age. For the most part, the practice involves marrying adolescent girls to men who are usually significantly older than they are. According to international advocacy organizations, there are 60 million child brides worldwide. Research into the practice of early marriage has revealed that getting married at such a young age limits young girls' skills, resources, knowledge, social support, mobility, and autonomy. Compared to women who marry later, young married girls have little power in relation to their husband and in-laws, making them extremely vulnerable to domestic violence and abandonment (WHO, 2008; ICRW, 2009).

Most of these girls will also give birth at an early age. Worldwide, about 16 million young women and girls, aged 15–19 years old, give birth each year. These adolescent pregnancies account for about 11 percent of all births worldwide. Ninety-five percent of these births occur in low- and middle-income countries. According to the World Health Organization, the average adolescent birth rate in middle-income countries is more than twice as high as that in high-income countries, with the rate in low-income countries being five times as high. Today, half of all adolescent births occur in just seven countries: Bangladesh, Brazil, the Democratic Republic of the Congo, Ethiopia, India, Nigeria and the United States (WHO, 2008; WHO, 2009). In addition, recent research on the Indian subcontinent indicates that young women who marry at age 18 or older are less likely to be subjected to domestic violence. They are also more likely to use contraceptives and delay their first pregnancy (Santhya et al., 2010).

Becoming pregnant and giving birth at too early of an age can severely compromise a girl's health, and sometimes can also jeopardize her life (Rycel et al., 2009). In addition, very young mothers are more likely to give birth to stillborn infants, or to have their babies die in the first few days after delivery. Studies have shown that babies born to mothers younger than 20 are 50 percent more likely to suffer stillbirth or death in the first week of life compared to babies born to mothers 20–29 years old. Infant deaths during the first month of life are 50-100 percent higher if the mother is an adolescent, as compared with older mothers. In general, the younger the mother, the higher the risk.

and the woman may never suspect she was pregnant at all. Complications occur because the fallopian tubes cannot stretch enough to permit growth of the embryo. The embryo, therefore, must be removed before the tube bursts and causes severe hemorrhage and infection in the abdominal cavity. In very rare instances, a fertilized ovum escapes through the opening of the fimbriated end of the fallopian tube and implants itself and begins developing outside of the uterus, but within the abdominal cavity. Very rarely, these pregnancies have actually been successful, and a nearly full-term baby can be surgically delivered (Yildizhan et al., 2009). Difficulty and delay in diagnosis and treatment have made ectopic pregnancy the major cause of death during the first three months of pregnancy (Majhi et al., 2007).

Causes of Ectopic Pregnancy   Although there is often no clear explanation for why an ectopic pregnancy has developed, there are risk factors that make some women more susceptible to this condition than others. Any condition which interferes with transport of the embryo through the tube increases the risk of a tubal pregnancy. This includes tubal damage from an STI or surgery, smoking, or in vitro fertilization. Exposure to cigarette smoke alters the chemistry of the fluids within the fallopian tube, making it more likely that a tubal pregnancy will occur (Shaw et al.,

2010). The STIs chlamydia and gonorrhea can lead to pelvic inflammatory disease, which often results in the scarring of the fallopian tubes. This scarring interferes with the normal movement of the fertilized egg through the tube and to the uterus. Tubal pregnancy has also been associated with sterilization by tubal ligation and in tubal ligation reversal. The incidence is rare, however, and may be related to the method of tubal occlusion used. Women with endometriosis have been shown to be more likely to experience ectopic pregnancy as can medications used in fertility treatments that stimulate ovulation. Fertility treatments may alter the tubal environment and encourage early implantation (Shaw et al., 2010). While intrauterine devices (IUDs) were originally associated with higher rates of ectopic pregnancies, use of the newer copper or progestin IUDs actually results in lower rates of ectopic pregnancy than using no contraception.

Symptoms of an Ectopic Pregnancy   Early diagnosis of an ectopic pregnancy reduces the risks to the woman's fertility. Unfortunately, the early detection of tubal pregnancy can be difficult because the early symptoms mimic those of a normal uterine pregnancy. If the tubal implantation is situated so that fetal tissue is in contact with maternal blood vessels, human chorionic gonadotropin will appear in maternal blood and will yield a positive pregnancy test result. A tender and distended fallopian tube which can sometimes be felt during a pelvic examination is a classic symptom, but it is not always detectable. The first indications of an ectopic pregnancy are lower abdominal or pelvic pain, and cramps on one side of the pelvis. Sharp, stabbing pain in the pelvis or abdomen, accompanied by dizziness or light headedness may be an indication that the tube has ruptured and that there is hemorrhage into the uterus and body cavity and warrants immediate medical attention. If the internal bleeding irritates the peritoneal lining of the body cavity, the pain may be referred to the shoulder.

Laparoscopy, ultrasound, and MRI have made earlier determination of ectopic pregnancies possible. Ultrasound can rule out a tubal pregnancy if a placenta or a fetal beating heart is clearly seen in the uterus. If a pregnancy test is positive, and there is no uterine pregnancy visible with ultrasonography,

laparoscopic examination to permit visualization of the internal organs can make it possible to diagnose ectopic pregnancy before a rupture occurs. One other marker is the serum progesterone level, which may also be checked, since the concentration of this hormone is considerably lower in an ectopic pregnancy than in a normal pregnancy.

Treatments for Ectopic Pregnancy   Before 1975, nearly 80 percent of ectopic pregnancies ruptured before diagnosis. As a result of the newer diagnostic techniques, currently fewer than 30 percent rupture before they are recognized, despite the increased incidence of tubal pregnancies. Treatment options for an ectopic pregnancy will depend on the stage of the pregnancy when it is detected. If rupture has not occurred, a nonsurgical treatment is injection with drugs, such as methotrexate, that will stop embryonic development and end the pregnancy. In a study of ectopic pregnancy treatments, methotrexate was successful in 85 percent of cases (Hoover, 2010). This treatment can be done on an outpatient basis, and has the best chance of saving the fallopian tube and preserving fertility. If the fallopian tube has ruptured, emergency surgery is required to prevent death of the woman from hemorrhage. If surgery is required, two procedures that may be used are salpingostomy and salpingectomy. In the case of salpingostomy, a small incision is made in the tube and the contents are removed. This conservative treatment may preserve the function of the fallopian tube for future fertility. Salpingectomy involves removing the fallopian tube, and sometimes the ovary. In this case, fertility would be reduced, since only one ovary and fallopian tube would be left after the procedure. Despite attempts to preserve the tube, women who have had an ectopic pregnancy have a 12 percent incidence of recurrence, and 40 percent are unable to conceive again. Of the 60 percent who do become pregnant, approximately 15–20 percent will miscarry (Deutchman, 2009).

A tubal pregnancy must be terminated because it is not possible for the embryo to develop to full term without rupturing the fallopian tube and causing life-threatening hemorrhage. If the isthmus of the tube is the site of the implantation, an early rupture is more likely to take place because the thicker muscle of the tubal wall does not permit much stretching.

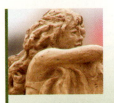

Economic Considerations
ECTOPIC PREGNANCY IN INSURED WOMEN

In recent years, insurance data has become a method of estimating the rates of ectopic pregnancies, at least in populations of women with health insurance. Two studies—one covering 1997 to 2000 (van den Eeden et al., 2005) and a second covering 2002 to 2007 (Hover et al., 2010)—used claims information from United States commercial insurance companies to determine that rates of ectopic pregnancy remained unchanged over the sample periods. However, treatments changed. While the rates between 1997 and 2000 indicated that the frequency of ectopic pregnancy did not increase, the number of women who received medical treatment for the condition did (van den Eeden et al., 2005). The nonsurgical methotrexate treatment, usually an outpatient treatment, increased from 11 percent of cases in 2002 to 35 percent by 2007. This corresponded with a decrease in more expensive surgical treatment from 40 percent to 33 percent (Hover et al., 2010).

Case Study

It is not Appendicitis

Gina is 23 years old. She and her partner have been trying to get pregnant, and she is delighted when her period is finally late. She is concerned, however, because she has been experiencing occasional sharp pain on the left side of her abdomen. Her first concern is that she may be having an appendicitis attack, but then she remembers that pain from appendicitis usually occurs on the right side of the body. She decides to ignore the pain, but a couple of hours later she finds herself doubled over on the bathroom floor experiencing excruciating pain and nausea. Her partner rushes her to the hospital, where an ultrasound identifies ectopic pregnancy. The doctor tells her that it is a good thing that she was brought to the hospital when she was because her fallopian tube was beginning to rupture, and if that had occurred, she could easily have died of severe hemorrhage.

1. Which treatment is most common for an ectopic pregnancy?

2. Why can't the embryo continue to grow in the fallopian tube?

3. What factors may be contributing to the increased frequency of ectopic pregnancies?

In the infundibular part of the fallopian tube or in the ampulla portion, it is possible for the pregnancy to continue longer, but it ultimately ruptures, usually into the pelvic cavity.

Placental Bleeding

Some women experience a small amount of bleeding, or spotting, throughout their pregnancies, with no negative consequences. Approximately 20 percent of women experience vaginal bleeding in the first 28 weeks of pregnancy (Snell, 2009). Bleeding may indicate a miscarriage, an ectopic pregnancy, or other complications and should be investigated. Fifty percent of women who have bleeding retain their pregnancy with no adverse consequences. Vaginal bleeding in the last trimester may be due to other complications of late pregnancy such as placenta previa, placental abruption, or preterm labor.

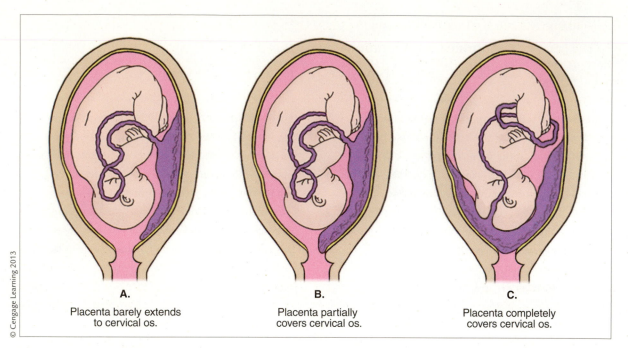

© Cengage Learning 2013

| A. | B. | C. |
| Placenta barely extends to cervical os. | Placenta partially covers cervical os. | Placenta completely covers cervical os. |

FIGURE 12-3: Placenta previa. A. Placenta extends toward cervix. B. Placenta partially covers cervix. C. Placenta completely covers cervix.

Placenta Previa   Placenta previa occurs in approximately 4 out of 1000 pregnancies (Faiz & Ananth, 2003). It is the result of implantation of the zygote in the lower part of the uterus instead of the more usual site higher up in the fundus. The placenta extends over the internal os of the cervix (Figure 12-3). Late in pregnancy or at the time of delivery, the placenta may separate from its attachment in the uterus causing characteristically painless bleeding that is bright red in color. Bleeding can be light or heavy with possible cramping, and it may stop for a few days or weeks, only to begin again. Placenta previa can cause preterm delivery of the fetus and post delivery hemorrhage in the mother (Zlatnik et al., 2007). If bleeding has occurred as early as 32 weeks, steps may be taken to prevent preterm delivery. If placenta previa is diagnosed at the time of labor, the baby may be delivered by cesarean section. In some cases, the neonate may need to be resuscitated and may require a blood transfusion immediately after delivery (Gagnon et al., 2009). Older mothers are more likely to experience this complication, as are mothers who have had previous abortion or cesarean section. Smoking and cocaine use can also contribute to the risk of developing this condition. Carrying a male fetus can also be a factor (Faiz & Ananth, 2003).

Placental Abruption   When the placenta begins to separate from the uterus before the birth of the baby, the condition is called **placental abruption** (Figure 12-4). Placental abruption is often fatal to the fetus because it results in an interruption of the supply of oxygen from the mother. This form of birth asphyxiation can result in neurological problems, low birth weight, and a low APGAR score, when the infant does survive (Zupan-Simunek, 2010).

Some risk factors that may contribute to placental abruption include maternal hypertension, prior C-section, and maternal age (Pariente et al., 2010).

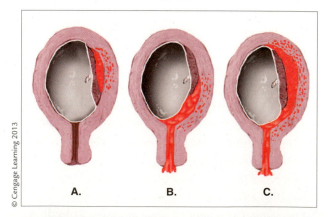

© Cengage Learning 2013

A.   B.   C.

FIGURE 12-4: Placental abruption. A. Central abruption with concealed hemorrhage. B. Marginal abruption with hemorrhage C. Complete abruption with hemorrhage.

This condition occurs most frequently in women who have had at least one prior pregnancy. Women who experience violence are also more likely to develop placental abruption (Leone et al., 2010), as are women who drink alcohol. In fact, as alcohol consumption increases, so does a woman's risk of this condition (Silihu et al., 2010). The chance of developing placental abruption dramatically increases when a pregnant woman uses cocaine. Even if the woman abstains from the drug during the second and third trimesters, cocaine use apparently causes early damage to the placental and uterine vessels and places the pregnancy at continued risk (Chasnoff et al., 1989). Other factors that may contribute to the risk of placental abruption include anemia (Bibi et al., 2009) and thyroid disorders (Krassas et al., 2010) and depression or stress (de Paz et al., 2010).

Miscarriage

The medical term for **miscarriage** is spontaneous abortion. Of all recognized pregnancies, about 25 percent end in a miscarriage (ASRM, 2008). Eighty percent of miscarriages occur in the first 12 weeks of pregnancy. There may be many more that occur before the diagnosis of pregnancy and are considered to be only delayed menstrual periods. In a study to determine the frequency of early miscarriages, women's hormone levels were measured every day to detect very early pregnancy. The researchers found that when these early pregnancies are included, about a third of pregnancies do not continue to term. Early miscarriages may be the result of genetic defects in the fetus, which prevent further development. Between five and ten percent of embryos and fetuses have chromosome abnormalities and these usually result in a miscarriage (Suzumari & Sugiura-Ogasawara, 2010). Late miscarriages which occur after the second trimester are much rarer. These are more likely to be caused by problems with the structure of the cervix, uterine abnormalities, preeclampsia, or preexisting diseases of the mother.

The first sign of the possibility of miscarriage is vaginal bleeding, with or without cramping. If painless uterine bleeding is occurring without any dilatation of the cervix, it is termed a threatened miscarriage. Sometimes the symptoms subside within several days and the pregnancy continues with no complications.

Continued bleeding accompanied by uterine cramps and dilatation of the cervix indicates progression to inevitable miscarriage. In most instances, the death of the fetus has taken place several weeks before the first symptoms of a miscarriage. Without the stimulus of the growing embryo, the placenta stops producing hormones that maintain the integrity of the endometrium. Once a miscarriage is underway, it can result in complete or incomplete abortion. In the case of a complete abortion, the placenta and the embryo leave the uterus, and the bleeding and cramping stop. More often, the abortion is incomplete. Some placental tissue remains in the uterus and may have to be removed by curettage to prevent infection. Occasionally, long after fetal death, the fetal and placental tissue are retained in the uterus, and there are no signs of abortion. This is called missed abortion. The signs and symptoms of pregnancy gradually disappear, and curettage is usually necessary to remove tissue. Eventually the uterine contents will spontaneously be expelled, but it could take several months.

Recurrent Pregnancy Loss

Having an early miscarriage during the first three months of pregnancy does not necessarily mean that a woman will have another one if she becomes pregnant again. Recurrent pregnancy loss is the condition when a woman experiences two or more consecutive miscarriages. This is a relatively rare condition with less than five percent of women experiencing two consecutive miscarriages, and only one percent experiencing three or more. When miscarriage is recurrent, genetic counseling and chromosome analysis of both parents is advised because it may indicate a chromosomal abnormality. Nutritional deficiencies, reproductive tract abnormalities, endocrine disturbances, and exposure to environmental agents have all been recognized as factors that contribute to miscarriage. Obesity, poorly controlled diabetes, and polycystic ovarian syndrome also increase the chances of miscarriage. Evidence is accumulating that links chemicals and other hazards in the home, environment, and the workplace with the growing incidence of miscarriage, stillbirths, and birth defects. There is also preliminary data that suggests that abnormalities in DNA packaging in sperm cells can influence the chances of miscarriage (ASRM, 2008). In many cases, a specific explanation is unknown. Once detected, correction and elimination of known conditions in women who have had successive miscarriages can often produce pregnancies with successful outcomes. Even when an explanation is not found, 60 to 70 percent of women who have experienced recurrent pregnancy loss are able to carry their pregnancies to term the next time they become pregnant (ASRM, 2008).

Hemolytic Disease of the Newborn

The condition, hemolytic disease of the newborn, is a pregnancy complication that originates from an incompatibility between the blood types of the mother and the fetus. In addition to the familiar ABO blood types, humans also have another blood type classification of positive or negative, depending on the presence or absence of a protein marker on the surface of the red blood cells called the Rh antigen. Rh positive individuals have the marker; Rh negative individuals lack the marker. Rh status becomes a concern if a woman is Rh negative and her developing fetus is Rh positive. In that case, the mother's body can create antibodies that destroy the blood of her fetus. This condition is called hemolytic disease of the newborn. The antibody attack on the fetal red blood cells can cause serious complications and even death of the fetus. The mother will not develop antibodies against the fetus's blood unless she has previously been exposed to Rh positive blood. This can happen through a blood transfusion or because of placental bleeding during labor and delivery of a previous Rh positive baby. Development of the anti-Rh antibodies can be prevented if the Rh negative woman is given an injection of RhoGam in situations where she might be exposed to Rh positive blood. RhoGam can also be given by injection to Rh negative mothers who are carrying an Rh positive fetus to prevent the formation of antibodies. Injections are usually given at 28 weeks and again at 34 weeks, a few weeks prior to labor.

Maternal Complications

Pregnancy alters a woman's physiology, and some of these alterations can lead to complications, some of which can be life threatening to her or her fetus. The risks of complications increase for women who are at either end of their reproductive years (Figure 12-5). Very young women who are at increased

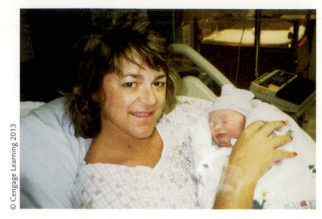

© Cengage Learning 2013

FIGURE 12-5: Many women over 35 are now giving birth for the first time.

risk of complication because their body has not had sufficient time to mature. Older mothers are more likely to have preexisting conditions, such as diabetes or hypertension, myomas or chromosome abnormalities that can adversely affect their pregnancies. Older mothers are also more likely to develop gestational diabetes, pregnancy induced hypertension, and other complications while pregnant. These factors contribute to the greater risk for mothers over 35 to experience a stillbirth, deliver a low birth weight baby, or require a cesarean section for delivery (Franz & Husslein, 2010).

Obesity is also a significant risk factor for developing complications, including hypertension, preeclampsia, and gestational diabetes. Obese women are more likely to require a cesarean section than are non-obese women (Bayrompour & Heaman, 2010). However, there is increasing evidence that exercise during pregnancy can attenuate some of the negative effects of obesity on pregnancy (Davies et al., 2010).

Hyperemesis Gravidarum

In about one percent of pregnancies, morning sickness can develop into **hyperemesis gravidarum**, a severe and persistent vomiting. While milder forms of morning sickness are associated with a reduced chance of miscarriage (Chan et al., 2010), severe nausea and vomiting can become a danger to the expectant mother's health. Women who experience persistent vomiting, more than four times per day, vomit blood, lose more than two pounds in one day, or are unable to keep down fluids for one day or more should seek medical assistance. This serious condition produces dehydration and disturbances in the body's acid-base balance and can lead to coma or even death for the mother (Pepper & Roberts, 2006; Einerson et al., 2007; Flaxman & Sherman, 2008). Testing for thyroid, liver, or gallbladder problems, which can also cause persistent vomiting, should be done before treating hyperemesis gravidarum. Hospitalization for intravenous feeding and other measures to relieve it are sometimes required (Badell et al., 2006 ; Verberg et al., 2005). A new method of treatment for extreme cases involves surgically implanting a feeding tube directly into the jejunum of the small intestine to avoid the nausea caused by food moving through the stomach and duodenum (Saha et al., 2009).

Gestational Diabetes

In three to six percent of pregnancies, placental hormones combined with metabolic changes can produce gestational diabetes. The condition results in dangerously high blood sugar levels. Although this condition subsides after giving birth, women who develop gestational diabetes are at greater risk to develop Type 2 diabetes later in life. The chronic high blood sugar associated with gestational diabetes can cause nerve and kidney damage. In addition to the potential harm that high blood sugar can have on expectant mothers, uncontrolled blood sugar can have several adverse effects on the developing fetus, including causing congenital abnormalities (Allen et al., 2007) and a condition called macrosomia, or large size for gestational age (Dietz et al., 2009; Vetr, 2005; Jaruratanasirikul et al., 2009). Large babies are more likely to require a cesarean section or suffer birth injuries when delivered vaginally. They can be born with respiratory distress syndrome. They often suffer from hypoglycemia, or abnormally low blood sugar, right after they are born because their insulin levels are too high. Babies born to women with gestational diabetes have a higher risk of developing Type 2 diabetes as well as obesity later in life (Gillman et al., 2010). Gestational diabetes can be controlled by monitoring the mother's blood sugar levels, modifying her diet (Monroy et al., 2008), and getting sufficient exercise. In some cases, medications such as insulin will be prescribed. Research indicates that successfully managing gestational diabetes can decrease the negative maternal and fetal outcomes associated with this condition (Alwan et al., 2009; Dennedy and Dunne, 2010; Tieu et al., 2010).

Preeclampsia-Eclampsia

The disorder known as **preeclampsia** is a combination of symptoms that includes pregnancy-induced hypertension (PIH), protein in the urine, and edema. This condition is a leading cause of maternal and fetal illness and death worldwide (Gleicher, 2007). If preeclampsia progresses, it can develop into a condition known as **eclampsia** which is a life-threatening complication involving seizures (Figure 12-6). Some women who have preeclampsia also develop an inadequate blood supply to the placenta. In the past, preeclampsia was called toxemia because it was believed to be caused by a toxin in the blood, a theory that turned out to be false. Preeclampsia is a risk factor for both preterm delivery and intrauterine growth restriction (IUGR) which contributes to a low birth weight for the infant. Children born with IUGR are more likely to develop hypertension and metabolic disorder in adulthood (Zupan-Simunek, 2010). There is some evidence that children who are born to mothers who experienced preeclampsia are also more likely to develop respiratory disorders later in life (Wu et al., 2010).

Several mechanisms have been suggested to explain how preeclampsia develops. Genetic factors have been suggested as a possible cause, and so has the breakdown of maternal immunologic tolerance to the fetus. Early research (Ezkanazi et al., 1991) identified

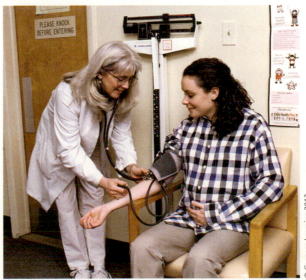

FIGURE 12-6: Regular blood pressure monitoring can detect gestational hypertension and early signs of preeclampsia.

© Cengage Learning 2013

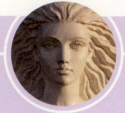

focus on

EXERCISE

Can Exercise Reduce the Risk of Gestational Diabetes, Gestational Hypertension, and Preeclampsia?

Moderate exercise, both before and during pregnancy, offers significant benefits to both the mother and fetus, and may even reduce the risk of such pregnancy complications as gestational diabetes, gestational hypertension, and preeclampsia (Yeo, 2010; Tobias et al., 2010; Falcao et al., 2010; Fortner et al., 2010; Stutzman et al., 2010). Some of the potential benefits for pregnant women who exercise include: improved cardiovascular health (Davies et al., 2010), reduced muscle cramping, reduced edema, less weight gain during pregnancy, and improved emotional well being. Fetal benefits include reduced fat mass, improved stress tolerance, and enhanced neuro-behavioral development (Meizer et al., 2010). Exercise during pregnancy has also been associated with shorter labor and less risk of cesarean section or assisted vaginal birth. Contrary to concerns that exercise might increase the chance of preterm delivery and low birth weight infants, recent studies have found that when comparing sedentary women with women who engaged in moderate exercise, there were no differences in terms of their risk of preterm delivery, low birth weight babies, or low APGAR scores (Barkat et al., 2009a; Barakat et al., 2009b; Barakat et al., 2008).

the following characteristics as risk factors for developing preeclampsia:

- never having borne a child (nulliparity)
- having a previous history of eclampsia
- being obese prior to pregnancy compared with the control women
- being of African descent (compared with women of European descent)
- being over 35
- having gestational diabetes
- working during pregnancy regardless of the kind of job

Recent research is exploring similarities between preeclampsia and autoimmune disorders to understand how preeclampsia develops (Gleicher, 2007). Since

inflammation, which leads to the hypertension, protourea, and edema of preeclampsia, is an important component of this condition developing, some researchers are suggesting that treatments that address inflammation may be developed in the future (Dusse et al., 2010; Borzychowski et al., 2006). Researchers are also exploring the possible links between vitamin D deficiencies and the development of preeclampsia (Shin et al., 2010; Powe et al., 2010; Bodnar et al., 2007).

The first in the triad of symptoms associated with preeclampsia is a rapid weight gain of at least 1 Kg (2 lb) in one week. Since the weekly gain normally should be less than a pound each week during the last six months of pregnancy, a greater gain can indicate water retention that causes edema. The edema of preeclampsia is the deeply pitting type; an indentation or pit remains for a period of time when a finger is poked into the swollen tissue. The second symptom is a rise in systolic blood pressure to 30 mm Hg above the normal readings and a diastolic pressure of at least 15 mm Hg above normal. A woman who is not having her weight, blood pressure, and urine routinely checked may not notice the symptoms. As preeclampsia becomes more severe, headache, dizziness, and blurred vision occur. Pain under the sternum, an indication of liver enlargement, is a serious sign. When this is accompanied by vomiting and scanty urination, there is a risk of convulsions and, possibly, death. Research is currently underway to identify biomarkers that can be tested early in a pregnancy to identify women who are most at risk of developing this condition (Reslan & Khalil, 2010).

The prognosis for a mild preeclampsia is best if it is detected early. Because the only definitive cure is the delivery of the baby, treatment involves reducing the symptoms, preventing progression to the more severe stages, and trying to maintain the pregnancy until the fetus is able to live independently. With mild preeclampsia, bed rest at home and a high protein diet with vitamin supplements may result in improvement. More severe preeclampsia requires hospitalization. In severe preeclampsia, as soon as it is practical, labor is induced or a cesarean section is performed. Careful monitoring and treatment of early symptoms can limit the progression of preeclampsia to the more severe, life-threatening form.

Preterm Labor and Preterm Delivery

Preterm labor is defined as labor that begins before 37 weeks gestation (Figure 12-7). The rate of premature delivery has increased in the United States by 36 percent between 1980 and 2007 and now represents 12.7 percent of births (March of Dimes, 2010). Complications associated with preterm deliveries are a leading cause of death for babies during their first month of life. Because their organ systems have not had time to develop fully, premature infants face a number of potential complications. Respiratory distress syndrome is a problem for babies born before 34 weeks gestation. The lungs are one of the last organs to mature and will not function adequately if the baby is born before they have completed enough of their development. Another potential complication is bleeding in the brain. This condition is also called intraventricular hemorrhage (IVH), and it results in brain damage. If the heart has not developed completely, the condition patent ductus arteriosus can result. This condition is an incomplete readjustment of the heart to life outside of the womb, and it leads to inefficient blood flow through the circulatory system. If not corrected, this condition can lead to heart failure. Necrotizing enterocolitis (NEC) results from the underdeveloped state of the intestine. Finally, retinopathy of prematurity (ROP) is a condition that can result in blindness if left untreated. It occurs mainly in babies born before 32 weeks gestation.

Premature birth also contributes to many long-term health problems such as cerebral palsy, mental retardation, blindness, and chronic lung problems. Additional problems with the central nervous system resulting in emotional, behavioral, and cognitive difficulties have also been reported (Kinney, 2006). Most babies that are born prematurely are also low birth weight babies.

One of the reasons that preterm delivery is such a difficult problem to predict or prevent is that there appear to be multiple factors that contribute to it. The March of Dimes (2009) has identified several triggers that may lead to premature labor and delivery. Certain bacterial infections of the mother's genital or urinary tract, as well as infections elsewhere in the body, especially when they cause inflammation, can initiate an immune response that can trigger labor prematurely. Chronic stress in the mother can result in the production of the hormone corticotropin-releasing hormone (CRH), which can trigger a cascade of additional hormones that stimulate uterine contractions. If the fetus is not receiving sufficient blood flow from the placenta, it too can release CRH and trigger contractions. If a woman is experiencing uterine bleeding during pregnancy, it can trigger the release of blood clotting proteins that have the effect of stimulating uterine contractions. Finally, any condition that leads to excessive stretching of the uterus can cause the release of chemicals that stimulate contractions. Carrying multiple fetuses can contribute to this stretching.

It appears that any of these conditions or a combination of them can lead to premature labor. Although preterm labor can happen to any pregnant woman, women are considered especially at risk if they have had a previous preterm birth, are pregnant with multiples (ASRM, 2009; ASRM, 2008), or have certain uterine or cervical abnormalities. Women of African descent have the highest rate of preterm

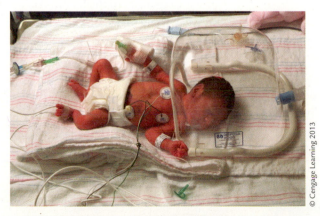

© Cengage Learning 2013

FIGURE 12-7: Premature infants often need help breathing because their lungs are not yet fully developed.

delivery in the United States, at 17.8 percent. Women of Asian and Pacific Island descent have the lowest rate at 10.5 percent (AGOG, 2006).

Although it is common to experience Braxton-Hicks contractions, especially during the last weeks of pregnancy, there are symptoms that may indicate the onset of premature labor. These include:

- Pelvic pressure and lower back pain
- An increase in vaginal discharge
- A change in the frequency of uterine contractions

It is important to seek medical help if these symptoms appear, since it may be possible to administer medications to stop the contractions and delay labor for a few days to help the baby's lungs to mature more quickly. In some cases the administration of progesterone hormone can successfully stop preterm contractions and prolong the pregnancy (Petrini et al., 2005).

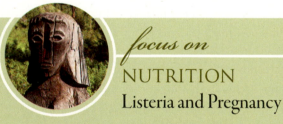

focus on
NUTRITION
Listeria and Pregnancy

Listeria monocytogenes is a common environmental bacterium that produces infections when people eat foods contaminated with the organism. Recent outbreaks have involved cold cuts, fresh cheeses, and beef and bean burritos. Unpasteurized milk has a reputation as a common source of infection. While anyone who eats contaminated products can develop an infection, pregnant women are up to 20 times as likely to develop the flu-like symptoms, fever, and digestive system upset characteristic of an infection (CDC, 2010). However, the greatest risk is to the embryo. The bacterium can cross the placenta producing severe fetal infections. This infection may result in stillbirth, miscarriage, or premature labor. A study of pregnancy-associated listeriosis cases between 2004 and 2007 found that 20 percent of the women miscarried. Of the infants who survived to birth, 33 percent developed meningitis and 36.5 percent developed blood infections (Jackson, et al., 2010). To minimize the risk of infection, pregnant women should avoid potential sources of contamination including fresh pâté, soft cheeses, uncooked deli meats and hotdogs, and cold smoked fish (CDC, 2010).

Complications after Delivery

The amount of pain experienced by new mothers and degree of care they need after delivery depends on their birth experience, procedures used during delivery, number of previous deliveries, and the condition of the mother. In general, women who have a spontaneous vaginal birth may have some soreness in the perineal area, although pain is likely to be more acute if an episiotomy was done or if the birth was assisted with instruments. Women who delivered by cesarean section usually require a longer hospital stay to recover from the abdominal surgery.

Streptococcus Infection

Infection has always been a potential complication of pregnancy, and historically it leads to deaths in both mother and child. Group B streptococci are part of the group of bacteria that causes strep throat, rheumatic fever, scarlet fever, and a type of pneumonia. Group B strep, however, are found in the urogenital and digestive tracts of nearly a third of all healthy adults and normally cause neither symptoms nor harm. However, in pregnant women, the bacterium can produce both maternal and newborn infection. Ninety-eight percent of infants who are infected with Group B strep will have no problem. If unrecognized and untreated in the other two percent, however, permanent brain or lung damage or death can occur. One in five pregnant women harbors Group B strep at the time of delivery and can pass the organism to the infant. Babies are more likely to become infected under the following conditions:

- When there is premature rupture of membranes and labor does not start within 12 hours
- When the newborn is premature or of low birth weight
- When the mother has a fever before or during labor and delivery, or within 48 hours after delivery
- If a woman has already delivered a baby with Group B strep

The symptoms of Group B infection—fever over 100°F, respiratory difficulty, irritability, and then lethargy—usually occur during the first week of life but can occur in an infant up to two months of age. The only protection against Group B strep infection is identification of the organisms in pregnant women by a screening test. If she is found to be a carrier, she should be monitored and may be treated with antibiotics if she is in a high-risk category. In view of the potentially devastating effects on newborns and infants, some obstetricians and pediatricians have recommended a public education campaign to test all pregnant women for carrier status. A group of parents whose babies died of the infection has formed a national organization to alert the public and health professionals to the disease and to spur research efforts and the development of a vaccine.

Postpartum Depression

Postpartum depression affects one in seven new mothers and may last for many months. The World Health Organization (2008) reports that women are twice as prone to depression as men (five percent compared to 2.5 percent) and that depression rates increase during pregnancy (eight-10 percent) and especially in the year following delivery (18 percent). Symptoms usually appear within the first six months after the birth of a child. Although the precise cause of postpartum depression is unknown, it has been suggested that fluctuations in gonadal hormones as the body readjusts after pregnancy may play a role. Many of the symptoms of postpartum depression, including changes in sleep patterns, energy level, and appetite, are easy to misinterpret as normal experiences during and immediately after pregnancy. Other symptoms include: difficulty concentrating, irritability, heightened anxiety, and obsessive thoughts, as well as a disinterest in daily activities. There are potential complications associated with postpartum depression including difficulty bonding with the baby, which can lead to emotional, social, and cognitive problems in the child later on (ACOG, 2007). In addition, recent evidence suggests that women suffering from postpartum depression are less likely to successfully initiate and maintain breast-feeding of their infants (Dennis & MCQueen, 2009). Treatments include psychotherapy in mild cases and psychotherapy plus short-term use of medications in moderate and severe cases.

MONITORING THE MOTHER AND BABY'S PROGRESS DURING PREGNANCY

There are a number of methods available for monitoring the progress of the developing fetus during pregnancy. These methods are often used to test for genetic and developmental disorders such as Down syndrome or neural tube defects. New methods are periodically being developed. Some of the techniques used to monitor the fetus's progress in the womb include nuchal translucency test (NT), blood tests, amniocentesis, chorionic villi testing, ultrasound, and fetoscopy. In 2007, the American College of Obstetricians and Gynecologists issued guidelines recommending that all women, regardless of age, have access to diagnostic testing, and that pregnant women should consider the least invasive screening options for assessing the risk of Down syndrome (ACOG, 2007). The benefits of testing must be weighed against the risks of the tests themselves.

Diagnostic Ultrasound

The ultrasound scanner consists of a small handheld transducer or scanner that converts electrical energy into sound waves. As the waves, emitted in the form of pulses or short bursts, encounter blood, bones, and organs of different densities, they are reflected back toward the source. These bounced-back echoes of sound waves are shown as a pattern on a viewing screen (Figure 12-8). Ultrasound, or sonography, has dramatically increased diagnostic capabilities. Ultrasound can assist in accurately dating the age of the fetus. Knowledge of gestational age is important for amniocentesis, for determining whether preterm labor should be stopped with drugs or the delivery allowed to take place, and for assessing the status of an alleged post due-date fetus before induction of labor. Determining the age of the fetus is essential when a repeat cesarean is scheduled. Ultrasound can also confirm a suspected multiple pregnancy, evaluate the reason for bleeding during pregnancy, and determine a variety of fetal abnormalities. Ultrasonography can also help detect ectopic pregnancy. The nuchal translucency (NT) test is performed by using ultrasound

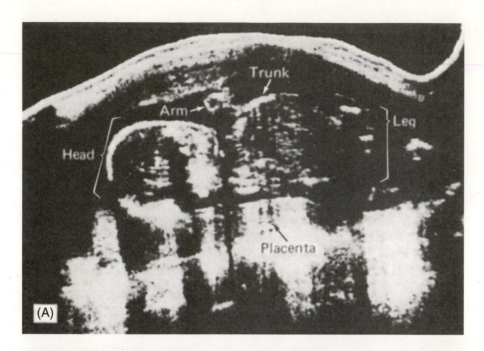

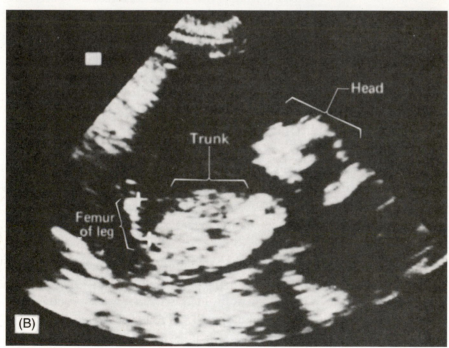

FIGURE 12-8: Ultrasonography of fetus. A. 25-week Fetus B. 15-Week Fetus. *(Courtesy of Sinai-Samaritan Medical Center, Milwaukee, WI)*

to measure the fluid filled area of the baby's neck at 10–14 weeks gestation. This test is used to detect Down syndrome in the fetus. The American College of Obstetricians and Gynecologists (2007) has recommended that NT testing plus a blood test during the first trimester is more effective than NT alone and together constitute an effective screening test for the general public. If screening suggests Down syndrome,

amniocentesis or chorionic villi sampling can confirm the results.

Ultrasound is currently considered safe (Figure 12-9). As yet, there is no evidence of any dangerous effects of ultrasound to humans, but neither is there sufficient evidence to state for certain that it is completely harmless. Ultrasound energy is not ionizing radiation like X-rays with known

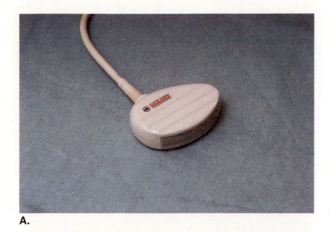

A.

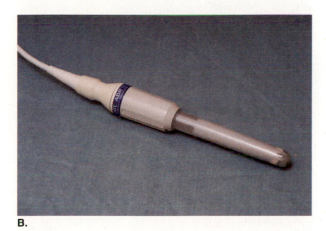

B.

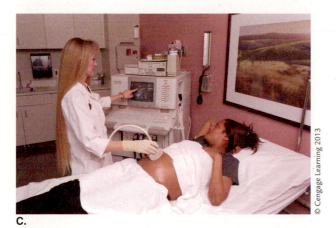

C.

© Cengage Learning 2013

FIGURE 12-9: Transabdominal Ultrasonography.
A. Transabdominal ultrasound transducer. B. Transvaginal ultrasound transducer. C. Transabdominal ultrasonography.

harmful effects. There are, however, at least two ways that ultrasound could cause damage to tissues. One is the production of heat, which can be appreciable in some of the newer, more powerful ultrasound equipment, particularly Doppler ultrasound. At present, some researchers discourage the use of Doppler ultrasound during the first trimester of fetal development (Houston et al., 2009). A second mechanism is mechanical vibrations, which can lead to a phenomenon called cavitations. With cavitations, gas microbubbles form, increase in size, and burst in the tissues in response to sound waves, potentially disrupting fetal cells. Although damage to insect eggs and some mammalian tissue has been produced by ultrasound-induced cavitations, the implications for human tissue are still unknown. Several long-term follow-up investigations of children exposed to prenatal diagnostic ultrasound, have produced reassuring results concerning detrimental consequences such as miscarriage, congenital abnormalities, communicative disorders, or cancer. However, many of these studies were based on older less powerful ultrasound technology and further study is needed to understand the effects of more powerful technologies currently in use (Houston et al., 2009). There have been, however, several reports of a curious association between routine ultrasound screening in utero and subsequent left-handedness, especially in boys, but researchers found no evidence of impaired neurological development or attention deficit (Salvesen et al., 1993; Kieler et al., 1998). Of particular concern, however, are commercial services that provide "keepsake" images for purchase. These services are usually not overseen by trained medical personnel and often use powerful imaging technologies that can cause thermal and mechanical damage to the fetus. Both the American College of Obstetrics and Gynecologists (ACOG) and the United States Department of Agriculture (USDA), advise against the use of these imaging services (ACOG, 2004; Phillips et al., 2010).

Amniocentesis

It is possible to detect chromosomal abnormalities, neural tube disorders, and over 70 hereditary biochemical disorders in the fetus before birth by amniocentesis. The cells in the amniotic fluid have sloughed off from the fetus or from the amniotic membrane and are genetically identical to those of the fetus. On an outpatient basis, an amniotic fluid tap can be performed between the 14th and 16th weeks of pregnancy. Using an ultrasound image as a guide, a needle is inserted through the abdominal

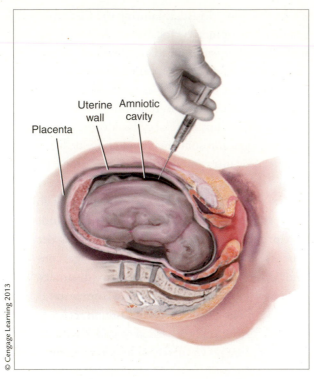

FIGURE 12-10: Amniocentesis. A sample of amniotic fluid is withdrawn for analysis.

wall and a small sample of amniotic fluid is withdrawn (Figure 12-10). The sample is then tested for chromosomal abnormalities, biochemical traits and immunoassays.

Although complications of the procedure are infrequent, amniocentesis is not without some danger to the fetus and to the mother. Fetal risks can include rupture of the membranes and a subsequent

miscarriage. The estimated increased risk of miscarriage as a result of amniocentesis is 0.08–2.5 percent. The risk of miscarriage is greater in twin pregnancies. Other complications include bleeding as a result of the needle hitting a fetal blood vessel or puncture of the fetus leading to scars, depressions, or dimples. Maternal risks include puncture of the bladder, intestine, or a blood vessel, but the likelihood of serious injury is quite small. Risks for the fetus and mother appear to increase when amniocentesis is performed during the last three months of pregnancy.

Chorionic Villi Sampling

Another method of prenatal detection of genetic abnormalities that can be performed in the first trimester of pregnancy is called chorionic villi sampling (CVS). This method typically yields results faster than amniocentesis. Performed between the eighth and 10th weeks of pregnancy, the technique involves the insertion, under ultrasound guidance, of a small plastic catheter through the cervix or trans abdominally into the uterus in order to withdraw a sample of chorionic villi tissue, the fetal contribution to the early placenta (Figure 12-11). The tissue sample is processed for chromosome studies, and preliminary results of the chorionic cell analyses can be obtained within 24 hours. The chorionic sampling procedure has the advantage of earlier detection over amniocentesis, but there are increased risks. The miscarriage rate, although small, currently is estimated to

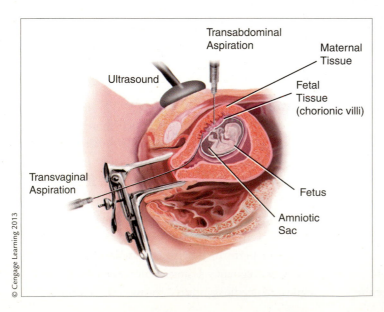

FIGURE 12-11: Chorionic Villi Sampling. A sample of the placenta is removed for analysis.

be greater than that associated with amniocentesis performed at 15–18 weeks of gestation. Cramping and vaginal bleeding may occur, and there have been some reports of uterine infection with serious complications.

Fetalscopy

Fetoscopy is the technique of directly viewing the fetus within the uterus using fiber-optics. This allows visualization of anatomical abnormalities such as limb defects or facial clefts. The technique is currently performed to confirm or exclude a genetic defect found through amniocentesis, or a congenital anomaly detected by ultrasonography. The procedure has also been used to provide fetal therapy or to obtain a fetal biopsy. Fetoscopy is a higher risk procedure than other techniques used to assess the fetus. There is a chance of complications, including bleeding, amniotic fluid leakage, or pregnancy loss through infection or miscarriage. Fetoscopy is also associated with premature delivery. Because of the risks associated with this procedure, it is rarely employed as the primary prenatal diagnostic method.

Contraction Stress Test and Nonstress Test prior to Labor

The **contraction stress test (CST)** tries to duplicate the stresses of labor in order to determine how well the placenta can circulate blood to the fetus during contractions and how well the fetus can tolerate labor. Usually this test is performed when a placental insufficiency is suspected, as in the cases of preeclampsia, intrauterine growth retardation, diabetes mellitus, or a previous stillbirth. This test may also be warranted when an irregularity of fetal heart rate has been observed. The test involves stimulating contractions with oxytocin and monitoring the fetal heart rate and the pattern of contractions.

Originally prescribed only for high-risk pregnancies, the CST has become widely used as a general screening for a successful labor and delivery, despite some of the inherent risks of the test itself. This test has some serious limitations, however, and is prone to a large percentage of false positives and occasional false negatives. One of the reasons for the high percentage of false positives is that the injection of oxytocin can stimulate the kind of uterine contractions that

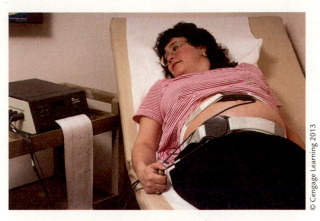

FIGURE 12-12: An expectant mother undergoing a nonstress test.

can themselves compromise the oxygen supply of the fetus enough to produce a "positive" interpretation of the results. This result can then lead to an unnecessary cesarean section.

A fetal nonstress test (NST) is based on the premise that a fetus's well-being can be assessed by the increase in fetal heart rate in response to fetal movement. During this test, an external monitor is used to record the fetal heartbeat as the fetus spontaneously moves around after the mother drinks a sweet drink (Figure 12-12). After 20–40 minutes of recording, the results are classified as "reactive" or "nonreactive," based on its baseline heart rate compared to the heart rate during movement. If the heart rate increases in response to movement the fetus is said to be "reactive." A nonreactive test has been correlated to a higher incidence of fetal distress during labor, fetal mortality, and intrauterine growth retardation, and is seen as an indication for a contraction stress test as a follow-up procedure. Like the CST, this test is also prone to a high rate of false positives.

MEDICAL PROCEDURES AND INTERVENTIONS DURING LABOR AND DELIVERY

Labor is a normal physiological process. However the process does have potential risks and medical interventions -from simple pain management to surgery - have been a part of labor and delivery throughout history. Low-risk pregnancies should require few if any interventions. The use of interventions varies widely around the world and, as women's health has become increasingly medicalized, interventions have become common in low risk pregnancies.

The practice of applying medical interventions to low risk deliveries has raised important questions about commonly used interventions. These questions have led to research on the long-term effects of some of the commonly used childbirth interventions, and the results are now appearing in scientific and professional journals. An increasing number of studies link commonly used childbirth interventions such as episiotomy and cesarean section with long-term postpartum health problems. These problems include urinary stress incontinence, urinary urge incontinence, fecal incontinence, and sexual dysfunction (Borders, 2006; van Brummen et al., 2006). While it is impossible to predict what will happen during each labor and delivery, and emergencies can necessitate interventions even when they are not planned for, women and healthcare providers should consider the long-term effects of some of these commonly used procedures. There is also concern that the use of one medical intervention can make it more likely that additional interventions will be needed.

Lithotomy Position

In the lithotomy position, a woman gives birth while lying on her back with her feet in stirrups. This position gained popularity with obstetricians in the middle of the twentieth century because it allows easy access to a birthing mother's vagina if the obstetrician determines that medical procedures are needed. Unfortunately, the lithotomy position requires a woman to push against gravity while in labor and puts undue stress on her pelvic floor. In addition, the weight of the baby in this position puts pressure on the blood vessels in the mother's abdomen and can cause the laboring mother to feel light-headed. When women give birth in positions that are more comfortable, these problems can be alleviated.

Induction of Labor

Labor can be induced or a slow labor can be sped up by the administration of the drug pitocin, a synthetic form of oxytocin. Other common methods of inducing labor include breaking the fetal membranes and applying prostaglandins to the cervix to stimulate contractions (Sakala & Corry, 2008). Often a combination of methods is used to induce labor (Declereq et al., 2006). Induction of labor

should rarely be necessary in a typical pregnancy and delivery. However, the percentage of births that result from induced labor has increased dramatically in the United States in recent decades. In 1990, 9.5 percent of labors were induced and by 2005, the percentage had risen to 22.3 percent (Hamilton et al., 2007; Martin et al., 2006). Some researchers argue that the numbers may be even higher (Yasmeen et al., 2006). Inducing labor may be required when an early delivery is necessary, as in severe preeclampsia, Rh incompatibility, or diabetes mellitus, or when the membranes have ruptured prematurely and infection could occur. Labor may also be induced in the case of a pregnancy that is prolonged past the due date. Some researchers have suggested that for overdue pregnancies at 41 weeks, the risks of induction are offset by the benefits of potentially avoiding a cesarean section, although more research is needed (Coughey, 2009).

The Listening to Mothers II Survey (DeClereq et al., 2006), conducted by the nonprofit organization, Childbirth Connection, found that mothers gave the following reasons, or combinations of reasons, for why they experienced induction of labor: caregiver's concern that the baby was overdue (25 percent), maternal health problems that called for quick delivery (19 percent), mother's desire to end the pregnancy (19 percent), a desire to control the timing of the birth either by the mother or the caregiver (18 percent), and caregiver's concern about the size of the baby (17 percent). Other, less common reasons given for labor induction were concern about infection after membranes had broken (nine percent), and concern for the baby's health (nine percent). Inducing labor to control the timing of delivery is considered to be primarily for convenience. The safety of purely elective induction is questionable, and the United States Food and Drug Administration restricts the use of pitocin for inducing labor to medical reasons only. There are some potential drawbacks to using pitocin to induce labor. Pitocin is a highly potent drug and difficult to control. Overdosage can result in uterine contractions that are too strong or too frequent, and if the uterus is hypersensitive, the results could be disastrous. In addition, fetal heart rate abnormalities during labor and a significant increase in the incidence of neonatal jaundice have been directly attributed to the use of pitocin to induce labor (Conner & Seaton, 1982). Finally, pitocin interferes with a laboring mother's receptors for her own oxytocin hormone, and this can disrupt the effectiveness of her natural oxytocin to accomplish other important functions during labor and delivery such as reducing postpartum hemorrhage when the placenta is delivered (Phaeuf, 2000). Oxytocin hormone is also important for establishing feelings of attachment in the mother for the infant and it plays an important role in breast-feeding (Buckley, 2004b). While there may be circumstances when the induction of labor is needed to preserve the health of the mother or infant, it is important to consider that there are costs to bypassing the physiological events that constitute spontaneous labor and delivery. Research indicates that spontaneous labor is triggered by the interplay of signals between the mother and the fetus; signals which may indicate that the fetus is mature enough and ready to be born. Determining gestational age by ultrasound and other means is not always accurate, so a high incidence of labor inductions may be contributing to a significant number of premature infants.

Fetal Heart Rate Monitoring

Since its development in the 1980s, the use of continuous or intermittent electronic fetal heart rate monitoring (EFM) during labor has become routine in almost all United States hospitals. EFM has replaced the stethoscope as the primary method of observing changes that would indicate fetal distress (Figure 12-13). The normal fetal heart rate is between 110 and 160 beats per minute, although it is normal for the rate to slow during contractions. A heart rate that does not vary, or remains too slow or too fast is considered abnormal (ACOG, 2009). Abnormal fetal heartbeat combined with an abnormally low fetal blood pH is indication that the fetus is suffering from lack of oxygen, indicating fetal distress. When brain cells are deprived of oxygen, they undergo irreversible injury, and brain damage or death can be the result. EFM was created to detect asphyxiation in the infant that could lead to cerebral palsy. In the 20 plus years since its introduction, it has been found that only 0.2 percent of children with cerebral palsy had abnormal EFM reading

during delivery. In that time period, there has been no decline in cerebral palsy. One study (Graham et al., 2006) showed a decrease in neonatal seizures with continuous use of EFM, but no other significant benefits.

Recently, there has been increasing controversy about the overall benefit of using EFM, especially in the case of low risk deliveries. John M Freeman (2007) of Johns Hopkins University School of Medicine has pointed out that the use of fetal heart rate monitoring during normal deliveries has led to the creation of a pseudo disease, namely the abnormalities of fetal heart rate during the birth process. Reacting to these supposed abnormalities has led to an increased tendency to interfere with the birth process and to use medical interventions, when there is not good scientific evidence that they are needed and beneficial. In some cases, interventions are potentially harmful.

One of the disadvantages of EFM is that the position necessary for EFM, lying flat on the back, is the worst possible position for labor and delivery. It adversely affects comfort, lowers uterine activity, and causes what can be a dangerous drop in the mother's blood pressure. In some women, blood pressure falls by more than a third and fetal oxygen deprivation results. Furthermore, to attach the electrodes for internal monitoring, the fetal membranes have to be artificially ruptured (amniotomy) early in labor (Figure 12-14). Because the protection afforded by the amniotic fluid is now lost, the fetal head is more vulnerable. The uterine contractions produce uneven pressure on the head, which can result in decreased cerebral blood flow and a decrease in fetal heart rate. Both the position and the procedure for EFM, designed to indicate fetal distress, can actually cause fetal distress.

Additional adverse effects of fetal monitoring include an increased incidence of uterine infections as a result of the leads introduced into the uterus and the fetal complication of scalp abscess and infection. For the woman in labor, the electronic fetal heart rate monitor can be disconcerting, if not frightening. It may be impossible to concentrate on relaxation techniques while hooked up to a machine with flashing lights and heartbeat sounds. Finally, there are large inconsistencies in how individual doctors interpret

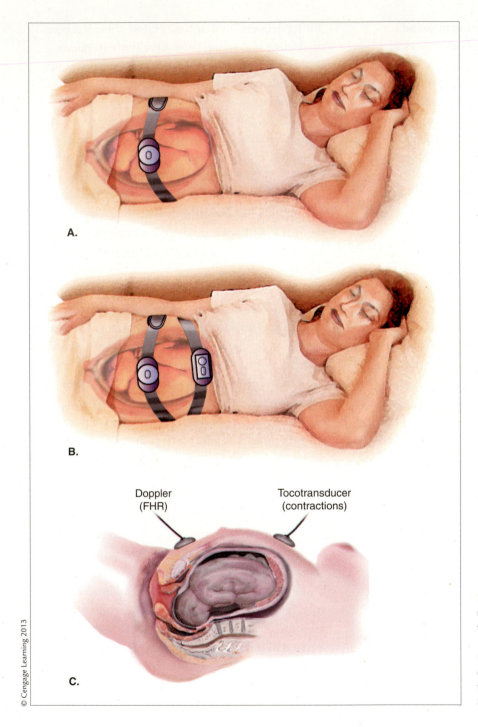

A.

B.

Doppler (FHR)   Tocotransducer (contractions)

C.

© Cengage Learning 2013

FIGURE 12-13: External fetal heart rate monitoring. A. Ultrasound transducer in place over fetal heart. B. Tocotransducer in place over the uterine fundus. C. Lateral view of the correct placement of Doppler and the tocotransducer on the maternal abdomen.

the numbers produced by EFM signals and misinterpretations have tended to lead to increases in medical interventions during childbirth. Widespread inconsistencies in the interpretation of EFM signals have prompted the American College of Obstetricians and Gynecologists to refine their Guidelines for Fetal Heart Rate Monitoring (AGOG, 2009). It is without question that during the past decades the substitution of cesarean section for a vaginal delivery has increased tremendously in association with electronic fetal heart rate monitoring. This shift toward more C-sections has been at the cost of increased maternal mortality and morbidity. Recent research on EFM has continued to provide somewhat ambiguous conclusions regarding its benefits, although it has now been very widely adopted.

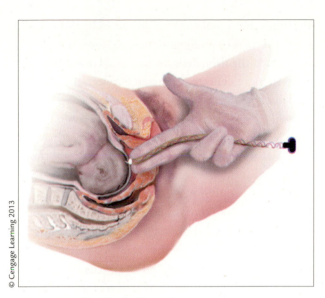

FIGURE 12-14: Fetal Scalp Electrode.

Pain Medications

There are two major categories of pain medications that are used during childbirth, and these are regional anesthetics and systemic analgesics. Both categories have advantages and disadvantages that must be weighed carefully by a woman and her doctor to minimize harmful effects on either herself or her baby. All drugs, whether they are given systemically, inhaled as gases, or injected for a local nerve block, carry some risks. Medications move into the bloodstream; cross the placenta; and depending on the time of administration, the kind of drug, and the dosage, can affect the fetus and the newborn baby. Because a baby is unable to metabolize or excrete the drug as rapidly or effectively as an adult, the infant may be born with a varying amount of respiratory and nervous system depression, resulting in a lowered APGAR score. Medications can cross the placenta and cause the fetus and neonate to be less alert and less active. This change in the newborn's alertness can interfere with establishing breast-feeding (Reynolds, 2010). Because using modern pain medications during childbirth is a relatively recent phenomenon, there has not yet been enough time to conduct many scientific studies to evaluate the long-term effects of these medications on infants who are exposed to them. Recent studies, however, suggest a link between exposure to pain medications during birth and the increased risk of developing drug addiction later in life. Until more is known about the long-term effects of pain medications during

childbirth, common sense dictates that avoiding pain medications all together or using the least depressing drug in the lowest possible dosage is best.

Regional Blocks

Regional pain relief means that the sensory nerve impulses from the pelvic area are blocked by the injection of a local anesthetic in the same way that the dentist treats a tooth before drilling. The most common technique in the United States is epidural anesthesia which has replaced other types of local anesthetics. Other regional anesthetics include the paracervical, pudendal, and the "spinals"—subarachnoid, saddle, and continuous caudal blocks. All have advantages and disadvantages.

A paracervical block is an injection that deadens the sensations arising from the dilating cervix during the first stage of labor (Figure 12-15). When the cervix has dilated to 4 or 5 cm, a local anesthetic is injected into the lateral fornix on either side. The anesthesia does not last very long and may have to be repeated after an hour or two. Transitory slowing of the fetal heart rate as a result of repeated injections

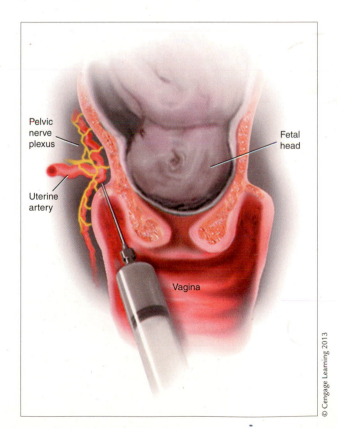

Pelvic
nerve
plexus

Fetal
head

Uterine
artery

Vagina

FIGURE 12-15: Paracervical block.

has been observed, so the total drug dosage must be monitored.

A pudendal block anesthetizes the nerve supply to the perineum, the vulva, and the vagina. The injection can be made directly through the perineal tissue or, as is more frequent, through the vagina (transvaginally). The nerve block takes effect in five minutes and lasts about an hour. If given, it is usually injected late in the second stage of labor when the cervix is completely dilated; it decreases the vaginal and perineal discomfort of the actual delivery. The pudendal block does not decrease the pain of contractions, however, so it is sometimes supplemented by another pain medication.

The remaining regional anesthetics are called spinals because the injections are made into the coverings around the spinal cord itself (Figure 12-16).

The brain and spinal cord are protected by three complete coverings or meninges: the outermost tough dura mater, the thin, delicate arachnoid mater, and the even more delicate pia mater. Between the arachnoid mater and the pia mater is the subarachnoid space filled with cerebrospinal fluid that cushions the brain and spinal cord. The sensory nerves that carry pain impulses from the pelvic organs enter the spinal cord at the level of the 11th and 12th thoracic vertebrae. The motor nerves that cause uterine contractions exit from the cord higher up, at the level of the seventh and eighth thoracic vertebrae. Therefore, injections of an anesthetic that are made below the eighth thoracic vertebra will block all sensations but should, theoretically, not interfere with uterine contractions. However, this is not always the case.

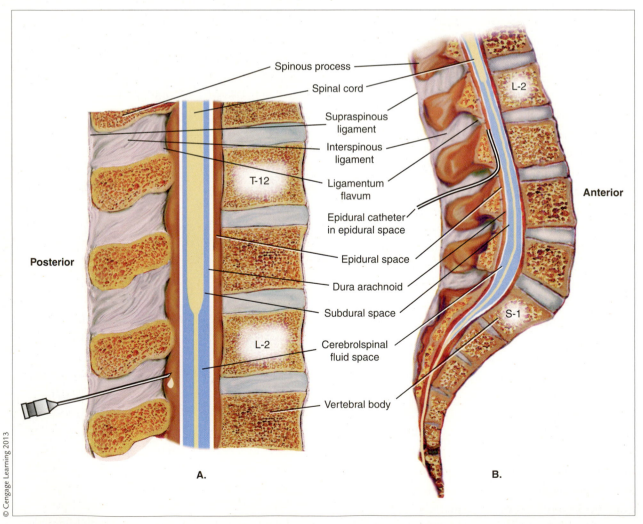

FIGURE 12-16: Epidural Block. A. Placement of the epidural needle in the epidural space. B. Placement of a catheter in the epidural space.

Epidural anesthesia is achieved by an injection into the epidural space, which lies just outside the meninges, specialized membranes that protect the spinal cord. Lumbar epidural analgesia has become the most popular anesthetic during labor and delivery. It gives complete relief from pain with fewer effects on the mother and infant than most other types of medication. It may be given as a single dose just before delivery, but, more commonly, continuous administration is started during the first stage of labor. With the woman lying on her left side, a needle is introduced between the third and fourth lumbar vertebrae until it reaches the epidural space. A plastic catheter is then threaded through the needle, the needle is withdrawn, and the catheter is taped into place on the skin so that appropriate doses of the local anesthetic drug can be given at intervals.

Continuous epidural block is popular because of the high degree of pain relief and the reduction of fetal depression compared to other pain killing medications. There are, however, several disadvantages to its use. It requires an experienced anesthesiologist to time it properly and perform it safely and effectively. It slows labor in the first stage and causes the pushing reflex in the second stage to be reduced or lost so that the baby may have to be delivered by forceps. A reduction in the mother's blood pressure is an ever-present complication. Uncontrollable shaking of the legs or a temporary paralysis may occur. Neither is significant or lasts very long but can certainly be alarming if a woman is unprepared. And finally, if the dura mater is accidentally perforated, the result will be a subarachnoid anesthesia which increases the chance of a post spinal headache. For a cesarean section, a larger volume of drug is administered to produce greater blocking of pain higher up in the cord. The subarachnoid spinal and the caudal block are similar to an epidural block except that the site of the needle insertion is different.

Systemic Analgesics

Systemic analgesia was once the preferred technique of pain relief in the United States and still is in those hospitals where the trained personnel needed to administer the currently popular lumbar epidural analgesia are unavailable. These drugs include tranquilizers, sedatives, narcotics, and barbiturates. Tranquilizers and sedatives have been used in early labor if a woman is particularly tense and anxious. They do not relieve pain but diminish anxiety. Sedatives and tranquilizers can slow labor, cause drowsiness or sleep, and occasionally result in dizziness, nausea, and vomiting. In some women, their use results in paradoxical effects, and mood elevation, excitement, restlessness, or even delirium may occur. The closer to delivery the drugs are given, the more likely that they will cause central nervous system depression in the newborn.

Narcotic pain reliever increases a laboring woman's tolerance to pain. It easily crosses the placenta, so the amount and timing of administration are very important. If labor takes less time than expected, the adverse effects of the drug on the fetus/newborn are evidenced by respiratory depression. Adverse effects on the mother may include nausea, vomiting, and rapid heartbeat, so the drug should be used cautiously in women with cardiac disease.

Inhaling gas through a mask to provide complete anesthesia or loss of consciousness is virtually nonexistent nowadays, but whiffs of low-concentration nitrous oxide-oxygen mixtures in a self-administered vaporizer can be used intermittently during the second stage of labor. Because there is a time lag of several seconds before the gas can get from the lungs into the bloodstream and to the brain, the inhalation has to be started before the contraction begins for maximum pain relief. Fetal depression is possible, but rare, with low concentrations of gas.

Relief of Pain without Medication

There are mechanical and physical reasons for discomfort in childbirth; no one invents or imagines it. But there is evidence from laboratory studies that while everyone probably feels pain in the same way physiologically, there is enormous variation in the way that different individuals perceive and respond to pain. The degree and quality of pain during labor and delivery can be greatly influenced by a woman's attitude and preconceived notions toward the birth process. Prepared childbirth techniques such as Lamaze and other relaxation techniques can help to reduce the stress and pain of childbirth (Figure 12-17).

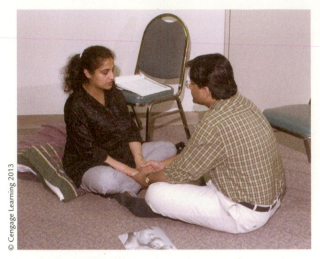

© Cengage Learning 2013

FIGURE 12-17: Childbirth preparation classes teach breathing and relaxation techniques for pain relief during labor.

There are many alternatives available for women who want to eliminate or minimize their use of pain medications during labor. Acupuncture, a thousand-year-old Chinese method of anesthesia, performed by placing slender needles in acupuncture points on the body, has been used for cesarean deliveries in China, and in labor and vaginal deliveries in the West. After the needles are inserted, they may be stimulated by rotation or electric current. Hypnosis, an altered state of consciousness, is reportedly effective when the woman has had previous training sessions with a skilled hypnotist who is, preferably, also skilled in obstetrics. Transcutaneous electrical nerve stimulation, also known as TENS, utilizes the application of a mild electric current to the skin to enhance the body's production of the pain-relieving endorphins. The device is placed on the chest area at specific points. The frequency and intensity of the stimulation is ordinarily hand-controlled by the laboring mother, who can increase the amount during contractions.

Another way of shortening labor, reducing the need for epidural anesthesia, and significantly reducing cesarean section rates could be a very old-fashioned method—the reliance on a birthing companion. Pediatricians Kennell and Klaus (1991) conducted a controlled, randomized, clinical trial with 616 women who gave birth in a technologically sophisticated hospital in Texas. Of the women studied, one-third, or 216, received emotional support that included continuous talking and touching from a "doula," a Greek term that means an experienced woman who guides and helps a new mother in infant care. The doula met the laboring woman at the time of hospital admission and remained at her bedside—soothing and encouraging her throughout delivery. The doulas in the study were from 22–55 years of age, had each delivered at least one child vaginally, and had taken eight weeks of training. The second group of 200 women was observed in the delivery room, and the remaining women constituted the control group and received no special treatment. The researchers reported that the women with doulas had labors about two hours shorter than those who received no special care, that epidural block was used in 7.8 percent of the supported women as compared to 22.6 percent in the observed group and 55.3 percent of the control group, and that only eight percent of the doula-attended women had cesarean deliveries compared with 13 percent of the observed and 18 percent of the control women (Kennell et al., 1991).

Episiotomy

An **episiotomy** is a surgical cut through the perineum to enlarge the vagina during childbirth. In rare cases episiotomy may be necessary to prevent damage to the infant or to prevent more serious injury to the posterior wall of the mother's vagina or rectum during delivery. An episiotomy may be extended in a lateral direction at about a 45° angle to the left or to the right, or more rarely it may be midline and extended from the vagina directly down toward the anus (Figure 12-18). The timing of the cut is important: if it is done too early, the normal blood loss will increase; if it is performed too late, lacerations may have already taken place. Both the World Health Organization (Liljestrand, 2003) and the American College of Obstetricians and Gynecologists (ACOG, 2003) have issued statements that it is undesirable for episiotomy to be performed routinely, and its use in the United States has been declining in the past decades from 60.9 percent in 1979 (Frankman, 2009) to 25 percent in 2005 (DeClereq, 2006). It should be noted, however, that there is tremendous regional variation in the United States in the rate

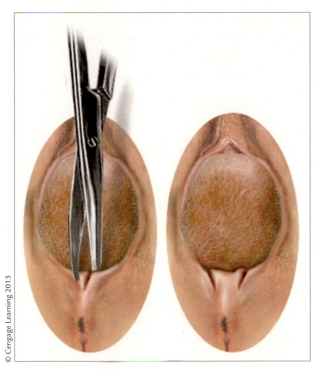

FIGURE 12-18: Episiotomy.

of episiotomy, even variation from one hospital to another. Episiotomy is still very common though in some parts of the world.

Originally, episiotomy was thought to prevent pelvic floor relaxation after the baby was born. Pelvic floor relaxation can lead to both short- and long-term problems with urinary and fecal incontinence. Recent scientific evidence, however, indicates that episiotomy does not prevent pelvic floor relaxation and increases a women's chance of experiencing long-term urinary incontinence (Kudish et al., 2008; Cohain, 2008; Hartman, et al., 2005). Episiotomy also increases the chances of anal sphincter tears during childbirth (Frankman et al., 2009; Baydock et al., 2009, Wheeler and Richter, 2007), which can lead to fecal incontinence. Furthermore, cutting through the tissues of the perineum can result in damage to erectile tissues in the vicinity of the vagina. Damaged erectile tissues can be replaced with fibrotic scar tissue, resulting in diminished sexual function (Williams et al., 2007; Signorello et al., 2001). Episiotomies have to be sutured after the baby and the placenta are delivered, when the perineum is still extremely sensitive. Even with a local anesthetic, the repair is usually quite painful. As the stitches heal and are absorbed

in the postpartum period, there is also considerable discomfort.

There are birthing practices that can help the laboring mother avoid the need for an episiotomy. Perineal massage practiced at home for a month before delivery and then performed by the birth attendant during the second stage of labor is advocated by some nurse-midwives and may help to prevent perineal tearing. The lithotomy position in which a woman lies on her back during delivery may also make it more likely that an episiotomy will be needed because of the increased tension on the pelvic floor. Alternative birth positions, such as those used in home deliveries or nontraditional settings, appear to lessen the strain on the perineum and reduce the need for an episiotomy. Additional medical procedures such as inducing labor and the use of forceps or vacuum extraction are often done in conjunction with episiotomy, so avoiding these procedures also decreases a woman's chances of having an episiotomy. Because the routine use of episiotomy varies so much between practitioners, it is important for women to discuss their preferences regarding episiotomy with their caregiver.

Assisted Vaginal Births

Assisted vaginal births, also called operative vaginal births, rely on the use of forceps or vacuum extraction. These tools are used to pull on the fetus's head while the mother pushes during labor (Figure 12-19 and Figure 12-20). Forceps and vacuum extraction are often used in conjunction with an episiotomy. These methods are usually used when progress moving the baby through the birth canal during the pushing stage has ceased or if the baby is close to being delivered and an urgent problem has developed requiring the head to be shifted to a better position for birth. About 8.7 percent of babies in the United States were born by assisted vaginal delivery in 1979, and that rate declined to five percent in 2009. Some researchers have suggested that the number of assisted vaginal births has declined as obstetricians began to favor cesarean section as the preferred method for difficult births (Frankman et al., 2009). As with episiotomy, there is wide geographic variation in the United States in the use of assisted vaginal birth (Clark et al., 2007). It is estimated that the rate of operative vaginal

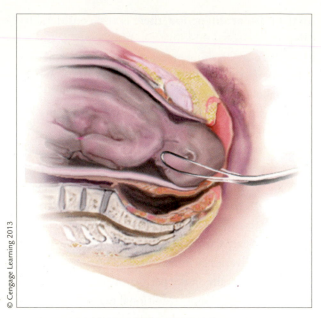

© Cengage Learning 2013

FIGURE 12-19: Assisted vaginal birth using forceps.

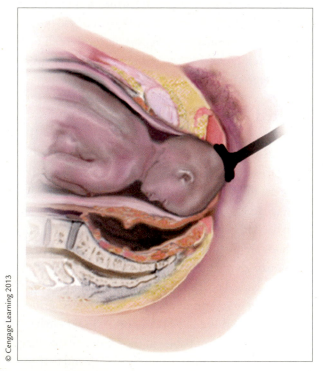

© Cengage Learning 2013

FIGURE 12-20: Assisted vaginal birth using vacuum extraction.

births ranges between five percent and 20 percent in industrialized nations (Majoko & Gardener, 2008). The need for these interventions is more likely if the mother is lying on her back in the lithotomy position as she pushes. The use of epidural anesthesia may also

contribute to slowing the progress of the second stage of labor because it diminishes the Ferguson reflex that triggers the laboring mother to push. If progress is slowed too much, forceps or vacuum extraction may be used.

The use of forceps or vacuum extraction does pose some short- and long-term risks to mothers and infants, and these risks must to be weighed when deciding if and when these methods are necessary. There is an increased risk of damage to the mother's perineum and pelvic floor, especially when forceps are used, when compared to spontaneous or unassisted vaginal birth (Prapas et al., 2009; Caughey et al., 2005; Kudish et al., 2008; Benedetto et al., 2007). Pelvic floor damage can increase the chances of short- or long-term urinary or fecal incontinence (Baydock, 2009; Pretlove et al., 2008; Dudding et al., 2008; Wheeler and Richter, 2007). Perineal injuries can also contribute to pain during intercourse. Some studies have found that vacuum extraction is associated with fewer incidences of pelvic floor damage than forceps assisted births (Vacca, 2002). Some risks to the infant include retinal hemorrhages, intracranial hemorrhage and hematomas, clavicle fractures, shoulder nerve injuries, low APGAR score, and respiratory distress (Prapas et al., 2009; Caughey et al., 2005; Lurie et al., 2005; Demissie et al., 2004). In cases where help is needed to deliver the baby, these risks must be weighed against the short- and long-term risks of cesarean section to both the mother and the infant.

Cesarean Sections

A **cesarean section** (C-section) is the surgical removal of a fetus through an incision in the mother's abdomen (Figure 12-21). Cesarean section was developed to remove a baby from the uterus if it became impossible for it to be delivered vaginally. Although relatively safe, cesarean sections do pose risks to both mothers and their infants. The World Health Organization has determined that a five percent rate of Cesarean section births in a country's population is a healthy average rate (Althabe & Belizan, 2006). This means that for five out of every 100 deliveries, a complication or emergency may arise in which a cesarean section is the best alternative available to preserve the health of the mother or her infant. However, in cases without

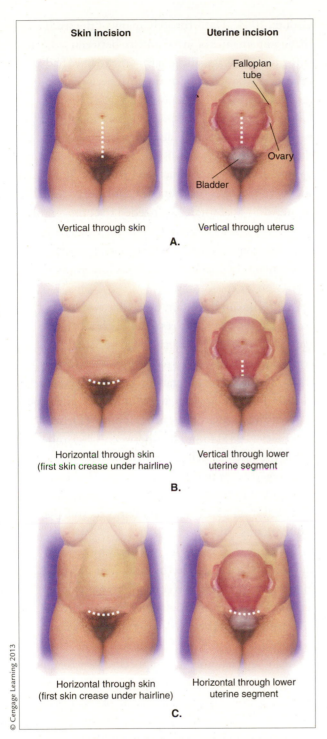

Skin incision | **Uterine incision**

Fallopian tube

Ovary

Bladder

Vertical through skin | Vertical through uterus

A.

Horizontal through skin (first skin crease under hairline) | Vertical through lower uterine segment

B.

Horizontal through skin (first skin crease under hairline) | Horizontal through lower uterine segment

C.

© Cengage Learning 2013

FIGURE 12-21: Cesarean section incisions. A. Skin and uterine incisions are both vertical. This type of incision is most often used in emergency situations. B. Horizontal skin and low vertical uterine incision. C. Horizontal skin and uterine incision.

in countries where cesarean section rates are over five percent, mothers and their infants are being placed under unnecessary risk of negative health effects. In spite of this guideline, the rate of cesarean section is rising dramatically in some parts of the world, especially in the United States. In 1965, only 4.5 percent of deliveries in the United States were cesarean births. By the end of 1996, the number had almost quadrupled to 20.7 percent and by 2006 the rate jumped to over 31 percent. By 2008, for every 100 babies born, 33 were delivered by cesarean section. This statistic is even more startling when one realizes that one in three women in the United States experiences childbirth as a surgical procedure (Sakala & Corry, 2008).

A number of explanations have been suggested for the precipitous increase in cesareans in the United States. Fetal distress, dystocia, and breech presentation are the other major indications for cesarean delivery. Currently, most breech presentations are delivered by cesarean before labor begins to avoid any risk of fetal asphyxia, even though it is sometimes possible to reposition a breech baby. Although older physicians were trained in the delivery of breech babies, many younger doctors lack experience in vaginal delivery. Forceps deliveries, because of potential risks to the mother and infant, are often avoided in favor of surgical delivery. An additional factor contributing to the greater incidence of cesarean sections is the older age of first-time mothers, those who have delayed childbearing and, hence, are seen as being at greater risk for complications after age 30. However, the cesarean rate has also increased for women under 30, and this may lead to even greater numbers in the future because of the dictum, "once a cesarean, always a cesarean." More than one-third of all cesareans are performed on women who have had a previous cesarean.

A review of studies from 1950 to 1980 (Lavin et al., 1982) presented data to show that vaginal delivery is safe in 74.2 percent of women who have had a previous C-section. It may even be a safe alternative in 33.3 percent of women whose previous cesarean was the result of dystocia (fetal pelvic disproportion, difficult and prolonged labor). During that time, there was a growing consensus that the policy of routine repeat cesareans should be abandoned

complications or emergency, cesarean sections pose more short- and long-term risk to the mother and baby than a spontaneous vaginal birth. It follows that and the national rates for vaginal birth after cesarean (VBAC) rose from 3.4 percent in 1980 to 18.5 percent in 1989. A number of large studies and reviews have since demonstrated the safety of VBAC (Flamm et al., 1990; Rosen & Dickinson, 1990), but in recent years the number has declined. Some barriers to routine availability of VBAC may include: (1) a hospital's inability to meet the American College of Obstetricians and Gynecologists guidelines for VBAC, which include 24-hour blood banking, continuous EFM, an anesthetist, and the on-site presence of a physician capable of performing a cesarean; (2) a doctor or a woman's preference for a scheduled cesarean delivery; and (3) fear of malpractice suits by the obstetrician (Taffel, Placek, Moien, & Kasary, 1991). Women who are interested in VBAC should consult with their doctor to see if VBAC is a safe option for them.

The Childhood Connection, a non-profit organization that has provided information about pregnancy since 1918, urges women and healthcare providers to consider some of the long-term risks that have been shown to accompany cesarean section. For the mother, these include a high risk of subsequent infertility, increased chance of ectopic pregnancy, placenta previa, placental abruption, and rupture of the uterus during future pregnancies. Women who deliver by C-section are more likely to experience problems breast-feeding. Babies born by cesarean suffer a high risk of surgical cuts and injuries during the procedure, respiratory problems at birth, and a higher risk of developing asthma later in childhood or adulthood (Jain et al., 2009; Zanardo, 2004).

There is an increasingly held perception, at least in the United States, that the reason for the dramatic rise in cesarean deliveries is that they are requested by expectant mothers as elective procedures. Recent analysis indicates however, that the number of women who are urged to have cesarean sections by their healthcare providers far outnumber women who request it (Declereq, 2006). There is another perception that having a cesarean section, rather than going through labor and vaginal delivery, prevents pelvic floor damage that can result in urinary and anal incontinence later in life (Victrup et al., 2006;

Groutz, 2004). Unfortunately, many of the studies that compare rates of incontinence between women who give birth vaginally and those who have had a cesarean section, do not distinguish between spontaneous vaginal birth and assisted vaginal births. Combining the data for spontaneous and assisted vaginal birth confounds the results because several of the procedures used in assisted vaginal birth, such as episiotomy, forceps and vacuum extraction, have been shown to increases the chance of damage to the pelvic floor. Additional studies are needed to compare the incidence of postpartum problems for women who have cesarean sections with women who experience spontaneous vaginal births, without forceps, vacuum extraction, or episiotomy.

A decline in the infant mortality rate has paralleled the rise in the cesarean birth rate in the United States, a statistic that could encourage complacency with regard to the increased surgeries. Similar declines in fetal mortality have taken place in Europe, however, without the accompanying increase in cesareans. For example, O'Driscoll and Foley (1983) found that between 1965 and 1980, the cesarean delivery rate remained virtually unchanged at about 4.5 percent at the National Maternity Hospital in Dublin, while perinatal mortality fell from 42.1 per 1,000 infants to 16.8 per 1,000 infants.

Because the reasons for a delivery by cesarean section have expanded beyond their previous indications, the surgery is conceivably a possibility for every pregnant woman. It should, therefore, be discussed with the physician well in advance of delivery. In countries like the United States, where cesareans are common, it is important for women to know their doctor's criteria for emergency cesarean birth. She should get an explanation of the procedure that would be used, the anesthetic, the after effects, whether she could have her partner in the operating room with her, and whether subsequent pregnancies would also require abdominal surgery.

Medical Procedures to Deliver the Placenta

Some physicians prefer not to wait for the placenta to be expelled, and they speed up the process by applying external pressure to the abdomen to restart

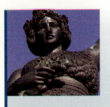

Historical Considerations
CESAREAN SECTIONS IN ANTIQUITY

Despite being a common modern surgery, the origin of the C-section is lost in the depths of history. Artwork from cultures as distant as Ancient China and medieval Europe depict C-sections. The Torah contains references to twins delivered by C-section and the procedure also appears in Hindu, Greek, and Egyptian mythology. In Greek mythology, the god Apollo performed a C-section to deliver his son, Asclepius, from the dead body of his human mother. In most cases, the procedure was carried out to save the child's life. Ancient Roman law required a child be delivered by C-section if the mother was dying, and the term "cesarean" possibly refers to the laws of Caesar. A case of a woman surviving a C-section occurs in fourteenth century Switzerland, although for the next several centuries, a woman's chance of surviving the procedure remained slight, due to both the lack of anatomical knowledge and the risk of infection (Sewell, 1993).

contractions. The rationale behind the assistance is that for some women there is a significant amount of bleeding that occurs if the placenta is allowed to be delivered spontaneously. After the placenta is expelled, the massage of the uterus is continued because the continued contractions constrict the uterine blood vessels and minimize the possibility of hemorrhage. In some cases, a uterotonic drug is given to stimulate firm contractions and reduce blood loss. Breast-feeding the new infant immediately after delivery also triggers a release of oxytocin, which has the same effect on stimulating uterine contractions.

CONCLUSION

In a small percentage of pregnancies, the medical interventions described in this chapter can be essential to saving the life of a mother or infant. There is increasing evidence, however, that the routine use of some of these procedures, especially during labor and delivery, interrupts the normal sequence of physiological events that can take place to bring a new baby into the world. Expectant mothers must take an active role in discussing with their healthcare providers how they would like to approach their pregnancy and birth experience.

REVIEW QUESTIONS

1. Describe the techniques that can be used to monitor the health of a fetus during pregnancy.

2. What is preeclampsia-eclampsia? What causes this condition?

3. What is the role of a doula?

4. What are the potential complications to the mother associated with assisted vaginal birth?

5. What are the health risks associated with cesarean sections?

CRITICAL THINKING QUESTIONS

1. Should "elective cesarean sections" be available for reasons besides medical necessity?

2. Fetal heart monitoring is often cited as one of the major components of the "cascade of interventions" that lead to an increase in the number of cesarean sections. When is fetal heart monitoring useful? Are there situations where it may not be beneficial?

WEB LINKS

Childbirth Connection
www.childbirthconnection.org

Campaign to end Fistula
www.endfistula.org

REFERENCES

Aladjem, S. (Ed.). (1980). *Obstetrical practice.* St. Louis, MO: C. V. Mosby.

Allen, V. M., Armson, B. A., Wilson, R. D., Allen, V. M., Blight, C., Gagnon, A., Johnson, J. A., Langlois, S., Summers, A., Wyatt, P., Farine, D., Armson, B. A., Crane, J., Delisle, M. F., Keenan-Lindsay, L., Morin, V., Schneider, C. E., Van Aerde, J., & Society of Obstetricians and Gynecologists of Canada. (2007). Teratogenicity associated with pre-existing and gestational diabetes. *Journal of Obstetrics and Gynaecology Canada, 29*(11), 927–944.

Althabe, F., & Belizan, J. F. (2006). Cesarean section: The paradox. *Lancet, 368,* 1472-1473.

Alwan, N., Tuffnell, D. J., & West, J. (2009). Treatment for gestational diabetes. *Cochrane Database Systematic Review,* (3), CD003395.

American College of Obstetricians and Gynecologists. (1989). Intrapartum fetal heart rate monitoring. (Technical bulletin no. 132). Washington, DC: Author.

American College of Obstetricians and Gynecologists. (2001). Fetal heart rate monitoring during labor. Washington, DC: Author.

American College of Obstetricians and Gynecologists. (2004). Committee opinion no. 297: Nonmedical use of obstetric ultrasonography. *Obstetrics & Gynecology, 104,* 423–424.

American College of Obstetricians and Gynecologists. (2004). Committee opinion no. 299: Guidelines for diagnostic imaging during pregnancy. *Obstetrics & Gynecology, 104,* 647–651.

American College of Obstetricians and Gynecologists. (2005, September). Committee opinion no. 315: Obesity in pregnancy. *Obstetrics & Gynecology, 106*(3), 671–675.

American College of Obstetricians and Gynecologists. (2005, November). Committee opinion no. 324:

Perinatal risks associated with assisted reproductive technology. *Obstetrics & Gynecology, 106*(5, Part 1), 1143–1146.

American College of Obstetricians and Gynecologists. (2006, April). Practice bulletin no. 71: Episiotomy. *Obstetrics & Gynecology, 107*(4), 956–962.

American College of Obstetricians and Gynecologists. (2006, April). What to expect after your due date. Retrieved January 16, 2008 from http://www.medem.com/MedLB/article_detaillb.cfm?article_ID=ZZZRDLPH97C&sub_cat=2005.

American College of Obstetricians and Gynecologists. (2006, July 13). ACOG statement in support of IOM report, "Preterm birth: Causes, consequences, and prevention. Retrieved on January 17, 2008 from http://www.acog.org/from_home/publications/press_releases/nr07-13-06.cfm.

American College of Obstetricians and Gynecologists. (2007, January). Practice bulletin no. 77: Screening for fetal chromosomal abnormalities. *Obstetrics & Gynecology, 109*(1), 217–228.

American College of Obstetricians and Gynecologists. (2007, January 2). New recommendations for Down syndrome: Screening should be offered to all pregnant women. Retrieved on January 17, 2008 from http://www.acog.org/from_home/publications/press_releases/nr01-02-07-1.cfm.

American College of Obstetricians and Gynecologists. (2007, May 7). The challenges of diagnosing and treating maternal depression: Women's health experts weigh in. Retrieved from http://www.acog.org/from_home/publications/press_releases/nr05-07-07-2.cfm.

American College of Obstetricians and Gynecologists (2009, June 22). ACOG refines fetal heart rate monitoring guidelines. Retrieved from http://www.acog.org/from_home/publications/press_releases/nr06-22-09-2.cfm.

American Society for Reproductive Medicine, Patient Education Committee and Publications Committee. (2004). *Multiple pregnancy and birth: Twins, triplets, and higher order multiples. A guide for patients.* Birmingham, AL: Author.

American Society for Reproductive Medicine. (2009). New SART data posted; Triplet and higher order multiples from ART are below two percent. *ASRM Bulletin, 11*(11).

American Society for Reproductive Medicine. (2008). Complications and problems associated with multiple births. Patient fact sheet. Retrieved from http://www.asrm.org/uploadedFiles/ASRM_Content/Resources/Patient_Resources/Fact_Sheets_and_Info_Booklets/complications_multiplebirths.pdf.

American Society for Reproductive Medicine. (2008). Recurrent pregnancy loss. Patient fact sheet. Retrieved from http://www.asrm.org/uploadedFiles/ASRM_Content/Resources/Patient_Resources/Fact_Sheets_and_Info_Booklets/recurrent_preg_loss.pdf.

Badell, M. L., Ramin, S. M., & Smith, J. A. (2006). Treatment options for nausea and vomiting during pregnancy. *Pharmacotherapy, 26*(9), 1273–1287.

Barakat, R., Ruiz, J. R., Stirling, J. R., Zakynthinaki, M., & Lucia, A. (2009a). Type of delivery is not affected by light resistance and toning exercise training during pregnancy: A randomized controlled trial. *American Journal of Obstetrics and Gynecology, 201*(6), 590, e1-6.

Barakat, R., Lucia, A., & Ruiz, J. R. (2009b). Resistance exercise training during pregnancy and newborn's birth size: A randomized controlled trial. *International Journal of Obesity (London), 33*(9), 1048–1057.

Barakat, R., Stirling, J. R., & Lucia, A. (2008). Does exercise training during pregnancy affect gestational age? A randomized controlled trial. *British Journal of Sports Medicine, 42*(8), 674–678.

Baydock, S. A., Flood, C., Schulz, J. A., MacDonald, D., Esau, D., Jones, S., & Hiltz, C. B. (2009). Prevalence and risk factors for urinary and fecal incontinence four months after vaginal delivery. *Journal of Obstetrics and Gynaecology Canada, 31*(1), 36–41.

Bayrampour, H., & Heaman, M. (2010). Advanced maternal age and the risk of cesarean birth: A systematic review. *Birth, 37*(3), 219–226.

Bendetto, C., Morozio, L., Prandi, G., Roccia, A., Blefari, S., & Fabris, C. (2007). Short-term maternal and neonatal outcomes by mode of delivery. A case-controlled study. *European Journal of Obstetrics & Gynecology and Reproductive Biology,, 135*(1), 35–40.

Bibi, S., Ghaffer, S., Pir, M. A., & Yousfani, S. (2009). Risk factors and clinical outcome of placental abruption: A retrospective analysis. *Journal of Pakistan Medical Association, 59*(10), 672–674.

Birnbach, D. J., Bucklin, B. A., & Dexter, F. (2010). Impact of anesthesiologists on the incidence of vaginal birth after cesarean in the United States: A role of anesthesia availability, productivity, guidelines, and patient safety. *Seminars in Perinatology, 34*(5), 318–324.

Bodner, L. M., Catov, J. M., Simhan, H. N., Holick, M. F., Powers, R. W., & Roberts, J. M. (2007). Maternal vitamin D deficiency increases the risk of preeclampsia. *Journal of Clinical Endocrinology and Metabolism, 92*(9), 3517–3522.

Borders, N. (2006). After the afterbirth: A critical review of postpartum health relative to method of delivery. *Journal of Midwifery & Women's Health, 51*(4), 242–248.

Borzychowski, A. M., Sargent, I. L., & Redman, C. W. (2006). Inflammation and pre-eclampsia. *Seminars in Fetal & Neonatal Medicine, 11*(5), 309–316.

Buckley, S. J. (2004). Drugs in labor: An overview. *Midwifery Today: International Midwife,* (71), 13-20, 65, 67.

Byrne, M., Agerbo, E., Bennedsen, B., Eaton, W. W., & Mortensen, P. B. (2007). Obstetric conditions and risk of first admission with schizophrenia: A Danish national register based study. *Schizophrenia, 97*(1–3), 51–59.

Caughey, A. B., Sundaram, V., Kaimal, A. J., Cheng, Y. W., Gieger, A., Little, S. E., Lee, J. F., Wong, L., Shaffer, B. L., Tran, S. H, Padula, A., McDonald, K. M., Long, E. F., Owens, D. K., & Bravata, D. M. (2009). Maternal and neonatal outcomes of elective induction of labor. *Evidence Report: Technology Assessment (Full Report),* (176), 1–257.

Caughey, A. B., Sandberg, P. L., Zlatnik, M. G., Thiet, M. P., Parer, J. T., & Laros, R. K., Jr. (2005). Forceps compared with vacuum: Rates of neonatal and maternal morbidity. *Obstetrics & Gynecology, 106*(5 Pt 1), 908–912.

Centers of Disease Control. (2010). Listeriosis and pregnancy. Retrieved March 18, 2010 from http://www.cdc.gov/ncbddd/pregnancy_gateway/infections-Listeria.html.

Chan, R. L., Olshan, A. F., Savitz, D. A., Herring, A. H., Daniels, J. L., Peterson, H. B., & Martin, S. L. (2010). Severity and duration of nausea and vomiting symptoms in pregnancy and spontaneous abortion. *Human Reproduction, 25*(11), 2907–2912.

Chasnoff, I. J., Griffith, D. R., McGregor, S., et al. (1989). Temporal patterns of cocaine use in pregnancy. Perinatal outcome. *Journal of the American Medical Association, 261*(12), 1741–1744.

Childbirth Connection. (2006). *What every pregnant woman should know about cesarean section* (2nd ed). New York, NY: Childbirth Connection. Available at http://www.childbirthconnection.org/cesareanbooklet/.

Clapp, J. F. (2006). Influence of endurance exercise and diet on human placental development and fetal growth. *Placenta, 27*(6-7), 527–534.

Clapp, J. F. (2006). Effects of diet and exercise on insulin resistance during pregnancy. *Metabolic Syndrome and Related Disorders, 4*(2), 84–90.

Clark, S. L., Belfort, M. A., Dildy, G. A., Herbst, M. A., Mayers, J. A., & Hankins, G. D. (2008). Maternal death in the 21st century: Causes, prevention, and relationship to cesarean section. *American Journal of Obstetrics and Gynecology, 199*(1), 36.e1-5, 91-92, e7–11.

Clark, S. L., Belfort, M. A., Hankins, G. D., Meyers, J. A., & Houser, F. M. (2007). Variation in the rates of operative delivery in the United States. *American Journal of Obstetrics and Gynecology, 196*(6), 526, e1–5.

Cohain, J. S. (2008). Episiotomy, hospital birth and cesarean section: Technology gone haywire--What is the sutured tear rate at first births supposed to be? (2008). *Midwifery Today International Midwife,* (85), 24–25.

Conner, B. H., & Seaton, P. G. (1982). Birth weight and use of oxytocin and analgesic agents in labor in relation to neonatal jaundice. *Medical Journal of Australia, 2,* 466–469.

Davidoff, M. J., Dias, T., Damus, K., Russell, R., Bettegowda, V. R., Dolan, S., Schwarz, R. H., Green, N. S., & Petrini, J. (2006). Changes in the gestational age distribution among U.S. singleton births: Impact on rates of late preterm birth, 1992 to 2002. *Seminars in Perinatology, 30*(1), 8–15.

Davies, G. A., Maxwell, C., McLeod, L., Gagnon, R., Basso, M., Bos, H., Delisle, M. F., Farine, D., Hudon, L., Menticoglou, S., Mundle, W., Murphy-Kaulbeck, L., Oullet, A., Pressey, T., Roggensack, A., Leduc, D., Ballerman, C., Biringer, L., Jones, D., Lee, L. S., Shepherd, D., Wilson, K., & Society of Obstetricians and Gynecologists of Canada. (2010). Obesity in pregnancy. *Journal of Obstetrics and Gynaecology Canada, 32*(2), 165–173.

De Chateau, P. (1980). Parent–neonate interaction and its long-term effects. In E. G. Simmel (Ed.), *Early experience and early behavior.* New York, NY: Academic Press.

Declercq, E., Cunningham, D. K., Johnson, C., & Sakela, C. (2008). Mother's reports of postpartum pain associated with vaginal and cesarean deliveries: Results of a national survey. *Birth, 35*(1), 16–24.

Declercq, E., Menacker, F., & MacDorman, M. (2006). Maternal risk profiles and the primary cesarean rate in the United States, 1991–2002. *American Journal of Public Health, 96,* 867–872.

Declercq, E. R., Sakela, C., Correy, M. P., & Applebaum, S. (2006) Listening to mothers II: Report of the second national survey of women's childbearing experiences. New York, NY: Childbirth Connection, October 2006a. Available at http://www.childbirthconnection.org/listeningtomothers/.

Declercq, E. R., Sakela, C., Correy, M. P., & Applebaum, S. (2008). New mothers speak out: National survey results highlight women's postpartum experiences. New York, NY Childbirth Connection.

Declercq, E., Menacker, F., MacDorman, M., Maternal risk profiles and the primary cesarean rate in the United States, 1991–2002. Am J Public Health 2006b;96:867–72.

Demissie, K., Rhoads, G. G., Smulian, J. C., Balasubramanian, B. A., Gandhi, K., Joseph, K.

S., & Kramer, M. (2004). Operative vaginal delivery and neonatal and infant adverse outcomes: Population based retrospective analysis. *British Medical Journal, 329*(7456), 24–29.

Dennedy, M. C., & Dunne, F. (2010). The maternal and fetal impacts of obesity and gestational diabetes on pregnancy outcome. *Best Practices & Research: Clinical Endocrinology & Metabolism, 24*(4), 573–589.

Dennis, C. L., & McQueen, K. (2009). The relationship between infant-feeding outcomes and postpartum depression: A qualitative systematic review. *Pediatrics, 123*(4), e736–751.

De Paz, N. C., Sanchez, S. E., Huaman, L. E., Chang, G. D., Pacora, P. N., Garcia, P. J., Ananth, C. V., Qiu, C., & Williams, M. A. (2010). Risk of placental abruption in relation to maternal depressive, anxiety and stress symptoms. *Journal of Affective Disorders, 130*(1–2), 280-284.

Deutchman, M., Tubay, A. T., & Turok, D. (2009). First trimester bleeding. *American Family Physician, 79*(11), 985–992.

Dietz, P. M., Callaghan, W. M., & Sharma, A. J. (2009). High pregnancy weight gain and risk of excessive fetal growth. *American Journal of Obstetrics and Gynecology,201*(1), 51.e1–6.

Dudding, T. C., Vaizey, C. J., & Kamm, M. A. (2008). Obstetric anal sphincter injury: Incidence, risk factors, and management. *Annals of Surgery, 247*(2), 224–237.

Dunnihoo, D. R. (1990). *Fundamentals of gynecology & obstetrics* (p. 445). Philadelphia, PA: J. B. Lippincott.

Dusse, L. M., Rios, D. R., Pinheiro, M. B., Cooper, A. J., & Lwaleed, B. A. (2010). Pre-eclampsia: Relationship between coagulation, fibrinoloysis and inflammation. *Clinica Chimica Acta, 412*(1–2), 17-21.

Eerdekens, A., Debeer, A., Van Hoey, G., DeBorger, C., Sachar, V., Gudlinckx, I., Devlieger, R., Hanssens, M., & Vanhole, C. (2009). Maternal bariatric surgery: Adverse outcomes in neonates. *European Journal of Pediatrics, 169*(2), 191–196.

Einarson, T. R., Navioz, Y., Maltepe, C., Einarson, A., & Koren, G. (2007). Existence and severity of nausea and vomiting in pregnancy (NVP) with different partners. *Journal of Obstetrics & Gynaecology, 27*(4), 360–362.

Erkolla, R., Gronroos, M., Punnonen, R., et al. (1984). Analysis of intrapartum fetal deaths: Their decline with increasing electronic fetal monitoring. *Acta Obstetrica et Gynaecologica Scandinavica, 63,* 459.

Eskanazi, B., & Bracken, M. B. (1982). Bendectin (Debendox) as a risk factor for pyloric stenosis. *American Journal of Obstetrics and Gynecology, 144*(8), 919–924.

Eskanazi, B., Fenster, L., & Sidney, S. (1991). A multivariate analysis of risk factors for preeclampsia. *Journal of the American Medical Association, 266*(2), 237–241.

Ettner, F. M. (1977). Hospital technology breeds pathology. *Women and Health, 2*(2), 17–22.

Faiz, A. S., & Ananth, C. V. (2003). Etiology and risk factors for placenta previa: An overview and meta-analysis of observational studies. *Journal of Maternal-Fetal and Neonatal Medicine, 13*(3), 175–190.

Fabro, S., & Sieber, S. M. (1969). Caffeine and nicotine penetrate the pre-implantation blastocyst. *Nature, 223*(204), 410–411.

Falcao, S., Bisotto, S., Michel, C., Lacasse, A. A., Vaillancourt, C., Gutkowska, J., & Lavoie, J. L. (2010). Exercise training can attenuate preeclampsia-like features in an animal model. *Journal of Hypertension, 28*(12), 2384–2385.

Farina, A., Hasegawa, J., Raffaelli, S., Ceccarini, C., Rapacchia, G., Pittalis, M. C., Brondelli, L., & Rizzo, N. (2010). The association between preeclampsia and placental disruption induced by chorionic villous sampling. *Prenatal Diagnosis, 30*(6), :571–574.

Flamm, B. L., Newman, L. A., Thomas, S. J., et al. (1990). Vaginal birth after cesarean delivery: Results of a 5-year multicenter collaborative study. *Obstetrics and Gynecology, 76*(5), 750–754.

Flaxman, S. M., & Sherman, P. W. (2008). Morning sickness: Adaptive cause or nonadaptive consequence of embryo viability? *American Naturalist, 172*(1), 54–62.

Forfar, J., & Nelson, M. M. (1973). Epidemiology of drugs taken by pregnant women: Drugs that may affect the fetus adversely. *Clinical Pharmacologies and Therapeutics, 14,* 632.

Fortner, R. T., Pekow, P. S., Whitcomb, B. W., Sievert, L. L., Markenson, G., & Chasen-Taber,

L. (2010). Physical activity and hypertensive disorders of pregnancy among Hispanic women. *Medicine & Science in Sports & Exercise, 43*(4), 636–646.

Fowler, S. (1991, June 23). Coach makes birth easier and reduces cesarean rate. *Chicago Tribune.*

Frankman, E. A., Wang, L., Bunker, C. H., & Lowder, J. L. (2009). Episiotomy in the United States: Has anything changed? *American Journal of Obstetrics and Gynecology, 200*(5), 573.e1-7.

Franz, M. B., & Husslein, P. W. (2010). Obstetrical management of the older gravida. *Women's Health (London, England), 6*(3), 463–468.

Freeman, J. M. (2007). Beware: The misuse of technology and the law of unintended consequences. *Neurotherapeutics, 4*(3), 549–554.

Gagnon, R., Morin, L., Bly, S., Butt, K., Cargill, Y. M., Denis, N., Hietala-Coyle, M. A., Lim, K. I., Ouellet, A., Raciot, M. H., Salem, S., Diagnostic Imaging Committee, Hudon, L., Basso, M., Bos, H., Delisle, M. F., Farine, D., Grabowska, K., Meticoglou, S., Mundle, W., Murphy-Kaulbeck, L., Pressey, T., Roggensack, A., & Maternal Fetal Medicine Committee. (2009). Guidelines for management of vasa previa. *Journal of Obstetrics and Gynaecology Canada, 31*(8), 748–760.

Gardner, M. J., Snee, M. P., Hall, A. J., et al. (1990). Results of case-control study of leukemia and lymphoma among young people near Sellafield nuclear plant in West Cumbria. *British Medical Journal, 300*(6722), 423–429.

Gavin, L., et al. (2009). Sexual and reproductive health of persons aged 10-24 years – United States 2002 – 2007. *Morbidity and Mortality Weekly Report Surveillance Summaries, 58*(SS06), 1–18.

Geller, D. A., Wieland, N., Carey, K., Vivas, F., Petty, C. R., Johnson, J., Reichert, E., Pauls, D., & Biederman, J. (2008). Perinatal factors affecting expression of obsessive compulsive disorder in children and adolescents. *Journal of Child and Adolescent Psychopharmacology, 18*(4), 373–379.

Gill, S. K., & Einarson, A. (2007). The safety of drugs for the treatment of nausea and vomiting in pregnancy. *Expert Opinion on Drug Safety, 6*(6), 685–694.

Gillman, M. W., Rifas-Shiman, S., Berkey, C. S., Field, A. E., & Colditz, G.. A. (2003). Maternal gestational diabetes, birth weight, and adolescent obesity. *Pediatrics, 111*(30), 221–226.

Gillman, M. W., Oakey, H., Baghurst, P. A., Volkmer, R. E., Robinson, J. S., & Crowther, C. A. (2010). Effect of treatment of gestational diabetes mellitus on obesity in the next generation. *Diabetes Care,. 33*(5), 964–968.

Gleicher, N. (2007). Why much of the pathophysiology of preeclampsia-eclampsia must be of an autoimmune nature. *American Journal of Obstetrics and Gynecology, 196*(1), 5.e1–7.

Golding, J., Vivian, S., & Baldwin, J. A. (1983). Maternal antinauseants and clefts of lip and palate. *Human Toxicology, 2,* 63–73.

Gosik, A. (2007, October 12). U.S. ranks 41st in maternal mortality: New report will be discussed at London meeting. Cox News Service. Retrieved from http://www.seattlepi.com/default/article/U-S-ranks-41st-in-maternal-mortality-1252472.php.

Graham, E.M., Petersen, S.M., Christo, D.K., & Fox, H.E. (2006). Intrapartum electronic fetal heart rate monitoring and the prevention of perinatal brain injury. *Obstetrics and Gynecology, 108*(3 Pt 1), 656–666.

Grant, A., O'Brien, N., Joy, M., et al. (1989). Cerebral palsy among children born during the Dublin randomized trial of intrapartum monitoring. *Lancet, ii,* 1233–1236.

Grantham-McGregor, S. M., & Fernald, L. C. (1997). Nutritional deficiencies and subsequent effects on mental and behavioral development in children. *Southeast Asian Journal of Tropical Medicine and Public Health, 28*(Suppl. 2), 50–68.

Groutz, A., Rimon, E., Peled, S., Gold, R., Pauzner, D., Lessing, J. B., & Gordon, D. (2004). Cesarean section: Does it really prevent the development of postpartum stress urinary incontinence? A prospective study of 363 women one year after their first delivery. *Neurourol Urodyn, 23*(1), 2–6.

Guelinckx, I., Devlieger, R., & Vansant, G.. (2009). Reproductive outcomes after bariatric surgery: A critical review. *Human Reproductive Update, 15*(2), 189–201.

Guise, J. M., Eden, K., Emeis, C., Denman, M. A., Marshall, N., Fu, R. R., Janik, R., Nygren, P., Walker, M., & McDonagh, M. (2010). Vaginal birth after cesarean: New insights. *Evidence Report/Technology Assessment (Full Report),* (191),1–397.

Haire, D. (1977). *The cultural warping of childbirth.* Seattle WA: International Childbirth Education Association (rev.).

Hamilton, B. E., Martin, J. A., & Ventura, S. J. (2007). Births: Preliminary data for 2006. *National Vital Statistics Reports, 56*(7).

Harrison, M. R., Filly, R. A., Golbus, M. S., et al. (1982). Fetal treatment. *New England Journal of Medicine, 307*(26), 1651–1652.

Hartmann, K., Viswanathan, M., Palmieri, R., Gertlehner, G., Thorp, J., & Lohr, K. N. (2005). Outcomes of routine episiotomy: A systematic review. *Journal of the American Medical Association, 293,* 2141–2148.

Haverkamp, A. D., & Orleans, M. (1983). An assessment of electronic fetal monitoring. *Women's Health, 7*(3), 115–133.

Hibbard, L. T. (1976). Changing trends in cesarean section. *American Journal of Obstetrics and Gynecology, 125,* 798–804.

Hill, R. M., Craig, J. P., & Chaney, M. D. (1977). Utilization of over-the-counter drugs during pregnancy. *Clinical Obstetrics and Gynecology, 20*(2), 381–394.

Hincz, P., Borowski, D., Krekora, M., Podciechowski, L., Horzelski, W., & Wilczynski, J. (2009). Maternal obesity as a perinatal risk factor. *Ginekologia Polska, 80*(5), 334–337.

Hoover, K. W., Tao, G., & Kent, C. K. (2010). Trends in the diagnosis and treatment of ectopic pregnancy in the United States. *Obstetrics & Gynecology, 115*(3), 495–502.

Hoosain, N., Khan, N., Sultana, S. S., & Khan, N. (2010). Abruptio placentae and adverse pregnancy outcomes. *Journal of the Pakistan Medical Association, 60*(6), 443–446.

Houston, L. E., Odibo, A. O., & Macones, G. A. (2009). The safety of obstetrical ultrasound: A review. *Prenatal Diagnosis, 29,* 1204–1212.

Imperiale, T. F., & Petrulis, A. S. (1991). A meta-analysis of low-dose aspirin for the prevention of pregnancy-induced hypertensive disease. *Journal of the American Medical Association, 266*(2), 260–264.

International Center for Research on Women (ICRW). About child marriage. Retrieved June 1, 2009 from http://www.icrw.org/what-we-do/adolescents/child-marriage.

Intrauterine devices: An effective alternative to oral hormonal contraception. (2009). *Prescrire International, 18*(101), 125–130.

Jackson, K. A., Iwamoto, M., & Swerdlow, D. (2010). Pregnancy-associated listeriosis. *Epidemiology and Infection, 17,* 1–7.

Jahromi, B. N., & Husseini, Z. (2008). Pregnancy outcome at maternal age 40 and older. *Taiwanese Journal of Obstetrics and Gynecology, 47*(3), 318–321.

Jain, N. J., Kruse, L. K., Demissie, K., & Khandelwal, M. (2009). Impact of mode of delivery on neonatal complications: Trends between 1997 and 2005. *Journal of Maternal-Fetal and Neonatal Medicine, 22*(6), 491–500.

Jaruratanasirikul, S., Sangsupawanich, P., Koranantakul, O., Chanvitan, P., Sriplung, H., & Patanasin, T. (2009). Influence of maternal nutrient intake and weight gain on neonatal birth weight: A prospective cohort study in southern Thailand. *Journal of Maternal-Fetal Neonatal Medicine, 22*(11), 1045–1050.

John, E. M., Savitz, D. A., & Sandler, D. P. (1991). Prenatal exposure to parents' smoking and childhood cancer. *American Journal of Epidemiology, 133*(2), 123–132.

Kaupp, U. B., Kashikar, N. D., & Weyand, I. (2008). Mechanisms of sperm chemotaxis. *Annual Review of Physiology, 70,* 93–117.

Kennell, J., Klaus, M., McGrath, S., et al. (1991). Continuous emotional support during labor in a US hospital. *Journal of the American Medical Association, 265*(17), 2197–2201.

Kettering, H. S., & Wolter, D. F. (1977). Complications of cesarean section. *Transactions of the Pacific Coast Obstetrical and Gynecological Society, 44,* 29–34.

Kieler, H., Axellson, O., Haglund, B., et al. (1998). Routine ultrasound screening in pregnancy and the children's subsequent handedness. *Early Human Development, 50*(2), 233–245.

King, J. C., & Fabro, S. (1982). Alcohol consumption and cigarette smoking: Effect on pregnancy. *Clinical Obstetrics and Gynecology, 26*(2), 437–448.

Kinney, H. C. (2006). The near-term human brain and risk for periventricular leukomalacia: A review. *Seminars in Perinatyology, 30*(2), 81–88.

Klaus, M., Jerauld, R., & Kreger, N. (1972). Maternal attachment. *New England Journal of Medicine, 286*(9), 460–463.

Klaus, M., & Kennell, J. (1983). Parent to infant bonding: Setting the record straight. *Journal of Pediatrics, 102*(4), 575–576.

Klaus, M., & Kennell, J. H. (1976). *Maternal-infant bonding.* St. Louis, MO: C. V. Mosby.

Klaus, M., & Kennell, J. H. (1993). *Mothering the mother: How a doula can help you have a shorter, easier, and healthier birth.* Old Tappan, NJ: Addison Wesley Longman.

Krassas, G. E., Poppe, K., & Glinoer, D. (2010). Thyroid function and human reproductive health. *Endocrine Reviews, 31*(5), 701–755. doi:10.1210/er.2009-0041.

Kudish, B., Blackwell, S., McNeeley, S. G., Bujold, E., Kruger, M., Hendrix, S. L., & Sokol, R. (2006). Operative vaginal delivery and the midline episiotomy: A bad combination for the perineum. *American Journal of Obstetrics and Gynecology, 195*(3), 749–754.

Kudish, B., Sokol, R. J., & Kruger, M. (2008). Trends in major modifiable risk factors for severe perineal trauma, 1996- 2006. *International Journal of Obstetrics and Gynecology, 102*(2), 165–170. doi:10.1016/J.IJGO2008.02.017.

Lavin, J. P., Stephens, R. F., Miodovnik, M., & Barden, T. P. (1982). Vaginal delivery in patients with a prior cesarean section. *Obstetrics and Gynecology, 59*(2), 135–148.

Lent, M. (1999). The medical and legal risks of the electronic fetal monitor. *Stanford Law Review, 51*(4), 807–837.

Leone, J. M., Lane, S. D., Koumans, E. H., DeMott, K., Wojtowycz, M. A., Jensen, J., & Aubry, R. H. (2010). Effects of intimate partner violence on pregnancy trauma and placental abruption. *Journal of Women's Health (Larchmont), 19*(8), 1501–1509.

Liljestrand, J. (2003). Episiotomy for vaginal birth: RHL commentary. *WHO Reproductive Health Library.* Geneva, Switzerland: World Health Organization.

Lurie, S., Glezerman, M., & Sadan, O. (2005). Maternal and neonatal effects of forceps versus vacuum operative vaginal delivery. *International Journal of Gynaecology & Obstetrics, 89*(3), 293–294.

Lydon-Rochelle, M. T., Holt, V. L., Nelson, J. C., Cardenas, V., Gardella, C., Easterling, T. R., & Callaghan, W. M. (2005). Accuracy of reporting of maternal in-hospital diagnosis and intrapartum procedures of Washington state linked birth records. *Pediatric and Perinatal Epidemiology, 19*(6), 460–471.

Majhi, A. K., Roy, N., Karmakar, K. S., & Banerjee, P. K. (2007). Ectopic pregnancy-An analysis of 180 cases. *Journal of the Indian Medical Association, 105*(6), 308, 310, 312.

Majoko, F., & Gardener, G. (2008). Trial of instrumental delivery in theatre versus immediate cesarean section for anticipated difficult assisted births. *Cochrane Database Systematic Review,* (4), CD005545.

March of Dimes. Preterm labor Retrieved from http://www.marchofdimes.com/pnhec/188_1080.asp.

Martin, J. A., Hamilton, B. E., Sutton, P. D., Ventura, S. J., Meacker, F., & Kirmeyer, S. (2006). Births: Final data for 2004. *National Vital Statistics Reports, 55*(1).

Martin, J. A., Hamilton, B. E., Sutton, P D., Ventura, S. J., Meacker, F., Kirmeyer, S., & Munson, M. L. (2007). Births: Final data for 2005. *National Vital Statistics Reports, 56*(6).

Martin, J. A., et al. (2009). Births: Final data for 2006. *National Vital Statistics Reports, 57*(7).

Mathews, T. J., & MacDorman, M. F. (2006). Infant mortality statistics from the 2003 period linked birth/infant death data set. *National Vital Statistics Reports, 54*(15).

McCourt, C., Weaver, J., Statham, H., Beake, S., Gamble J., & Creedy, D. K. (2007). Elective cesarean section and decision making: A critical review of the literature. *Birth, 34,* 65–79.

Retrieved from http://www.blackwell-synergy.com/toc/bir/34/1.

Melzer, K., Schultz, Y., Boulvain, M., & Kayser, B. (2010). Physical activity and pregnancy: Cardiovascular adaptations, recommendations and pregnancy outcomes. *Sports Medicine, 40*(6), 493–507.

Michaelis, J., Michaelis, H., Gluck, E., & Koller, S. (1983). Prospective study of suspected associations between certain drugs administered during early pregnancy and congenital malformations. *Teratology, 27,* 57–64.

Miller, M. W., Brayman, A. A., & Abramowicz, J. S. (1998). Obstetric ultrasonography: A biophysical consideration of patient safety—The "rules" have changed. *American Journal of Obstetrics and Gynecology, 179*(1), 241–254.

Milunsky, A., Jick, H., Jick, S., et al. (1989). Multivitamin/folic acid supplementation in early pregnancy reduces the prevalence of neural tube defects. *Journal of the American Medical Association, 262*(20), 2847–2852.

Monroy, T. R., Reeves, A. C. C., Naves Sanchez, J., & Macias, A. E. (2008). Influence of an individualized diet on control of gestational diabetes mellitus. *Ginecologia Y Obstetricia de Mexico, 76*(12), 722–729.

Nyberg, K., Buka, S., & Lipsett, L. (2000). Perinatal medication as a potential risk factor for adult drug abuse in a North American cohort. *Epidemiology, 11*(6), 715–716.

Mulinare, J., Cordereo, J. F., Erickson, J. D., & Berry, R. J. (1988). Periconceptional use of multivitamins and the occurrence of neural tube defects. *Journal of the American Medical Association, 260*(21), 3141–3145.

Niebyl, J. R. (1990). Teratology and drugs in pregnancy and lactation. In J. R. Scott, et al. (Eds.), *Danforth's obstetrics and gynecology* (6th ed.). Boston, MA: J. B. Lippincott.

Niswander, K. (1976). *Obstetrics: Essentials of clinical practice* (p. 267). Boston, MA: Little, Brown.

Niswander, K., Henson, G., Elbourne, D., et al. (1984). Adverse outcome of pregnancy and the quality of obstetric care. *Lancet, ii,* 827–831.

O'Driscoll, K., & Foley, M. (1983). Correction of decrease in perinatal mortality and increase in cesarean section rates. *Obstetrics and Gynecology, 61*(1), 1–5.

Page, E. W., Villee, C. A., & Villee, D. B. (1976). *Human reproduction* (2nd ed.). Philadelphia, PA: W. B. Saunders. Pariente, G., Wiznitzer, A., Sergienko, R., Mazor, M., Holcberg, G., & Sheiner, E. (2010). Placental abruption: Critical analysis of risk factors and perinatal outcomes. *Journal of Maternal-Fetal and Neonatal Medicine, 24*(5), 696–702.

Pepper, G. V., & Craig Roberts, S. (2006). Rates of nausea and vomiting in pregnancy and dietary characteristics across populations. *Proceedings: Biological Science, 273*(1601), 2675–2679.

Petrini, J. R., Callaghan, W. M., Klebanoff, M., Green, N. S., Lackritz, E. M., Howse, J. L., Schwarz, R. H., & Damus, K. (2005). Estimated effect of 17 alpha-hydroxyprogesterone caproate on preterm birth in the United States. *American College of Obstetricians and Gynecologists, 105*(2), 267–272.

Phaneuf, S., Rodriguez Linares, B., TambyRaja, R. L., MacKenzie, I. Z., & Lopez Bernal, A. (2000). Loss of myometrial oxytocin receptors during oxytocin-induced and oxytocin-augmented labor. *Journal of Reproductive Fertility, 120*(1), 91–97.

Phillips, R. A., Stratmeyer, M. E., & Harris, G. R. (2010). Safety and U.S. regulatory considerations in the non-clinical use of medical ultrasound devices. *Ultrasound in Medicine & Biology, 36*(8), 1224-1228.

Placek, P. J., Taffel, S., & Moien, M. (1983). Cesarean section delivery rates: United States, 1981. *American Journal of Public Health, 73*(8), 861–862.

Owe, C. E., Seely, E. W., Rana, S., Bhan, I., Ecker, J., Karumanchi, S. A., & Thadhani, R. (2010). First trimester vitamin D, vitamin binding protein, and subsequent preeclampsia. *Hypertension, 56*(4), 758–763.

Prapas, N., Kalogiannidis, I., Prapas, I., Xiromeritis, P., Kalogiannidis, P., & Makedos, G. (2006). Twin gestation in older women, intrapartum complications, and perinatal outcomes. *Archives of Gynecology and Obstetrics, 273*(5), 293–297.

Prapas, N., Kalogiannidis, I., Masoura, S., Diamanti, E., & Makedos, G.. (2009). Operative vaginal delivery in singleton term pregnancies:

Short-term maternal and neonatal outcomes. *Hippokratia, 13*(1), 41–45.

Pretlove, S. J., Thompson, P. J., Tooza-Hobson, P. M., Radley, S., & Knan, K. S. (2008). Does the mode of delivery predispose women to anal incontinence in the first year postpartum? A comparative systematic review. *British Journal of Obstetrics & Gynaeology, 115*(4), 421–434.

Ralt, D., Goldenberg, M., Fetterolf, P., et al. (1991). Sperm attraction to a follicular factor(s) correlates with human egg fertilizability. *Proceedings of the National Academy of Sciences, 88,* 2840–2844.

Resian, O. M., & Khalil, R. A. (2010). Molecular and vascular targets in the pathogenesis and management of the hypertension associated with preeclampsia. *Cardiovascular & Hematological Agents in Medicinal Chemistry, 8*(4), 204–226.

Rimawi, L. (2006). Premature infant. In *Disease and conditions encyclopedia.* Retrieved January 16, 2008, from http://health.discovery.com/encyclopedias/illnesses.html?article=2728.

Rosen, M. G., & Dickinson, J. C. (1990). Vaginal birth after cesarean: A meta-analysis of indicators for success. *Obstetrics and Gynecology, 76*(5), 865–869.

Rosenberg, L., Mitchell, A. A., Shapiro, S., & Slone, D. (1982). Selected birth defects in relation to caffeine-containing beverages. *Journal of the American Medical Association, 247,* 1429–1432.

Rossett, H., Quellette, E. M., Weiner, L., & Owens, E. (1978). Therapy of heavy drinking during pregnancy. *Obstetrics and Gynecology, 51*(1), 41–46.

Russell, M. (1991). Clinical implications of recent research on the fetal alcohol syndrome. *Bulletin of the New York Academy of Medicine, 67*(3), 207–222.

Rycel, M., Wilczynski, J., Sobala, W., & Nowakowska, D. (2009). Analysis of teenage pregnancy outcomes and delivery between 2000 and 2006. *Ginekologia Polska,79*(12), 867–870.

Reynolds, F. (2010). The effects of maternal labor analgesia on the fetus. *Best Practices & Research: Clinical Obstetrics & Gynaecology, 24*(3), 289–302.

Ruager-Martin, R., Hyde, M. J., & Modi, N. (2010). Maternal obesity and infant outcomes. *Early Human Development, 86*(11),

715–722.- Saha, S., Loranger, D., Pricolo, V., & Degli-Esposti, S. (2009). Feeding jejunostomy for the treatment of severe hyperemesis gravidarum: A case series. *Journal of Parenteral & Enteral Nutrition, 33*(5), 529–534. doi:10.1177/0148607109333000.

Sakela, C. (2006a). Carol Sakela's letter from North America: An uncontrolled experiment: Elective delivery predominates in the United States. *Birth, 33*(4), 332–335.

Sakela, C., & Corry, M. P. (2008). Achieving the Institute of Medicine's six aims for improvement of maternity care. *Women's Health Issues, 18*(2), 75–78.

Salihu, H. M., Kornosky, J. L., Lynch, O., Alio, A. P., August, E. M., & Marty, P. J. (2010). Impact of prenatal alcohol consumption on placenta-associated syndromes. *Alcohol, 45*(1), 73–79.

Salvesen, K. A., Vatten, L. J., Eik-Nes, S. H., et al. (1993). Routine ultrasonography in utero and subsequent handedness and neurological development. *British Medical Journal, 307*(6897), 159–164.

Santhya, K. G., Ram, U., Acharya, R., Jejeebhoy, S. J., Ram, F., & Singh, A. (2010). Associations between early marriage and young women's marital and reproductive health outcomes: Evidence from India. *International Perspectives on Sexual and Reproductive Health, 36*(3), 132–139.

Satpathy, H. K., Fleming, A., Frey, D., Barsoom, M., Satpathy, C., & Khandalavala, J. (2008). Maternal obesity and pregnancy. *Postgraduate Medicine, 120*(3), E01-9.

Sewell, J. (1993). *Cesarean section: A brief history.* A brochure to accompany an exhibition on the history of cesarean section at the National Library of Medicine. Washington, DC: American College of Obstetricians and Gynecologists.

Schieve, L. A., Coqswell, M. E., & Scanlon, K. S. (1998). Trends in pregnancy weight gain within and outside ranges recommended by the Institute of Medicine in a WIC population. *Maternal and Child Health Journal, 2*(2), 111–116.

Schifrin, B. S. (1990). Electronic fetal monitoring and malpractice. *Female Patient, 15,* 79–82.

Seidman, D. S., Ever-Hadani, P., & Gale, R. (1990). Effect of maternal smoking and age on congenital anomalies. *Obstetrics and Gynecology, 76*(6), 1046–1049.

Shaw, J. L., Dey, S. K., Critchley, H. O., & Horne, A. W. (2010). Current knowledge of the aetiology of human tubal ectopic pregnancy. *Human Reproduction Update, 16*(4), 432–444. doi:10.1093/humupd/dmp057.

Shaw, J. L., Oliver, E., Lee, K. F., Entrican, G., Jabbour, H. N., Critchley, H. O., & Horne, A. W. (2010). Cotinine exposure increases fallopian tube PROKR1 expression via nicotinic AChR{alpha}-7: A potential mechanism explaining the link between smoking and tubal ectopic pregnancy. *American Journal of Pathology, 177*(5), 2509–2515.

Shields, J. R., & Schifrin, B. S. (1988). Perinatal antecedents of cerebral palsy. *Obstetrics and Gynecology, 71,* 899.

Shin, J. S., Choi, M. Y., Longtine, M. S., & Nelson, D. M. (2010). Vitamin D effects on pregnancy and the placenta. *Placenta, 31*(12), 1027–1034.

Shy, K., Luthy, D., Bennett, F., et al. (1990). Effects of electronic fetal-heart-rate monitoring, as compared with periodic auscultation, on the neurological development of premature infants. *New England Journal of Medicine, 322,* 588–593.

Signorello, L. B., Harlow, B. L., Chekos, A. K., & Repke, J. T. (2001). Postpartum sexual functioning and its relationship to perinea l trauma: A retrospective cohort study of primiparous women. *American Journal of Obstetrics and Gynecology, 184*(5), 881–890.

Snell, B. J. (2009). Assessment and management of bleeding in the first trimester of pregnancy. *Journal of Midwifery & Women's Health, 54*(6), 483–491.

Sørensen, H. G., Mortensen, E. L., Reinisch, J. M., & Mednick, S. A. (2003). Do hypertension and diuretic treatment in pregnancy increase the risk of schizophrenia in offspring? *American Journal of Psychiatry, 160,* 464–468.

Stafford, R. S. (1991). The impact of nonclinical factors on repeat cesarean section. *Journal of the American Medical Association, 265*(1), 59–63.

State of the world's mothers 2008: Closing the survival gap for children under 5. Retrieved from http://www.savethechildren.org/atf/cf/%7B9def2ebe-10ae-432c-9bd0-df91d2eba74a%7D/SOWM-2008-FULL-REPORT.PDF.

Stutzman, S. S., Brown, C. A., Hains, S. M., Godwin, M., Smith, G. N., Parlow, J. L., & Kisilevsky, B. S. (2010). The effects of exercise conditioning in normal and overweight pregnant women on blood pressure and heart rate variability. *Biological Research for Nursing, 12*(2), 137–148.

Streissguth, A. P., Aase, J. M., Clarren, S. K., et al. (1991). Fetal alcohol syndrome in adolescents and adults. *Journal of the American Medical Association, 265*(15), 1961–1967.

Streissguth, A. P., Barr, H. M., & Sampson, P. D. (1990). Moderate prenatal alcohol exposure: Effects on child IQ and learning problems at age 7 and 1/2 years. *Alcoholism, 14*(5), 662–669.

Suzumori, N., & Sugiura-Ogasawara, M. (2010). Genetic factors as a cause of miscarriage. *Current Topics in Medicinal Chemistry, 17*(29), 3431–3437.

Taffel, S. M., Placek, P. J., Moien, M., & Kasary, C. L. (1991). 1989 U.S. cesarean section rate steadies—VBAC rate raises to nearly one in five. *Birth, 18*(2), 73–77.

Thacker, S. B., & Stroup, D. F. (2000). Continuous electronic heart rate monitoring for fetal assessment during labor. *Cochrane Database Systematic Reviews, 2,* CD 000063.

Tieu, J., Middleton, P., McPhee, A. J., & Crowther, C. A. (2010). Screening and subsequent management for gestational diabetes for improving maternal and infant health. *Cochrane Database Systematic Review, 7,* CD007222.

Tobias, D. K., Zhang, C., van Dam, R. M., Bowers, K., & Hu, F. B. (2010). Physical activity before and during pregnancy and risk of gestational diabetes mellitus: a meta-analysis. *Diabetes Care, 34*(3), 221–229. doi:10.2337/dc10–1368.

Unterman, R. R., Posner, N. A., & Williams, K. N. (1990). Postpartum depressive disorders: Changing trends. *Birth, 17*(3), 131–137.

U.S. Department of Health and Human Services. Maternal, infant and child health. (2000). In *Healthy people 2010* (2nd ed.). Washington, DC: U.S. Government Printing Office (pp. 16,

30-31). Available at http://www.healthypeople.gov/2020/topicsobjectives2020/overview.aspx?topicid=26.

Vacca, A. (2002). Vacuum-assisted delivery. *Best Practices & Research: Clinical Obstetrics & Gynaecology, 16*(1), 17–30.

van Brummen, H. J., Bruinse, H. W., van de Pol, G., Heintz, A. P., & van der Vaart, C. H. (2006). Bothersome lower urinary tract symptoms 1 year after first delivery: Prevalence and effect of childbirth. *British Journal of Urology International, 98*(1), 89–95.

Van Den Eeden, S. K., Shan, J., Bruce, C., & Glasser, M. (2005). Ectopic pregnancy rate and treatment utilization in a large managed care organization. *Obstetrics & Gynecology, 105*(5 Pt 1), 1052–1057.

Verberg, M. F., Gillott, D. J., Al-Fardan, N., & Grudzinskas, J. G. (2005). Hyperemesis gravidarum, a literature review. *Human Reproduction Update, 11,* 527–539.

Vetr, M. (2005). Risk l factors associated with high birth weight deliveries. *Ceská Gynekologie, 70*(5), 347–354.

Viktrup, L. (2002). The risk of urinary tract symptoms five years after the first delivery. *Neurourol Urodyn, 21*(1), 2–29.

Viktrup, L., Rortveit, G., & Lose, G. (2006). Risk of stress urinary incontinence twelve years after the first pregnancy and delivery. *Obstetrics and Gynecology, 108*(2), 248–254.

Viswanathan, M., Siega-Riz, A. M., Moos, M. K., Deirlein, A., Mumford, S., Knaack, J., Thieda, P., Lux, L. J., & Lohr, K. N. (2008). Outcomes of maternal weight gain. *Evidence Report/Technology Assessment (Full Report),* (168), 1–223.

Wanyonyl, S., Sequeira, E., & Obura, T. (2006). Cesarean section rates and perinatal outcome at the Aga Khan University Hospital, Nairobi. *East African Medical Journal, 83*(12), 651–658.

Weigel, M. M., & Weigel, R. M. (1989). Nausea and vomiting of early pregnancy and pregnancy outcome. An epidemiological study. *British Journal of Obstetrics and Gynecology, 96,* 1304–1311.

Wheeler, T. L., 2nd, & Richter, H. E. (2007). Delivery method, anal sphincter tears and fecal incontinence: New information on a persistent problem. *Current Opinion in Obstetrics and Gynecology, 19*(5), 474–479.

Williams, A., Herron-Marx, S., & Knibb R. (2007). The prevalence of enduring postnatal morbidity and its relationship to type of birth and birth risk factors. *Journal of Clinical Nursing, 16*(3), 549–561.

Williams, A., Herron-Marx, S., & Carolyn, H. (2007). The prevalence of enduring postnatal perineal morbidity and its relationship to perineal trauma. *Midwifery, 23*(4), 392–403.

Wilson, R. D., Johnson, J. A., Allen, V., Gagnon, A., Langlois, S., Blight, C., Audibert, F., Desilets, V., Brock, J. A., Koren, G., Goh, I., Nyuyen, P., Kapur, B., Genetics Committee of the Society of Obstetricians and Gynaecologists of Canada, & the Motherrisk Program. (2007). Re-conceptional vitamin/folic acid supplementation 2007: The use of folic acid in combination with a multivitamin supplement for the prevention of neural tube defects and other congenital abnormalities. *Journal of Obstetrics and Gynaecology Canada, 29*(12), 1003–1026.

Woodward, L., Brackbill, Y., McManus, K., et al. (1982). Exposure to drugs with possible adverse effects during pregnancy and birth. *Birth, 9*(3), 165–171.

World Health Organization. (2005). The world health report 2005: Make every mother and child count. Geneva, Switzerland: Author.

World Health Organization. (2008). Adolescent pregnancy fact sheet.

World Health Organization. (2008). Maternal mental health and child health and development in low and middle income countries. Report to WHO meeting. Geneva, Switzerland: Author.

World Health Organization. Adolescent pregnancy: The facts. Retrieved June 1, 2009 from http://www.who.int/making_pregnancy_safer/topics/adolescent_pregnancy/en/index.html.

World Health Organization, Regional Office for South-East Asia. Introduction to the 'making pregnancy safer' initiative. Retrieved June 1, 2009 from http://www.searo.who.int/EN/Section13/Section36/Section129/Section396_1450.htm.

World Health Organization. Making pregnancy safer. Fact sheet. Retrieved June 1, 2009 from http://www.who.int/making_pregnancy_safer/en/.

Wu, C. S., Nohr, E. A., Bech, B. H., Vestergaard, M., Catov, J. M., & Olsen, J. (2010). Diseases in children born to mothers with preeclampsia: A population-based sibling cohort study. *American Journal of Obstetrics and Gynecology, 204*(2), 157.e1–5.

Yasmeen, S., Romano, P. S., Schembri, M. E., Keyzer, J. M., & Gilbert, W. M. (2006). Accuracy of obstetric diagnosis and procedures in hospital discharge data. *American Journal of Obstetrics and Gynecology, 194*(4), 992–1001.

Yeo, S. (2010). Prenatal stretching exercise and autonomic responses: Preliminary data and a model for reducing preeclampsia. *Journal of Nursing Scholarship, 42*(2), 113–121.

Yildizhan, R., Kolusari, A., Adali, F., Adali, E., Kurdoglu, M., Ozgokce, C., & Cim, N. (2009). Primary abdominal ectopic pregnancy: A case report. *Cases Journal, 2,* 84–85.

Zanardo, V., Simibi, K. A., Vedovato, S., & Trevisanuto, D. (2004). The influence of elective cesarean section on neonatal resuscitation risk. *Pediatric Critical Care Medicine, 5*(6), 566–570.

Zlatnik, M. G., Cheng, Y. W., Norton, M. E., Thiet, M. P., & Caughey, A. B. (2007). Placenta previa and the risk of preterm delivery. *Journal of Maternal-Fetal and Neonatal Medicine, 20*(10), 719–723.

Zupan-Simunek, V. (2010). Prognosis in newborns after mother's preeclampsia. *Annales francaises d'anesthesie et de reanimation, 29*(5), e135–139.

chapter 13

BIRTH CONTROL

CHAPTER COMPETENCIES

Upon completion of this chapter, the reader will be able to:

- Explain the difference between theoretical effectiveness and use effectiveness
- Identify and describe the major contraceptive methods available

- Explain how barrier contraceptives work
- Explain how hormonal contraceptives work
- Identify the risks and benefits of each method of birth control

KEY TERMS

abortion	condom	intrauterine device	spermicide
barrier contraceptive	diaphragm	(IUD)	tubal ligation
cervical cap	emergency contraception	oral contraceptive	vasectomy

INTRODUCTION

During her reproductive years, a woman engaging in sexual intercourse runs the risk of pregnancy (Figure 13-1). If the prevention of pregnancy is important, she can take steps to avoid it. Contraception, the prevention of a pregnancy, is an ancient practice. From the crocodile dung spermicides of ancient Egypt (Jütte, 2005) to the recent experimentation with male hormonal birth control methods (Page et al., 2008), the perfect contraceptive has proven elusive. Ideally, it would be completely safe, have no side effects, and be 100 percent effective at preventing an unwanted pregnancy. The method would be completely reversible; fertility would be

fully restored when the method was discontinued. It would be cheap enough for anyone to afford, distributed and marketed so that anyone could easily obtain it, and simple enough for anyone to use. It would require no medical intervention or prescription. The responsibility for using the method would be shared by both men and women, and it would meet everyone's cultural, religious, political, and philosophical requirements for controlling fertility. Because no one method meets all these criteria for every person, a variety of methods now exist, providing people options. There is no "best" birth control. Contraceptive techniques all have advantages and disadvantages. The choice between safety and

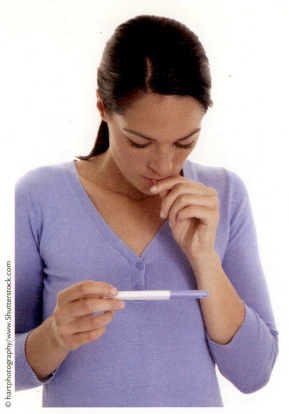

FIGURE 13-1: Properly using contraception is a necessary step to preventing pregnancy.

effectiveness should not have to be made by any woman or man. Every woman has to decide, based on her lifestyle and needs, which method is best for her current situation.

A woman does not have to commit to a single contraceptive method throughout her lifetime. As circumstances change, so may her choice of contraceptive. When intercourse is infrequent, it may not be necessary to use a method that provides continual protection. A couple who is delaying or spacing their family may be more concerned about the reversibility of a birth control method rather than it effectiveness. For those who have completed their family or have no desire to have children, sterilization is a permanent option.

A woman's ability to obtain contraceptives may be limited by cost, healthcare provider bias, and access. In the United States, refusal by some pharmacists to fill legal prescriptions can limit options even further (Wicclair, 2006). A study of over 650 Nevada pharmacists found that six percent refused to fill a prescription for a birth control method,

or transfer that prescription to another pharmacy that would fill it, based on religious objections (Davidson et al., 2010). The debate between conscientious objection laws and laws governing the duty to provide services continues with patients caught in the middle (Pope, 2010). Added to the mix is the amount of incomplete information, and misinformation, available on the different birth control methods. Women need to understand the effectiveness, the benefits, and the potential risks of different contraceptive methods if they are going to make an informed choice.

THEORETICAL EFFECTIVENESS AND USE EFFECTIVENESS

The effectiveness of any method of birth control refers to its ability to prevent pregnancy. Ranking the effectiveness depends on the method itself and how correctly it is used. The theoretical effectiveness of a method is its maximum success rate when it is used correctly, without error, every time intercourse occurs. The use effectiveness of a method refers to the success rate in actual practice by real people under real circumstances—including not using the method correctly or consistently. Use effectiveness rates include women or men to whom proper use has not been fully explained or understood. It also includes women whose partners may be unwilling to comply.

Comparisons between methods of birth control can be very misleading because what is being quoted may be the use effectiveness for some methods and the theoretical effectiveness for other methods. Measurements of contraceptive effectiveness are based on statistics gathered from major studies published in the scientific literature. These studies have been conducted at various times in many different countries on groups of women who varied in age, marital status, income, education, and motivation to use the method. When all of the results are lumped together, a wide range of effectiveness for a contraceptive method is possible. In most cases, the use effectiveness of a method gives the truest picture for a woman. Table 13-1 illustrates the theoretical effectiveness and the use effectiveness of the various methods of contraception.

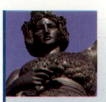

Historical Considerations
THE CURIOUS HISTORY OF CONTRACEPTION

Women's ways of regulating their fertility have been as diverse as women themselves. We will probably never know about some of the historic methods because contraceptive information was not always freely shared. In fact, in the United States up until a landmark court decision in 1936, it was illegal for anyone to import contraceptive supplies. By 1940, all states except Massachusetts and Connecticut allowed doctors to give contraceptive information to their patients. But doctors were not the original experts on contraception: women were. Ancient Egyptian women in 1900 BC made a vaginal suppository of plants, honey, and acacia gum to prevent pregnancy. In ancient India, women chewed seeds of Queen Anne's Lace to prevent or terminate pregnancy (Riddle, 1994). Women in Egypt and India also used animal dung, especially elephant and crocodile dung, to make contraceptive suppositories (Skuy, 1995). Starting around 700 BC, women in Cyrene on the coast of Libya mixed a potion containing silphium, a plant in the giant fennel family, to control reproduction. They harvested and exported so much silphium to Syria and Greece that the plant became extinct in 300 BC (Riddle, 1994). Women throughout Africa used an extract from the seeds of the prayer bead plant as a long-term contraceptive, with a dose effective over 13 menstrual cycles (Iwu, 1993). Japanese women used bamboo, and the women of Easter Island used seaweed as contraceptives (Tone, 2001). Some ferns have contraceptive properties and are known to have been used in ancient China, Hungary, and New Guinea (Bullough, 2001).

While there is ample evidence of contraceptive use throughout much of human history, there has also been controversy. The midwives who passed on contraceptive secrets during the Medieval Inquisition were burned at the stake for practicing medicine without a license. This practice effectively silenced midwives and others who had such knowledge. This attempt to control reproductive knowledge continued into modern times. In the United States, the Comstock Act of 1873 defined contraceptives as obscene and outlawed the dissemination of birth control information through the United States mail or across state lines (Tone, 2001). This law was an obstacle for birth control pioneers in the United States like Emma Goldman who smuggled contraceptives from Europe in 1890 and Margaret Sanger who published "illegal" information on "family limitation" in her magazine *The Woman Rebel* in 1914. Both women stood trial under the Comstock law.

Anthony Comstock, for whom the law was named, was the head of the New York Society for the Suppression of Vice, and he lead the crusade against contraception. Curiously, established companies such as Sears, Roebuck and Co. and Goodyear, who made and distributed contraceptives, were not prosecuted under this law (Tone, 2001). Other distributors had to disguise their contraceptive products in order to avoid Comstock's scrutiny. At the time, publically advocating contraception, especially for poor women, was out of the question. The courts, however, weren't particularly supportive of the Comstock laws and, eventually, it was the courts that established a broader right to birth control information. However, this process took decades.

For example, in theory, if 100 women use the hormone patch for a year, less than one should become pregnant. The use effectiveness has proven less successful; out of 100 women, eight should become pregnant. The same difference holds true for other methods. Periodic abstinence looks fairly effective—in theory—with only five women out of 100 becoming pregnant in a year. In actual practice, 25 per 100 will become pregnant, illustrating that theory and practice can be quite different. No method

Table 13-1 A comparison of the theoretical and use effectiveness of different contraceptive methods showing the number of unintentional pregnancies expected in a year per 100 users.

Contraceptive Method	Theoretical Effectiveness	Use Effectiveness
Male sterilization	0. 1	Less than 1
Female sterilization	0. 1	Less than 1
Injected hormones	0.3	3
Implanted hormones	0.1	Less than 1
IUD with hormones	0.2	Less than 1
Copper IUD	0.6	Less than 1
Nuvaring	0.3	5
Hormone patch	0.3	5
Oral contraceptives	0.3	5
Female condom	5	20
Male condom	2	11-16
Diaphragm	6	15
Cervical cap	9	16
Sponge	9-20	16-32
Periodic abstinence	5	25
Withdrawal	4	27
Spermicide	18	30
No contraception	85	85

Data taken from Trussell et al., 2007; Women's Health Information Center (2009) http://www.womenshealth.gov/faq/birth-control-methods.cfm#d; and California Family Health Council 2009 http://teensource.org/pages/4259/FemCap.htm#4262

is perfect, and the success of a specific method varies, based on the correctness and consistency of use and a woman's own unique biology.

CHOOSING A CONTRACEPTIVE METHOD

The contraceptive choices a woman makes are between her and her partner. Not all methods are equally effective with all women. In addition, there may be health risks with some contraceptives that may put the woman's health at risk. The choice needs to be an informed decision. Points to consider include:

- Does the method fit a woman's lifestyle? Partners may be unwilling to cooperate. Behaviors may make the method less effective or unsafe. For example, a woman may be uncomfortable inserting a ring or diaphragm.

- How effective is the method? Is the risk of pregnancy acceptable?

- How safe is the method? For example, women who smoke are at higher risk for forming a blood clot while using hormonal contraceptives.

- Will it be used consistently? A method that will not be used consistently is ineffective.

- How expensive is it? Some contraceptive methods may be too expensive. No matter how effective a method is, it doesn't work if a woman cannot afford it.

- Is it reversible? Sterilization works well, but if a person wants children at a later date, it is not a viable option.

- Will it protect against STIs? Many people think contraceptives protect against STIs. Condoms and abstinence do, but any method which allows an exchange of fluids or skin-to-skin contact carries a risk of transmitting an STI.
- Are there contraindications—medical conditions or medications that would interact with the method and lessen the effectiveness or increase the risks?

Women need to take these questions into consideration when making contraceptive choices. A woman's healthcare provider, someone who should be familiar with her health history, is a resource for helping her make a choice. The CDC, WHO, and Planned Parenthood offer additional information. Most colleges have health services, many offering reproductive health services at reduced costs. Local clinics and community health centers may also provide reproductive health services on a sliding scale.

CONTRACEPTIVE METHODS

Contraceptive methods fall under several major categories, and two or more methods can be combined to improve effectiveness. The categories include forms of abstinence, spermicides, barrier methods, hormonal methods, intrauterine devices, and surgical methods. Each method has its benefits and its risks.

Forms of Abstinence—Contraception Without Contraceptives

Avoiding intercourse either completely (continuous abstinence) or during fertile periods (periodic abstinence) can be effective methods of contraception, if followed correctly and consistently. The methods work by preventing the egg and sperm from coming in contact with one another.

Continuous Abstinence

Continuous abstinence—avoiding vaginal intercourse—is one of the oldest methods of preventing pregnancy. In theory, this method should be 100 percent effective; because sperm are never introduced into the vagina, pregnancy cannot occur. However, abstinence-only education programs have proven ineffective at changing teenage behavior (Harper et al., 2010). One recent study found that teens who received abstinence-only sex education were half as likely to use a reliable birth

control method when they did become sexually active compared to other members of the cohort educated in other birth control methods (Isley, et al., 2010). Another drawback of abstinence is that it requires a strong commitment and strict adherence to avoiding vaginal intercourse. Many individuals are unable to maintain the level of self-control necessary and, for that reason, the use effectiveness is not 100 percent. On the benefit side, the method is free, requires no medical intervention, and has no physiological side effects.

Periodic Abstinence—Fertility Awareness

There are several methods of periodic abstinence called variously natural birth control, natural family planning, basal body temperature monitoring (BBT), or fertility awareness methods. Observations of physical changes and calculations are used to determine the fertile and the nonfertile periods of the reproductive cycle. The couple abstains from vaginal intercourse during the fertile times. In its most sophisticated form, using a combination of several procedures, only five pregnancies per 100 women should occur. However, in actual practice, the method is less effective—25 pregnancies

Critical Thinking

Comprehensive Sexual Education versus Abstinence-Only

The Bush Administration spent over 175 million dollars annually on abstinence-only sex education programs. These programs could only discuss the failure rates of other methods, nothing more (Ott and Santelli, 2007). Comprehensive programs educate students on a range of contraceptive options—including abstinence. Two separate studies now indicate that comprehensive programs delay the start of sexual activity and cut teen pregnancy when compared to abstinence-only education programs (Ott and Santelli, 2007; Center for the Advancement of Health, 2008).

What program should school children be taught? Why?

per 100 women—most likely due to the variations in women's fertile times and potential problems interpreting the observations necessary to identify fertile periods.

Techniques for the use of periodic abstinence for contraception are based on several assumptions:

- That ovulation occurs once per cycle about 14 days before the onset of the next menstrual period;
- That the ovum is viable and capable of being fertilized for about 72 hours;
- That sperm are able to survive in the female reproductive tract to fertilize an ovum for about 72 hours.

Identification of the fertile period can be accomplished by using a calendar if the reproductive cycles are consistently regular. The calendar method of calculating the fertile period, during which sexual intercourse cannot take place, requires keeping track of the length of each of the menstrual cycles over several months (Figure 13-2). This method of calculation presumes that ovulation occurred 14 days before menstruation. However, because of the variability of cycles, ovulation cannot be pinpointed exactly. Inclusion of changes in basal body temperature (BBT) and cervical mucus can help refine the determination of fertile times.

The use of the basal body temperature (BBT) chart can enhance the effectiveness of periodic abstinence. BBT relies on a visible, measurable indication of ovulation—the slight elevation of the body temperature under basal conditions that occurs at the time of, or shortly before, the egg is released from the ovary. To use BBT to avoid pregnancy, a woman must have cycles in which an obvious rise in temperature occurs—only then can this method be used to determine ovulation. Sexual intercourse is restricted until three consecutive days after the elevation of temperature has occurred—that is, until the postovulatory phase when conception is biologically impossible. A major drawback to the BBT method is that it does not predict ovulation. It merely indicates when it has occurred. For complete safety, sexual intercourse is limited to the 10 or 12 days before the next menstrual period.

The cervical mucus produced by the endocervical glands undergoes changes during the

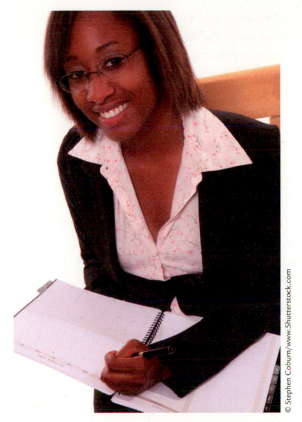

FIGURE 13-2: The calendar method of calculating fertility as a means to preventing pregnancy requires careful tracking of the menstrual cycles over several months.

reproductive cycle. Between the end of menstruation and the beginning of the fertile period, the cervical mucus is opaque white or yellow, and its consistency is described as tacky or gummy. This thick mucus creates a mucus plug, temporarily sealing the cervix, and this period is considered a safe time. Estrogen levels are high just prior to ovulation, and the cervical discharge increases in amount, becomes clear, and has a higher salt content. At the time of ovulation, the mucus becomes very profuse, has the consistency of egg white, and at the peak production during the time of ovulation, has spinnbarkeit. This is the ability of the mucus to be stretched between the thumb and forefinger into a long, clear, thin strand. If this clear mucus is smeared onto a glass slide and permitted to dry, it can be seen under the microscope to fern, forming a highly branched pattern because of the salt content. These signs indicate very fertile mucus—a very unsafe time for intercourse if a woman does not want to become pregnant—and persist for several days after ovulation. Postovulatory mucus is sticky and thick under the influence of progesterone. The thick mucus indicates a return to the infertile part of the cycle. This viscous mucus may become clear and watery just before menstruation, but this stage occurs inconsistently.

Withdrawal

The withdrawal of the penis from the vagina before ejaculation occurs is called by the Latin term, coitus interruptus. As a method of contraception, it is probably the oldest, best known, and most widely used means of preventing pregnancy in the world. It requires no device or preparation, costs nothing, and is always available, safe, and reversible, but it does have one obvious disadvantage—for most couples it is less effective than most other methods, with a use effectiveness far below other methods. While often not considered a true form of abstinence, withdrawal uses the same principles—keeping sperm out of the vagina.

The method requires that the male withdraw his penis completely from the vagina before ejaculation and to ejaculate well away from the vagina. The first few drops of the true ejaculate contain the greatest concentration of sperm, and if some pre-ejaculatory fluid escapes from the urethra before orgasm, conception may result. When a couple uses withdrawal consistently, they are likely to develop their own techniques to make the method mutually satisfactory. It does require self-control during an activity in which loss of control is usually considered to be more pleasurable. A woman may find it more difficult to

relax when she is concerned about the man's ability to withdraw in time.

Spermicides

Spermicides are chemicals that are placed in the vagina to stop the movement of sperm, block the cervix, and, over the course of several hours, kill the sperm. When used as the only method of birth control, spermicides are relatively ineffective (see Table 13-1). In combination with other barrier methods their effectiveness increases. With spermicides, consistent use each and every time there is sexual intercourse is the main factor that determines their effectiveness. Most spermicides contain nonylphenoxypolyethoxyethanol (nonoxynol-9). Despite early lab results that suggested nonoxynol-9 acted as a microbiocide, killing sexually-transmitted pathogens, more recent data suggests that in actual use the spermicide may increase the risk of STI transmission (Baptista and Ramalho-Santos, 2009). Allergic reactions to nonoxynol-9 occur in some individuals, and some women find the spermicides messy. Spermicides must be inserted into the vagina near the cervix before intercourse to be effective and must be reapplied if intercourse is repeated (Hatcher et al., 2008). Not using enough spermicide, placing it too low in the vagina, or forgetting to reapply spermicide can diminish its effectiveness. In its favor, this method is available over the counter, is relatively inexpensive, and is completely reversible.

Spermicides are available in several forms—foam, creams, gels, and solid films (Figure 13-3).

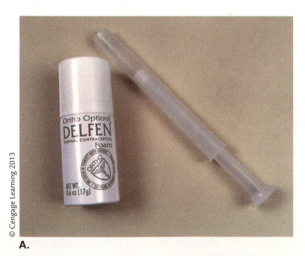

© Cengage Learning 2013

A.   **B.**

FIGURE 13-3: Spermicides come in several forms. A. Foams. B. Films.

Contraceptive foam consists of an oil-in-water emulsion medium which provides a mechanical cervical barrier and the chemical spermicide. The foam is packaged in a pressurized container. It may be released into an applicator from the can, or may be purchased in packets of disposable applicators for direct discharge into the vagina. A foaming tablet form is also available. Although contraceptive creams and gels are also available, they are not recommended for use without diaphragms or cervical caps because they are less likely to cover the cervix rapidly and evenly to block sperm.

A contraceptive film consists of a 2-by-2-inch thin sheet of film of nonoxynol-9. The square is folded and must be inserted near the cervix not less than five minutes before intercourse to allow enough time for the sheet to dissolve and release the spermicide. This method is effective for about two hours and has failure rates equivalent to other spermicide barrier preparations.

Barrier Contraceptives

Barrier contraceptives prevent pregnancy by physically blocking the passage of sperm throughout the cervix, preventing the sperm from getting to the egg. They include condoms, diaphragms, cervical caps, and sponges. Because barrier contraceptives are used only when they are needed, the body is not subjected to a daily dose of hormones, as with hormonal forms of birth control. Disadvantages include occasional allergies to a particular product, a slightly increased risk of UTI and other infections, a broad range of reliability, and what some perceive as their inconvenience.

Male Condoms

A male condom, probably the most widely used contraceptive in the world, is the only kind of birth control device used by the male. A **condom** is a thin, flexible sheath made of latex, flexible plastic, or animal membrane that is closed on one end and open at the other. The condom is rolled over an erect penis to fit tightly during intercourse in order to trap the ejaculate and prevent semen from entering the vagina.

The origin of the condom is unknown. The first recorded account of condom use appeared in 1564 in the writings of Italian anatomist Gabrielli Fallopius and described a linen sheath to cover the penis in order to protect males from syphilis, although no mention of its use as a contraceptive was made. Historically, condoms made of fabric, fish skin, and intestinal membranes were used to prevent transmission of STIs and were commonly used in the brothels during the eighteenth century. Recently, evidence that condoms can prevent most STIs and cervical cancer has increased their use.

Condoms today are usually made of latex or a flexible plastic and come in a variety of colors, textures, and even flavors (Figure 13-4). Condoms designed to prevent pregnancy have expiration dates printed on the individual package. Strictly decorative condoms are also available. Some come prelubricated with spermicide. Condoms can be purchased with a plain tip or with a reservoir to collect the semen. In condoms without the reservoir, semen is more likely to be pushed along the sides of the condom and leak into the vagina during intercourse.

To be effective, a condom must be used correctly. The condom is rolled over an erect penis before it enters the vagina and is worn throughout sexual intercourse. If the condom has no reservoir to hold the semen, the first half inch of the condom should be pinched with the fingers while unrolling to keep out the air and leave a space to catch the ejaculate. Condoms can be used with a water-based lubricant, but oil-based lubricants can deteriorate the latex and lead to breakage. An objection to condom use has been that it interrupts sexual intercourse. Some couples have found that a condom need not detract from sexual enjoyment by incorporating the activity of putting on the condom as part of their foreplay. Soon

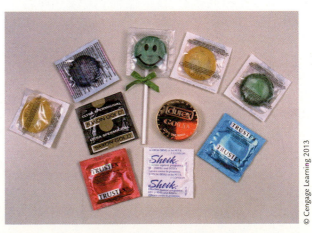

FIGURE 13-4: Male condoms come in a variety of types.

© Cengage Learning 2013

after ejaculation, the condom should be held tightly by the rim at the base while the penis is withdrawn from the vagina. If the penis becomes flaccid in the vagina, sperm can spill over the open end. If the condom tears or comes off in the vagina, a spermicide should immediately be applied inside the vagina.

Condoms are moderately effective in preventing pregnancy with a use effectiveness of 15 pregnancies per 100 women. The condom is relatively inexpensive, designed for one time use, and needs no prescription to obtain. It gives males a chance to participate in the responsibility for birth control, and it has the added important advantage of protecting both partners against HIV and other sexually transmitted infections. For individuals with latex allergies, plastic condoms are available.

Female Condom

A condom that a woman can wear was approved by the United States Food and Drug Administration in 1993. The female condom consists of a polyurethane sheath with a flexible ring at each end (Figure 13-5). To insert a female condom, the ring at the closed end of the condom is pinched together and inserted into the vagina until it reaches the cervix, then the ring is released. When properly positioned, the inner ring fits behind the pubic bone, and the outer ring surrounds and covers the labia (Figure 13-6). Like the male condom, care must be taken when removing the female condom after intercourse to prevent spilling semen into the vagina. Female condoms are slightly less effective at preventing pregnancy than male

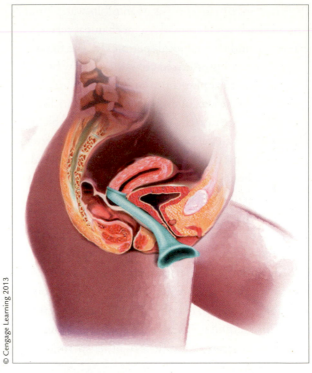

FIGURE 13-6: Proper placement of a female condom.

condoms, with 21 in 100 women becoming pregnant when using this method of birth control. The lower use effectiveness of the female condom may be because it does not fit as tightly as a male condom and is more likely to slip into the vagina, allowing semen to leak in.

Diaphragm

A **diaphragm** is a soft rubber dome surrounded by a flexible, metal spring that is inserted into the vagina to cover the cervix (Figure 13–7). The diaphragm itself is a good mechanical barrier to sperm, but alone it cannot completely bar the passage of sperm. For this reason, the diaphragm must always be used with spermicide and can be viewed as a cup that holds spermicide against the cervix. Diaphragms vary in both type and size. A woman must be properly fitted by a healthcare provider with the specific type and size diaphragm suited to her.

There are some contraindications to diaphragm use. A woman who is sensitive to the spermicide or has a latex allergy cannot use a diaphragm. Diaphragms should not be used during menstruation. Diaphragms must initially be fitted by a health professional and refitted after childbirth or substantial

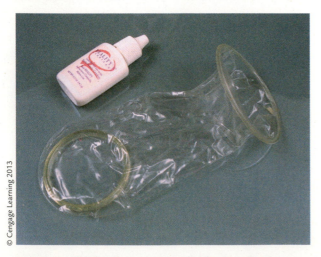

© Cengage Learning 2013

FIGURE 13-5: The female condom made of polyurethane.

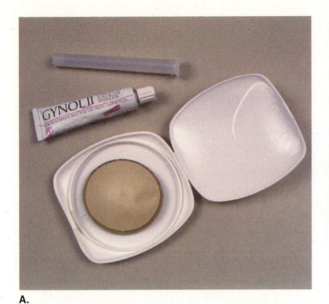

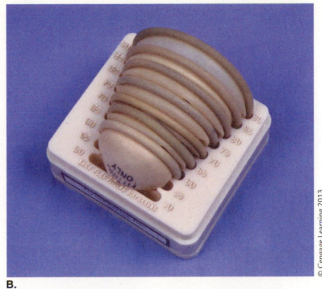

A.

B.

© Cengage Learning 2013

FIGURE 13-7: A. A diaphragm with spermicide; B. Size range of diaphragms.

weight loss or gain of 10 kg (roughly 20 pounds) or more. The use effectiveness is roughly equivalent to that of a male condom, with 16 women per 100 users becoming pregnant while using this form of contraception.

When being fitted for a diaphragm, a woman will be instructed how to correctly insert and remove her diaphragm. For maximum effectiveness, the diaphragm is filled with about 15 mL (1 tablespoon) of spermicide with additional spermicide spread around the rim. The sides are pinched together, and it is inserted into the vagina against the cervix. In its proper position, the diaphragm should completely cover the cervix and the upper portion of the vagina. The diaphragm can be inserted several hours before intercourse, but additional spermicide should be inserted into the vagina for repeated intercourse. After intercourse, the diaphragm must not be removed for a minimum of six hours.

One disadvantage of diaphragm use is its association in epidemiological studies with urinary tract infections (UTIs). Several studies have shown that a mild and transient increase in the number of *Escherichia coli* (normal intestinal flora) in the urine and in the vagina normally occurs as a result of sexual intercourse. Hooten and colleagues (1991) found, however, that while the increase in bacteria disappears within 24 hours in women who use oral contraceptives, both the prevalence and the persistence of these

bacteria in the urine and the vagina is significantly increased in women who use a diaphragm with spermicide. These increases are also found in those using a condom with spermicidal foam. In addition, vaginal flora have the ability to form biofilms on intravaginal devices (Chassot et al., 2010), and a diaphragm must be washed after use with mild soap to limit microbial growth.

Cervical Cap

In contrast to the diaphragm, which covers the entire upper part of the vaginal canal between the pubic bone and the posterior fornix, a **cervical cap** as indicated by its name, is a smaller, thimble-shaped latex cup which covers only the cervix. Cervical caps are made of rubber and are used with spermicide in the same way diaphragms are. They must be fitted individually so that the rim of the cap surrounds the base of the cervix while the dome of the cap does not actually touch the cervical os (Figure 13-8). The device remains in place through suction and is removed by tilting the rim away from the cervix with the index finger to break the suction.

One disadvantage of the cervical cap is that it can be more difficult to learn the proper technique of insertion and removal, partially because the cap must be placed deep in the vaginal canal. Because the cap can stick by suction to any part of the vaginal walls or to the side of the cervix, it must be checked

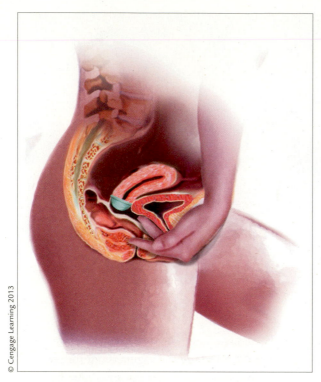

© Cengage Learning 2013

FIGURE 13-8: Proper insertion of a cervical cap.

with the finger to confirm that the cervix is covered. Cervical caps can also be dislodged during intercourse, although this is less likely to occur than with a diaphragm. Dislodgement may result from changes in size or position of the cervix that normally occur during a woman's monthly cycle or sexual excitement or during sexual activity itself. Like the diaphragm, the cap must remain in place for at least six hours after intercourse. In contrast to the diaphragm, additional spermicide does not have to be added to the vagina if multiple intercourse occurs, unless the cap is accidentally dislodged. The effectiveness of the cap appears to be about the same as the diaphragm.

The safety record of the cap also is similar to that of the diaphragm. Although several cases of toxic shock syndrome (TSS) have been reported in diaphragm users, there have been no occurrences of TSS as a result of using a cervical cap. One matter of concern has been the possibility of cervical changes resulting from the suction that the cap exerts on the cervix. A study by Bernstein and colleagues (1986) found that four percent of cervical cap users had abnormal pap smears after three months of use compared with only 1.7 percent of diaphragm users. However, this result was not substantiated by other

cap researchers investigating cervical cap use (Gollub & Sivin, 1989; Richwald et al., 1989).

An additional safety issue concerns the amount of time the cap can stay in place. Historically, when cervical caps were made of rigid materials such as silver, ivory, aluminum, or plastic, women were advised that they could safely leave them inserted for the entire month, removing them only for their menstrual period. Current recommendations are far more conservative. The cap should be inserted for a maximum of 48 hours to minimize the risk of irritation, vaginal infection, or cervical abrasion.

Vaginal Sponge

In April 1983, the FDA approved a synthetic foam contraceptive sponge that could be inserted into the vagina for up to 24 hours as an over-the-counter contraceptive. The sponge was approximately 2 inches in diameter, 1 1/2-inches thick, and contained the spermicide nonoxynol-9. The spermicide was activated with water before inserting the sponge into the vagina. The sponge has a small depression on one surface to aid in positioning it over the cervix and a loop on the other surface to help with its removal from the vagina (Figure 13-9). Several brands of contraceptive sponges are now available over the counter.

Contraceptive sponges vary in their effectiveness depending on whether or not a woman has delivered a child. In nulliparous women (women who have not given birth), 16 out of 100 become pregnant, however, the failure rate doubles to 32 out of 100 in parous women (women who have previously given birth).

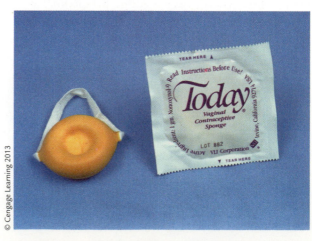

© Cengage Learning 2013

FIGURE 13-9: An example of a contraceptive sponge.

Hormonal Methods of Birth Control

Hormonal contraceptives work by altering the reproductive hormones in a woman's body. This prevents development and release of eggs from the ovary. In addition, the hormonal changes limit the development of the endometrium, making them effective for treating some cases of dysmenorrhea and abnormal uterine bleeding. Contrary to popular notion, hormonal contraceptives do not make the body think it is pregnant. During pregnancy, the levels of estrogen and progesterone soar both from the maternal increase and production by the placenta. With hormonal contraceptives, hormone levels remain low. Hormonal contraceptives are available in several hormone combinations and several delivery methods including oral contraceptives, injected hormones, implants, contraceptive patches, and a contraceptive vaginal ring.

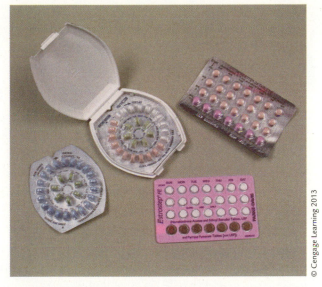

FIGURE 13-10: Several types of oral contraceptives.

© Cengage Learning 2013

Oral Contraceptive

The first **oral contraceptive** was approved by the Food and Drug Administration (FDA) in 1960. It had actually been on the market for several years, prescribed to prevent miscarriage and menstrual disorders, but its introduction as an oral contraceptive was the start of a new era in birth control - hormonal contraception. Other brands soon appeared, and what generically became known as "The Pill" rapidly achieved enormous popularity. The social impact of what was hailed as a breakthrough in effective, easy, and safe contraception was so far-reaching that people began to speak of a "sexual revolution."

It was not surprising that many women needed little encouragement to use oral contraceptives. For centuries, the idea of swallowing something to prevent pregnancy had caused women to dose themselves with potions and poisons many of which were ineffective at best, and deadly at worst. Oral contraceptives provided almost perfect effectiveness with the added benefit of the elimination of menstrual pain and bleeding for many users. The introduction of contraceptive pills also gave a woman complete control of her reproductive capacity without having to worry about her partner.

Although oral contraceptives are commonly referred to as "the pill," there are many different versions which differ in their composition, their

effectiveness, and the side effects that they produce (Figure 13-10). Natural estrogen and progesterone are inactivated by the digestive system when they are taken orally. Synthetic versions of these steroids are modified forms of the natural hormones and are used as medications. Combined oral contraceptive pills (COCs) are composed of a synthetic estrogen and progestin. Most of these are available in both 21- and 28-tablet packages. The progestin-only pills, or minipills, contain a low dose of progestins and have a lower theoretical effectiveness rate than the combined pills. They are supplied in 28- and 42-tablet packages. Low-dose and ultralow-dose contraceptive pills became available in the late 1970s, followed by, "biphasic" and "triphasic" combinations that step up the dose of the progestin at intervals through the pill-taking cycle. Currently, the most commonly used contraceptive pills have about one-fifth the level of estrogen that was present in the pills of the 1960s and about one-twentieth the dose of progestin.

Oral contraceptives work primarily by suppressing the production of FSH and LH. As a result, normal follicle growth and ovulation do not occur. The synthetic steroids in the pills provide a constant amount of reproductive hormones, which are metabolized within 24 hours and which replace the normal cyclic production of a woman's own estrogen and progesterone. If, for some reason, the midcycle surge of LH is not completely inhibited, it is possible that an "escape" ovulation may occur.

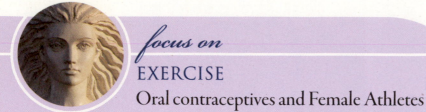

focus on

EXERCISE
Oral contraceptives and Female Athletes

Concerns have been raised that the hormones in oral contraceptives could have an effect on women's performances during athletic competition (Burrows and Peters, 2007). The number of female athletes using oral contraceptives now matches their use in the general population. An Australian study found that, at least for rowers, low estrogen and progesterone levels found in women using oral contraceptives coincided with better performance (Redman and Weatherby, 2004). This research was based on a small sample size, but it raises interesting questions concerning the use of female steroids during competition.

Secondary contraception is provided by the progestational activity of the pills. Sperm penetration into the uterus is prevented by a thickening of the cervical mucus, and the endometrium undergoes changes that inhibit implantation. Progestin-only pills—the minipills—do not necessarily prevent ovulation and exert their function primarily through these secondary effects.

The monthly bleeding that occurs while taking oral contraceptives is a false menstruation produced by estrogen and progesterone stimulation of the endometrium, followed by withdrawal of the hormones for the last seven days of the cycle. This is accomplished either though placebo pills or by taking no pills for seven days. For many years, women quietly shared the information with other women that skipping the placebo week and starting in on the next cycle of pills would prevent their monthly periods. This is the basis behind some of the newer oral contraceptives which cause menstrual suppression of up to a year.

To be most effective, oral contraceptives must be taken every day, at the same time of day. This maintains consistent levels of hormones in the body. Oral contraceptives are highly effective with a failure rate of eight women per 100 users becoming pregnant over a one year time frame. There are a number of drugs that interact with oral contraceptives and may reduce the efficacy or increase the side effects of either the oral contraceptives or the drugs taken. A woman should discuss any medication with her healthcare provider before beginning oral contraceptives.

Despite their effectiveness, there are a number of side effects associated with oral contraceptive use (Table 13-2). Weight gain and migraines are common side effects. Some researchers have reported that the incidence of gallstones (cholelithiasis) and inflammation of the gallbladder (cholecystitis) is higher in women who are taking oral contraceptives than in those who are not. This association appears to be greater only in the first few years of pill use, but women who have had previous gallbladder disease or who have had their gallbladders removed should choose another form of contraception.

Blood clots, stroke, and heart attack pose the most serious risks, particularly in women over age 35 (La Vecchia, 1990). Some of the newer COC use the synthetic progestin drospirenone. A recent study found drospirenone oral contraceptive users had nearly twice the rate of blood clots compared with users of other COC and a six-fold increase over women who did not use oral contraceptives ("Drospirenone: high risk of venous thrombosis, 2011).

There are some women who should not use oral contraceptives. The absolute contraindications to pill usage are pregnancy, current or past history of blood clotting disorders, current or past history of cerebrovascular or coronary artery disease, known or suspected estrogen-dependent cancers, any undiagnosed vaginal bleeding, or any current or past liver disease. When, for example, a woman already has an underlying risk of developing heart disease or cancer, the superimposition of oral contraceptives on those predisposing factors could increase her odds of developing pill-associated diseases. Behaviors such as smoking increase the risk of clot formation and women who smoke should discuss other methods of birth control with their healthcare provider.

Table 13-2 Side Effects of Combined Oral Contraceptive Related to Hormones and Dosage.

General Side Effects

Estrogen Excess	Estrogen Deficiency	Progestin Excess	Androgen Excess
Chloasma	Nervousness	Appetite increase	Acne
Chronic nasopharyngitis	Vasomotor	Depression	Cholestatic jaundice
Gastric influenza	symptoms	Fatigue	Hirsutism
Hay fever and allergic rhinitis		Hypoglycemia	Increased libido
Urinary tract infection		Decreased libido	Oily skin and scalp
		Neurodermatitis	Rash and pruritis
		Weight gain	Edema

Reproductive Side Effects

Estrogen Excess	Estrogen Deficiency	Progestin Excess	Progestin Deficiency
Breast changes	Absence of	Cervicitis	Breakthrough bleeding
Cervical extrophy	withdrawal	Decreased flow	Delayed withdrawal
Dysmenorrhea	bleeding	Moniliasis	bleeding
Hypermenorrhea	Continuous		Dysmenorrhea
Menorrhagia	bleeding		Heavy flow with clots
Clotting with menses	Hypomenorrhea		
Increased breast size	Pelvic relaxation		
Mucorrhea (mucus discharge)	Atropic vaginitis		
Uterine enlargement			
Uterine fibroid growth			

Cardiovascular Side Effects

Estrogen Excess		Progestin Excess	
Capillary fragility		Hypertension	
Cerebrovascular accident		Leg vein dilation	
Deep vein thrombosis			
Telangiectasis			
Thromboembolic disease			

Premenstrual Side Effects

Estrogen Excess or Progestin Deficiency
Bloating
Dizziness
Edema
Headache
Irritability
Leg cramps
Nausea and vomiting
Visual changes
Weight gain

Data adapted by Littleton & Engebretson (2005) from Managing Contraceptive Pill Patients, by R. P. Dickey, 2001, Durant, OK: Essential Medical Information Systems.

Implanted Hormonal Contraceptives

Implantable hormonal contraceptives were introduced in the early 1990s. Norplant, the first hormonal implant, consisted of silicone rubber capsules filled with a synthetic progestin, levonorgestrel, also found in many oral contraceptives. The soft, flexible tubes (Figure 13-11), each about the size of a matchstick, are inserted with a large-bore needle under

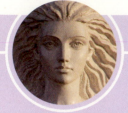

focus on

EXERCISE
Oral Contraceptive-Induced Vitamin Deficiencies

For years, there have been questions about whether oral contraceptives cause vitamin deficiencies. A Belgian study of over 200 women compared users of oral contraceptives with IUD users and women using no form of contraception. According to their results, oral contraceptives significantly lower beta-carotene levels and raise selenium levels in women who use them. However, vitamin C and zinc levels were not different between the test groups (Pincemail et al., 2007). This research suggests that a woman on oral contraceptives should eat foods rich in beta-carotene or discuss taking a supplement with her healthcare provider

(Waknine, 2006), and provides up to three years of protection. It slowly releases etonogestrel, another form of progestin. It has the advantage of providing rapid protection once implanted and a rapid return to fertility when removed (Fischer, 2008). Unlike Norplant, Implanon is a single rod, small enough that it rarely scars, and is not visible under the skin. Other implants, including Jadelle, Nesterone, Capronor, and Anuelle, contain varying forms of synthetic progesterone and use a variety of delivery methods. Capronor and Anuelle have biodegradable capsules and do not require a return visit to a health professional for removal.

Implantable contraceptives are highly effective, with less than one pregnancy per 100 women occurring per year. They provide contraceptive protection for one to seven years depending on the specific implant. They also have the advantage of being reversible; fertility can be restored by removing the implants. After removal of the Norplant contraceptive, 20 percent of women trying to become pregnant succeed during the first month, 49 percent by the fourth month, 73 percent after the sixth month, and 86 percent by the end of a year (Shoupe & Mishell, 1989).

Implantable contraceptives do require a visit to a medical professional for insertion. Side effects include menstrual disruptions, inflammation at the implant site, and scar tissue. Rarer side effects include headaches, weight changes, mood swings, and an increased risk of ovarian cysts. As with oral contraceptives, the use of implantable contraceptives is contraindicated in women with acute liver disease, a history of breast cancer, heart attacks, blood clots, stroke, or unexplained vaginal bleeding, and for women who smoke.

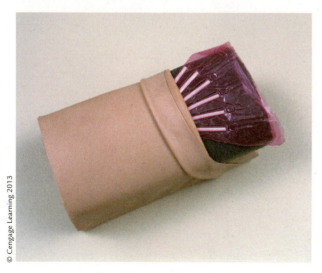

© Cengage Learning 2013

FIGURE 13-11: Implantable contraceptives.

the skin of the inside of the woman's upper arm. The procedure requires local anesthesia, takes about 10 minutes, and requires no stitches. Over a period of several years, the capsules release constant low levels of hormone, thickening cervical mucus so sperm cannot enter the cervix, and decreasing the thickness of the endometrial lining of the uterus, making it unreceptive to implantation. When the hormones have all been released, the implant tubes are removed.

In addition to Norplant, several newer implantable contraceptives are available around the world. Implanon has replaced Norplant in the United States

The Depo-Provera Injectable Contraceptives

For women who feel uncomfortable with implants, injectable contraceptives provide an alternative for long-term hormonal birth control. Depo-Provera, also known as "the shot", is the trade name for the synthetic progestin medroxyprogesterone and

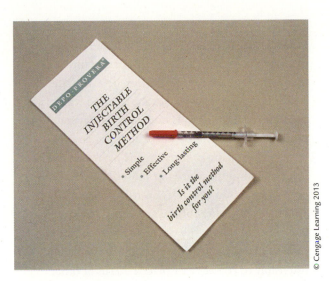

FIGURE 13-12: Injectable contraceptive.

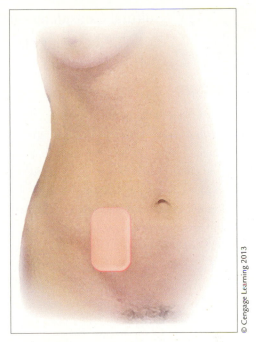

FIGURE 13-13: The contraceptive patch is placed on the skin and the hormones diffuse into the system.

consists of a single injection of hormone into the arm or hip muscle (Figure 13-12). It acts like other progestin-only preparations to prevent pregnancy for three months. Depo-Provera has an effective rate of three pregnancies per 100 users. The injections are given under medical supervision and need to be repeated every three months.

Many women on Depo-Provera have menstrual irregularities ranging from spotting to occasional episodes of very heavy vaginal bleeding during the first cycle of this contraceptive. After the first month of use, amenorrhea is more common. The method is not reversible between injections; the hormones must be gradually metabolized by the body to be removed. Side effects associated with Depo-Provera use are similar to those associated with hormonal contraception—headaches, weight gain, abdominal bloating, depression, dizziness, and fatigue. Studies also show that Depo-Provera can decrease bone density in young women (Johnson et al., 2008; Scholes et al., 2005), but the effect is reversible upon stoppage of the drug. One report (Skegg and Spears, 1989) suggested that Depo-Provera may increase the risk of breast cancer in young women by encouraging proliferation of pre-existing cancer cells. Contraindications are similar to those of other hormonal contraceptives.

The Contraceptive Patch

The contraceptive patch is a combined estrogen-progestin contraceptive (Figure 13-13). The hormones are embedded in a gel within the patch, the patch is attached to the skin, and the hormones diffuse at low levels into the bloodstream. The patch must be replaced weekly. Because the hormones need to diffuse across the skin and subcutaneous adipose tissue, women who weigh more than 198 pounds may find the method less effective or require a higher dose patch. The placement of the patch also impacts the rates of hormone delivery.

Research indicates that the patch is as effective as oral contraceptives, but patch users reported increased incidence of dysmenorrhea, nausea, and breast discomfort leading to discontinuation of use (Lopez et al., 2008). The patch, like combination oral contraceptives, increases the risk of blood clots (Kluft et al., 2008). Contraindications are the same as with oral contraceptives.

Vaginal Contraceptive Ring

NuvaRing is a flexible ring with embedded estrogens and progestin that is inserted deep into the vagina to encircle the cervix. The ring is left in place for three weeks and removed for one week before beginning the next cycle. Once in place, the ring slowly releases hormones which, just like oral contraceptive, inhibit ovulation and thicken the cervical mucus to prevent sperm from passing through the

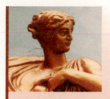

Cultural Considerations
CONTRACEPTIVE CHOICES

A woman's choice of contraceptive method depends on a variety of factors—availability, cost, familiarity with the method, partner attitudes, and cultural attitudes, to name a few. A study by the University of Alabama showed distinct differences between Hispanic immigrants and non-Hispanics with regard to knowledge of contraceptives and reproductive biology and choice of contraceptive. Hispanic women were less familiar with contraceptive choices, had lower rates of contraceptive use, and preferred injectable contraception when they used one. Non-Hispanics were more likely to use contraceptives, but preferred oral contraceptives to injectable contraceptives (Garcés-Palacio et al., 2008). Although the sample examined only women in Memphis, Tennessee, the study suggests that women of different cultural backgrounds may have very different knowledge bases and different attitudes toward contraceptive methods. Outreach programs need to be familiar with cultural preferences and work within those differences to educate women about the contraceptive options that are available to them.

caravan journeys. The writings of Hippocrates, the Greek physician who is called the father of medicine, describe the use of a hollow tube passed into a human uterus through which medication or a small device would be inserted. Whether the method was actually used for contraception is not clear. For several thousand years after Hippocrates, there was no further historical mention of intrauterine devices, although intravaginal suppositories or pessaries were widely used as a method of birth control.

The forerunners of the modern IUDs were most likely the stem pessaries of the late nineteenth and early twentieth centuries. Placed into the vagina ostensibly to correct a displaced uterus or other "female disorders," stem pessaries were small caps or buttons made of wood, ivory, pewter, or precious metal that fit over the cervix and were attached to stems that led into the cervical canal or even farther into the uterine cavity.

The modern history of IUDs began in the 1920s, when a German physician, Ernst Grafenberg, developed the Grafenberg ring. Composed of silver, and silkworm gut, the ring was the first IUD with published success rate data. However, the Grafenberg ring was not well accepted by the medical community due to concerns about infection and fell into disrepute. During the 1960s, two independent workers, Oppenheimer in Israel and Ishihama in Japan, who had earlier rediscovered the Grafenberg rings, published their reports of the successful use of intrauterine devices. These reports lead to the initiation of several clinical trials and two international conferences which publicized the positive results of the trials. This resulted in another shift in medical opinion. IUDs were now believed to be closest to the "ideal" contraceptive. Although they had the drawback of requiring a clinical procedure for insertion, once in place, IUDs required only periodic checking by the user. They provided long-term protection against pregnancy that was completely reversible once the device was removed.

However, side effects—particularly infection, pelvic inflammatory disease (PID), ectopic pregnancy, sterility, and death—became serious problems with one specific design, the Dalkon shield. This device, which had pointed projections that clung to the uterine lining, was especially favored in the early 1970s because it appeared to resist expulsion,

cervix. It is more effective than oral contraceptives, with six pregnancies per 100 users per year. The contraindications for the ring are the same as other combination estrogen/progestin contraceptives. Side effects with the ring are minimal, although it is associated with an increase in the rates of vaginosis (Lopez et al., 2008).

Intrauterine Devices (IUDs)

A small object placed in the uterus to prevent pregnancy is called an **intrauterine device (IUD)**. Many forms of IUDs have been used to prevent pregnancy since ancient times. One frequently told story concerns the Arabian practice of inserting a small pebble into a camel's uterus to avoid pregnancy during long a particular problem in young nulliparous women. The problems linked to the Dalkon shield lead to its removal from the market and a discrediting of all IUDs for many years.

The history of the Dalkon Shield still influences opinions about IUDs despite research that supports the safety of current IUD models. The newer IUDs are associated with neither PID nor ectopic pregnancies (Stubbs and Schamp, 2008). Some additional monthly bleeding and pain is commonplace in IUD users, especially during the first few months after insertion. While the additional blood loss has been found to persist for some time, pain that continues past the first couple of months after insertion is not normal and requires examination and reevaluation by a healthcare provider.

Worldwide, more than 150 million women are using IUDs for contraception (Kaneshiro & Aeby, 2010). Currently, there are two types of IUD approved in the United States—ParaGard and Mirena (Fantasia, 2008). ParaGard is a copper-containing, T-shaped piece of plastic. It releases low levels of copper, which acts as a spermicide, and is effective for up to 12 years. Mirena releases low levels of levonorgestrel, a form of progestin, and is effective for up to five years (Figure 13-14). Both work by inhibiting sperm movement through the uterus. In addition, the levonorgestrel released from Mirena inhibits ovulation and thickens cervical mucus (Ortiz & Croxatto, 2007). IUDs have the advantage of high level efficacy—less than one woman per 100 users becomes pregnant while using the device—and provide years of protection. Once removed, fertility is restored, and as an added benefit, IUDs can be used by women who are nursing.

An IUD needs to be inserted by a medical professional using an instrument to introduce the IUD through the cervix. Some women will feel slight cramping during the procedure. Once in place, the IUD fits into the lumen of the uterus with the string extending through the cervix into the vagina (Figure 13-15). The strings are used to check that the IUD is still in place and has not been expelled. Spontaneous expulsion of IUDs is most frequent during the first few months after insertion and usually occurs during menstruation. A 1995 study (Bahamondes et al.,) reported that a woman who has expelled one IUD has a 30 percent chance of expelling subsequent insertions. It is important to check for the IUD's presence after each period by palpating for the end of the string that extends out of the cervix. If it is not there, or if the string appears to be longer than it was originally, an office or clinic visit to check the location of the IUD is necessary.

Contraindications for using an IUD include cervical inflammation, an abnormal uterine shape, cervical and uterine cancers, unexplained vaginal bleeding, or an STI (Nelson, 2000). Women with sensitivity to any of the components of the IUD should also avoid using this form of birth control. Side effects for IUDs include cramping following insertion, heavier menstrual flow, infection, and dysmenorrhea. However, the risk of side effects is very low (Kaneshiro & Aeby, 2010). Copper IUDs have been in use for a relatively short period of time and some concern has been expressed about the copper toxicity, but meta-analysis of studies of copper

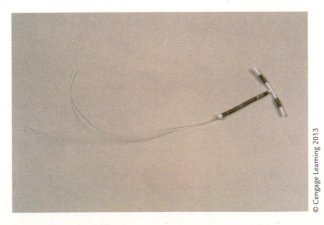

© Cengage Learning 2013

FIGURE 13-14: An IUD.

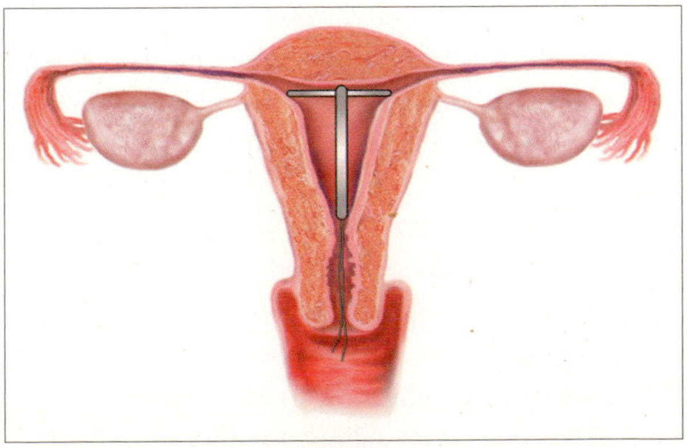

© Cengage Learning 2013

FIGURE 13-15: Proper placement of an IUD.

Changing Contraceptive with Age

Mina is a 35-year-old woman in a long-term, monogamous relationship. She and her partner have just relocated across country. She's been taking birth control pills for the last seven years, but her new doctor explains that it is time to switch to another method because of her age and family history of heart disease. Her partner has a latex allergy, so condoms or a diaphragm are not good options. Besides, they both would prefer a more convenient method that allows for more spontaneity. She looks at the patch, the vaginal ring, and Depo-Provera (medroxy-progesterone), but decides to use a copper IUD instead.

1. Why did her doctor advise her to stop taking birth control pills?

2. Why did she pick the IUD instead of one of the other options she investigated?

3. What possible side effects or complications should she be aware of?

IUDs finds few problems (O'Brien et al., 2008). The amount of copper released is small and most remains in the uterus to be expelled with the menstrual fluid. The amount of copper that is absorbed into the bloodstream has been calculated as being only five percent of that which is normally absorbed from the diet (Hasson, 1978). While most women will have no problems with this level of the metal, women with sensitivity to copper should avoid this IUD.

Surgical Sterilization

Sterilization is an effective method of contraception for those who are certain that they do not want children. It is a one-time process, providing almost 100 percent protection against pregnancy. Prior to 1973, the number of male sterilizations, or vasectomies, exceeded the female sterilizations, or tubal ligations. After 1973, the popularity of the female procedure increased rapidly, partly because of the introduction of newer techniques, and partly because of the Supreme Court's ruling on abortion, affirming a woman's right to control her own body, extended to voluntary sterilization.

Female Sterilization

Female sterilization involves interrupting the movement of sperm and eggs through the fallopian tubes. **Tubal ligation** is the classic operation for female sterilization. Simple ligation, or tying a suture around the loop of the fallopian tube without cutting it, is rarely performed today because of its high failure rate, which was due to the sutures tendency to slip off the loop. Today, surgeons performing a tubal ligation may electrically cauterize the tube in several places and use a clip to pinch the tube closed. Alternately, the surgeon may remove a piece of the tube and seal the cut ends. Laparoscopic sterilization is the technique of tubal ligation most frequently used in the United States. A long, slender tube with a fiber-optic light source, a laparoscope, is inserted through a tiny incision in the abdomen, and the fallopian tube is then sealed (Figure 13–16). Another technique uses small plugs which are placed in the fallopian tubes from within the uterus, using access through the vagina. Tissue grows around the plugs, firmly holding them in place and sealing the tubes.

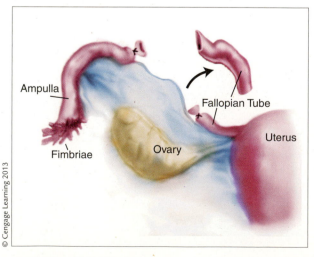

© Cengage Learning 2013

FIGURE 13-16: Tubal ligation.

The advantage of this technique is that no abdominal cutting is required.

Sterilization is highly effective, with less than one woman per 100 becoming pregnant. The method is not considered reversible, and for that reason some physicians try to dissuade women from having the surgery (Lawrence et al., 2010). In addition, because tubal ligation involves surgery, there are risks of postoperative pain and postoperative infection, as well as the risks associated with anesthesia. In addition, tubal ligation costs more than other methods.

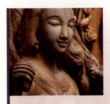

Social Considerations
COERCIVE AND FORCED STERILIZATION OF WOMEN

A woman's reproductive rights are critical aspects of a broader autonomy, yet, many times these rights are at risk, and women from ethnic minority groups oftentimes face even greater obstacles. Worldwide, the ugly practice of coerced and forced sterilization has been used to oppress women of various racial and ethnic groups. Coerced or forced sterilization is the process of permanently ending someone's ability to reproduce without her free consent. In women, this is often done through tubal ligation or hysterectomy.

There are several examples of situations where particular groups of women have been targeted with coerced or forced sterilization. In the United States, according to General Accounting Office (GAO) reports, some 3,406 Native American women between the ages of 15–44 were sterilized between 1973 and 1976 by Indian Health Service medical personnel (Lex & Norris, 1992). However, the true numbers may be much higher, as the investigation was initially limited to four Indian Health Service hospitals, so the total number of women sterilized remains unknown. The GAO's report listed many violations of the rights of Native American women undergoing sterilization procedures, such as inadequate consent forms, medical personnel ignoring a wide range of professional requirements, and the sterilization of girls (Jarrell, 1992).

Peru is another example. In the mid to late 1990s in Peru, some 200,000 to 300,000 women were coercively sterilized (Liberated Latina, 2009). In 2002, Peru's Minister of Health issued a national apology for the forced sterilization of indigenous women. According to Peruvian rights advocate Maria Esther Mogollon, sterilizations focused on poor and indigenous women (Liberated Latina, 2009). The majority of these women never signed informed consent statements for their sterilization, and many were subjected to threats, coercion, and other violations of their rights. In some cases, when women went into the hospital to give birth, doctors sterilized them without their consent. Many would not find out until several years later that they had in fact been sterilized.

In more recent years, Romani women in the Czech Republic, Slovakia, and Hungary have also faced forced and coercive sterilization. In 2005, the Czech Public Defender of Rights issued a report which found more than 80 cases of coerced sterilizations where doctors failed to ensure informed consent (European Roma Rights Center, 2006). The illegal performance of tubal ligation or related sterilizing procedures affected mostly women of Roma origin. In Slovakia, doctors have coercively sterilized Romani women as recently as 2003 (Human Rights Watch, 2003). As in Peru, sterilizations were performed on Romani women during their deliveries without their prior informed consent. Other Romani women gave their written consent to sterilization, but were coerced into doing so at the time when their delivery was in progress and they were in the midst of regular contractions. Others were not of legal age when sterilization was performed on them, meaning they could not have given their legal consent. As in Peru, many Romani women did not know they had been sterilized. Only after reviewing their medical record did some women find out that the reason for their infertility was because of sterilization.

Vasectomy

In males, sterilization is most often produced through a **vasectomy** (Figure 13-17). The procedure is usually carried out in the healthcare provider's office using local anesthesia. The portion of the vas deferens that is located in the scrotum is surrounded by a sheath of connective tissue called the spermatic cord, which contains nerves and blood vessels. With a vasectomy, local anesthetic is injected into the scrotum and a small incision is made. The spermatic cord is drawn out, opened, and a small segment of the vas deferens is removed. The cut ends of the vas deferens are sealed and the incision is then sutured. A no-incision vasectomy technique has also been developed which involves a specialized needle puncturing the vas deferens and cauterizing or blocking the tubes. Both methods block the transportation of sperm through the reproductive tract. Because some viable sperm remain in the tubes of the reproductive tract, sterility is not immediate with either method. Another contraceptive method must be used until two semen samples, taken to a lab, test negative for viable sperm.

Vasectomies are usually a permanent method of sterilization and are a highly effective contraceptive method. There is discomfort immediately after the procedure and a slight risk of infection immediately following the procedure, but no other side effects are associated with the procedure.

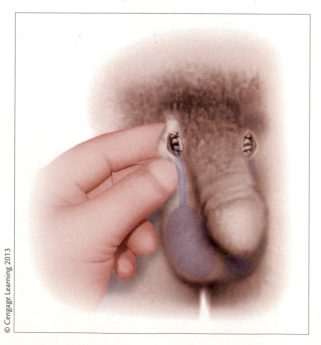

FIGURE 13-17: Vasectomy.

© Cengage Learning 2013

EMERGENCY CONTRACEPTION (EC)

Despite the best intentions and planning, contraceptive methods can fail—a condom can break, patches can come off, a diaphragm can slip—and an alternative emergency method is needed. Rape victims may need an emergency option to prevent pregnancy. **Emergency contraception** (EC), also called the morning after pill, reduces the risk of pregnancy after unexpected or unprotected intercourse or contraceptive failure. Various methods of EC are available in different parts of the world. In the United States, the most common form is called Plan B. This method consists of two tablets of levonorgestrel and is available in pharmacies without a prescription.

If taken within 72 hours of unprotected intercourse, EC is 89 percent effective at preventing pregnancy. Plan B can be used up to five days after unprotected intercourse, but it becomes less effective. The level of hormone in Plan B prevents ovulation and disrupts the reproductive cycle. Without ovulation, egg and sperm cannot meet and fertilization cannot occur. Follow-up testing to confirm that there is no pregnancy is recommended if a woman does not menstruate within three weeks of using EC or if she shows any signs of pregnancy.

EVIDENCE BASED PRACTICE

Plan B and Teen Contraceptive Choices

When Plan B emergency contraception was approved as an over-the-counter (OTC) medication rather than prescription medication, concerns were raised that teens, particularly younger teens, would be using Plan B as their primary birth control. However, a study of teens from age 13 to 19 indicates that Plan B is not being used as a primary contraceptive method. According to the research, young women chose to use Plan B as it was intended—for emergency contraception when another method failed (Krishnamurti, Eggers, & Fischoff, 2008).

Prompt access to EC is important to prevent pregnancy. However, 23–35 percent of pharmacies surveyed in one study were unable to supply EC within 24 hours of a request due to a lack of supply (Davidson et al., 2010). In addition, emergency contraception is sometimes confused with abortion even though emergency contraception does not terminate an existing pregnancy. The confusion has led some pharmacies to refuse to sell emergency contraception. A study of the availability of EC in three large metropolitan areas found that four percent of the pharmacists refused to sell Plan B because of religious concerns (Davidson et al., 2010).

ABORTION

Abortion, the termination of a pregnancy, has been practiced throughout history, yet the procedure has created legal, social, and religious debate which continues to this day in the United States. Political campaigns often highlight a candidate's position on this issue, and confirmation hearings for Supreme Court justices frequently raise the issue. Weitz (2010) refers to abortion as the "most contested social issue of our time". The induced termination of a pregnancy is legal and safe and, based on the Roe v. Wade Supreme Court case, is a woman's right under the United States Constitution based on the fundamental right to privacy. Since the legalization of abortion in 1973, there have been multiple campaigns to restrict women's decisions concerning their bodies. Laws have been enacted that deny equal access to abortion for all women. Federal and state funding for abortions has been limited. Significant restrictions on abortion were implemented through provisions of a Missouri law upheld by the Supreme Court in 1989. The decision in Webster vs. Reproductive Health Services barred abortions at a "public facility" even if no public funds were used and the woman paid for the full cost of the procedure. Because private hospitals associated with medical schools or community hospitals often receive public funding in the form of grants or accept Medicaid payments, public facilities can be broadly interpreted to include most private institutions. The Missouri law also banned public employees, including doctors, nurses, and other health providers, from performing or assisting an abortion not necessary to save a woman's life and mandated medical tests to determine whether a fetus could live outside the uterus. By upholding the restrictions in the Missouri law, the Supreme Court provided the states with new authority to limit the right to abortion. Age requirements, waiting periods, and parental notification laws have been proposed or adopted in many states. Despite these limits, legal abortions continue. According to the Planned Parenthood Federation, one in three women in the United States has an abortion by the time they are 45. Fifty percent of those women have already had one or more prior abortions (Kavanaugh et al., 2010).

Methods of Abortion

The earlier in pregnancy an abortion is performed, the less complex and safer the procedure is. In the United States, two types of abortions are performed. Medication-induced abortions rely on the drug mifepristone, sometimes referred to as the abortion pill. Surgical abortions require an in-clinic procedure. The two most common forms of surgical abortion are aspiration, and dilation and evacuation (D and E).

Medication-induced Abortion

In the 1980s, a team of French researchers developed a synthetic steroid that could cause expulsion of the embryo from the uterus of a pregnant woman. The drug, mifepristone, was designated as RU-486, after the manufacturer, Roussel-Uclaf. Mifepristone is a progesterone antagonist that binds tightly to progesterone receptors and, by competing with progesterone, successfully blocks the action of the hormone. When the progesterone is blocked by mifepristone, it provokes a miscarriage. The endometrium begins to erode and the implanted embryo is expelled along with the endometrial tissue. The drug is taken orally in a single dose, followed by a second drug, a form of prostaglandin, which causes uterine contractions. When administered during the first nine weeks of pregnancy, mifepristone in combination with the prostaglandin has a 97 percent success rate in causing a miscarriage. In most instances, the expulsion occurs within 24 hours of receiving prostaglandin. If the abortion is incomplete, the pregnancy must be terminated by surgical abortion. The rate of complications of heavy bleeding and infection with mifepristone are similar to that in surgical abortions, about one percent. Most women experience some uterine pain, but side effects of nausea, vomiting, and diarrhea also may appear after the prostaglandin administration.

On the basis of several large multicenter studies in France and England, mifepristone is a proven safe and effective abortifacient. Mifepristone was approved for use in the United States by the FDA in September 2000. Despite its FDA approval, considerable controversy continues regarding the use of mifepristone.

Surgical Abortion

Surgical abortions are performed in a medical facility. The choice of technique depends on how advanced the pregnancy is. Before a procedure, a woman is given a medical exam, information about the procedure, and preliminary instructions.

Aspiration abortions are the most common type of surgical abortion performed during the first 16 weeks of pregnancy. Prior to the procedure, pain medications and antibiotics are usually administered. During the procedure, the cervix is dilated and a tube is introduced into the uterus to suction out the contents. A curette may be used to remove any remaining tissue after the aspiration is completed.

For terminations after 16 weeks, a D and E procedure is used. In this case, a woman is given pain medication, antibiotics, and medications to produce light sedation. The cervix is dilated, and a combination of instruments and suction is used to empty the uterus.

During and after either procedure, the uterine muscles contract to prevent hemorrhage and reduce the uterus to its original size. These contractions may cause strong cramps for 10–20 minutes after the abortion. A period of rest and recovery follows, during which the woman usually receives instructions on aftercare and contraception. She may then leave and return to her normal routine, but most women prefer to rest for the remainder of that day, and to avoid particularly strenuous activities for a few days. It is usual to experience cramps and bleeding for the first two weeks after an abortion, and it is not unusual for spotting to occur for another two weeks after that. The next normal menstrual period is likely to start four to six weeks after surgery, and most women ovulate within the first three weeks. Intercourse should be avoided for a week after abortion, and to avoid getting pregnant again immediately, a method of contraception must be used after that.

Legal abortion during the first 16 weeks of pregnancy is statistically safer than continuing the pregnancy and delivering a child. When abortion is delayed beyond the 12th week, however, the risk of both major and minor complications is increased. In a 1998 comprehensive review article, Gans Epner et al. reported, using 1991 data, that the risk of abortion-related mortality from legal abortions was 0. 8 per 1000 procedures. The morbidity risk at eight gestational weeks or less was 0.2 per 100,000 procedures and rose to 5.9 per 100,000 procedures at 16–20 gestational weeks. At 21 gestational weeks or more, mortality rates rose to 16.7 per 100,000 procedures, exceeding the risk of maternal death from childbirth (6.7 per 100,000 deliveries). The risks associated with abortion are primarily infection and excessive bleeding. Illegal abortions, performed outside medical settings, pose a much greater risk and resulted in thousands of women's deaths and injury prior to the legalization of abortion.

Several studies have been conducted to determine whether prior abortion has any affects on subsequent pregnancies. The findings of investigations in Seattle, Boston, Hawaii, and New York indicated that there was no link between a previously induced abortion and a later complication or unfavorable outcome of pregnancy. The researchers found that abortion had no association with infertility, ectopic pregnancy, miscarriage, early delivery, low birth weight babies, or greater infant morbidity or mortality.

CONCLUSION

For a woman wishing to control her fertility, several methods exist. To make an informed choice, a woman needs to understand her options, the benefits of each method and its risks. She needs to determine what she considers an acceptable level of pregnancy risk and which method she is comfortable with. Today's contraceptive methods are not perfect. New methods are continually being explored. Male contraceptives, microbiocides/spermicide combinations, and contraceptive vaccines are all methods that are currently under investigation and may become the contraceptives of the future. Contraceptive needs and preferences change thoughout a woman's life, and a woman who stays informed about the latest options will be able to determine which methods may be the best choice for her.

REVIEW QUESTIONS

1. How do barrier contraceptive methods work?

2. How do hormonal contraceptive methods work?

3. What contraindications exist for hormonal methods?

4. What factors should a woman consider when making contraceptive choices?

5. Why is the withdrawal method not very effective?

CRITICAL THINKING QUESTIONS

1. Compare the risks of taking a pregnancy to full term with the risks on different contraceptive methods. How do they compare?

2. Why does contraception polarize communities?

3. Where should people get their contraceptive information?

WEBLINKS

World Health Organization
www.who.int

Planned Parenthood International
www.plannedparenthood.org

REFERENCES

American College of Obstetricians and Gynecologists. (1987). Oral contraceptives. (Technical Bulletin No. 106.) Washington, DC: Author.

Amory, J. K. (2008). Progress and prospects in male hormonal contraception. *Current Opinion in Endocrinology, Diabetes and Obesity, 15*(3), 255–260.

Bahamondes, L., Diaz, J., Marchi, N., et al. (1995). Performance of copper intrauterine devices when inserted after an expulsion. *Human Reproduction, 10*, 2917–2918.

Baptista, M., & Ramalho-Santos, J. (2009). Spermicides, microbicides and antiviral agents: Recent advances in the development of novel multi-functional compounds. *Mini-Reviews in Medicinal Chemistry, 9*(13), 1556–1567.

Beral, V., Hermon, C., Kay, C., Hannaford, P., et al. (1999). Mortality associated with oral contraceptive use: 25 year follow up of cohort of 46,000 women from Royal College of General Practitioners' oral contraception study. *British Medical Journal, 318*(7176), 96–100.

Bernstein, G. S., Clark, V. S., Coulson, A. H., et al. (1986). Use effectiveness of cervical caps. Final Report to NICHD, Contract No. 1-HD-1-2804.

Bullough, V. L. (2001). *Encyclopedia of birth control.* Santa Barbara, CA: ABC-CLIO.

Burrows, M., & Peters, C. E. (2007). The influence of oral contraceptives on athletic performance in female athletes. *Sports Medicine, 37*(7), 557–574.

Cale, A. R., Farouk, M., Prescott, R. J., et al. (1990). Does vasectomy accelerate testicular tumor? Importance of testicular examination before and after vasectomy. *British Medical Journal, 300*(6721), 370.

Center for the Advancement of Health. (2008, March 20). Comprehensive sex education might reduce teen pregnancies. *Science Daily.* Retrieved April 30, 2011, from http://www.sciencedaily.com/releases/2008/03/080319151225.htm.

Chassot, F., Camacho, D. P., Patussi, E. V., Donatti, L., Svidzinski, T. I., & Consolaro, M. E. (2010). Can Lactobacillus acidophilus influence the adhesion capacity of *Candida albicans* on the combined contraceptive vaginal ring? *Contraception, 81*(4), 331–335.

Davidson, L. A., Pettis, C. T., Joiner, A. J., Cook, D. M., & Klugman, C. M. (2010). Religion and conscientious objection: A survey of pharmacists' willingness to dispense medications. *Social Science & Medicine, 71*(1),161–165.

Drospirenone: High risk of venous thrombosis. (2011). *Prescrire International, 20*(113), 43–45.

Eisenberg, M. L., & Lipshultz, L. I. (2010). Estimating the number of vasectomies performed annually in the United States: Data from the National Survey of Family Growth. *Urology, 184*(5), 2068–2072.

Epner, J. E., Jonas, H. S., & Seckinger, D. L. (1998). Late-term abortion. *Journal of the American Medical Association, 280*(8), 724–729.

European Roma Rights Centre. (2006, March 14). Czech report on coercive sterilisation of Romani women published in English translation: Civil society organisations throughout Europe urge government follow-up. Retrieved from http://www.errc.org/cikk.php?cikk=2528.

Fantasia, H. C. (2008). Options for intrauterine contraception. *Journal of Obstetric, Gynecologic, & Neonatal Nursing, 37*(3), 375–383.

Fischer, M. A. (2008). Implanon: A new contraceptive implant. *Journal of Obstetric, Gynecologic, & Neonatal Nursing, 37*(3), 361–368.

Gallegos, A. J. (1983). The zoapatle—A traditional remedy from Mexico emerges to modern times. *Contraception, 27*(3), 211–221.

Garcés-Palacio, I. C., Altarac, M., & Scarinci, I. C. (2008). Contraceptive knowledge and use among low-income Hispanic immigrant women and non-Hispanic women. *Contraception, 77*(4), 270–275.

Glasier, A., Thong, K. J., Dewar, M., et al. (1992). Mifepristone (RU-486) compared with high-dose estrogen and progestogen for emergency post coital contraception. *New England Journal of Medicine, 327*(15), 1041–1044.

Godsland, I. F., Crook, D., & Wynn, V. (1991). Coronary heart disease risk markers in users of low-dose oral contraceptives. *Journal of Reproductive Medicine, 36*(3) (Suppl.), 226–237.

Gollub, E. L., & Sivin, I. (1989). The Prentif cervical cap and Pap smear results: A critical appraisal. *Contraception, 40*(3), 343–349.

Harper, C. C., Henderson, J. T., Schalet, A., Becker, D., Stratton, L., & Raine, T. R. (2010). Abstinence and teenagers: Prevention counseling practices of healthcare providers serving high-risk patients in the United States. *Perspectives on Sexual and Reproductive Health, 42*(2), 125–132.

Hasson, H. M. (1978). Copper IUDs. *Journal of Reproductive Medicine, 20*(3), 139–154.

Hatcher, R., Trussell, J., Nelson, A., Cates, W., & Stewart, F. (2008). *Contraceptive technology* (19th ed.). New York, NY: Ardent Media.

Henshaw, S. K., & Van Vort, J. (1990). Abortion services in the United States, 1987 and 1988. *Family Planning Perspectives, 22*(3), 102–110.

Hooten, T. M., Hillier, S., Johnson, C., et al. (1991). *Escherichia coli* bacteriuria and contraceptive method. *Journal of the American Medical Association, 265*(1), 64–67.

Human Rights Watch. (2003). Joint NGO statement on the issue of illegal sterilization of Romani women in Slovakia. Retrieved from http://www.hrw.org/en/news/2003/07/21/joint-ngo-statement-issue-illegal-sterilization-romani-women-slovakia.

Isley, M. M., Edelman, A., Kaneshiro, B., Peters, D., Nichols, M. D., & Jensen, J. T. (2010). Sex education and contraceptive use at coital debut in the United States: Results from Cycle 6 of the National Survey of Family Growth. *Contraception, 82*(3), 236–242.

Iwu, M. M. (1993). *Handbook of African medicinal plants.* Boca Raton, FL: CRC Press.

JAMA Women's Health Contraception Information Center. (1997). ParaGard T 380A intrauterine copper contraceptive. Retrieved from http://www.ama-assn.org/special/contra/ortho/paragard.htm.

Jarrell, R. H. (1992). Native American women and forced sterilization, 1973–1976. *Caduceus, 8.* 45–58.

Johnson, C. C., Burkman, R. T., Gold, M. A., Brown, R. T., Harel, Z., Bruner, A., Stager, M., Bachrach, L. K., Hertweck, S. P., Nelson, A. L., Nelson, D. A., Coupey, S. M., McLeod, A., & Bone, H. G. (2008). Longitudinal study of depot medroxyprogesterone acetate (Depo-Provera) effects on bone health in adolescents: Study design, population characteristics and baseline bone mineral density. *Contraception, 77*(4), 239–248.

Jütte, R. (2010). The longue durée of contraceptive methods. *History & Philosophy of the Life Sciences, 27*(1), 71–79.

Kaneshiro, B., & Aeby, T. (2010). Long-term safety, efficacy, and patient acceptability of the intrauterine Copper T-380A contraceptive device. *International Journal of Women's Health, 2,* 211–220.

Kavanaugh, M. L., Jones, R. K., & Finer, L. B. (2010). How commonly do US abortion clinics offer contraceptive services? *Contraception, 82*(4), 331–336.

Kluft, C., Meijer, P., LaGuardia, K. D., & Fisher, A. C. (2008). Comparison of a transdermal contraceptive patch vs. oral contraceptives on hemostasis variables. *Contraception, 77*(2), 77–83.

Krishnamurti, T., Eggers, S. L., & Fischhoff, B. (2008). The impact of over-the-counter availability of "Plan B" on teens' contraceptive decision making. *Social Science & Medicine, 67*(4), 618–627.

La Vecchia, C., Franceschi, S., Bruzzi, P., Parazzini, F., & Boyle, P. (1990). The relationship between oral contraceptive use, cancer and vascular disease. *Drug Safety, 5,* 436–446.

Lawrence, R. E., Rasinski, K. A., Yoon, J. D., & Curlin, F. A. (2010). Factors influencing physicians' advice about female sterilization in USA: A national survey. *Human Reproduction, 26*(1), 106–111.

Lex, B. W., & Norris, J. R. (1999). Health status of American Indian and Alaska native women. In *Women and health research: Ethical and legal issues of including women in clinical studies* (vol. 2). Workshop and Commissioned Papers, Institute of Medicine (IOM).

Libertad Latina (2009). The forced sterilization of Latina and indigenous women and youth in Canada, the United States and across Latin America. Retrieved June 1, 2009, from http://www.libertadlatina.org/Crisis_Forced_Sterilization.htm.

Lopez, L. M., Grimes, D. A., Gallo, M. F., & Schulz, K. F. Skin patch and vaginal ring versus combined oral contraceptives for contraception. *Cochrane Database Systematic Review,* (1), CD003552.

Moghissi, K. S. (1976). Accuracy of basal body temperature for ovulation detection. *Fertility and Sterility, 27*(12), 1415–1421.

Nelson, A. L. (2000). The intrauterine contraceptive device. *Obstetrics and Gynecology Clinics of North America, 27*(4), 723–740.

O'Brien, P. A., Kulier, R., Helmerhorst, F. M., Usher-Patel, M., & d'Arcangues, C. (2008). Copper-containing, framed intrauterine devices for contraception: A systematic review of randomized controlled trials. *Contraception, 77*(5), 318–327.

Ortiz, M. E., & Croxatto, H. B. (2007). Copper-T intrauterine device and levonorgestrel intrauterine system: Biological bases of their mechanism of action. *Contraception, 75*(6 Suppl), S16–30.

Ott, M. A., & Santelli, J. S. (2007). Abstinence and abstinence-only education. *Current Opinion in Obstetrics and Gynecology, 19*(5), 446–452.

Page, S. T., Amory, J. K., & Bremner, W. J. (2008). Advances in male contraception. *Endocrine Reviews, 29,* 465-493. doi:10.1210/er.2007-0041.

Phillips, J., Hulka, J., Hulka, B., et al. (1981). American Association of Gynecological Laparoscopists. Membership survey. *Journal of Reproductive Medicine, 26*(10), 527–537.

Pincemail, J., Vanbelle, S., Gaspard, U., Collette, G., Haleng, J., Cheramy-Bien, J. P., Charlier, C., Chapelle, J. P., Giet, D., Albert, A., Limet, R., & Defraigne, J. O. (2007). Effect of different contraceptive methods on the oxidative stress status in women aged 40- 48 years from the ELAN study in the province of Liege, Belgium. *Human Reproduction, 22*(8), 2335–2343.

Planned Parenthood Federation of America. (1998). Diaphragms and cervical caps. Retrieved from http://www.plannedparenthood.org/birth-control/diaphragms.htm.

Pope, T. M. (2010). Legal briefing: Conscience clauses and conscientious refusal. *Journal of Clinical Ethics, 21*(2), 163–176.

Redman, L. M., & Weatherby, R. P. (2004). Measuring performance during the menstrual cycle: A model using oral contraceptives. *Medicine & Science in Sports & Exercise, 36*(1), 130–136.

Reproductive Health Online. (2000, January 31). Recommendations for contraceptive use. Retrieved from http://www.reproline.jhu.edu/.

Richwald, G. A., Greenland, S., Gerber, M. M., et al. (1989). Effectiveness of the cavity-rim cervical cap: Results of a large clinical study. *Obstetrics and Gynecology, 74*(2), 143–148.

Riddle, J. M., Estes, J. W., & Russell, J. C. (1994). Birth control in the ancient world. *Archaeology. 47*(2), 29–35.

Scholes, D., LaCroix, A. Z., Ichikawa, L. E., Barlow, W. E., & Ott, S. M. (2005). Change in bone mineral density among adolescent women using and discontinuing depot medroxyprogesterone acetate contraception. *Archives of Pediatrics and Adolescent Medicine, 159*(2), 139–144.

Shoupe, D., & Mishell, D. R. (1989). Norplant: Subdermal implant system for long-term contraception. *American Journal of Obstetrics and Gynecology, 160*(5, Pt. 2), 1286–1292.

Skegg, D., & Spears, G. (1989). Depot medroxyprogesterone (Depo-Provera) and the risk of breast cancer. *British Medical Journal, 299,* 759–762.

Skuy, P. (1995). *Tales of contraception: A museum of discovery.* Toronto, Ontario: History of Contraception Museum.

Stadel, B. V. (1988). Oral contraceptives and premenopausal breast cancer in nulliparous women. *Contraception, 38*(3), 287–299.

Stubbs, E., & Schamp, A. (2008). The evidence is in. Why are IUDs still out?: Family physicians'

perceptions of risk and indications. *Canadian Family Physician, 54*(4), 560–566.

Tietze, C. (1973). Intrauterine devices: Clinical aspects. In E. S. Hafez & T. N. Evans (Eds.), *Human reproduction.* Hagerstown, MD: Harper & Row.

Tone, A. (2001). *Devices & desires: A history of contraceptives in America.* New York, NY: Hill & Wang.

Trussell, J. (2004). Contraceptive efficacy. In R. A. Hatcher, J. Trussell, F. Stewart, A. Nelson, W. Cates, F. Guest, & D. Kowal. *Contraceptive technology* (18th rev. ed.). New York, NY: Ardent Media.

Trussell, J. (2007). Contraceptive efficacy. In R. A. Hatcher, J. Trussell, A. L. Nelson, W. Cates, F. H. Stewart, & D. Kowal. *Contraceptive technology* (19th rev. ed.). New York, NY: Ardent Media.

Vessey, M. P. (1989). Epidemiological studies of oral contraception. *International Journal of Fertility, 34* (Suppl), 64–70.

Wakine, Y. (2006, July 20). FDA approvals: Implanon and Exelon. Retrieved May 5 from http://www.medscape.com/viewarticle/541244.

Weitz, T. A. (2010). Rethinking the mantra that abortion should be "safe, legal, and rare." *Journal of Women's History, 22*(3), 161–172.

Wicclair, M. R. (2006). Pharmacies, pharmacists, and conscientious objection. *Kennedy Institute of Ethics Journal, 16*(3), 225–250.

Yuzpe, A. A. (1979). Post-coital contraception. *International Journal of Gynecology and Obstetrics, 16,* 497–505.

chapter 14

INFERTILITY: CAUSES AND TREATMENTS

CHAPTER COMPETENCIES

Upon completion of this chapter the reader will be able to:

- Define infertility and understand the different types of infertility found in both women and men
- Identify factors that contribute to infertility in males and females

- Identify ways to protect fertility if future parenthood is desired
- Identify and describe current methods for treating infertility, including their success/failure rates, and potential health risks

KEY TERMS

artificial insemination

assisted reproductive technologies (ART)

endocrine disruptors

fallopian tube sperm profusion (FSP)

gamete intrafallopian transfer (GIFT)

higher order multiple pregnancies

infertility

intracytoplasmic sperm injection (ICSI)

intrauterine insemination (IUI)

in vitro fertilization (IVF)

superovulation

surrogate mother

varicocele

zygote intrafallopian transfer (ZIFT)

INTRODUCTION

Infertility is medically defined as the inability to conceive a child during the course of one year of regular sexual intercourse unprotected by contraception (Kamel, 2010) or the inability to carry a pregnancy to birth. This term can either apply to individuals who are not able to reproduce or to couples who are unable to produce offspring together (Figure 14-1). Between 13-15 percent of couples are infertile worldwide. Subfertility refers to reduced fertility when compared to the average and can involve either problems conceiving or carrying a baby to term. For women, primary infertility occurs when she has never been able to conceive or carry a pregnancy to term. Secondary infertility occurs when she has difficulty getting pregnant after already having conceived and carried a full-term pregnancy. On average, 20-25 percent of heterosexual couples having regular sexual intercourse without birth control will conceive within one month, and 60 percent will conceive within six months (Kamel, 2010). Statistically, however, if conception has not occurred by the

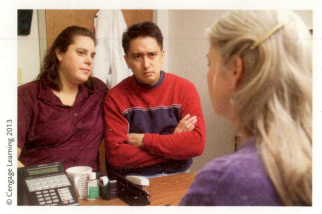

FIGURE 14-1: Fertility applies to couples who are unable to produce offspring together, as well as individuals who are not able to reproduce.

end of one year, the chances of becoming pregnant decrease. The American College of Obstetrics and Gynecologists (ACOG, 2007) recommends seeking fertility assistance after six months to one year of attempting to conceive. In the United States, infertility is recognized as a disease by both the American Society for Reproductive Medicine (ASRM) and the American College of Obstetricians and Gynecologists (ACOG). However, infertility treatments are expensive and may not be covered by insurance. This may limit treatment options and is especially a problem for single women or homosexual couples who are seeking treatment for infertility.

After puberty, fertility declines throughout a person's lifetime and the older an individual is, the more difficulty they may have conceiving a child. Biological factors associated with the normal aging process are responsible. In women, atresia of eggs as she approaches menopause, along with other changes in the reproductive system, decreases the chances of conception. The older a woman is, the greater her potential of risk from exposure to infections or chemicals that reduce fertility. A woman's peak fertility occurs between the ages of 20 and 25, declines through her 30s, and drops directly after 40. A woman ceases being fertile when she reaches menopause and stops ovulating. Similarly, male fertility peaks in the mid-20s, decreases in the 30s, and declines markedly after age 40. Male fertility does not terminate completely as it does in postmenopausal women, but it can decline to levels that make reproduction unlikely.

WORLDWIDE TRENDS IN INFERTILITY

There is growing concern that rates of human infertility are rising. The United Nations has reported a drop in the world birthrate from 2.65 children per woman of childbearing age in 2005 down to 2.55 by 2010 (UN, 2007). Social and behavioral factors play a role in declining birth rates; the availability of contraceptives, decisions to limit family size, or to space children all have an impact on the overall birthrate. However, there is increasing scientific evidence that along with these behavioral trends, there has also been an actual drop in fertility rates, and that more couples or individuals who want to have children are faced with reduced fertility (Skakkebaek et al., 2006; Jorgensen et al., 2006; Jensen et al., 2008). This is not just a problem faced by older individuals who have postponed starting a family; the problems are showing up in increasingly younger individuals of both sexes. There is strong evidence that semen quality and sperm counts have declined dramatically in the last 50 years. Merzenich et al. (2010) indicate that sperm densities may have dropped by as much as 50 percent since 1934, though the rates vary geographically and by study method. In the 1940s, an average sperm count for a young man was around 100 million sperm per milliliter of ejaculate, or 100 million/mL. Recent research shows the average sperm count for young men in Copenhagen, Denmark to now be around 45 million/mL, and in Singapore, 44.7 million/mL. American and European researchers have suggested that 48-55 million/mL should be considered the lowest cutoff for normal sperm counts, so many men now have sperm counts that are in the sub-fertile or infertile range. It is estimated that one in eight couples in the United States are infertile, and the statistic is now one in six in the U.K. (Andersson et al., 2008).

FACTORS THAT CONTRIBUTE TO INFERTILITY

Most infertility is caused by sperm abnormalities, problems with ovulation, or obstruction of the fallopian tubes (Kamel, 2010). In many cases, the causes of infertility in a couple are the result of both male and female subfertility, or its cause can be unexplained. The reasons for the increase in infertility rates are not entirely understood, and it probably results from a combination of factors. In many industrialized nations, there has been a trend to postpone having children until later in life, when fertility naturally declines. In many countries, increases in obesity rates have also contributed to declines in fertility. Obesity can lead to a host of problems such as high blood pressure, high triglyceride levels in the blood, and insulin resistance, often indicating a condition called metabolic syndrome. In women, metabolic syndrome is often associated with another condition polycystic ovary syndrome (PCOS), which can contribute to infertility. Dramatic increases in some types of sexually transmitted infections, chlamydia and gonorrhea in particular, produce pelvic inflammatory disease (PID) and scarring of the fallopian tubes, both conditions which reduce fertility.

There is growing scientific evidence that many man-made chemicals used to make plastics, pesticides, fire retardants, and other products can mimic sex hormones in the body and affect both development and reproductive function. Many of these chemicals mimic or alter the effects of estrogen, testosterone, and other hormones interfering with the endocrine system. The effects of these **endocrine disruptors** have been studied in wildlife species since the early 1990s. Studies in the United States and Europe have shown that even small doses of these chemicals can cause reproductive failure in a variety of animal species, including humans (Gray et al., 2006; Foster et al., 2008; Mendola et al., 2008; Welshons et al., 2006). In some cases, sex reversal has been observed in fish living in water containing these chemicals (Jobling et al., 2009; Tyler et al., 2009). Endocrine disrupting chemicals have also been shown to interfere with human development and reproduction, and may also be partially responsible for recent dramatic increases in reproductive cancers, especially testicular, prostate, and breast cancers (Maffini et al., 2006). In 2007, leading researchers, medical doctors, and research scientists gathered for the Summit on Environmental Challenges to Reproductive Health and Fertility to discuss the impact of these persistent pollutants. The executive summary from these meetings is available as a Weblink at the end of this chapter (Woodruff et al., 2008).

EVALUATION OF INFERTILITY

In order for a pregnancy to become established, a complex orchestration of events must take place. There are many points in this process where things can go wrong. A man's testes must produce a sufficient number of mature active sperm able to move through unobstructed ducts so that they can be ejaculated in the appropriate concentration. These sperm must be deposited in a woman's vagina, reach and penetrate the cervical mucus, and ascend into the uterus and through the fallopian tubes. A woman has to produce a fertilizable egg that enters the fallopian tube so that it can be fertilized by a sperm within a period of several hours after ovulation. The resulting zygote must then move down the fallopian tube and implant in the receptive endometrium for a pregnancy to occur and for development to continue. In both sexes, there must be appropriate levels of secretion of hormones to sustain these reproductive processes.

Any restriction or impairment of these processes can reduce fertility. Among 30–40 percent of infertile couples, problems with the man's reproductive tract are the cause. Likewise, in about 30 percent of infertile couples, the problem resides with the woman's infertility. The remaining cases are attributed to a combination of infertility or subfertility issues in both partners, or to unexplained infertility. Investigations of infertility are geared to systematic assessment of all the factors involved in the passage of the sperm and ova toward each other. They include tests aimed at diagnosing problems in semen quality, vaginal, cervical, uterine, and ovarian problems. Male factor infertility is usually the easiest to diagnose so semen quality is often evaluated first, in the case of heterosexual couples.

Diagnosing Male Infertility

Male infertility accounts for approximately 35-40 percent of infertility within couples. The evaluation of male infertility will usually begin with a general physical exam, including a discussion of medical history, illnesses, disabilities, medications, and sexual habits (Figure 14-2). Male infertility can have many causes—nutritional, endocrinological, developmental, pharmacological, occupational, immunological, or anatomical. Semen quality can be evaluated by

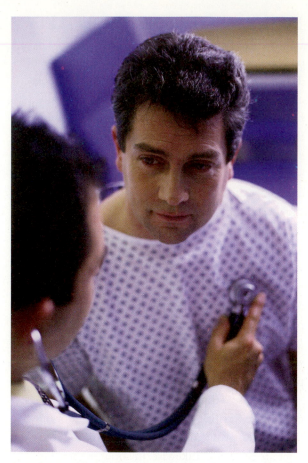

FIGURE 14-2: Evaluation of male infertility starts with a physical examination. *(Courtesy of Photodisc)*

conducting a laboratory test called a semen analysis or sperm count. For a semen examination, a man is asked to produce a specimen by ejaculating into a container after two–three days of sexual abstinence.

This specimen is analyzed for volume, viscosity, number of sperm, sperm viability, motility, and sperm shape. The average volume of ejaculate is 3.5 mL, but it can vary from 2–10 mL. A low volume (1 mL or less) may not be enough to come in contact with the cervix when it is deposited into the vagina. For unknown reasons, a volume higher than 8 mL is also associated with infertility. After determining volume, the specimen is examined under the microscope, and the numbers of sperm in a sample are counted. To be considered fertile, the specimen should contain at least 20 million sperm per milliliter. The shape and activity level of the sperm in the semen correlates to fertility as well. For there to be a strong probability of pregnancy, the semen should contain 50–70 percent live sperm that move rapidly forward across the microscopic

field and retain their motility for several hours. A low sperm count with highly motile sperm usually represents greater fertility than a high sperm count with poor motility (Aitkin, 2006; Lewis, 2007). Sperm which are deformed, have extra tails, or are immature are much less likely to be able to fertilize an egg.

Thyroid and testosterone hormone levels may also be tested to make sure that they are adequate to support healthy sperm production. In some cases, transrectal and scrotal ultrasounds may be performed to check for obstructions of the ejaculatory duct or for evidence of retrograde ejaculation. With retrograde ejaculation, semen is ejaculated into the bladder rather than out through the penis. In some cases, a genetic evaluation may also be required.

Factors that Can Negatively Affect Semen Quality

About 25 percent of infertile males have a condition called **varicocele**, which are varicose veins located around one or both of the testicles. These varicose veins cause blood to backflow into the scrotum from the abdomen, raising the average temperature around the testicle. The increased temperature adversely affects the structure of the sperm made in the testicle, as well as their motility (Andre-Rocha, 2007). Varicocele can be repaired with outpatient surgery that usually results in improvements in sperm concentration, morphology, and motility (Agarwal et al., 2007). Testicular heating also adversely affects sperm production. Scrotal temperature is ordinarily 2.2°C less than body temperature and optimum for sperm. Exposing the testes to heat by taking a sauna or steam bath; wearing tight pants or thermal underwear; or even having the kind of occupation (truck driver on cross-country hauls) that results in scrotal heating can reduce fertility.

Research has found that sons born to women who smoked while they were pregnant have reduced sperm counts and testicular volume compared to men born to non smokers (Jensen et al., 2004; Ramiau-Hansen, 2007). Other studies have detected a direct effect of smoking on the sperm concentrations and levels of follicle stimulating hormones of male smokers (Kalyani et al., 2007; Ozgur et al., 2005). In fact, non-smokers were found to have a 49 percent higher sperm count than smokers (Richthoff et al., 2008). Some factors are known to have a temporary effect on male fertility. Infectious such as mononucleosis, hepatitis, and other infections (Wang et al., 2006) can depress sperm production for several months. Certain tranquilizers or mood-elevating drugs may not only produce impotence but also suppress growth and production of sperm. Heavy marijuana smoking depresses sperm counts and testosterone production (Kumar et al., 2009). A number of therapeutic drugs are known to produce temporary infertility. In addition, exposure to chemicals such as dioxins, PCBs, pesticides, and other endocrine disruptors found in plastics, detergents, and other industrial chemicals can reduce sperm motility (Philips and Tanphaichiter, 2008; Hauser et al., 2005; Hauser 2006; and Swan, 2006).

Sometimes in an effort to become pregnant, a couple may try to increase the frequency of intercourse. However, increasing the frequency of coitus beyond four times a week may actually be lowering the sperm count to the point where pregnancy is unlikely. Even in a very fertile male, 12–24 hours should elapse between ejaculations for the sperm quality to have good fertilizing capacity. If a man is less than optimally fertile, it can take at least 48 hours to regain an appropriate sperm concentration.

Diagnosing Female Infertility

An evaluation of female infertility will usually begin with a general physical exam and a regular gynecological exam, and the doctor may ask questions about medical history, menstrual cycles, and sexual habits. The most common causes of female infertility are problems with ovulation, hormone secretion from the ovaries, and blockages of the fallopian tubes. However, problems can also arise with the vagina, cervix, uterus, and immune system, so these may also be examined. In addition to tests specific to these organs, laparoscopy or pelvic ultrasound can be used to look for problems with the uterus, fallopian tubes, or ovaries. With laparoscopy, an illuminated fiber optic telescope is used to view the organs in the abdomen (Figure 14-3). Laparoscopy is especially useful for detecting endometriosis, scarring, and blockages of the fallopian tubes, and other structural problems. Pelvic ultrasound can also be used to detect irregularities in the fallopian tubes and the uterus. Genetic testing may also be required.

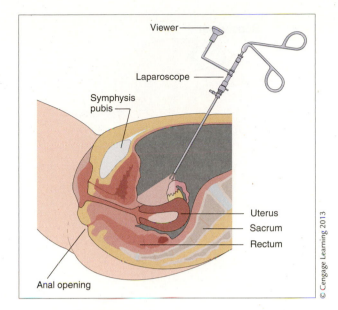

FIGURE 14-3: Laparoscopy.

© Cengage Learning 2013

Vaginal and Cervical Factors that Affect Fertility

Infections that cause vaginitis can affect fertility because changes in vaginal pH can hamper sperm motility. A recent study has found that *Candida albicans*, the organism that causes yeast infections, can adversely affect the motility and membrane characteristics of otherwise healthy sperm (Tain et al., 2007). Even if there are no symptoms or clinical signs of vaginitis, a microscopic examination of vaginal discharge is an important part of an infertility investigation. To enter the uterus, sperm must pass through the cervix. The properties of the cervical mucus determine whether the sperm can pass through or whether they are blocked. Around the time of ovulation, the cervical mucus is clear, watery, and less viscous, more alkaline and most receptive to sperm traveling through. Within a day or two after ovulation, the cervical mucus, now influenced by progesterone, becomes thick and viscous, impeding the passage of sperm. If the cervical mucus does not change consistency to allow sperm entrance through the cervix, then fertility will be impaired. Since the consistency of cervical mucus is primarily under hormonal control, hormone testing is also used to detect abnormalities.

Uterine Factors that Affect Fertility

Endometriosis, even when the fallopian tubes and ovaries are unaffected, can affect a women's ability to get pregnant. Women with endometriosis are also more

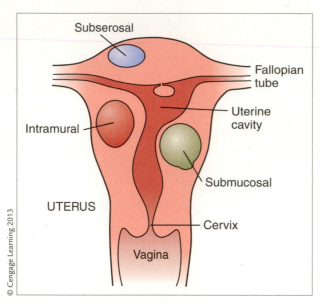

© Cengage Learning 2013

FIGURE 14-4: Three distinct types of uterine fibroids.

likely to suffer spontaneous abortion than infertile women without endometriosis, who have become pregnant through infertility treatments (Matalliotakis et al., 2008). Women who want to have children and who are aware that they have the disease may be advised to consider having children early and spacing them close together before the endometriosis becomes further advanced.

There has been some controversy in the scientific community about the impact of uterine fibroids on fertility. There are three distinct types of uterine fibroids, subserosal, intramural, and submucosal (Figure 14-4), and their classification is based on the location of the fibroid in the uterus. Recent reviews of scientific studies to date indicate that different types of uterine fibroids have different effects on fertility, with sub-mucosal fibroids having the most deleterious effect. Intramural fibroids also affect fertility, but to a lesser degree, and subserous fibroids do not seem to impair fertility. Removing submucosal fibroids increases the odds of becoming pregnant and carrying a baby to term. The benefit of removing intramural fibroids is less clear (Casini et al., 2006; Pritts et al., 2008; Klatsky et al., 2008).

Tubal Factors that Affect Fertility

If the fallopian tubes are partially blocked, the sperm may not be able to reach the egg, or the fertilized egg may not be able to pass through the tube into the uterus. Intrauterine devices (IUDs) have been associated with tubal damage (Merki-Feld et al., 2007) as have STIs. The Center for Disease Control (2008) has gathered data that indicates that one in four sexually active teenage girls in the United States is infected with an STI, a situation which poses a serious risk to their future fertility. It is possible to determine if the fallopian tubes are blocked. Two of these tests, the Rubins test and hysterosalpingography, use gas or fluids injected into the fallopian tubes to measure how open they are. Microsurgery can sometimes be performed on the fallopian tubes to remove blockages. Some of these surgeries can be done laparoscopically, avoiding the need for full abdominal surgery. Success rates vary between 20–60 percent depending on which part of the tube is blocked (ASRM, 2006). Another procedure, balloon tuboplasty, involves inserting a wire with a small balloon attached into the os of the cervix, through the uterus and into the blocked tube. Slowly inflating the balloon can sometimes remove the blockage.

Ovarian and Hormonal Factors that Affect Fertility

The ovaries serve two essential roles in fertility: they produce eggs and they secrete hormones essential to establishing and maintaining a pregnancy. In most cases, blood tests are performed to determine if ovulation is occurring. Ovarian reserve testing is often done to determine if the eggs available can be successfully fertilized. Blood tests can also reveal if hormone levels are interfering with conception and if hormone secretion is adequate to support a pregnancy. Elevated levels of the hormone prolactin can disrupt the synthesis or release of the hormones GnRH and progesterone and interfere with the establishment of pregnancy. Likewise, an increased androgen production due to an adrenal disorder can cause a disturbance in the feedback loop of hormones between the hypothalamus, pituitary gland, and ovary. Daily measurements of the amounts of hormone levels in the blood or of hormone metabolites in the urine can be made to check for these kinds of problems.

In some cases, a woman may ovulate but the resulting corpus luteum does not secrete enough progesterone to sufficiently prepare the endometrium for implantation. Blood tests can measure progesterone levels during the luteal phase of the menstrual cycle to determine both ovulation patterns and the function of the resulting corpus luteum. In some cases, an endometrial biopsy may be performed to determine if it is developing adequately under the influence of ovarian hormones. If the endometrium is underdeveloped, it indicates a condition called luteal phase defect. Endometrial biopsy is performed in the doctor's office, usually without anesthesia or with only a local numbing of the cervix. Recent overviews of infertility diagnosis techniques have suggested that endometrial biopsy is not as useful as other methods for evaluating fertility (deSutter, 2006).

Polycystic ovary syndrome (PCOS) is one of the most common causes of female infertility. Women who have PCOS often have difficulty conceiving because of irregular or absent ovulation. When women with the condition conceive, they are more prone to developing gestational diabetes and gestational hypertension and have more difficulty carrying their pregnancies to term. It has been suggested that the condition may result from a failure to use insulin properly. A recent small study with an investigational drug, D-chiro-inositol, which helps insulin to function more efficiently, showed that the drug

appeared to improve ovulation in women with polycystic ovary syndrome (Nestler et al., 1999).

Fertility problems result when a woman does not ovulate at all or ovulates very irregularly and infrequently. A woman can also determine if she is ovulating, and her ovaries' pattern of hormonal secretion, by charting her basal body temperature (BBT) to predict when she will be ovulating (Figure 14-5), especially when combined with observations of cervical mucus. It should be noted, however, that this method is less effective at determining the time of ovulation as a woman nears menopause. Timing intercourse to occur at the optimal time for conception can increase a couple's chances of getting pregnant. Home ovulation predictor kits which measure LH levels can also be used to time intercourse for conception. Ovulation normally occurs twelve hours after the luteinizing hormone peak.

Unexplained Infertility

In many infertile couples, no physical or physiological reasons for the difficulty can be detected in their reproductive systems. Women over 35 are more likely to be diagnosed with unexplained infertility. The problem may result from a combination

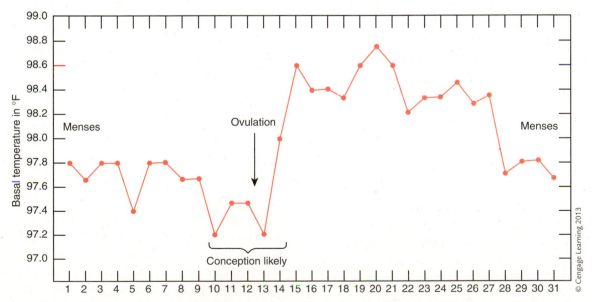

FIGURE 14-5: Basal body temperature (BBT) plotted during an ovulatory cycle is a biphasic curve. Daily temperatures tend to fluctuate in a pattern that is specific for every woman. Ovulation probably occurs the day before the elevation, which may be preceded by a drop in temperature of the cycle. Sperm retain fertilizing capacity for 24-48 hours, and eggs are able to be fertilized for 12-24 hours. Coitus every other day for about three to four days before and two to three days afterward would increase the probability of conception. Unfortunately, not all charts are as easily interpreted as this one.

© Cengage Learning 2013

of subfertility in both partners or from unknown reasons. Studies have pointed out that women with unexplained infertility often face increased risk of obstetric complications such as pre eclampsia, placental abruption, preterm labor, and emergency cesarean section when compared to the general population. These effects were present even after adjusting for age, parity, and fertility treatment (Padian et al., 2001). Future research may reveal some of the causes and possible treatments for some forms of unexplained infertility. Fertility treatments are more successful in individuals with unexplained infertility than in those with other types of infertility.

There is some evidence that mycoplasma infections are associated with infertility. Mycoplasmas bear similarities to both viruses and bacteria. One of the organisms belonging to this group, T-mycoplasma or *Ureaplasma urealyticum*, is believed to account for about half of the cases of nongonococcal urethritis in men and is frequently found in the vaginas of women where it produces no apparent symptoms (Figure 14-6). *Ureaplasma urealyticum* has been implicated by a number of investigators as the cause of repeated spontaneous abortion, stillbirths, and unexplained infertility, but its actual contribution is still unproven. When the infection has been discovered in the male partner of an infertile couple, however, and the man was

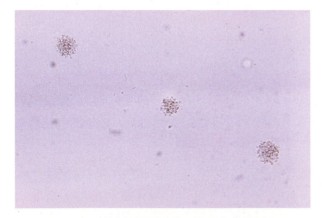

FIGURE 14-6: Magnified 500X, this photograph reveals some of the morphologic features exhibited by a number of medium-sized *Ureaplasm urealyticum* colonies, also known as T-strain mycoplasma. This bacterium is commonly found in both male and female urogenital tracts and normally causes no harm. Under adverse circumstances, however, this bacterium has been known to become pathogenic and has been linked to infertility and premature births. *(Courtesy of CDC/Dr. Francis Forrester)*

treated, pregnancy was achieved in a number of cases. Witkin and Toth (1983) noted that conception occurred in 60 percent of previously infertile couples once the *Ureaplasma urealyticum* infection was eradicated by therapy for both partners. These authors suggested that this kind of hidden but prevalent infection may play a role in infertility (Wang et al., 2006).

Immune system complications may contribute to some cases of unexplained infertility. Sperm-destroying antibodies have been demonstrated in the blood plasma of infertile men as well as in two-thirds of vasectomized men. This kind of autoimmune response has not been shown in the serum of partners of pregnant women. A similar autoimmune response in women is that of developing an antibody reaction to their own ova and has been suggested for some cases of unexplained infertility. Antibodies might bind to the zona pellucida, for example, and make it impossible for the sperm to penetrate the ovum. Treatment to reduce the level of antibodies in both men and women has been used with mixed results.

Rare cases have been reported in which women have suffered strong allergic reactions to semen—hives, hay fever symptoms, vulvovaginal swelling, and, in isolated instances, even anaphylactic shock. Less dramatically, a variety of sperm-immobilizing antibodies can be detected in the blood plasma and/or the cervical-vaginal secretions of a proportion of infertile women. Their significance for explaining infertility is unknown, however, because fertile women have also been found to have sperm antibodies circulating in their blood. There is evidence that treating a woman with unexplained infertility with anti-inflammatory medications in addition to other infertility treatments can increase the chances of becoming pregnant (Edelstam et al., 2008).

PRESERVING FERTILITY THROUGHOUT THE LIFETIME

A woman's long-term fertility is determined by many factors, including genetics and environmental influences that she is exposed to over the course of her lifetime. Some of these she will have control over and some she will not. If preserving fertility is a priority, then there are steps that can be taken to reduce the risk of losing fertility prematurely. Maintaining a healthy weight with adequate nutrition is an important step toward maintaining optimal fertility. Obesity can contribute to infertility, especially in women. Eating disorders and an unbalanced diet can also have an impact, as the body may be lacking essential nutrients needed for conception and successful continuation of a pregnancy. Activity level plays a role in fertility, with a sedentary lifestyle having a negative impact on fertility. On the other hand, too much exercise can interfere with ovulation.

Since pelvic infections can damage the fallopian tubes and reduce a woman's fertility, it is important to use safer sex practices including using a condom to prevent sexually transmitted infections. Two fertility damaging STIs, chlamydia and gonorrhea, are often symptomless in women until the damage is already done, so regular screening for these organisms is important. It is especially important to get early treatment to prevent damage.

The effects of many man-made chemicals and products on human reproduction are still not known, but there is mounting evidence that many chemicals can act as endocrine disruptors and have fertility reducing effects. While it would be difficult to avoid all such threats, it is important to be mindful of credible scientific information as it appears and to avoid exposure to endocrine disruptors when possible.

There have been recent advances in methods to preserve fertility for young women who must undergo radiation or chemotherapy to treat cancer (Letourneau et al., 2010). These therapies usually damage the ovaries, making it unlikely that they can continue producing eggs. Harvesting and freezing eggs before these treatments to preserve future fertility is a procedure that is showing some success. This practice is relatively new, and the long-term viability of frozen eggs is still being established. Another option that has been successful is the removal and cryopreservation of an entire ovary, and then

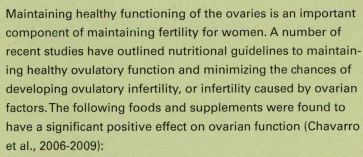
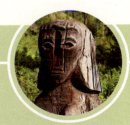

focus on

NUTRITION
The Fertility Diet

Maintaining healthy functioning of the ovaries is an important component of maintaining fertility for women. A number of recent studies have outlined nutritional guidelines to maintaining healthy ovulatory function and minimizing the chances of developing ovulatory infertility, or infertility caused by ovarian factors. The following foods and supplements were found to have a significant positive effect on ovarian function (Chavarro et al., 2006-2009):

- iron supplements
- multivitamin supplements that include folic acid
- high fat dairy products (Interestingly, low fat dairy products decreased ovarian function)
- low glycemic carbohydrates, such a whole grains

One study also suggested replacing animal protein sources in the diet with plant protein to maintain ovulatory function. Food that decreased fertility included:

- trans fats
- caffeine
- high glycemic carbohydrates such as foods high in sugar
- alcohol, especially for women over 30 years old

replacing it after the treatments have ended. As these techniques are further developed, they may offer some hope for women who simply want to bank some of their oocytes for future fertility. Feasibility would depend on the success rate of using frozen oocytes years after their harvest to establish a pregnancy.

INFERTILITY TREATMENTS

In the past, there was little recourse for childless couples. Today, advances in infertility research have made it possible with medical assistance for two-thirds of infertile couples to conceive and produce a baby. There are many different types of infertility treatments available, and the type of intervention selected depends, in part, on the cause of infertility. Although infertility treatments have been instrumental in allowing previously infertile people to have children, it must also be understood that some infertility treatments carry risks in terms of long-term cancer risk, birth defects, pregnancy complications, and problems associated with high order multiple pregnancies .

Medications that Increase Ovulation

Medications to increase ovulation are either used singly to treat infertility or in combination with other treatments such as artificial insemination and in vitro fertilization. These medications often cause several eggs to mature and ovulate, rather than just one, a condition called **superovulation**. There are a wide variety of fertility medications available, with some more effective at treating specific causes of infertility than others. Each medication will carry its own risks for side effects, which must be weighed when evaluating that drug for use. One of the most familiar fertility medications is clomiphene citrate. Clomiphene citrate in low doses is the safest and least expensive method of ovulation induction and is generally used first if conditions warrant it. Although its action is still not completely understood, it is believed to block the negative feedback effect of estrogen on the hypothalamus by occupying the estrogen receptor sites in the nuclei of hypothalamic cells. The hypothalamus is deceived into thinking that the body's circulating estrogen level is low and produces more GnRH to signal the pituitary production of FSH and LH in an attempt to increase more follicles to mature and produce estrogen. This process also triggers ovulation. According to several sources, 80–90 percent of women who meet the criteria for clomiphene therapy can be expected to ovulate and about half will get pregnant (Speroff, Glass, & Kase, 1989; Hutchinson-Williams, 1990). In some women, clomiphene's anti-estrogenic properties cause the production of less receptive cervical mucus. Even if ovulation occurs, conception may be hampered. Additional hormones may be administered to counteract this effect. Some side effects include hot flashes, breast soreness, nausea and vomiting, abdominal pain or soreness, visual disturbances, and hair loss. All of these symptoms occur infrequently and are reversible within a few days of discontinuing the drug. No evidence of a greater incidence of birth defects following ovulation induction has been documented. A more serious condition, ovarian hyperstimulation syndrome (OHSS), will be discussed later in this chapter.

Artificial Insemination

Artificial insemination is a process that places sperm into the female reproductive tract. This can be used when the source of infertility is poor semen quality. The technique can use either concentrated sperm from a male partner's semen or donor semen. Because infections can be transmitted to the prospective mother, and genetic diseases can be passed on to the baby, guidelines have been established by the American Society for Reproductive Medicine concerning the safety of donor semen. However, the guidelines are not binding and not every practitioner follows them. Reputable sperm banks screen donors for HIV, hepatitis, and other sexually transmitted infections and will test donors for genetic diseases such as cystic fibrosis, sickle cell carrier status, and Tay-Sachs carrier status. There is no formal policy in most states, however, that requires testing donors or even taking a medical history or keeping accurate records. After a year of artificial inseminations, the reported national success rate averages 57–70 percent, with the majority of pregnancies occurring in less than six months. Maternal age plays an important role in the success rate of this technique, with younger mothers having more success (Goldberg & Rodgers, 2009). Artificial insemination can be accomplished using a variety of different techniques.

Methods of Artificial Insemination

With intra-cervical insemination (ICI), semen is placed into the cervical mucus just prior to ovulation. A cervical cap or specially designed tampon is used to hold the semen against the cervix. Sperm must then swim through the cervical mucus into the uterus and to the fallopian tube to meet the egg. When a concentrated sperm sample is placed directly into the uterus by means of a sterile trans-cervical catheter, the procedure is called **intrauterine insemination**, or IUI. With intrauterine insemination, the sperm are capacitated and washed to eliminate the seminal fluid and concentrate the sperm. Capacitation, or the changes in the sperm plasma membrane that allow interaction with the egg, normally occurs in the female reproductive tract but, in this case, takes place when the sperm are incubated in an artificial culture medium. Sperm are sorted, and the most motile sperm are then placed into the uterus near the tubal openings using a catheter directed by ultrasound. Studies have indicated an overall pregnancy rate of about 25 percent using IUI (Bensdrop et al., 2007). Some researchers have suggested that IUI has a higher success ratio than does ICI (Goldberg & Rodgers, 2009). In both cases, insemination is timed to coincide with ovulation.

Artificial insemination is usually accompanied with fertility medications to stimulate ovulation. A recent review of the scientific literature on these procedures found that for cycles in which fertility medications were not used, IUI was no more successful than intercourse timed to favorably coincide with ovulation. The study also found that the success rates of IUI with fertility medications (ie. stimulated cycles) did not differ significantly from IUI alone. This data is in contrast to earlier studies that tended to support the use of IUI with fertility medications. However, the study points out the need for further research using controlled, randomized trials to further understand which practices are best for treating infertility with artificial insemination (Bensdrop et al., 2007).

Finally, **fallopian tube sperm profusion (FSP)** involves placing sperm directly into the fallopian tubes and bypassing the cervix and uterus all together. It is more complicated than IUI and involves placing the semen in a catheter that is passed through the cervix, through the uterine cavity, and into the fallopian tube. The catheter is guided with ultrasound. A recent review of the scientific literature has found that FSP is more effective than IUI for treating unexplained infertility (Cantineau et al., 2004; Bensdorp et al., 2007).

Assisted Reproductive Technologies (ART)

While artificial insemination is primarily used to treat male infertility, **assisted reproductive technologies (ART)** are used when female reproductive function is impaired. With ART, both egg and sperm are collected, combined, and the resulting embryo placed into the female reproductive tract. In vitro fertilization (IVF) is the most common form of ART, comprising 99 percent of the ART procedures, but other forms of ART are becoming more available.

A Short History of Assisted Reproductive Technologies

The birth of a baby girl to a British woman whose fallopian tubes were irreparably obstructed signaled the beginning of a new era in infertility therapy. Although millions of cattle had been produced by a combination of artificial insemination with embryo transfer, the first fertilization of a human egg outside of the mother's body and placement into the uterus to complete its embryonic development did not occur until 1978 when researchers successfully established a pregnancy in 30-year-old Lesley Brown through **in vitro fertilization (IVF)**. Her egg was combined with her husband's sperm in a petri dish and the fertilized egg nurtured to the 8-cell stage before being returned to the uterus for implantation. Nine months later, the first "test-tube baby" was born. Since Louise Joy Brown's birth, IVF has become a widely used method of infertility therapy. The success rate, initially very low, has improved.

Originally, IVF treatment was limited to women with tubal abnormalities, but during the 1980s, the therapy was extended to include those with unexplained infertility, endometriosis, pelvic adhesions, congenital or DES-induced anomalies of the reproductive tract, immunologic causes for infertility, women whose partners have low sperm count, and women age 40 or older. Early in its history, IVF was to some extent viewed as a way for almost anyone to have a baby, no matter what their age or the cause of their infertility. However, it has become clear the IVF does have limitations, and like other infertility treatments, it is less effective for older individuals than it is for younger ones. A recent study has found that the success rate of IVF is only one percent for women aged 45 or older (Sullivan et al., 2008). Other researchers have proposed that IVF does not have a reasonable success rate in women over 45 (Wang et al., 2008: Klipstein et al., 2005; Leridon & Slama, 2008).

InVitro Fertilization Procedure

The fundamentals of IVF appear straightforward. Although different IVF programs vary in their protocols, the first step of IVF involves stimulating the ovaries to induce multiple follicle formation. Follicle

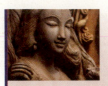

Social Considerations
BECOMING AN EGG DONOR

As ART has become more common in the treatment of infertility, the demand for donated eggs to be used in these procedures has increased. The age of the egg is important, so eggs from younger women are more likely to result in successful pregnancies than are older eggs. In some cases, younger women might be asked to donate eggs to help an older family member or friend become pregnant. This process is called oocyte donation. The amount of money that a woman can be compensated for donating oocytes depends on where she lives because payment for oocyte donation is allowed in some countries and not in others. In the United States, the ASRM has established that egg donors can ethically be paid between $5000 and $10,000 per donation (Luk and Petrozza, 2008).

The decision of whether or not to donate eggs is an important one. The rewards, in some cases financial, and in others emotional, can be substantial. However, it is important to consider that oocyte donation is a complicated, time-consuming process, and that it does carry some risks. While the process of the egg donation will vary from program to program, there will usually be several physical and psychological exams conducted to screen potential donors. If selected, an oocyte donor will undergo the same procedures to harvest eggs as a woman preparing to undergo IVF, including treatment with fertility medications to stimulate superovulation, including OHSS, which can lead to blood clots and kidney failure.

Oocytes donors carry some additional risks as well. If the oocyte donor has unprotected intercourse during the donor cycle, they can become pregnant with twins or a higher order pregnancy. The long-term effects of egg harvesting on future fertility have not yet been determined. Complications such as bleeding, infections, or removal of an ovary can reduce fertility.

development is monitored daily, and the ovum is removed from the ovary just prior to ovulation. The ovum is fertilized in vitro, and then it is placed into the uterine cavity for implantation. IVF procedures may use a woman's own eggs or donor eggs. For older women wishing to become pregnant with IVF, using donor eggs from younger women increases the chance of success (Sullivan et al., 2008).

Ovulation Induction and Retrieval   Usually, superovulation is stimulated using fertility medications. Follicular development is monitored by the daily measurement of serum estrogen levels and ultrasound imaging of the growing follicles. When several follicles are at least 14 mm or greater in diameter and the estrogen level reaches an acceptable threshold, a single injection of an LH mimic is given to stimulate the LH surge and induce the final maturation of the follicles. The ova are harvested by laparoscopy under general anesthesia, but ultrasound-guided techniques have largely replaced the laparoscopic method at most IVF centers. The harvested oocytes are microscopically evaluated for their maturation. Mature oocytes are incubated in culture medium for four to six hours before the sperm are added; immature oocytes are incubated for a minimum of 24 hours to ensure that they are likely to be fertilized.

Fertilization   While the oocytes are incubating, a semen specimen is procured. The sperm are washed and concentrated, and the most motile are capacitated. The capacitated sperm are added to petri dishes of culture medium that each contains an oocyte. Sixteen to 17 hours later, each oocyte is examined for signs of fertilization. Once a sperm enters an oocyte, it completes its second meiotic division, so the presence of a second polar body and two pronuclei indicates that fertilization has occurred. When the sperm count is very low, or when previously frozen oocytes are used, the zona pellucida may be slit, partially dissected, or lasered, or the sperm may be microinjected into the oocyte (Hill et al., 1991). This process is called intracytoplasmic sperm injection (ICSI). The technique enables a man who produces sperm, even though the sperm have not been ejaculated and have been removed from the testes by the physician, to father a child if the procedure works. Some infertility researchers have raised questions about this technique, citing concerns about the possibility of chromosomal defects in the ICSI babies (Kolata, 1999). Some infertility specialists recommend that all men with severe sperm production problems be offered genetic counseling before attempting either IVF or ICSI, since the problems that are hindering sperm production may also endanger a pregnancy. In those cases, donor sperm may be considered.

Embryo Transfer   Embryos are most often transferred between 48 and 80 hours after fertilization when they are at the four to eight cell stages. Although the transfer of more than one embryo increases the chances of implantation and pregnancy, the placement of more than two embryos increases the risk of a multiples pregnancy. A catheter is used to introduce the embryos into a woman's uterus through the cervical os. When more than two eggs are fertilized, most programs offer the option of cryopreserving (freezing) the resulting embryos. The survival rate of frozen embryos is estimated at about 50 percent, and these embryos can be used for successive transfers, if pregnancy is not established. If the transferred embryos implant, HCG levels will begin to rise. Because the drugs used to stimulate superovulation are believed to alter the estrogen-progesterone ratio, progesterone may be given to supplement the luteal phase of the uterine endometrium.

Results of IVF

It seems that it should be easy to determine the success rate of IVF by calculating the number of successful pregnancies established per attempt made. Unfortunately, what constitutes a successful pregnancy has not always been standardized, so some information is not reliable. Pregnancies that ended in a miscarriage may or may not be considered a success, depending on who is compiling the records. Of late, the outcome of a baby born, has become the more accepted criterion, and based on this, the success rates of IVF can be evaluated. In 2002, the CDC calculated the overall average success rate of IVF to be 28 percent. They noted that infertile couples with uterine factors or multiple infertility factors had a below average success rate, whereas couples with tubal factor, ovulatory dysfunction, male infertility, or unexplained infertility had above average success with IVF (CDC, 2002). If an individual or a couple is able to undergo more than three attempts at IVF, there is evidence that the chances of achieving a pregnancy increase. The group at the Jones Institute for Reproductive Medicine of the Eastern Virginia Medical School, one of the nation's oldest, largest, and most respected IVF programs, has reported that their cumulative pregnancy rates were 32.75 percent after one cycle of treatment, 50.75 percent after two cycles, and 63.75 percent after three cycles.

Critical Thinking

Extra Embryos

Assisted reproductive technologies often result in excess embryos. Options for what to do with these embryos range from freezing them for future use, donating them for scientific research, or disposing of them. What are the factors that must be considered when an individual or a couple must decide what to do with extra embryos? How might a couple's circumstances influence their decision? What would you decide?

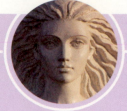

focus on

EXERCISE

Effects of Exercise on In Vitro Fertilization Success

Exercise may have a negative effect on in vitro fertilization success for women who exercise regularly. In a study of 2232 patients trying to become pregnant through in vitro fertilization, those who reported exercising four or more hours per week for one to nine years prior to treatments were 40 percent less likely to have a live birth. Those who participated in cardiovascular exercise were 30 percent less likely to have a live birth than those who reported no exercise. Women who exercised regularly were three times more likely to experience cycle cancellation during their treatments and twice as likely to experience implantation failure and pregnancy loss (Morris et al., 2007).

A variety of researchers have studied the effect of a woman's age on her chances of having a baby through IVF. In a large Australian study of IVF from 2002-2005, the highest success rates were found in women from 22 years old to 36 years old. Interestingly, their study found that for each year a woman waited past the age of 30, her chances of conceiving decreased by 11 percent, and her chance of carrying the pregnancy to term decreased by 13 percent. They concluded that women aged 35 or older should be advised to seek fertility assessment and treatment earlier rather than waiting (Wang et al., 2008).

Gamete Intrafallopian Transfer (GIFT) and Zygote Intrafallopian Transfer (ZIFT)

Although IVF is the most common form of ART, other techniques are available. GIFT is similar to IVF in that superovulation induction and the aspiration of oocytes take place, but fertilization by the sperm does not take place in vitro in the laboratory. With **gamete intrafallopian transfer (GIFT)**, the mixture of sperm and the oocytes are loaded into a catheter and, through laparoscopy, two oocytes and about 100,000 motile sperm are introduced into each fallopian tube. Thus, fertilization takes place in the body (in vivo), which distinguishes the procedure from IVF. The advantage of GIFT is that it is less complicated; there is

---

Case Study

Unexplained Infertility

Cody, age 28, and Angelia, age 26, have been trying to conceive. Angelia went off the pill a year and a half ago, and despite regular sex, they are having no luck. They have been using the ovulation predictor kits, and despite the kits indicating Angelia is ovulating, they still haven't been able to get pregnant. They decide to consult a fertility specialist who orders a semen analysis for Cody. All his lab values are within normal ranges. Motility, volume, and sperm numbers are fine. Angelia's evaluation also shows no abnormalities. She is ovulating, her fallopian tubes are open, and her endometrium is receptive. Post-coital testing also indicates no problem. The doctor informs them that they have unexplained infertility. For reasons that cannot be identified, they simply cannot get pregnant. However, he explains that they are good candidates for assistive reproductive technologies.

1. What might be factors that could contribute to unexplained infertility?

2. What are some of the assisted technologies they and their doctor might consider in order to get pregnant?

no need for embryo transfer, so the procedure is less expensive. A major disadvantage is the necessity for laparoscopy under general anesthesia, which increases risk, potential complications, and discomfort. **Zygote intrafallopian transfer** (ZIFT) is similar to GIFT in that the transfer is made into the fallopian tubes but fertilization takes place in vitro as in IVF and it is the fertilized eggs, or zygotes, that are transferred. ZIFT is a variation used when it is deemed important to get direct evidence of the fertilizing capacity of the oocytes and sperm.

Risks Associated with Fertility Medications and Assisted Reproductive Technologies (ART)

When treatment with fertility medications is prolonged and large amounts of medication are taken, the ovaries can be overly stimulated, resulting in ovarian hyperstimulation syndrome (OHSS) (Lobo, 2007). This condition results in enlarged and painful ovaries and, often, the formation of ovarian cysts. Symptoms of this condition include bloating, abdominal discomfort, nausea, and diarrhea. These symptoms usually resolve when the next period arrives, but if a pregnancy is established, the symptoms may last longer. In some cases, OHSS can cause extensive fluid accumulations in the chest and abdomen, leading to swelling, shortness of breath and low blood pressure. This syndrome can result in blood clots, kidney failure, fluid build-up in the lungs, and shock. In severe cases, this syndrome can result in complications that

require the surgical removal of an ovary in order to prevent complications that can become life threatening. Some research has linked fertility medications with the development of reproductive cancers, but other studies have not shown an association. The long-term safety or cancer risks of using fertility medications are not known at present, because the widespread use of these medications is a relatively recent phenomenon.

Another risk associated with using fertility medications, and with ART, is the increased chance of **higher order multiple pregnancies**. When more than one egg is stimulated to ovulate, there is a greater risk that multiple eggs will become fertilized and implant in the uterus. About seven to ten percent of the pregnancies after clomiphene use are multiple; primarily twins, but triplets may occur as frequently as one in 400 live births and quadruplets as frequently as one in 800 (Brandes et al., 2010). The risk of multiple births after fertility medications in general depends on a number of factors, including the type of medication, the woman's age, the quality of the sperm, and the dosage and duration of treatment, but it is usually 10–20 percent (Figure 14-7). Transfer of multiple embryos during IVF and ZIFT procedures can also result in a multiple pregnancy. The incidence of high-order multiple gestations, defined as giving birth to three or more infants, is fortunately still relatively small but has quadrupled since the mid-1980s. These babies are likely to be born prematurely and are at risk for a range of problems. Inevitably born prematurely,

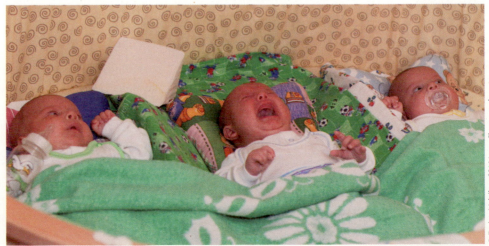

FIGURE 14-7: Fertility medications and ART technologies have a higher risk of multiple births.

© Dmitry Melnikov, 2011/www.Shutterstock.com

they have increased possibilities of lung and intestinal problems. If they survive, the infants may face cerebral palsy and developmental and physical disabilities. One option to prevent a high-order multiple gestation is selective reduction, or removal of one or more fetuses in the uterus, leaving others to develop normally. Because selective reduction could imperil the entire pregnancy, it is generally viewed as a last resort. Guidelines have been established in the United States and in Canada with recommendations about the optimal number of embryos that should be transferred to maximize the chance of establishing a pregnancy and minimize the chance of too many embryos implanting (Joint SOGC-CFS, 2008; ASRM, 2009; Borahay & Phelps, 2010; Practice Committee of the American Society for Reproductive Medicine; Practice Committee of the Society for Assisted Reproduction Technology, (2009).

Finally, there have been concerns raised about whether or not IVF pregnancies carry higher risks to mother and fetus than do other pregnancies. There is evidence that pregnancies resulting from IVF faced a higher risk of placenta previa, placental abruption, gestational hypertension, preterm delivery, low birth weight, and an unusually high rate of emergency cesarian section. There are some indications that children conceived as a result of ART, especially ICSI, face increased health risks compared to other children. In addition, Ludwig et al. (2008) found an increased incidence of birth defects. However, other researchers have countered that the conditions that lead to infertility in the first place, and not IVF itself, may be more important in contributing to complications in IVF pregnancies. ART is still a relatively new development in human reproduction, and additional research is needed to more fully understand the possible risks.

Surrogate Mothers

When an infertile woman is not able to carry a pregnancy to term, a **surrogate mother** may be employed. In this case, a fertile woman is paid by an individual or a couple to undergo a pregnancy achieved by either artificial insemination with donor semen or through IVF. In the case of gestational surrogacy, a woman with functional ovaries but a nonfunctional uterus contributes the egg to be fertilized and transferred by IVF to the surrogate. Gestational surrogacy can also be used if the pregnancy would be too great a health risk to a woman who wants a child. Usually, a surrogate mother is paid for undergoing the pregnancy, but in some cases, a woman may carry the child to term as an altruistic act for a friend or relative. The use of a surrogate can raise legal dilemmas, since few states have passed laws to regulate this process.

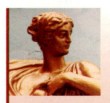

Cultural Considerations
SURROGATE MOTHERS IN INDIA

For infertile couples in the West who want to hire a surrogate mother in order to have a child, the costs can be prohibitive. In the United States, for example, surrogate mothers are typically paid around $15,000. Agencies that set up the agreement between the infertile couple and the surrogate add to the costs for the IVF treatments, which can double the cost. In contrast, it is possible to travel to an infertility clinic in Anand, India where the entire cost ranges between $2500 and $6500. Controversy arises as to whether or not the practice of going abroad to hire a surrogate for less than it would cost at home is a form of exploitation. The issue is complicated, since the money earned by the surrogate mothers far exceeds what they can earn through jobs that are currently available to them where they live. They are able to use the money to invest in their own children's educations or to buy a home.

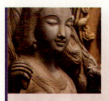

Social Considerations
GLOBAL ADOPTIONS

Through inter-country adoption, the legal transfer of parental rights from the birth parent/parents to another parent, or other parents, takes place. Over the last decade, United States families have adopted on average 20,000 children from foreign nations, each year. United States families pay an average $30,000 for an international adoption, including at least one visit to the country of their adopted child's birth (US Department of State, Office of Children's Issues, 2009).

While international adoptions can be filled with great joy, they sometimes also have a more menacing side. Human rights abuses, including the abduction of children within the context of international adoptions, are frequently reported and are a significant issue of concern. Unfortunately, there are many examples of children being taken from their home countries under dubious circumstances.

While UNICEF does not strictly oppose international adoption, it has stated that it believes international adoption should be considered only when the child cannot be suitably cared for in his or her home country (UNICEF, 2003). UNICEF's position has been that if a child has been abandoned, biological parents or extended family should be located. If that is not possible, placement for the child with a foster or in-country adoptive family should be looked into. Only when all other options have been exhausted, should inter-country adoption be considered.

By adhering to this policy, UNICEF has said that it seeks to ensure that international adoptions are conducted under a legal framework that protects the best interests of the child (UNICEF, 2003). While UNICEF has noted that many international adoptions are completed in good faith, they have also warned that a lack of legal oversight has resulted in child trafficking and kidnappings (UNICEF, 2003).

On April 1st, 2008, a new international treaty called the Hague Convention on Protection of Children and Co-operation in Respect of Inter-country Adoption entered into force in the United States. The Convention establishes important standards and safeguards to protect children in the process of inter-country adoptions, and adoptions are unable to proceed if such standards and safeguards are not met. As of early 2009, for example, the United States Department of State has issued adoption alerts on Vietnam and Guatemala, noting that United States citizens are not able to register new adoptions in those countries due to lack of sufficient safeguards at this time (United States Department of State, Office of Children's Issues, 2009).

ADOPTION

Adoption is one way for infertile couples or individuals to become parents. It is estimated that 250,000 children worldwide are adopted each year. In the United States, about 120,000 children per year are adopted. Of these about half are adopted by family members such as grandparents or stepparents. Adoption takes many forms. Older children and special needs children are often adopted out of foster care. International adoption accounts for about 20 percent of adoptions in the United States. Adoptions can be open or closed depending on whether the birth parents' identities are disclosed or not.

CONCLUSION

While there have been tremendous advances in infertility treatment in recent years, there are still limitations to what is possible in overcoming infertility. For this reason, it is important to evaluate lifestyle decisions in light of their potential effect on future fertility. This is true for the individual and throughout society as the effects of endocrine disruptors and other pollutants become clearer. Finally, it is important to consider that age plays a significant role in fertility and in the chances of success of infertility treatments.

REVIEW QUESTIONS

1. How is infertility defined medically?

2. What are the factors that can contribute to infertility?

3. What factors would be examined to evaluate a woman for infertility?

4. Contrast intracervical insemination (ICI), intrauterine insemination (IUI) and fallopian tube sperm profusion (FSP).

5. Explain the process of in vitro fertilization.

6. What are the differences between GIFT and ZIFT?

7. What are some of the risks associated with ART?

CRITICAL THINKING QUESTIONS

1. Should infertility treatments be covered by medical insurance?

2. What kinds of guidelines would have to be in place to ensure that women are not exploited when they serve as surrogate mothers for other individuals or couples?

WEBLINKS

American Society for Reproductive Medicine
www.asrm.org

International Council on Infertility Information Dissemination, Inc.
www.inciid.org

REFERENCES

Agarwal, A., Deepinder, F., Coxuzza, M., Agarwal, R., Short, R. A., & Sabanegh, E. (2007). Efficacy of varicocelectomy in improving semen parameters: New meta-analytical approach. *Urology, 70*(3), 352–358.

Aitken, R. J. (2006). Sperm function tests and fertility. *International Journal of Andrology, 29*(1), 69–75.

American College of Obstetricians and Gynecologists. (2007). Evaluating infertility. Retrieved from http://www.acog.org/publications/patient_education/bp136.cfm.

American Society for Reproductive Medicine Practice Committee. (2006). Salpingectomy for hydrosalpinx prior to in vitro fertilization. *Fertility and Sterility, 86*(Suppl 4), S200–S201.

Andersson, A. M., Jorgensen, N., Main, K. M., Toppari, J., Rajpert-De Meyts, E., Leffers, H., Juul, A., Jensen, T. K., & Skakkebaek, N. E. (2008). Adverse trends in male reproductive health: We may have reached a crucial 'tipping point.' *International Journal of Andrology, 31*(2), 74–80.

Andrade-Rocha, F. T. (2007). Significance of sperm characteristics in the evaluation of adolescents, adults and older men with varicocele. *Journal of Postgraduate Medicine, 53*(1), 8–13.

Bensdorp, A. J., Cohen, B. J., Heineman, M. J., & Vanderkerckhove, P. (2007). Intra-uterine insemination for male subfertility. *Cochrane Database Systematic Review, Oct 17*(4), CD000360.

Borahay, M., & Phelps, J. (2010). Potential liability of reproductive endocrinologists for high order multiple gestation. *Journal of Assisted Reproduction Genetics, 27*(4), 157–159.

Brandes, M., Hamilton, C. J., Bergevoet, K. A., de Bruin, J. P., Nelen, W. L., & Kremer, J. A. (2010). Origin of multiple pregnancies in a subfertile population. *Acta Obstetricia et Gynecologica Scandinavica, 89*(9),1149–1154.

Cantineau, A. E., Heineman, M. J., Al-Inany, H., & Cohlen, B. J. (2004). Intrauterine insemination versus Fallopian tube sperm profusion in non-tubal subfertility: A systematic review based on a Cochrane review. *Human Reproduction, 19*(12), 2721–2729.

Casini, M. L., Rossi, F., Agostini, R., & Unfer, V. (2006). Effects of the position of fibroids on fertility. *Gynecological Endocrinology, 22*(2), 106–109.

Centers for Disease Control. (2008, March 13). Prevalence of sexually transmitted infections and bacterial vaginosis among female adolescents in the United States: Data from the National Health and Nutritional Examination Survey (NHANES) 2003-2004. Delivered at the 2008 National STD Prevention Conference, Chicago, IL.

Chavarro, J. E., Rich-Edwards, J. W., Rosner, B. A., & Willett, W. C. (2006). Iron intake and risk of ovulatory infertility. *Obstetrics and Gynecology, 108*(5), 1145–1152.

Chavarro, J. E., Rich-Edwards, J. W., Rosner, B. A., & Willett, W. C. (2007). Dietary fatty acid intakes and the risk of ovulatory infertility. *American Journal of Clinical Nutrition, 85*(1), 231–237. doi:10.1038/sj.ejcn.1602904.

Chavarro, J. E., Rich-Edwards, J. W., Rosner, B. A., & Willett, W. C. (2007). Protein intake and ovulatory infertility. *American of Journal of Obstetrics and Gynecology, 198*(2), 210.e1–7.

Chavarro, J. E., Rich-Edwards, J. W., Rosner, B. A., & Willett, W. C. (2008). Diet and lifestyle in prevention of ovulatory disorder infertility. *Obstetrics and Gynecology, 110*(5), 1050–1058.

Chavarro, J. E., Rich-Edwards, J. W., Rosner, B. A., & Willett, W. C. (2008). Use of multivitamins, intake of B vitamins, and risk of ovulatory infertility. *Fertility and Sterility, 89*(3), 668–676.

Chavarro, J. E., Rich-Edwards, J. W., Rosner, B. A., & Willett, W. C. (2009). A prospective study of dietary carbohydrate quantity and quality in relation to risk of ovulatory infertility. *European Journal of Clinical Nutrition, 63*, 78–86. doi:10.1038/sj.ejcn.1602904.

de Sutter, P. (2006). Rational diagnosis and treatment of infertility. *Best Practices & Research: Clinical Obstetrics & Gynaecology, 20*(5), 647–664.

Edelstam, G., Sjösten, A., Bjuresten, K., Ek, I., Wånggren, K., & Spira, J. (2008). A new rapid and effective method for treatment of unexplained infertility. *Human Reproduction, 23*(4), 852–856.

Foster, W. G., Neal, M. S., Han, M. S., & Dominguez, M. M. (2008). Environmental contaminants and human infertility: Hypothesis or cause for concern? *Journal of Toxicology & Environmental Health, Part B, 11*(3–4), 162–176.

Gilbert, W. M., Nesbitt, T. S., & Danielsen, B. (1999). Childbearing beyond age 40: Pregnancy outcome in 24,032 cases. *Obstetrics and Gynecology, 93*(1), 9–14.

Goldberg, J. M., & Rodgers, A. K. (2009). Optimizing success with donor insemination. *Frontiers in Bioscience (Elite Ed.), 11*, 355–366.

Gray, Jr., L. E. Wilson, V. S., Stoker, T., Lambright, C., Furr, J., Noriega, N., Howdeshell, K., Abkley, G. T., & Guillette, L. (2006). Adverse effects of environmental antiandrogens and androgens on reproductive development in mammals. *International Journal of Andrology, 29*(1), 96–104.

Guzick, D. S., Carson, S. A., Contifaris, C., et al. (1999). Efficacy of superovulation and intra-uterine insemination in the treatment of infertility. *New England Journal of Medicine, 340*(3), 177–183.

Guzick, D. S., Wilkes, C., & Jones, H. W., Jr. (1986). Cumulative pregnancy rates for in vitro fertilization. *Fertility and Sterility, 46*, 663.

Hauser, R., Williams, P., Altshul, L., & Calafat, A. M. (2005). Evidence of interaction between polychlorinated biphenyls and phthalates in relation to human sperm motility. *Environmental Health Perspectives, 113*(4), 425–430.

Hauser, R. (2006). The environment and male fertility: Recent research on emerging chemicals and semen quality. *Seminars in Reproductive Medicine, 24*(3),156–167.

Hill, D. L., Adler, D., Rothman, C., et al. (1991). Micromanipulation in a center for reproductive medicine. *Fertility and Sterility, 55*(1), 36–38.

Hutchinson-Williams, K. A. (1990). Induction of ovulation. In N. G. Kase, A. B. Weingold, & D. M. Gershenson (Eds.), *Principles and practice of clinical gynecology* (2nd ed.). New York, NY: Churchill Livingstone.

Jensen, T. K., Jorgensen, N., Punab, M., Haugen, T. B., Suominen, J., Zilaitiene, B., Horte, A., Andersen, A. G., Carlsen, E., Magnus, O., Matulevicius, V., Nermoen, I., Vierula, M., Keiding, N., Toppari, J., & Skakkabaek, N. E. (2004). Association of in utero exposure to maternal smoking with reduced semen quality and testis size in adulthood: A cross-sectional study of 1,770 young men from the general population in five European countries. *American Journal of Epidemiology, 159*(1), 49–58.

Jensen, T. K., Sobotka, T., Hansen, M. A., Pedersens, A. T., Lutz, W., & Skakkabaek, N. E. (2008). Declining trends in conception rates in recent birth cohorts of native Danish women: A possible role of deteriorating male reproductive health. *International Journal of Andrology, 31*(2), 81–92.

Jobling, S., Burn, R. W., Thorpe, K., Williams, R., & Tyler, C. (2009). Statistical modeling suggests that anti-androgens in wastewater treatment works effluents are contributing causes of widespread sexual disruption in fish living in English rivers. *Environmental Health Perspectives, 117*(5). doi:10.1289/ehp.0800197.

Joint SOGC-CFAS. (2006). Guidelines for the number of embryos to transfer following in vitro fertilization. (No. 182). Ottawa, Canada: Author.

Jorgensen, N., Asklund, C., Carlsen, E., & Skakkabaek, N. E. (2006). Coordinated European investigations of semen quality: Results from studies of Scandinavian young men is a matter of concern. *International Journal of Andrology, 29*(1), 54–61.

Kalyani, R., Basavaraj, P. B., & Kumar, M. L. (2007). Factors influencing quality of semen: A two year prospective study. *Indian Journal of Pathology Microbiology, 50*(4), 890–895.

Kamel, R. M. (2010). Management of the infertile couple: An evidence-based protocol. *Reproductive Biology and Endocrinology, 8,* 21.

Klatsky, P. C., Tran, N. D., Caughey, A. B., & Fujimoto, V. Y. (2008). Fibroids and reproductive outcomes: A systematic review from conception to delivery. *American Journal of Obstetrics and Gynecology, 198*(4), 357–366.

Klipstein, S., Regan, M., Ryley, D. A., Goldman, M. B., Alper, M. M., & Reindollar, R. H. (2005). One last chance for pregnancy: A review of 2,705 in vitro fertilization cycles initiated in women age 40 years and above. *Fertility and Sterility, 84*(2), 435–445.

Kolata, G. (1999, March 30). New questions about popular fertilization technique. *The New York Times,* D10.

Kumar, S., Kumari, A., & Muraka, S. (2009). Lifestyle factors in deteriorating male reproductive health. *Indian Journal of Experimental Biology, 47*(8), 615–624.

Lentz, G. M., Lobo, R. A., & Gershenson, D. M. (Eds.). (2007). *Comprehensive gynecology* (5th ed.), Chapter 41. Philadelphia, PA: Mosby Elsevier; 2007.

Leridon, H., & Slama, R. (2008). The impact of a decline in fecundity and of pregnancy postponement on final number of children and demand for assisted reproduction technology. *Human Reproduction, 23*(6), 1312–1319.

Letourneau, J. M., Milisko, M. E., Cedars, M. I., & Rosen, M. P. (2010). A changing perspective: Improving access to fertility preservation. *Nature Reviews Clinical Oncology, 8,* 56–60. doi:10.1038/nrclinonc.2010.133.

Lewis, S. F. M. (2007). Is sperm evaluation useful in predicting human fertility? *Reproduction, 124,* 31–40.

Lobo, R. A. (2007). Infertility: Etiology, diagnostic evaluation, management, prognosis. In: V. L., Katz, G. M. Lentz, R. A. Lobo, & D. M. Gershenson.(Eds.). *Comprehensive gynecology* (5th ed.), Chapter 41. Philadelphia, PA: Mosby Elsevier.

Ludwig, A. K., Katalinic, A., Thyen, U., Sutcliffe, A. G., Diedrich, K., & Ludwig, M. (2009). Physical health at 5.5 years of age of term-born singletons after intracytoplasmic sperm injection: Results of a prospective, controlled, single-blinded study. *Fertility and Sterility, 91*(1), 115–124.

Luk, J., & Petrozza, J. C. (2008). Evaluation if compliance and range of fees among American Society for Reproductive Medicine-listed egg donor and surrogacy agencies. *Journal of Reproductive Medicine, 53*(11), 827–852.

Macklin, R. (1991, January/February). Artificial means of reproduction and our understanding of the family. *Hastings Center Report, 1,* 5–11.

Maffini, M. V., Rubin, B. S., Sonnenschein, C., & Soto, A. M. (2006). Endocrine disruptors and reproductive health: The case of bisphenol-A. *Molecular and Cellular Endocrinology, 254–255,* 179–186.

Matalliotakis, I., Cakmak, H., Dermitzaki, D., Zervoudis, S., Goumenou, A., & Fragouli, Y. (2008). Increased rate of endometriosis and spontaneous abortion in an in vitro fertilization program: No correlation with epidemiological factors. *Gynecology and Endocrinology, 24*(4), 194–198.

Mendola, P., Messer, L. C., & Rappazzo, K. (2008). Science linking environmental contaminant exposures with fertility and reproductive health impacts in the adult female. *Fertility and Sterility, 89*(2 Suppl), e81–94.

Menning, B. E. (1988). *Infertility: A guide for the childless couple* (2nd ed.). Englewood Cliffs, NJ: Prentice-Hall.

Merzenich, H., Zeeb, H., & Blettner, M. (2010). Decreasing sperm quality: A global problem? *BMC Public Health, 10,* 24.

Merki-Field, G. S., Gosewinkel, A., Imthurn, B., & Leeners, B. (2007). Tubal pathology: The role of hormonal contraception, intrauterine device use and chlamydia trachomatis infection. *Gynecologic and Obstetric Investigation, 63*(2), 114–120.

Morris, S. N., Missmer, S. A., Cramer, D. W., Powers, R. D., McShane, P. M., & Hornstein, M. D. (2007). Effects of lifetime exercise on the outcome of in vitro fertilization. *Obstet Gynecol Ocet, 108*(4), 938–945.

Nestler, J. E., Jakubowicz, D. J., Reamer, P., et al. (1999). Ovulatory and metabolic effects of D-chiro-inositol in the polycystic ovary syndrome. *New England Journal of Medicine, 340*(17), 1314–1320.

Ozgur, K., Isikoglu, M., Seleker, M., & Donmez, L. (2005). Semen quality of smoking and non-smoking men in infertile couples in a Turkish population. *Archives of Gynecology and Obstetrics, 271*(2), 109–112.

Pandian, Z., Bhattacharya, S., & Templeton, A. (2001). Review of unexplained infertility and obstetric outcome: A 10 year review. *Human Reproduction, 16*(12), 2593–2597.

Phillips, K. P., & Tanphaichitr, N. (2008). Human exposure to endocrine disrupters and semen quality. *Journal of Toxicological and Environmental Health, Part B: Critical Reviews, 11*(3–4), 188–220.

Practice Committee of the American Society for Reproductive Medicine; Practice Committee of the Society for Assisted Reproduction Technology (2009). Guidelines for the number of embryos transferred. *Fertility and Sterility, 92*(5), 1518–1519.

Pritts, E. A., Parker, W. H., & Olive, D. L. (2009). Fibroids and infertility: An updated and systematic review of the evidence. *Fertility and Sterility, 91*(4), 1215–1223.

Ramlau-Hansen, C. H., Thulstup, A. M., Storgaard, L., Toft, G., Olsen, J., & Bonde, J. P. (2007). Is prenatal exposure to tobacco smoking a cause of poor semen quality? A follow-up study. *American Journal of Epidemiology, 165*(12), 1372–1379.

Richthoff, J., Elzanaty, S., Rylander, L., Hagmar, L., & Giwercman, A. (2008). Association between tobacco exposure and reproductive parameters in adolescent males. *International Journal of Andrology, 31*(1), 31–39.

Schwartz, D., & Mayaux, M. (1982). Female fecundity as a function of age: Results of artificial insemination in 2193 nulliparous women with azoospermic husbands. Federation CECOS. *New England Journal of Medicine, 306*(7), 404–406.

Skakkebaek, N. E., Jorgenson, N., Main, K. M., Rajpert-Demeyts, E., Leffers, H., Anderron, A., Juul, A., Carlsen, E., Mortensen, G. K., Jensen, T.,K., & Toppari, J. (2006). Is human fecundity declining? *International Journal of Andrology, 29*(1), 2–11.

Speroff, L., Glass, R. H., & Kase, N. G. (1989). *Clinical gynecologic endocrinology and infertility* (4th ed.). Baltimore, MD: Williams & Wilkins.

Sullivan, E., Wang, Y., Chapman, M., & Chambers, G. (2008). Success rates and cost of a live birth following fresh assisted reproduction treatment in women aged 45 years and older, Australia 2002-2004. *Human Reproduction, 23*(7), 1639–1643.

Swan, S. H. (2006). Semen quality in fertile US men in relation to geographical area and pesticide exposure. *International Journal of Andrology, 29*(1), 62–68.

Tian, Y., Xiong, J., Hu, L., Huang, D., & Xiong, C. (2007). Candida albican and filtrates interfere with human spermatozoal motility and alter the ultrastructure of spermatozoa: An in vitro study. *International Journal of Andrology, 30*(5), 421–429.

Trounson, A. (1985). Clinical progress and new research developments in embryo and egg cryopreservation. Abstract presented at the Fourth World Congress on In Vitro Fertilization, Melbourne, Australia.

Tulandi, T., Plouffe, L., & McInnes, R. (1982). Effect of saliva on sperm motility and activity. *Fertility and Sterility, 38*(6), 581–589.

Tyler, C. R., Filby, A. L., Bickley, L. K., Cumming, R. I., Gibson, R., Labadie, P., Katsu, Y., Liney, K. E., Shears, J. A., Silva-Castro, V., Urushitani, H., Lange, A,. Winter, M. J., Iguchi, T., & Hill, E. M. (2009). Environmental health impacts of equine estrogens derived from hormone replacement therapy. *Environmental Science & Technology, 43*(10), 3897–3904. doi:10.1021/es803135q.

UNICEF. (2003). UNICEF statement on inter-country adoption. Retrieved from http://www.unicef.org/media/media_41118.html.

United Nations Department of Economic and Social Affairs, Population Division. (2007). World population prospects: The 2006 revision: Highlights. Working paper No. ESA/P/WP.202. Retrieved from http://www.un.org/esa/population/publications/wpp2006/wpp2006.htm.

U. S. Department of State, Office of Children's Issues. (2009). Inter-country adoptions. Retrieved June 1, 2009 from http://adoption.state.gov/.

van Noord-Zaadstra, B. M., Looman, C. W. N., Alsbach, H., et al. (1991). Delaying childbearing: Effect of age on fecundity and outcome of pregnancy. *British Medical Journal, 302,* 1361–1365.

Ventura, S. J., Martin, J. A., Curtin, S. C., Mathews, T. J., & Park, M. M. (2000). Births: Final data for 1998. *National Vital Statistics Report, 48*(3), 1–100.

Wang, Y., Liang, C. L., Wu, J. Q., Qin, S. X., & Gao, E. S. (2006). Do ureaplasma unrealyticum infections in the genital tract affect semen quality? *Asian Journal of Andrology, 8*(5), 562–568.

Wang, Y. A., Healy, D., Black, D., & Sullivan, E. A. (2008). Age-specific success rate for women undertaking their first assisted reproductive technology treatment using their own oocytes in Australia, 2002-2005. *Human Reproduction, 23*(7), 1633–1638.

Welshons, W. V., Nagel, S. C., & vom Saal, F. S. (2006). Large effects from small exposures. III. Endocrine mechanisms mediating effects of bisphenol A levels of human exposure. *Endocrinology, 147*(6 Suppl), S56–69.

Witkin, S. S., & Toth, A. (1983). Relationship between genital tract infections, sperm antibodies in seminal fluid, and infertility. *Fertility and Sterility, 40*(6), 805–808.

Woodruff, T. J., Carlson, A., Schwartz, J. M., & Giudice, L. C. (2008). Proceedings of the Summit on Environmental Challenges to Reproductive Health and Fertility: Executive summary. *Fertility and Sterility, 89*(2), 281–300.

Yanagimachi, R., Yanagimachi, H., & Roberts, F. J. (1976). The use of zona-free animal ova as a test system for the assessment of the fertilizing capacity of the human spermatozoa. *Biology of Reproduction, 15,* 471–476.

MENOPAUSE

Upon completion of this chapter, the reader will be able to:

- Describe the causes of menopause
- Describe the physiological changes associated with perimenopause and menopause
- Explain how and why fertility declines with menopause
- Describe the changes in sex hormone production that take place in a woman's body as she experiences menopause
- Describe the health concerns that become more prevalent in postmenopausal women, including osteoporosis, cardiovascular diseases, breast cancer and dementia
- Delineate the history and effects of hormone therapies for menopause

KEY TERMS

bone mass density (BMD)

estrogen replacement therapy (ERT)

hormone replacement therapy (HRT)

menopause

perimenopause
osteoporosis

selective estrogen receptor modulators (SERMs)

INTRODUCTION

Menopause, or climacteric, is the final phase of a woman's reproductive ability. Medically speaking, the term menopause refers to the cessation of the menses, and a woman is considered to be postmenopausal 12 months after her last menstrual period. It is common, however, for the months and years surrounding the last period to be referred to as menopause. In light of these two definitions, menopause is both an event and a process. To complicate matters further, the time leading up to menopause is also referred to as **perimenopause.** Perimenopause generally begins in the 40s and is believed to be influenced by factors similar to those that affect menarche: race, heredity, climate, nutrition, general health, and socioeconomic status. Reproductive hormone levels begin to fluctuate during perimenopause, and women may notice irregularities in their menstrual cycles during this time. Fluctuations in hormone levels may lead to physiological changes such as hot flashes, night sweats, vaginal dryness, changes in libido, forgetfulness, and trouble sleeping, although not all women experience these changes.

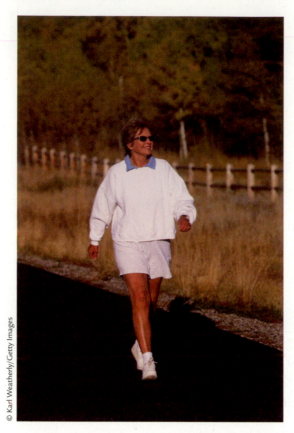

© Karl Weatherly/Getty Images

FIGURE 15-1: The age a woman can experience menopause varies, but in the United States, the average age of menopause is 51.

One-half of all women experience menopause between the ages of 45 and 50, one-fourth before age 45, and one-fourth after age 50 (Figure 15-1). In the United States, the average age of menopause is 51. About eight percent of women experience premature menopause before age 40. Factors contributing to early menopause include cigarette smoking (Willett et al., 1983), not having had children (Kato et al., 1999), and medically treated depression (Harlow et al., 1995). Menopause is said to be delayed when it occurs after age 55.

DECLINE IN FERTILITY AND THE CESSATION OF MENSTRUATION

Menopause is usually a gradual process, with menstrual irregularity making it very difficult to tell precisely when ovulation and menstruation have stopped. As menopause approaches, an increasing number of the menstrual cycles are anovulatory, producing no egg. Between the ages of 40 and 45,

an estimated 75 percent of the cycles are ovulatory. After age 46, the percentage drops to 60 percent. Pregnancy after menopause is extremely rare. It is assumed that such a conception must have resulted from the random ovulation of a surviving follicle and was not associated with a menstrual cycle. For women who want to avoid pregnancy and who are in perimenopause, determining when contraception is no longer needed can be complicated. For woman over 45, the longer the period of amenorrhea, the more likely it is that menopause has occurred. Between age 45 and 49, a six month interval without menstruation means a 45 percent probability of menopause, but in a woman 53 or older, the probability is 70 percent. After an amenorrhea of six months, 55 percent of women in their late 40s, and 30 percent of women in their early 50s still could expect to have one or more additional episodes of menstruation. Even after one year of no menstrual periods, 10.5 percent of women ages 45–49, 6.4 percent of women ages 50–52, and 4.5 percent of women 53 or older could have another menstrual cycle, possibly accompanied by ovulation. The probability of menopause is greater when amenorrhea has been preceded by prior irregularity, but if avoidance of pregnancy is important to a woman, it would be prudent to use contraceptives for a full year after the last menstrual period (Wallace et al., 1979). Blood tests are currently being developed to help women predict when menopause will occur for them.

Humans are one of the few animal species to regularly outlive their reproductive capacities, a trait that humans share with elephants, pilot whales, as well as some monkeys and the great apes. In addition, human females usually have a longer post-reproductive period than human males do. Several explanations have been proposed for this phenomenon. One explanation addresses the significant energetic costs of reproduction for females. This theory proposes that as they age, the effort that women expend helping their children and their grandchildren to survive and reproduce benefits their evolutionary fitness more than continuing to have their own additional children would (Figure 15-2) (Hrdy, 1999). Another explanation points out that on average, human life

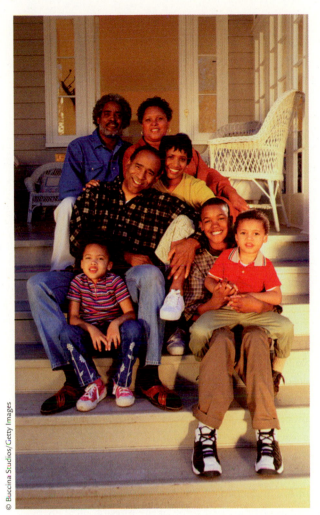

© Buccina Studios/Getty Images

FIGURE 15-2: One possible reason human females have a longer post-reproductive period than human males is that the energy they expend helping their children and grandchildren survive provides greater benefit to their evolutionary fitness than continuing to have additional children.

spans are now longer than they have typically been throughout any point in human evolution, so it is a relatively recent development that women regularly outlive their reproductive years.

CHANGES IN HORMONE LEVELS THAT ACCOMPANY MENOPAUSE

Menopause can occur either as a natural process as a woman ages or it can be induced suddenly as a result of medical procedures at any age after puberty. Women are born with an average of one to two million ovarian follicles. Through childhood, adolescence, and maturity, follicles are lost by ovulation and atresia. As the number of follicles decline the

ovaries produce less estrogen. Eventually, there is not sufficient estrogen to inhibit the pituitary gonadotropins, such as follicle-stimulating hormone (FSH) and luteinizing hormone (LH), whose levels begin to increase. In the first years after menopause, the FSH levels in the blood and urine rise 10–20 times above what they were during the reproductive years. LH levels also significantly increase, and measuring these hormones in the blood can provide information about a woman's menopausal status. Secretion of the other pituitary hormones (prolactin, growth hormone, adrenocorticotropic hormone, thyroid-stimulating hormone) appears to be unaffected by menopause. When the level of estrogen secreted by the ovaries falls below a critical level, the hormonal feedback system that facilitates menstruation is altered. Eventually the reduced level of estrogen secretion is not enough to cause cells of the endometrium to proliferate, and the menstrual cycles stop. Menopause is a normal physiological consequence of the aging of the ovary.

Estrogen takes several forms in the body. Between puberty and menopause, the majority of estrogen is secreted by the ovaries in a form called estradiol. Other steroid hormones, including some androgens that are secreted by the adrenal glands can be converted into estrogen, usually in a form called estrone. This conversion takes place in the blood and in the adipose tissues. Estrone is the most common form of estrogen in postmenopausal women. As menopause proceeds, the ovaries diminish their production of estradiol. The adrenal secretion of steroid hormones and the conversion to estrone begins to take over as the main source of estrogen. Postmenopausal estrogen levels depend primarily on this non-ovarian production of estrone. Because much of this production takes place in adipose tissues, women with more adipose tissues tend to have higher estrogen levels after menopause than do women with less. Estradiol is more biologically active than estrone. The shift from estradiol to the less potent estrone and the general reduction in both estrogen and progesterone during the premenopausal and the postmenopausal years can result in a variety of physical changes, some of which can be uncomfortable. The extent and rate of postmenopausal estrogen production varies from woman to woman. In some postmenopausal women, estrogen is maintained at a moderate level for the rest of their lives.

In addition to estrogen, other hormone levels change during menopause. As menopause approaches and women experience more anovulatory cycles, their progesterone levels also decline. Without ovulation of an egg, no corpus luteum forms, and no progesterone is secreted from the ovary. This lack of progesterone alters the secretory phase of the uterine cycle and can begin to change the pattern of the menstrual cycle. At first anovulatory cycles are likely to be shorter, and 21-day cycles are not unusual. As ovarian function decreases further, cycles may eventually become longer. This occurs because without progesterone, the endometrium is only stimulated by estrogen, and proliferation of the endometrium takes longer. In the years preceding and after menopause, the adrenal glands continue to make and secrete some progesterone. However, there is evidence that chronic stress can decrease their ability to do so. The combination of depleted estrogen and progesterone, as well as changes in the ratio of estrogen to progesterone in the body is thought to contribute to some of the physical changes that many women experience during menopause. In addition to menstrual cycle length irregularities, many women experience alterations in the menses itself. In some cases, there is a shift toward shorter menses with a light flow. Heavy bleeding and longer flow may also occur. Heavy bleeding in postmenopausal women can be a symptom of uterine cancer, or other problems. If bleeding takes place after 12 months of amenorrhea, it is important to consult with a medical professional.

Medical menopause occurs when the function of the ovaries is disrupted due to disease or a medical procedure. Surgical removal of the ovaries will cause medical menopause, as will cancer treatments such as chemotherapy which can impair ovarian function. In the case of ooectomy, or removal of the ovaries, menopause will be sudden and permanent. In the case of chemotherapy, menopause may be either permanent or temporary. Medical menopause is usually accompanied by the same set of physical changes as natural menopause, but these changes can be more intense. Their onset can be abrupt following the medical procedure that induced the menopause. Hormone replacement therapy is often proscribed to women who undergo medical menopause.

TREATING MENOPAUSE AS AN ENDOCRINE DISORDER: A HISTORY OF HORMONE REPLACEMENT THERAPY

In many societies, especially those that value youth over age and wisdom, menopause has been depicted as a change to be dreaded and even as a medical disorder. From about the 1950s to the early part of the twenty-first century, there was a trend in many industrialized nations to treat menopause as a hormone deficiency disease rather than as a natural process. In fact, some researchers referred to menopause as an edocrine disorder, similar to diabetes or hypothyroidism, with hormone replacement as the most logical treatment (Edgren, 1988). However, menopause is not a disease but a normal event, like menarche and menstruation. Beginning in the 1960s, women were prescribed various forms of hormone treatment to preserve their youth and femininity and to prevent the changes that accompany menopause. In the early 1960s, pharmaceutical companies and some physicians started to promote the administration of estrogen at menopause as a way for women to remain healthy, young, and sexy. These medications were called **estrogen replacement therapy (ERT)** and are sometimes now referred to as unopposed estrogen treatments. Estrogen replacement therapy diminished some of the physiological changes that can accompany menopause, so it is not surprising that the sales of the drug quadrupled in 10 years as millions of women were encouraged routinely to take it. By the mid-1970s, there were some urban areas of the country where more than half of the menopausal women were receiving ERT (Stadel & Weiss, 1975). The majority of annual prescriptions written for postmenopausal women were for conjugated equine estrogens, which are obtained from the urine of pregnant horses and are also called natural estrogens. When synthetic progesterone is added to ERT the medication is then called hormone replacement therapy (HRT).

Medical Risks Associated with Estrogen Replacement Therapy (ERT) and Hormone Replacement Therapy (HRT)

Early in 1975, scientific studies began to appear that suggested ERT increased a woman's risk of developing uterine cancer. These studies found that the risk of getting endometrial cancer was increased by 5–14 times by taking ERT, and that the risk was increased after only a year of cyclic ERT. The likelihood of developing endometrial cancer was increased with the duration of use and dosage of the medication. While cessation of ERT diminished the risk of developing endometrial cancer, reports showed that the risk remained elevated for as long as 10–14 years after discontinuing therapy (Shapiro et al., 1985; Paganini-Hill et al., 1989). Research has also found a link between ERT and an increased risk for breast cancer, primarily among women currently or recently on long-term ERT (Collaborative Group on Hormonal Factors in Breast Cancer, 1997; Jacobs, 2000).

By the late 1980s, a synthetic form of progesterone called progestin began to be combined with estrogen to form a new medication called **hormone replacement therapy (HRT)**. The progestin was added to decrease the risk of endometrial cancer. Hormone replacement therapy carried with it both benefits and risks. While the addition of progestin did counter the additional risk of uterine cancer, it still leads to abnormal cells in the endometrium (Lobo, 1999). HRT also contributes to high blood pressure and can also contribute to breast tenderness, bloating, and PMS-like side effects.

Throughout the 1990s, the greatest concern associated with HRT became the enhanced risk of developing breast cancer. Because the addition of progestin in HRT reduced the risk of endometrial cancers associated with ERT (or unopposed estrogen), it was hoped that the same benefit might also be true for breast cancer. However, scientific studies began to accumulate indicating that the addition of progestin not only failed to reduce risk, but instead increased the risk of developing breast cancer (Colditz et al., 1998; Schairer et al., 2000). Research supports a greater link for long-term (more than 10 years) than short-term (less than 5 years) estrogen use. A major study published in the Journal of the American Medical Association in early 2000 made headline news across the country by affirming, through analysis of data from 46,000 women who participated in the Breast Cancer Detection Demonstration Project that combined estrogen-progestin therapies were associated with greater risk

for breast cancer than estrogen alone, that such risk is particularly relevant for lean women, and that increased risk is directly related to duration of use, and the risk is largely limited to current or recent users. The researchers concluded that risk increases eight percent for each year of HRT use and one percent per year for estrogen alone (Schairer et al., 2000). Stated another way, a woman on hormone replacement therapy for 10 years doubles her risk of breast cancer. In 2002, the largest controlled study, the Women's Health Initiative, found that HRT increases a woman's risk of developing breast cancer by 26 percent.

In spite of the increased breast cancer risk, HRT was also originally thought to protect menopausal women from important health risks such as osteoporosis, cardiovascular disease, stroke, and dementia. The first large, long-term scientific study of the risks and benefits of HRT, the Women's Health Initiative (WHI), began in 1991. Only five years into the study, in an almost unprecedented move, the researchers stopped the trial because the data collected to that point so strongly indicated that HRT increased the risk of invasive breast cancer (Chlebowski et al., 2009), heart attack, strokes, and blood clots, including pulmonary embolism (Heiss et al., 2008). Since that time, the recommendation has been that HRT not be prescribed to prevent heart disease or dementia, and that it be prescribed for as short a period as possible to treat complaints associated with menopause. The Women's Health Initiative has provided invaluable information to women and their doctors about the risks and benefits of hormone replacement therapy. The United States Department of Health and Human Services has summarized the recommendations of the WHI as follows:

- Menopausal therapy should be used at the lowest dose for the shortest duration to reach treatment goals, although it is not known at what dose there may be less risk of serious side effect.
- Menopausal hormone therapy products are effective for treating moderate to severe hot flashes and night sweats, moderate-to-severe vaginal dryness, and the prevention of osteoporosis with menopause, but carry serious risks. Therefore,

postmenopausal women who use or are considering using estrogen or estrogen with progestin treatments should discuss with their healthcare providers whether the benefits outweigh the risks.

- If these products are prescribed solely for vaginal symptoms, healthcare providers are advised to consider the use of topical vaginal products (gel or cream applied locally).

- If menopausal hormone therapy is used for osteoporosis, the risks for osteoporosis must outweigh the risk of other cancers, heart disease, and other complications. Healthcare providers are encouraged to consider other treatments before providing HRT for osteoporosis.

- Menopausal hormone therapy has never been approved for prevention of cognitive disorders such as Alzheimer's disease or memory loss. In fact, the WHI found that women treated with menopausal hormone therapy have a greater risk of developing dementia.

PHYSIOLOGICAL CHANGES ASSOCIATED WITH HORMONAL CHANGES

Between 15–20 percent of women have, besides the cessation of menstrual periods, no other observable indications that they are approaching menopause. For these women, the hormonal and physiological changes that occur are so gradual that they are almost imperceptible. At the other end of the spectrum, another 15–20 percent of women suffer from physical complaints and psychological disturbances that can seriously disrupt their lives. The majority of women's experiences are between these extremes (Figure 15-3).

This variability of physiological responses to menopause may be the result of genetics, or it can be influenced by environmental and personal choices about diet, exercise or lifestyle. A woman's attitudes and feelings about menopause can also have a measurable effect on her experience, as can cultural expectations (Shea, 2006; Anderson and Yoshizawa, 2007; Lu et al., 2007; Karacam and Seker, 2007; Gupta et al., 2006). Women in cultures that view menopause and aging in a positive light tend to report fewer troubling effects as they make this transition.

Hot Flashes and Hot Flushes

Changes in hormones preceding menopause sometimes results in disturbances in the temperature-regulating center, called the vasomotor center, in the brain. This causes an abrupt change in body temperature, which is experienced as a hot flash. Hot flashes are a generalized

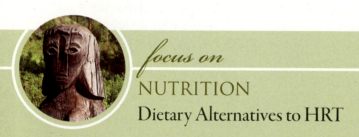

focus on

NUTRITION
Dietary Alternatives to HRT

When the Women's Health Initiative ended their study on the safety of HRT early, menopausal women were left suddenly confronted with a need to find alternative treatments for hot flashes, vaginal dryness, and loss of libido. Much hope was pinned on phytoestrogens, which are chemicals naturally found in plants that mimic the activities of estrogen in the body. These phytoestrogens are found in some herbs and in soy products. Many women began consuming these products to alleviate hot flashes and night sweats, as well as other changes that accompany menopause. Results from research into the effectiveness of phytoestrogens to relieve these symptoms have been mixed, which is not surprising since many different sources and concentrations have been tested (Lethaby, 2007; Chiechi et al., 2003; Pokaj et al., 2006; Green et al., 2007; Geller & Studee, 2005). Research has, however, found many important beneficial effects of some phytoestrogens, particularly on improving cardiovascular health, and on maintaining bone density (Borelli & Ernst, 2010). Kreijkamp-Kaspers et al. (2004) found that consuming even a small amount of dietary lignans, which are found in flaxseeds, had a protective effect on blood pressure and hypertension. Wong & Rabie (2008) have found that quercetin, a compound found in onions and apples, was able to stimulate bone formation grafts in rabbits and may stimulate osteoblasts in humans as well.

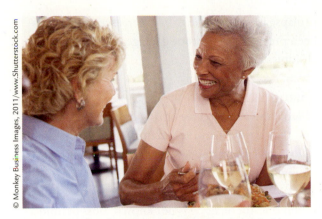

FIGURE 15-3: The physiological changes experienced with menopause vary widely for individual women.

phenomenon, however in most cases, the greatest rise in temperature occurs over the fingers and toes, and perspiration is most apparent on the upper body. The skin of the face and neck may redden and flush, but in some women only the hands and fingers are flushed. Hot flashes may occur during sleep and can provoke a night sweat. If severe, night sweats can interrupt sleep and cause insomnia which can contribute to the fatigue and mood swings that sometimes accompany menopause. Any factor that affects the temperature-regulating mechanism, such as being in a warm room, exercise, eating, or emotional stress can trigger hot flashes. Other factors such as caffeine, alcohol, and cigarette smoke may also trigger hot flashes. They may occur only once or twice a day, or many times a day; they may last for a few weeks or continue for years. Eventually, hot flashes will subside, but they can be a distressing and lifestyle disrupting experience for some women.

An estimated 75 percent of the women who enter menopause experience hot flashes. However, only a small minority experience vasomotor symptoms severe enough to require medical help. Since the hot flashes are mediated through the autonomic nervous system, drugs that work on the autonomic nervous system are sometimes prescribed. Phytoestrogens, which are estrogen-like molecules found in plants, may be a good option for countering hot flashes for some women (Green et al., 2007; Pockaj et al., 2006), and there are indications that traditional Chinese medicines may also be effective (Kwee et al., 2007). A short-term prescription of hormone replacement therapy is also effective, but carries significant increased risks of reproductive cancers and heart disease. Generally, while HRT is an effective treatment for hot flashes, short-term management of hot flashes may not be worth the risks associated with HRT.

Vaginal Dryness and Changes in Vaginal Tone

Another physical change that can accompany menopause that is experienced by some women is

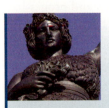

Historical Considerations
CRONE AS WISE WOMAN

Margaret Mead once said that "there is no greater power in the world than the zest of a postmenopausal woman." Yet, today's youth-obsessed culture is not one which is particularly supportive of women aging gracefully. Too often, societies do not revere older and elderly women. Many cultures, however, have embraced the 'crone as wise woman.' While 'crone' has taken on something of a pejorative connotation in some cultures (Merriam-Webster's Dictionary defines crone as "a withered old woman"), its roots have been said to be in the tradition of the Triple Goddess, depicting the three stages of a woman's development from birth to maiden to wise elder. For every woman, aging is a natural part of life to be embraced.

While women are exhorted not to grow old gracefully, but rather to fight it "every step of the way" (as some ad campaigns have suggested), turning the term 'crone' on its head can be an exercise in empowerment, self-definition, and joy.

the gradual decrease in the thickness of the skin layers lining the vagina. This thinning usually begins to appear 10–20 years after menopause, suggesting that it is more of a result of simple aging than it is of menopause itself. Thinning can be accompanied with a reduction of vaginal secretions that can result in vaginal dryness. In some cases, vaginal dryness can lead to dyspareunia, or pain during intercourse. In addition, as the epithelial cells begin to decrease their secretion of the carbohydrate glycogen, the beneficial bacteria that inhabit the vagina may begin to decline. These normal flora influence the pH of the vagina, and without them, the vaginal secretions become less acidic. This change in pH can leave the vagina more vulnerable to vaginitis and sexually transmitted infections.

Regular sexual activity is also effective for maintaining the health and tone of the vagina during the premenopausal and postmenopausal years. In a study of 52 postmenopausal women, they confirmed the earlier report of Masters and Johnson concerning the beneficial effect of sexual activity on vaginal atrophy. Women who had intercourse three or more times monthly or who masturbated experienced less vaginal atrophy than the women who engaged in less frequent sexual activity or did not masturbate (Leiblum et al., 1983). In addition Chiechi et al. (2003) found that a phytochemical-rich diet can increase the production of new cells in the vaginal lining and may be useful for preventing vaginal thinning. Local treatment with estrogen-containing suppositories or creams has been shown to be effective, and less estrogen is absorbed into the bloodstream when applied topically, than when taken in a pill form (Goldstein, 2010). When thinning is less severe, symptoms may be alleviated by the use of water-based lubricating gels.

Because the vulvar skin and underlying adipose tissues are more sensitive to decreases in estrogen (Mac Bride et al., 2010) than the skin and adipose tissues of the rest of the body, the labia majora, minora, and mons pubis shrink in size. Pubic hair may also become scant. In addition, the vagina itself can shrink in both length and width. The strength and elasticity of the muscles and ligaments of the pelvis may also be affected by the hormonal shifts accompanying menopause, so the risk of uterine prolapse increases. The risk is increased if there has been previous pelvic floor damage sustained during childbirth.

Changes in Libido

Menopause may alter a woman's libido. Some women find they are more interested in sex when pregnancy is no longer a possibility. Others experience a loss of libido during menopause (Nappi & Lachowsky, 2009). Whether this is truly a result of menopause or simply a result of aging is not known. Loss of libido is more likely caused by a decline in testosterone than estrogen. Between her 20s and her 40s, a woman's testosterone levels decrease by about 50 percent. If a woman takes HRT, her testosterone levels can decline even more dramatically. There is recent research that indicates that treatment with testosterone may help to improve libido in menopausal women, but the long-term effects are not yet understood (Panay et al., 2010; Krapf & Simon, 2009; Rymen et al., 2010).

SOME DISEASE RISKS INCREASE AFTER MENOPAUSE

At the time of menopause, the risk for serious diseases such as cardiovascular disease, osteoporosis, and Alzheimer's disease begins to increase. Part of the increased risks results from changes in hormone concentrations that accompany menopause, and part results from the cumulative effects of aging. As the protective effects of estrogen and progesterone decline, the importance of healthy lifestyle choices that reduce the risk of serious diseases increases. Fortunately, maintaining a healthy diet, smoking cessation, and getting adequate exercise can help to reduce the risks and impact of many of the serious diseases that affect postmenopausal women.

Coronary Heart Disease and Stroke

Heart disease is the number one killer of women 50–75 years of age, claiming five times as many lives as breast cancer (Vitale et al., 2007; Huston & Lanka, 1997). Cardiovascular disease can lead to heart attack and stroke. African American and Hispanic women are particularly at risk of dying from a heart attack after menopause (McSweeney et al., 2010). Higher levels of circulating estrogen and progesterone protect premenopausal women from cardiovascular disease, but after menopause a woman's risk catches up to that of men, and there is a steady increase in their rate of heart disease deaths after the age of 50. Within the first few years after menopause, the risk of cardiovascular disease is not appreciably greater, but it continues to increase with each passing year. By the age of 60, the rate of heart attacks in women equals that of men six to 10 years younger.

Although cardiovascular disease kills equal numbers of men and women worldwide, there are differences in how the disease develops and presents itself in males and females. The factors that contribute to cardiovascular disease include cholesterol levels, blood lipid profiles, and hypertension or high blood pressure. While all of these factors contribute to cardiovascular disease in both sexes, cholesterol levels appear to play a larger role in men in the development of heart disease than in women. For women, high blood pressure and diabetes play a larger role (Vitale et al., 2007). In addition, women are less likely than men to develop atherosclerosis, which results in the hardening and

narrowing of the arteries (Kuller, 2010). Symptoms of a heart attack also appear to differ somewhat between men and women, which can contribute to misdiagnosis of heart attack in women. Typical symptoms of a heart attack include: chest pain, shoulder or arm pain, shortness of breath, and unusual fatigue. Although symptoms overlap, women are less likely than men to experience chest pain and shoulder or arm pain (Lovlien et al., 2009). Women are more likely to experience unusual fatigue, sleep disturbances, and shortness of breath (McSweeney et al., 2003).

A woman's natural estrogen has a beneficial effect on cholesterol levels by promoting the production of "good" HDL cholesterol and inhibiting the production of "bad" LDL cholesterol. In addition to promoting HDL cholesterol levels, estrogen acts as an antioxidant in the blood, reducing damage by free radicals. Estrogen also promotes the dissolving of bloods clots and the dilation of blood vessels, two mechanisms that help to prevent heart attacks and strokes. Prior to the publication of the Women's Health Initiative study, it was assumed that administering synthetic estrogens in the form of HRT would

Case Study

What Do these Symptoms Mean?

Etta is 64 years old and she is enjoying her post-menopausal years. She is glad to be finished going through the transition of menopause and has found that it is a relief not to worry about the bother of hot flashes or night sweats anymore. A couple of recent changes are causing her concern, however. For the past two weeks she has felt unusually fatigued and she is not sure why, since her activity level has not changed. She has had a couple of sleepless nights, which is unusual for her, now that she is past the stage of menopause where she was experiencing occasional night sweats. She has also been noticing that she is suddenly prone to indigestion, even though her diet has not changed. While volunteering one day at a fund-raiser for her favorite non-profit organization, Etta was suddenly feeling progressively worse. By noon she was experiencing shortness of breath and she began to break out in a cold sweat. Another volunteer, who happened to also be an EMT, asked Etta about her symptoms and immediately called 911. What is happening to Etta?

1. How do heart attack symptoms present differently in women than in men?

2. Why are postmenopausal women at greater risk for heart attack than other women?

3. What can a woman do to reduce her risk of having a heart attack?

protect menopausal and postmenopausal women from heart disease and stroke. In fact, it was assumed that the protection from cardiovascular disease that HRT would provide, for many women outweighed the risks of developing breast or endometrial cancer associated with HRT. However, the WHI study was stopped early because of the overwhelming evidence that HRT increased a woman's chances of suffering a heart attack by 29 percent. HRT increases a woman's chances of suffering a stroke by 41 percent, and doubles a woman's chances of developing blood clots.

Osteoporosis

The term **osteoporosis** literally means "holes-in-the-bone." Osteoporosis is a chronic skeletal disorder and although it affects both sexes, women are more vulnerable to this condition than men. Osteoporosis is both a natural consequence of aging and a result of a variety of factors including the decline in estrogen and progesterone levels that accompany menopause. Throughout the lifetime, bones undergo constant remodeling and renewal. Specialized bone cells called osteoclasts dissolve older and more fragile bone tissues so that bone cells called osteoblasts can replace them with healthy new bone tissue. This constant remodeling allows repair and continually deposits new bone, even in the elderly. As individuals age, the activity levels of the osteoblasts begin to decline, while the pace of the osteoclasts usually does not. The shift in hormone levels that accompanies menopause can accelerate this process. As the osteoclasts begin to dissolve more bone than the osteoclasts produce, **bone mass density (BMD)** decreases and osteoporosis can result. In industrialized Western countries, more than one-third of the women older than 65 display some degree of osteoporosis. Interestingly, an analysis of the mineral density of skeletons buried in an English graveyard dating back to 1729 revealed better bone density in all ages of individuals compared with the average bone densities today. The differences were attributed to better diet and exercise level (Lees et al., 1993). Osteopenia is a term that describes a bone density that is lower than average, but that has not reached the level of osteoporosis.

About 85–90 percent of peak bone mass is acquired by women by the age of 18, after which bone density usually decreases. Women generally have a proportionately lower peak bone mass than men to start with, and their rate of bone loss throughout their lifetime is usually greater than that of men. Bone loss also accelerates temporarily

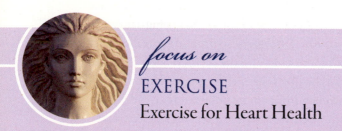

focus on

EXERCISE
Exercise for Heart Health

Scientific research is showing that it is never too late to start exercising. In a study involving 46 formerly sedentary postmenopausal women, Maesta et al. (2007) found that only 16 weeks of progressive resistance training, three times per week had a significant positive impact on the body composition of the participants verses control subjects who did not exercise. The women who engaged in resistance training gained muscle mass and lost abdominal fat. In another study involving 50 healthy, obese postmenopausal women, Aubertin-Leheudre et al. (2007) found that by combining aerobic exercise and daily isoflavone supplementation for six months, women were able to significantly improve their clinical risk factors for cardiovascular disease. Exercise, even in moderate amounts, will increase HDL levels. For example, a group of researchers at the Cooper Institute for Aerobics Research found that previously sedentary women who walked three miles a day, five days a week, for six months, regardless of the pace, had an increase of six percent in HDL levels. The women who walked at the fastest pace (a 12-minute mile) also increased their cardio respiratory fitness by 16 percent, about the same as that of women who jogged (Duncan, Gordon, & Scott, 1991). Walking or other cardiovascular exercise each day can aid the heart as well as build bone, improve mood, and help maintain a healthy weight.

with menopause. In the United States, a woman can lose up to 20 percent of her bone mass during the five to seven years after menopause. Then the bone loss percentage shifts back to a rate of one to two percent per year. Since women tend to live longer than men, they also have more opportunity to lose bone, which further contributes to their chances of developing osteoporosis. Petite women of Northern European or Asian descent are more prone to developing osteoporosis, however, women of all ethnic backgrounds are at risk. Genetics play a role, and a family history of osteoporosis can also increase one's risk. Other risk factors for osteoporosis include any condition that results in an estrogen deficiency, such as having had ovaries removed before the age of 40 or prolonged amenorrhea brought about by conditions such as anorexia or bulimia. Smoking and excessive consumption of caffeine or alcohol can contribute to osteoporosis, as can a dietary calcium or Vitamin D deficiency. Chronic alcoholism interferes with the body's ability to absorb calcium and build bone mass. Certain medications such as corticosteroids, thyroid hormone, or anticonvulsants, when taken on a long-term basis, appear to also increase the likelihood of developing osteoporosis. Finally, since weight-bearing exercise stimulates the osteoblasts to produce more bone tissue, long periods of immobilization or a general lack of exercise can also contribute to a woman's chances of developing osteoporosis (Wong & Rabie, 2008).

As osteoporosis progresses, bone density can decrease to the point where the bones can no longer support the body or sustain normal pressures. In its most serious form, osteoporosis results in a predisposition to fractures. In the United States, about half of all women will suffer from osteoporosis-related fractures at some point in their lifetimes. When fractures occur in the thinned and weakened vertebra that support most of the weight in the spinal column, the result is a progressive decrease in height and bending of the spine producing swayback or humpback (Figure 15-4). Approximately one of four women older than 60 years of age has such spinal compression fractures. Other types of fractures are more likely to lead to long-term disability and even death. Postmenopausal women are twice as likely to fracture a hip as premenopausal

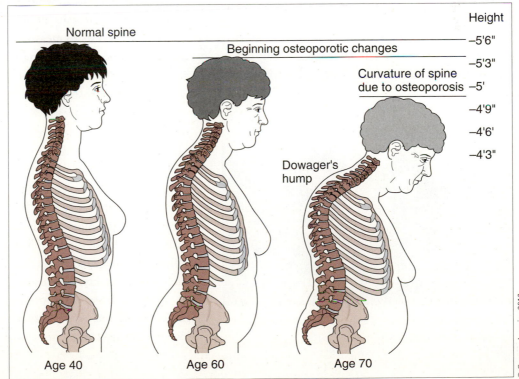

FIGURE 15-4: Osteoporosis can cause small fractures in the vertebrae which result in a loss of height and a Dowager's hump.

Normal spine

Beginning osteoporotic changes

Curvature of spine due to osteoporosis

Dowager's hump

Height
–5'6"
–5'3"
–5'
–4'9"
–4'6'
–4'3"

Age 40   Age 60   Age 70

© Cengage Learning 2013

women (Banks et al., 2009). Breaking a limb results in immobilization, which not only further aggravates osteoporosis, but may also result in lung collapse, pneumonia, and death. Women who have suffered a hip fracture have an increased risk of dying from other conditions during the months and years following their injury compared to women who have not experienced a hip fracture (Haentjens et al., 2010; Vestergaard et al., 2009; Kannegaard et al., 2010).

Osteoporosis is a painful, crippling, and potentially fatal condition that can be difficult to treat once it is established. There are, however, ways that a woman can maintain bone mass throughout her lifetime and potentially avoid or lessen the effects of osteoporosis. It is important to build bone health through weight-bearing exercise and a nutritious diet throughout childhood and adolescence. A woman who reaches a good peak bone mass in youth through good nutrition, exercise, and adequate calcium intake will be less likely to suffer from osteoporosis later in life. In fact, good nutrition, including calcium-rich foods and adequate vitamin D, as well as other vitamins, minerals, and phytochemicals play a role in bone health, so eating a balanced diet throughout the lifetime is important for preventing osteoporosis. There is evidence that a combination of factors associated with excess carbonated beverage consumption can diminish the peak bone mass achieved. Excess carbonated beverage consumption is especially of concern in young girls who are

still building bone mass and have not reached their peak bone density. Caffeine in the soda may interfere with calcium absorption. Caffeine acts as a diuretic, so an excess can have a flushing effect that can further increase mineral loss (Libuda et al., 2008; Tucker et al., 2006).

A combination of strength training and weight-bearing exercise has been found to be effective for not only preventing bone loss, but increasing bone density. Strength training, in addition to strengthening muscles, stimulates osteoblasts in the bones and results in an increase in bone density. It is especially helpful for protecting the bones of the arms and the upper spine. Weight-bearing exercises such as walking, jogging, and running help to improve the density of the bones of the legs, hips, and lower spine (Figure 15-5). Unfortunately, activities such as swimming, cycling, and elliptical trainers, while providing cardiovascular benefits, do not stress the bones enough to stimulate an increase in their density.

Screening Tests and Treating Osteoporosis

Two measurements are typically used by medical professionals to describe bone density. The T Score compares a woman's bone density to that of a young adult whose bones are at peak density. The Z score compares a woman's bone density to the average bone density of other women her own age. Screening tests to measure bone density have not been particularly informative for asymptomatic younger or middle-aged women to determine whether osteoporosis may develop in the future, but they can be used to establish a baseline level of bone mass. In addition, bone density measurement techniques can detect low bone mass in younger women with genetic risk factors and enable them to make changes in diet and exercise that can prevent further bone loss. Dual energy x-ray (DEXA) technologies are currently the most widely used method for measuring bone density in the United States, although ultrasound, magnetic resonance imagery (MRI), and single energy X-rays, can also be used.

In order to treat osteoporosis, it is important to minimize lifestyle practices that contribute to the loss of bone mass and to maximize lifestyle practices

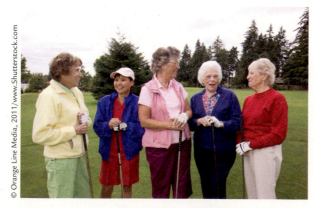

FIGURE 15-5: Weight-bearing exercises help improve bone density as women age.

that support healthy bone function. For this reason, smoking cessation and healthy nutrition, including a reduction in carbonated beverages, can be of benefit. Practices that reduce a woman's risk of falling are also important for reducing the potentially catastrophic effects of osteoporosis. There is increasing evidence that weight-bearing exercise, including walking, helps to reduce bone loss, and can even contribute to restoring bone density (Krustrup et al., 2010; Martyn-St James & Carroll, 2006, 2008, 2009; Rotstein et al., 2008; Kemmler et al., 2010). In addition to stimulating osteoblasts and increasing BMD, exercise can strengthen muscles and help women to maintain the flexibility and balance that they need to prevent debilitating falls (Hourigan et al., 2008; Kamide et al., 2009). If medications are prescribed, healthy lifestyle habits can increase the benefits observed.

At present, most medications to treat osteoporosis fall into one of two categories: those that inhibit osteoclasts and prevent bone reabsorption, and those that stimulate osteoblasts and encourage bone building. Most osteoporosis medications are relatively new, and evaluation of their long-term effects is still underway. Long-term effects are still relatively unknown. The benefits and risks of the different types of medications vary, depending on a woman's age, menopausal status, and other health risks. For this reason, care must be used in deciding whether to use medications at all, and if so, which ones are best suited to each woman's circumstances (Miller & Derman, 2010).

Previous to the findings of the Women's Health Initiative study, HRT was heavily promoted to prevent or reduce bone loss in menopausal women. Research indicates that hormone replacement therapy does reduce the risk of fractures due to osteoporosis. However, in light of the results of the Women's Health Initiative Study, the United States Food and Drug Administration recommends that HRT only be used to treat osteoporosis if the risks associated with osteoporosis outweigh the risks associated with HRT. They also recommend that other treatments be tried before HRT is prescribed. HRT works best to prevent bone loss during the first 5–10 years after menopause when bone loss is greatest.

Bisphosphonates are currently the most common type of medication given for osteoporosis. By inhibiting osteoclast activity, these medications can, at least temporarily, increase bone mineral density and reduce the risk of fractures. However, these medications have not been available long enough to gauge the long-term effects of suppressing normal bone physiology. While these drugs can reduce bone reabsorption, they cannot trigger the production of new bone, and may in fact lead to an overall reduction in bone formation. Disruption of normal bone re-modeling activity may have negative long-term effects on the bones. In fact, there have been a number of recent studies linking bisphosphonates with over-mineralization of bones, a condition that reduces their mechanical strength and makes them more brittle and prone to fracture (Goddard et al., 2009; Kwek et al., 2008). There is also concern that suppressing bone remodeling allows micro-fractures to accumulate in the bones, contributing to their increased vulnerability to breaking (Odvina et al., 2005). Bisphosphonates also have significant side effects to consider, including stomach cramps and heartburn in about one half of the women who use them.

The medications called **selective estrogen receptor modulators (SERMs)** provide alternatives to HRT and bisphosphonates for treating and preventing osteoporosis (Iwamoto, 2010). SERMS are synthetic hormones that can either mimic or block the effects of a woman's own estrogen, and offer some protection against osteoporosis. Because they compete with estrogen binding at estrogen receptor sites in breast tissue, SERMS are also often prescribed to decreases the risk for certain breast cancers. Unfortunately, some SERMS increase the risk of endometrial cancer, and at present, all SERMS increase the risk for blood clots.

Calcitonin, a hormone produced by the thyroid gland, increases calcium levels in the bones by encouraging osteoblast activity, and discouraging osteoclast activity. Thus, calcitonin can reduce the rate of bone loss and may even increase bone mass in postmenopausal osteoporotic women. Another hormone, parathyroid hormone, can have the effect of stimulating the production of new bone tissue, if carefully administered in the proper dosage. Prolonged high dosages of parathyroid hormone, however, can actually reduce bone density. This medication must be administered daily by injection or by nasal spray, and there are some indications that long-term use may increase the risk of developing bone tumors.

Osteopenia and Preventing Osteoporosis

The increased availability of bone mass scanning technologies has made it easier for premenopausal women to determine their bone mass density. If a woman's BMD is more than one standard deviation but less than 2.5 standard deviations below the average BMD of young woman at peak bone density, she will be diagnosed with osteopenia. Osteopenia is not a disease, rather it is a classification of a BMD that is less than average, but not indicative of osteoporosis. It should be noted that by the standard definition, 16 percent of young women have osteopenia. This information can be useful for women who may want to modify lifestyle habits that may be contributing to lower BMD. Some have suggested that women who are diagnosed with osteopenia should be prescribed osteoporosis medications, including bisphosphonates, to prevent future osteoporosis. There are three potential drawbacks to this approach. First, there is not clear evidence that the BMD cut off levels that define osteopenia are associated with a greater risk of developing osteoporosis later in life. Second, there is currently no evidence that osteoporosis medications, with the exception of HRT, which carries its own health risks, prevent the development of osteoporosis over the number of years that preventative treatments would be necessary. Finally, many osteoporosis medications have been available for 15 years or less, and the long-term effects of their use are not yet understood. Some of the potential risks may be substantial, and at present preventative medication for osteopenia is not recommended for women with osteopenia and no other risk factors for osteoporosis (Bhalla, 2010).

Dementia and Alzheimer's Disease

Since both men and women can develop dementia and Alzheimer's disease, it is clear that the natural effects of aging play a role in these conditions. However, women are more likely than men to develop Alzheimer's disease and dementia, and this has lead

researchers to wonder if the hormonal shifts that accompany menopause may contribute to these conditions. A woman's natural estrogen and progesterone hormones affect mood and cognition, including memory, but the mechanism of how these sex hormones interact with the nervous system to produce these effects is not yet fully understood (van Wingen et al., 2008; Andreen et al., 2009; Shechter et al., 2010; Mass et al., 2009; Bitzer, 2009). Decreases in estrogen and progesterone during menopause may account for some of the mood alterations and memory problems that can take place during this time, as the body adjusts to its new hormone regime. When considering the effects of reproductive hormones on mood, cognition, and memory, it is important to distinguish between a woman's own estrogen and progesterone and synthetic hormones that are administered as hormone replacement therapy, as the effects are often very different. For example, at one time it was believed that hormone replacement therapy at the time of menopause would help to protect women from developing dementia in old age. However, an ancillary study to the Women's Health Initiative called the Memory Study, found that estrogen plus synthetic progestin did not improve cognition, and in fact doubled a woman's risk of developing dementia (Coker et al., 2010).

CONCLUSION

Menopause is a natural stage of a woman's life that results in decreased levels of estrogen and progesterone that produce physiological changes. While the most obvious change is the end of menstruation, the loss of the protective effects of estrogen and progesterone can have an impact on a woman's susceptibility to many serious conditions, such as cardiovascular disease, osteoporosis, Alzheimer's disease, and dementia. While in the past it was believed that these risks could be averted with the administration of synthetic and derived hormones in the form of HRT medications, in most cases the risks of using these medications outweigh the potential benefits. Instead, adopting healthy lifestyle habits such as getting adequate exercise and maintaining a healthy diet can help to ameliorate some of the potential discomforts and increased health risks of the postmenopausal years.

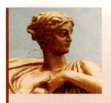

Cultural Considerations
WHAT CAN THE WORLD'S CENTURIONS TEACH US?

Menopause marks a time in a woman's life when a variety of health issues become more of a concern. The risks of heart disease, osteoporosis, and many types of cancer become more pronounced in the menopausal years. For some extraordinarily long-lived populations around the world however, the years between menopause and death are a time of vitality and activity. For example, the people of Okanowa, an island located off the southern tip of Japan, regularly live healthy, active lives into their 90s and even 100s. Older Okanowan women suffer much less from osteoporosis and have only half the hip fractures of women in the United States. They also have 80 percent less heart disease, and breast cancer is rare. Remarkably, when the estrogen levels of 100 year old Okanowans were tested, they had estrogen levels similar to an average 70 year old in the United States (Robbins, 2006). What contributes to their extraordinary health? Studies of the lifestyles of the Okanowan Centurions have found the following patterns:

- They consume fewer calories (by Western Standards) each day, but they are not undernourished.
- They consume only low glycemic index carbohydrates including whole grains, vegetables, and fruits.
- They eat a completely whole foods diet, with very little (if any) refined foods such as sugar, corn syrup, preservatives, artificial flavors, or other chemicals.
- They eat primarily fresh locally grown foods, in season rather than processed foods.
- Their diet is low in fat, but not extremely low in fat. The fats that they consume are from nuts, seeds, and fish rather than from bottled oils, margarine, or saturated animal fats.
- They derive their proteins primarily from plant sources such as beans, peas, whole grains, nuts, and seeds.

REVIEW QUESTIONS

1. Describe the physiological events that trigger menopause.

2. What is perimenopause?

3. Describe the physiological changes that can accompany menopause. Do all women experience these physiological changes?

4. Why was the Women's Health Initiative study on HRT stopped early?

5. Contrast ERT verses HRT in terms of what kinds of hormones they contain, their uses, and the risks of their use.

6. What is osteoporosis? What are the long-term effects of this disease?

7. Why does heart disease become more prevalent in postmenopausal women?

CRITICAL THINKING QUESTIONS

1. Are there circumstances under which a woman should use HRT? If so what are they?

2. What are the potential advantages and disadvantages to treating osteopenia with osteoporosis medications?

WEBLINKS

The North American Menopause Society
www.menopause.org

Mayo Clinic
www.mayoclinic.com (search for menopause)

REFERENCES

Anderson, D. J., & Yoshizawa, T. (2007). Cross-cultural comparisons of health-related quality of life in Australian and Japanese midlife women: The Australian and Japanese Midlife Women's Health Study. *Menopause, 14*(4), 697–707.

Andreen, L., Nyberg, S., Turkmen, S., van Wingen, G., Fernandez, G., & Backstrom, T. (2009). Sex steroid induced negative mood may be explained by the paradoxical effect mediated by GABAA modulators. *Psychoneuroendocrinology, 34*(8), 1121–1132.

Aubertin-Leheudre, M., Lord, C., Khalil, A., & Dionne, I. J. (2007). Effects of 6 months of exercise and isoflavone supplementation on clinical cardiovascular risk factors in obese postmenopausal women: A randomized, double-blind study. *Menopause, 14*(4), 624–629.

Banks, E., Reeves, G. K., Beral, V., Balkwill, A., Liu, B., & Roddam, A., for the Million Women Study Collaborators. (2009). Hip fracture incidence in relation to age, menopausal status, and age at menopause: Prospective analysis. *PLoS Medicine, 6*(11), e1000181.

Barrett-Conner, E., Wingard, D. L., & Criqui, M. H. (1989). Postmenopausal estrogen use and heart disease risk factors in the 1980s. *Journal of the American Medical Association, 261*(14), 2095–2100.

Bhalla, A. K. (2010). Management of osteoporosis in pre-menopausal women. *Best Practice & Research: Clinical Rheumatology, 24*(3), 313–327.

Bitzer, J. (2009). Progesterone, progestogens and psychosomatic health of the climacteric woman. *Maturitas, 62*(4), 330–333.

Borelli, F., & Ernst, E. (2010). Alternative and complementary therapies for menopause. *Maturitas, 66*(4), 333–343.

Chiechi, L. M., Putignano, G., Guerra, V., Schiavelli, M. P., Cisternino, A. M., & Carriero, C. (2003). The effect of a soy rich diet on the vaginal epithelium in postmenopause: A randomized double blind trial. *Maturitas, 45*(4), 241–246.

Chlebowski, R. T., Kuller, L. H., Prentice, R. L., Stefanick, M. L., Manson, J. E., Grass, M., Aragaki, A. K., Ockene, J. K., Lane, D. S., Sarto G. E., Rajkovic, A., Schenken, R., Hendrix, S. L., Ravdin, P. M., Rohan, T. E., Yasmeen, S., Andersen, G., & WHI Investigators. (2009). Breast cancer after use of estrogen plus progestin in postmenopausal women. *New England Journal of Medicine, 360*(6), 573–587.

Coker, L. H., Espeland, M. A., Rapp, S. R., Legault, C., Resnick, S. M., Hogan, P., Gaussoin, S., Dailey, M., & Shumaker, S. A. (2010). Postmenopausal hormone therapy and cognitive outcomes: The Woman's Health Initiative Memory Study (WHIMS). *Journal of Steroid Biochemistry and Molecular Biology, 118*(4–5), 304–310.

Colditz, G. A., & Rosner, B., for the Nurses' Health Study Research Group. (1998). Use of estrogen plus progestin is associated with greater increase in breast cancer risk than estrogen alone. *American Journal of Epidemiology, 147*(Suppl.), 645.

Collaborative Group on Hormonal Factors in Breast Cancer. (1997). Breast cancer and hormone replacement therapy: Collaborative reanalysis of data from 51 epidemiologic studies of 52,705 women with breast cancer and 108,411 women without breast cancer. *Lancet, 350*(9084), 1047–1059.

Duncan, J. J., Gordon, N. F., & Scott, C. B. (1991). Women walking for health and fitness. *Journal of the American Medical Association, 266*(3), 3295–3299.

Edgren, R. A. (1988). Pharmacology of hormonal therapeutic agents. In B. A. Eskin (Ed.), *The menopause: Comprehensive management* (2nd ed.). New York, NY: Macmillan.

Frodin, T., Alund, G., & Varenhurst, E. (1985). Measurement of skin blood-flow to assess hot flushes after orchiectomy. *Prostate, 7,* 203–209.

Geller, S. E., & Studee, L. (2005). Botanical and dietary supplements for menopausal symptoms: What works, what does not. *Journal of Women's Health (Larchmont), 14*(7), 634–649.

Goddard, M. S., Reid, K. R., Johnston, J. C., & Khanuja, H. S. (2009). Atraumatic bilateral femur fracture in long-term bisphosphonate use. *Orthopedics, 32*(8), 607. doi:10.3928/01477447–20090624–27

Goldstein, I. (2010). Recognizing and treating urogenital atrophy in postmenopausal women. *Journal of Women's Health (Larchmont), 19*(3), 425–432.

Green, J., Denham, A., Ingram, J., Hawkey, S., & Greenwood, R. (2007). Treatment of menopausal symptoms by qualified herbal practitioners: A prospective, randomized controlled trial. *Family Practice, 24*(5), 468–474.

Gupta, P., Sturdee, D.W., & Hunter, M. S. (2006). Mid-age health in women from the Indian subcontinent (MAHWIS): General health and the experience of menopause in women. *Climacteric, 9*(1), 13–22.

Haentjens, P., Magaziner, J., Colon-Emeric, C. S., Vanderschueren, D., Milisen, K., Velkeniers, B., & Boonen, S. (2010). Meta-analysis: Excess mortality after hip fracture among Older women and men. *Annals of Internal Medicine, 152*(6), 380–390.

Harlow, B. L., Cramer, D. W., & Annis, K. M. (1995). Association of medically treated depression and age at natural menopause. *American Journal of Epidemiology, 141*(12), 1170–1176.

Heiss, G., Wallace, R., Anderson, G. L., Aragaki, G. L., Beresford, S. A., Brzyski, R., Chlebowski, R. T., Gass, M., LaCroix, A., Manson, J. E., Prentice, R. L., Rossouw, J., Stefanick, M. L., & WHI Investigators. (2008). Health risks and benefits 3 years after stopping randomized treatment with estrogen and progestin. *Journal of the American Medical Association, 299*(9), 1036–1045.

Hourigan, S. R., Nitz, J. C., Brauer, S. G., O'Neill, S., Wong, J., & Richardson, C. A. (2008). Positive effects of exercise on falls and fracture risk in osteopenia women. *Osteoporosis International, 19*(7), 1077–1086.

Hrdy, S. (2000). *Mother Nature: Maternal instincts and how they shape the human species.* New York, NY: Ballantine Publishing Group.

Huston, J., & Lanka, L. (1997). *Perimenopause: Changes in women's health after 35.* Oakland, CA: New Harbinger.

Hutchinson, T. A., Polansky, S. M., & Feinstein, A. R. (1979). Postmenopausal oestrogens protect against fractures of hip and distal radius. *Lancet, 2,* 705–709.

Iwamoto, J. (2010). Effects of SERMs on bone health. Discrimination of SERMs from bisphosphonates in the treatment of postmenopausal osteoporosis. *Clinical Calcium, 20*(3), 396–407.

Jacobs, H. S. (2000). Postmenopausal hormone replacement therapy and breast cancer. *Medscape Women's Health, 5*(4). Retrieved January 15, 2011 from http://www.medscape.com/viewarticle/408925.

Kamide, N., Shiba, Y., Shiba, Y., & Shibata, H. (2009). Effects of balance, falls, and bone mineral density of a home-based exercise program without home visits in community-dwelling elderly women: a randomized controlled trial. *Journal of Physiological Anthropology, 28*(3), 115–122.

Kannegaard, P. N., van der Mark, S., Eiken, P., & Abrahamsen, B. (2010). Excess mortality in men compared to women following a hip fracture. National analysis of co-medications, comorbidity, and survival. *Age and Aging, 39*(2), 203–209.

Karacam, Z., & Seker, S. E. (2007). Factors associated with menopausal symptoms and their relationship with the quality of life among Turkish women. *Maturitas, 58*(1), 75–82.

Kato, I., Toniolo, P., Akmedkhanov, A., et al. (1999). Prospective study of factors influencing the onset of natural menopause. *Neurology, 53,* 308–314.

Kemmler, W., von Stengel, S., Engelke, K., Haberle, L., & Kalender, W. A. (2010). Exercise effects on bone mineral density, falls, coronary risk factors, and healthcare costs in older women: The randomized controlled senior fitness and prevention (SEFIP) study. *Archives of Internal Medicine, 170*(2), 17–185.

Krapf, J. M., & Simon, J. A. (2009). The role of testosterone in the management of hypoactive sexual desire disorder in post menopausal women. *Maturitas, 63*(3), 213–219.

Kreijkamp-Kaspers, S., Kok, L., Bots, M. L., Grobbee, D. E., & van der Schouw, Y. T. (2004). Dietary phytoestrogens and vascular function in postmenopausal women: A cross-sectional study. *Journal of Hypertension, 22*(7), 1381–1388.

Krustrup, P., Hansen, P. R., Andersen, L. J., Jakobsen, M. D., Sunstrup, E., Randers, M. B., Christiansen, L., Helge, E. W., Pedersen, M. T., Sogaard, P., Junge, A., Dvorak, J., Aagaard, P., & Bangsbo, J. (2010). Long-term musculoskeletal and cardiac health effects of recreational football and running for premenopausal women. *Scandinavian Journal of Medicine and Science in Sports, 20*(Suppl 1), 58–71.

Kuller, L. H. (2010). Cardiovascular disease is preventable among women. *Expert Review of Cardiovascular Therapy, 8*(2), 175–187.

Kwee, S. H., Tan, H. H., Marsman, A., & Wauters, C. (2007). The effect of Chinese herbal medicines (CHM) on menopausal symptoms compared to hormone replacement therapy (HRT) and placebo. *Maturitas, 58*(1), 83–90.

Kwek, E. B., Goh, S. K., Koh, J. S., Png, M. A., & Howe T. S. (2008). An emerging pattern of subtrochanteric stress fractures: A long-term complication of alendronate therapy? *Injury, 39*(2), 224–231.

Lee, J. R., & Hopkins, V. (2004). *What your doctor may not tell you about menopause.* New York, NY: Time Warner Book Group.

Lees, B., Molleson, T., Arnett, T. R., & Stevenson, J. C. (1993). Differences in proximal femur density over two centuries. *Lancet, 341,* 673–675.

Leiblum, S., Bachmann, G., Kemmann, E., et al. (1983). Vaginal atrophy in the postmenopausal woman. *Journal of the American Medical Association, 249*(16), 2195–2198.

Lethaby, A. E., Brown, J., Marjoribanks, J., Kronenberg, F., Roberts, H. & Eden, J. (2007). Phytoestrogens for vasomotor menopausal symptoms. *Cochraine Database Systematic Review, 17*(4), CD001395.

Libuda, L., Alexy, U., Remer, T., Stehle, P., Schoenau, E., & Kersting, M. (2008). Association between long-term consumption of soft drinks and variables of bone modeling and remodeling in a sample of healthy German children and adolescents. *American Journal of Clinical Nutrition, 88*(6), 1670–1677.

Lobo, R. A. (2001). Menopause management for the millennium. *Medscape Women's Health.* Retrieved January 15, 2011 from http://www.medscape.org/viewarticle/413064.

Lovlien, M., Johansson, I., Hole, T., & Schei, B. (2009). Early warning signs of an acute myocardial infarction and their influence on symptoms during the acute phase, with comparisons by gender. *Gender Medicine, 6*(3), 444–453.

Lu, J., Liu, J., & Eden, J. (2007). The experience of menopausal symptoms by Arabic women in Sidney. *Climacteric, 10*(1), 72–79.

Mac Bride, M. B., Rhodes, D. J., & Shuster, L. T. (2010). Vulvovaginal atrophy. *Mayo Clinic Proceedings, 85*(1), 87–94.

Maestra, N., Nahas, E. A., Nahas-Neto, J., Orsatti, F. L., Fernandes, C. E., Trainman, P., & Burini, R. C. (2007). Effects of soy protein and resistance exercise on body composition and blood lipids in postmenopausal women. *Maturitas, 56*(4), 350–358.

Martyn-St. James, M., & Carroll, S. (2006). Progressive high-intensity resistance training and bone mineral density changes among premenopausal women: Evidence of discordant site-specific skeletal effects. *Sports Medicine, 36*(8), 683–704.

Martyn-St. James, M., & Carroll, S. (2008). Meta-analysis of walking for preservation of bone mineral density in postmenopausal women. *Bone, 43*(3), 521–531.

Martyn-St. James, M., & Carroll, S. (2009). A meta-analysis of impact exercise on postmenopausal bone: The case for mixed loading exercise programmes. *British Journal of Sports Medicine, 43*(12), 898–908.

Mass, R., Holldorfer, M., Moll, B., Bauer, R., & Wolf, K. (2009). Why we haven't died out yet: Changes in women's mimic reactions to visual erotic stimuli during their menstrual cycles. *Hormones and Behavior, 55*(2), 267–271.

McSweeney, J. C., Cody, M., O'Sullivan, P., Elberson, K., Moser, D. K., & Garvin, B. J. (2003). Women's early warning symptoms of acute myocardial infarction. *Circulation, 108*(21), 2619–2623.

McSweeney, J. C., O'Sullivan, P., Cleaves, M. A., Lefler, L. L., Cody, M., Moser, D. K., Dunn, K., Kovacs, M., Crane, P. B., Ramer, L., Messmer, P. R., Garvin, B. J, & Zhao, W. (2010). Racial differences in women's prodromal and acute symptoms of myocardial infarction. *American Journal of Critical Care, 19*(1), 63–73.

Miller, P. D., & Derman, R. J. (2010). What is the best balance of benefits and risks among anti-resorptive therapies for postmenopausal osteoporosis. *Osteoporosis International, 21*(11), 1793–1802.

Naessen, T., Persson, I., Adami, H-O., et al. (1990). Hormone replacement therapy and the risk for hip fracture: A prospective, population-based cohort study. *Annals of Internal Medicine, 13,* 95–103. http://www.nia.nih.gov/healthinformation/publications/menopause.htm.

Nappi, R. E., & Lachowsky, M. (2009). Menopause and sexuality: prevalence of symptoms and impact on quality of life. *Maturitas, 63*(2), 138–141.

Odvina, C. V., Zerwekh, J. E., Rao, D. S., Maalouf, N., Gottschalk, F. A., & Pak, C. Y. C. (2005). Severely suppressed bone turnover: A potential complication of alendronate therapy. *Journal of Clinical Endocrinology & Metabolism, 90*(3), 1294–1301.

Paganini-Hill, A., Ross, R. K., & Henderson, B. E. (1989). Endometrial cancer and patterns of use of estrogen replacement therapy: A cohort study. *British Journal of Cancer, 59,* 445–447.

Panay, N., Al-Azzawi, F., Bouchard, C., Davis, S. R., Eden, J., Lodhi, I., Rees, M., Rodenberg, C.A.,

Pockaj, B. A., Gallagher, J. G., Loprinzi, C. L., Stella, P. J., Barton, D. L., Sloan, J. A., Lavasseur, B. I., Rao, R. M., Fitch, T. R., Rowland, K. M., Novotny, P. J., Richelson, E., & Fauq, A. H. (2006). Phase III double-blind, randomized, placebo-controlled crossover trial of black cohosh in the management of hot flashes: NCCTG Trial N01CC1. *Journal of Clinical Oncology, 24*(18), 2836–2841.

Prince, R. L., Smith, M., Dick, I. M., et al. (1991). Prevention of postmenopausal osteoporosis. A comparative study of exercise, calcium supplementation, and hormone-replacement therapy. *New England Journal of Medicine, 325*(17), 1189–1195.

Robbins, J. (2006). *Healthy at 100.* New York, NY: Random House Publishing Group.

Rosano, G. M., & Panina, G. (1999). Cardiovascular pharmacology of hormone replacement therapy. *Drugs and Aging, 15,* 219–234.

Rotstein, A., Harush, M., & Vaisman, N. (2008). The effect of a water exercise program on bone density of postmenopausal women. *Journal of Sports Medicine and Physical Fitness, 48*(3), 352–359.

Rymer, J., Schwenkhagen, A., & Sturdee, D. W. (2010). Testosterone treatment of HSDD in naturally menopausal women: The ADORE study. *Climacteric, 13*(2), 121–131.

Schairer, C., Lubin, J., Troisi, R., Sturgeon, S., Brinton, L., & Hoover, R. (2000). Menopausal estrogen and estrogen-progestin replacement therapy and breast cancer risk. *Journal of the American Medical Association, 283*(4), 485–491.

Shapiro, S., Kelly, J. P., Rosenberg, L., et al. (1985). Risk of localized and widespread endometrial cancer in relation to recent and discontinued use of conjugated estrogens. *New England Journal of Medicine, 313,* 969–972.

Shea, J. L. (2006). Parsing the ageing of Asian women: Symptoms results from the China study of midlife women. *Maturitas, 55*(1), 36–50.

Shechter, A., Varin, F., & Boivin, D. B. (2010). Circadian variation of sleep during the follicular and luteal phases of the menstrual cycle. *Sleep, 33*(5), 647–656.

Stadel, B. V., & Weiss, N. (1975). Characteristics of menopausal women: A survey of King and Pierce counties in Washington, 1973–74. *American Journal of Epidemiology, 102,* 209–216.

Steinberg, K. K., Thacker, S. B., Smith, J., et al. (1991). A meta-analysis of the effect of estrogen replacement therapy on the risk of breast cancer. *Journal of the American Medical Association, 265*(15), 1895–1990.

Studd, J., Pornel, B., Marton, I., et al. (1999). Efficacy and acceptability of intranasal 17 beta-oestradiol for menopause symptoms: Randomized dose-response study. *Lancet, 353*(9164), 1574–1578.

Tucker, K. L., Morita, K., Qiao, N., Hannan, M. T., Cupples, L. A., & Kiel, D. P. (2006). Colas, but not other carbonated beverages, are associated with low bone mineral density in older women: The Framingham Osteoporosis Study. *American Journal of Clinical Nutrition, 84*(4), 936–942.

U.S. Department of Health and Human Services, National Institutes of Health, National Heart, Lung and Blood Institute. (2005). Facts about menopausal hormone therapy. Retrieved January 15, 2011 from http://www.nhlbi.nih.gov/health/women/pht_facts.pdf.

Utian, W. H., & Boggs, P. P. (1999). 1998 Menopause survey: Part I. Postmenopausal women's perceptions about menopause and midlife. *Menopause, 6*(2), 122–128.

van Wingen, G. A., van Broekhoven, F., Verkes, R. J., Petersson, K. M., Backstrom, T., Buitelaar, J. K., & Fernandez, G. (2008). Progesterone selectively increases amygdala reactivity in women. *Molecular Psychiatry, 13*(3), 325–333.

Vestergaard, P., Rejnmark, L., & Mosekilde, L. (2009). Loss of life years after hip fracture. *Acta Orthopaedica, 80*(5), 525–530.

Vitale, C., Miceli, M., & Rosano, G. M. (2007). Gender-specific characteristics of atherosclerosis in menopausal women: Risk factors, clinical course and strategies for prevention. *Climacteric, 10, Suppl 2,* 16–20.

Wallace, R. B., Sherman, B. M., Bean, J. A., et al. (1979). The probabilities of menopause with increasing duration of amenorrhea in middle-aged women. *American Journal of Obstetrics and Gynecology, 135,* 1021–1024.

Weiss, N. S., Ure, C. L., Ballard, J. H., et al. (1980). Decreased risk of fractures of the hip and lower forearm with postmenopausal use of estrogen. *New England Journal of Medicine, 303,* 1195–1198.

Willett, W., Colditz, G., & Stampfer, M. (2000). Postmenopausal estrogens—opposed, unopposed, or none of the above. *Journal of the American Medical Association, 283*(4), 534–535.

Willett, W., Stampfer, M., Bain, C., et al. (1983). Cigarette smoking, relative weight, and menopause. *American Journal of Epidemiology, 117,* 651–658.

Williams, A. R., Weiss, N. S., Ure, C. L., et al. (1982). Effect of weight, smoking and estrogen use on the risk of hip and forearm fractures in postmenopausal women. *Obstetrics and Gynecology, 60*(6), 695–699.

Wong, R. W., & Rabie, A. B. (2008). Effect of quercetin on bone formation. *Journal of Orthopaedic Research, 26*(8), 1061–1066.

Yaffe, K., Sawaya, G., Lieberburg, I., & Grady, D. (1999). Estrogen therapy in postmenopausal women: Effects on cognitive function and dementia. *Journal of the American Medical Association, 279*(9), 688–695.

chapter 16

NUTRITION: FUEL FOR A WOMAN'S BODY

CHAPTER COMPETENCIES

Upon completion of this chapter, the reader will be able to:

- identify the major food groups and examples of foods within each
- differentiate between vitamins, minerals, and phytonutrients

- explain the functions of different nutrients in the body
- identify the specific nutritional needs of women over the lifespan

KEY TERMS

adenosine triphosphate (ATP)

amino acid

calorie

carbohydrate

fatty acids

lipid

mineral

phytonutrient

protein

vitamin

INTRODUCTION

Food provides energy for cellular metabolism as well as the raw materials necessary for tissue maintenance, growth, and repair. All of the chemical substances on which humans and other animals rely for the continuation of life, such as proteins, carbohydrates, lipids, vitamins, and minerals, are called nutrients. The nutritional demands of a woman's body depend on a combination of factors including her activity level, genetic factors, and changing hormone levels throughout her lifespan (Figure 16-1). A girl entering puberty requires additional energy to fuel cell division as well as increased levels of nutrients to provide the raw materials to build new cells. Menstruating

women require higher levels of iron than nonmenstruating women to replace the iron that is lost during menses. During pregnancy, hormonal changes and the metabolic demands of the fetus create additional nutritional demands. Breast-feeding also influences the nutritional demands of a woman. Menopause is accompanied by another metabolic shift, increasing a woman's need for calcium and other nutrients to combat the risk of osteoporosis and cardiovascular disease.

A woman's diet has an influence on her health (Figure 16-2). Cancer and cardiovascular disease—both conditions associated with obesity and food choices—are major causes of death. In

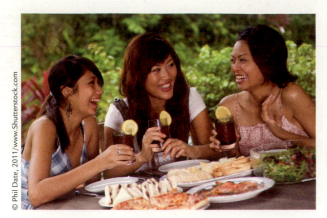

FIGURE 16-1: There are a number of factors that determine a woman's nutritional demands, including age, activity level, and genetics.

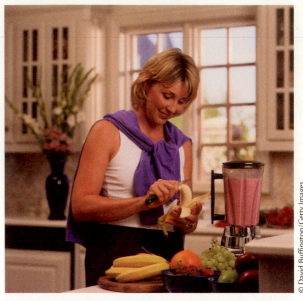

FIGURE 16-2: The foods that a woman eats can have a major impact on her health. A diet containing a variety of minimally processed foods appears to improve health.

2005, cardiovascular disease was responsible for 30 percent of deaths world wide, killing equal numbers of women and men. The majority of these deaths are linked to unhealthy diet and a lack of physical activity (WHO, 2007). A return to a diet composed of minimally processed foods appears to improve health. For example, recent research has found that the traditional Mediterranean diet reduced inflammation, cardiovascular disease, and type 2 diabetes (O'Keefe et al., 2008). In addition, plant-based compounds that are active in the human body, such as flavonoids, phytoestrogens, and other phytonutrients, have been the focus of increasing scientific research exploring their antioxidant, anticarcinogenic, and cardioprotective properties (Kris-Etherton et al., 2002). Antioxidants are compounds that deactivate harmful free radicals in the body formed as a side effect when the body cells use oxygen. Free radicals are unstable molecules that can damage cells, and research has suggested that a higher intake of antioxidants is related to a lower incidence of such diseases as cancer, heart disease, rheumatoid arthritis, or cataracts and also can slow the aging process. These nutrients are found in whole grains and a wide range of fruits and vegetables.

A woman can take personal responsibility for her health by understanding the biological basis of nutrition—what nutrients are, how the body processes them, what constitutes a healthy diet—and applying that knowledge to her own food choices (Figure 16-2). However, the current state of nutritional science does not address every aspect of the interactions between biology and nutrition. As food writer Michael Pollan points out in his 2008 book *In Defense of Food*, an understanding of nutrients alone does not make us healthier.

ENERGY PRODUCTION

Women get energy from the carbohydrates, proteins, and lipids in their diet. The energy value of food is expressed in terms of a unit called the kilocalorie or **Calorie** (with a capital C), usually identified on a food label as a calorie (with a small c). The scientific definition of a Calorie is the amount of heat that is required to raise the temperature of a kilogram of water (1,000 g) from 14.5 degrees celsius to 15.5 degrees celsius. In practical terms, it represents the amount of energy gained when cells convert the stored energy of foods into usable energy. Vitamins, minerals, and other nutrients are present in most foods and are essential for maintaining cell function, but they are not metabolized for energy.

Roughly, each gram of carbohydrate or protein provides four calories, while each gram of fat yields nine calories. Carbohydrates, proteins, and lipids

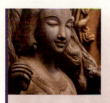

Social Considerations
THE DIET CRAZE

The grapefruit diet, the cabbage soup diet, or even the maple syrup diet—fad diets have been around for decades now, but unfortunately they usually do more harm than good. On any given day, anywhere between one-third to one-half of all Americans are on some kind of diet, but, as a nation, Americans are currently more overweight than they have ever been. Europe, Asia, and Central America are also facing increasing rates of obesity. The truth is that there is no silver bullet to weight loss. According to a 2006 study reported in *The New England Journal of Medicine*, most people who participate in weight-loss programs regain the weight lost within three to five years (Reisner, 2008).

For women in many cultures, the pressure to be thin is especially acute, with magazines, the Internet, and television infomercials exhorting women to banish the belly fat and obliterate cellulite on their thighs and hips. In the United States, dieting is a multi-billion dollar a year industry, with diet books, pills, powders, teas, advertisements, and advice nearly everywhere (Reisner, 2008). In some cases, these products contain ingredients which may be harmful or are untested.

The United States Federal Trade Commission (FTC) supplies useful tips to spot dieting scams, including false claims that people can eat their favorite high-calorie foods and still lose weight or that people can lose weight without diet or exercise (FTC, 2004). Other scam diets claim to block the absorption of fat, carbohydrates, or calories, or promise dramatic weight loss in the matter of a few days or weeks (FTC, 2004). If a woman needs to lose weight for health reasons, she may need to change some of her dietary habits, but she cannot rely on dieting alone. Instead, she should make a commitment to eating healthier, being more physically active, and taking better care of herself for the rest of her life.

---

are combined with oxygen within the body's cells to release energy by a process called cellular respiration. Cells capture the released energy to form a high-energy molecule called **adenosine triphosphate (ATP)**. Cells can then use ATP for energy to accomplish cellular activities such as making new proteins, dividing to make new cells, and transporting chemicals across their membranes to maintain homeostasis. Most cellular energy is obtained from the metabolism of glucose ($C_6H_{12}O_6$), a simple carbohydrate. In addition to ATP, cellular respiration produces carbon dioxide (CO_2) and water. The majority of the CO_2 is transported to the lungs to be exhaled as a waste product. The chemical reaction for the breakdown of one molecule of glucose is shown below:

$$C_6H_{12}O_6 + 6\,O_2 \ \rightarrow \ 6\,CO_2 + 6\,H_2O + 36\,ATP$$

Most foods are made up of a combination of carbohydrates, proteins, and lipids. Exceptions are highly refined products such as table sugar (a pure carbohydrate) and salad oil (a pure lipid). Even wheat flour, which is primarily carbohydrate, has up to 10 percent protein content. Foods such as peas and beans contain large amounts of carbohydrates and 20 percent or more of protein.

Carbohydrates

In the process called photosynthesis, green plants use solar energy to combine carbon dioxide and water into glucose, a six-carbon sugar that acts as the building blocks for most complex **carbohydrates**. Plant cells convert glucose into more complex carbohydrates and build additional compounds including lipids, proteins, and vitamins, utilizing the minerals

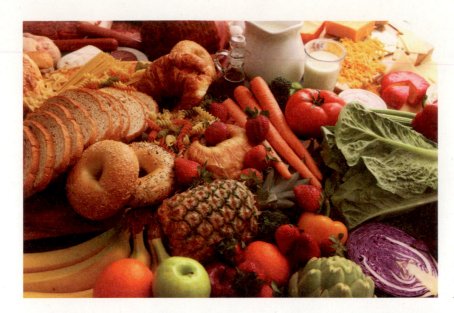

FIGURE 16-3: Fruits, vegetables, grains, and some dairy products are good sources of carbohydrates. *(Courtesy of Agricultural Research Service, USDA)*

and nitrogen. Important sources of carbohydrates in the diet are tuber and root vegetables, legumes (beans and peas), cereal grains, fruits, and products derived from them (Figure 16-3).

Carbohydrates are categorized on the basis of the size and complexity of the molecules into three groups—monosaccharides, disaccharides, and polysaccharides. Mono and disaccharides are referred to as simple sugars. Glucose is the best known and most prevalent monosaccharide and is the primary sugar of carbohydrate metabolism and energy production in the body. When diabetics test their blood sugar, they are measuring the amount of glucose traveling through their blood at that moment. Other common types of monosaccharides are fructose, or fruit sugar, and galactose, a component of milk sugar.

Disaccharides are formed from two monosaccharides linked together. Sucrose, or table sugar, is a disaccharide composed of glucose and fructose and is found in sugar cane, sugar beets, honey, and maple sap (Figure 16-4). The disaccharide lactose (milk sugar) is made of the simple sugars glucose and galactose. Individuals who are lactose intolerant lack the enzyme necessary to digest lactose down to the monosaccharides glucose and galactose. The undigested lactose passes to the large intestine where resident bacteria, the intestinal normal flora, can ferment it to gases and other products that produce intestinal irritation. Maltose, another disaccharide which is found in malted (sprouted) grains, consists of two glucose units.

Polysaccharides are composed of hundreds or thousands of monosaccharide units and are classified as complex carbohydrates. The most common polysaccharides are plant starch (amylose), pectin, cellulose, and glycogen (a complex carbohydrate stored in the skeletal muscles and liver as an energy reserve). Starches are derived from a variety of plant sources. Humans rely heavily on grains for their

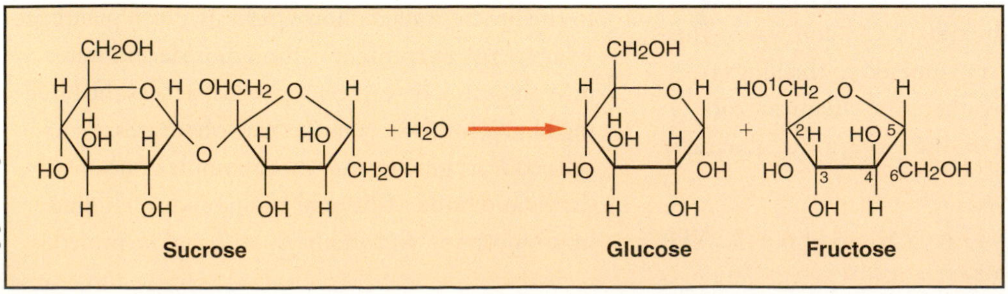

© Cengage Learning 2013

$$CH_2OH \quad OHCH_2 \qquad + H_2O \longrightarrow \qquad CH_2OH \quad HO^1CH_2$$

Sucrose   **Glucose**   **Fructose**

FIGURE 16-4: The chemical structure of the six-carbon sugars, glucose and fructose. When combined, they produce the disaccharide sucrose.

starch source. Millet, rice, buckwheat, barley, corn, and wheat are cultivated worldwide. Other grains such as quinoa, amaranth, and teff have a more localized distribution. Roots and tubers, such as manioc, taro, and potatoes, are additional sources of starch. Some fruits, such as plantain and breadfruit, also contain large amounts of starch. Cellulose forms the rigid walls around individual plant cells. Humans lack the enzymes required to convert cellulose to glucose and, therefore, cellulose passes through the digestive tract largely undigested. Foods high in cellulose are considered high-fiber, low-density foods. They have relatively few calories by volume because the body cannot utilize them for energy. Although cellulose cannot be digested, it does contribute to the mechanics of digestion by providing fiber and bulk. A moderate amount of cellulose and other indigestible materials is necessary for normal bowel activity and can be most easily obtained from whole-grain cereals, fruits, and vegetables. An increased incidence of diverticulitis (inflammation of small pockets in the wall of the colon), cancer of the colon, and heart disease has been correlated with a low fiber intake in the diet. Increasing the amount of fiber in the diet has additional benefits. Whole grains, especially oats, have been shown to reduce serum cholesterol levels and help control blood sugar levels (Sadiq Butt et al., 2008). Fiber also limits the recycling of estrogen from the colon, allowing it to be eliminated from the body. Finally, eating high fiber foods contributes to a feeling of fullness and can help prevent overeating.

Fats and Lipids

Fats and **lipids** are high energy molecules. The term "fat" refers to body fat, or the triglycerides stored in adipose tissue, as well as to fat in foods, such as butter, oils, and lard. "Lipid" is a broader term; it includes the phospholipids, which make up cell membranes, and the sterols such as cholesterol, in addition to the other fats. Although consuming too much can be unhealthy, fat is, in fact, necessary in the diet. Triglycerides provide both cellular energy and act as an energy storage reserve. During times when energy demands exceed the circulating sugar levels, the body can break down these stored fats for energy. Fat insulates the body, limiting heat loss, and

also supports and cushions the body's organs. The other lipids form parts of cellular membranes, transport molecules through the bloodstream, and act as hormones and other chemical messengers in the body. In addition to providing necessary fatty acids, fat in the diet is also required as a carrier molecule for the absorption of fat-soluble vitamins from the intestines.

Since lipids provide more than twice the calories per gram of either carbohydrates or proteins, foods containing lipids are generally higher in calories. Unfortunately, this high caloric density can contribute to consuming more calories than is necessary, leading to weight gain. Fat, much of it coming from animal sources, provides 35-45 percent of the calories in the typical American diet.

Triglycerides

Containing only carbon, hydrogen, and oxygen atoms, a triglyceride molecule consists of three molecules of **fatty acids** linked to one molecule of an alcohol called glycerol, commonly known as glycerin. A typical triglyceride is shown in Figure 16-5.

Palmitic, oleic, and stearic acids are the most common fatty acids found in nature. They are found frequently in food fats and are the common fatty acids in human body fat. Palmitic acid and stearic acid are examples of saturated fatty acids. A saturated fatty acid contains more hydrogen atoms than an unsaturated fatty acid. Typically, saturated fats are solid at room temperature. Cocoa butter (chocolate fat) and tropical oils such as palm kernel, palm, and coconut oil are saturated vegetable fats. Dairy foods, pork, beef, lamb, and poultry are also sources of saturated fats. Unsaturated fatty acids, such as linoleic, linolenic, and arachidonic, contain fewer hydrogen atoms and are usually liquid at room temperature. Unsaturated fats are found in olive oil, canola oil, avocados, sesame oil, corn oil, and fatty fish. Polyunsaturated fatty acids contain the fewest hydrogen atoms.

Trans Fats   Hydrogen atoms can be added to unsaturated fats by a process called hydrogenation. By this process, unsaturated vegetable oils can be transformed into solid shortening and margarine. Unfortunately, this process also produces molecules

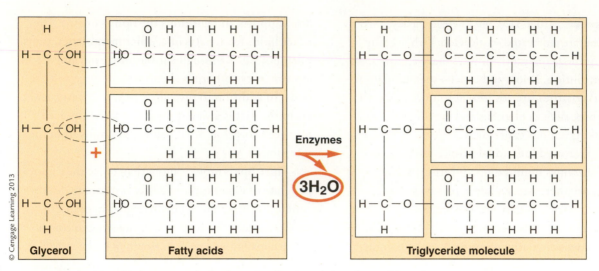

FIGURE 16-5: A triglyceride is composed of a glycerol molecule and three fatty acids.

called trans fats which are linked to increased risk of cardiovascular disease. While some trans fats occur naturally, the majority are produced from the hydrogenation process. Health concerns have lead to bans on the use of added trans fats in New York City, Boston, and California. Several manufacturers have now removed trans fats from their processed foods.

Omega Fatty Acids

Linoleic (an omega-6 fatty acid) and linolenic (an omega-3 fatty acid) acids are called the essential fatty acids because they cannot be synthesized by the body and must be obtained in the diet. Sources high in omega-6 fatty acids include corn and sunflower oils. Soybeans, cold-water fish, flax, and nuts are natural sources of omega-3 fatty acids. The essential fatty acids are necessary precursors in the synthesis of the chemical messenger prostaglandin by human tissue, and they contribute to the integrity of cell membranes.

Phospholipids

Phospholipids are structurally similar to triglycerides, however, one of the fatty acids in the molecule is replaced by a phosphate-containing compound. Cell membranes are composed of a double layer of phospholipid which creates a semi-permeable barrier. For this reason, phospholipids are important in maintaining healthy cells. The phospholipid lecithin,

found in egg yolk and soybeans, has been shown to play a role in reducing cardiovascular disease (Rousset, 2009). However, the majority of claims by lecithin supplement manufacturers remain unsupported by scientific research, and the body cells are able to synthesize adequate amounts of lecithin on their own.

Cholesterol

Cholesterol is a member of a class of lipids called sterols (Figure 16-6). Common foods that contain large amounts of cholesterol are those high in saturated fats, such as butter, whole milk, and full-fat cheeses, and meats that are heavily marbled with fat. Egg yolks and organ meats such as liver and kidney also contain appreciable amounts of cholesterol. Shellfish were once considered a high cholesterol food. However, refined techniques in

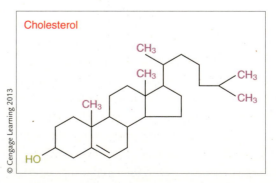

FIGURE 16-6: Chemical formula for cholesterol.

nutritional analysis now show that most shellfish are low in cholesterol and supply significant levels of the beneficial omega-3 fatty acids (Mayo Clinic, 2006). The liver converts cholesterol to cholic acid and combines it with other substances to form bile salts, which are necessary for the emulsion and digestion of dietary fats. Cholesterol is also essential for the synthesis of steroid hormones by the adrenal glands, the ovaries, and the testes. Steroid hormones include estrogen, progesterone, and testosterone. Along with phospholipids, cholesterol forms a component of cell membranes. After six months of age, dietary consumption of cholesterol is unnecessary because the body manufactures all the cholesterol it needs from other substances. Typically, adults produce about 200 mg of cholesterol daily. Most of this endogenous cholesterol is manufactured by the liver, but some is also synthesized by other tissues in the body. Research links high serum cholesterol levels with atherosclerosis, a condition in which fatty plaques of lipids, mostly cholesterol, are deposited on and in the artery walls. These cholesterol deposits build up, become fibrous and calcified, and eventually cause narrowing and hardening (arteriosclerosis) of the arteries. The narrowed vessels may become occluded, cutting off the supply of blood to a vital organ such as the heart or brain. Alternately, a plaque can break free and become a thrombus, or clot, that blocks a vessel, leading to a stroke, heart attack, or pulmonary embolism. In the United States, 39 percent of all female deaths are due to cardiovascular disease, making the implications of cholesterol in the diet all the more important (American Heart Association, 2008).

The body transports cholesterol through the blood attached to protein-based carrier molecules

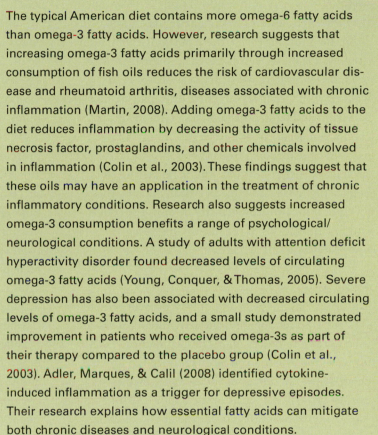

focus on
NUTRITION
Benefits of Omega-3 Fatty Acids

The typical American diet contains more omega-6 fatty acids than omega-3 fatty acids. However, research suggests that increasing omega-3 fatty acids primarily through increased consumption of fish oils reduces the risk of cardiovascular disease and rheumatoid arthritis, diseases associated with chronic inflammation (Martin, 2008). Adding omega-3 fatty acids to the diet reduces inflammation by decreasing the activity of tissue necrosis factor, prostaglandins, and other chemicals involved in inflammation (Colin et al., 2003). These findings suggest that these oils may have an application in the treatment of chronic inflammatory conditions. Research also suggests increased omega-3 consumption benefits a range of psychological/neurological conditions. A study of adults with attention deficit hyperactivity disorder found decreased levels of circulating omega-3 fatty acids (Young, Conquer, & Thomas, 2005). Severe depression has also been associated with decreased circulating levels of omega-3 fatty acids, and a small study demonstrated improvement in patients who received omega-3s as part of their therapy compared to the placebo group (Colin et al., 2003). Adler, Marques, & Calil (2008) identified cytokine-induced inflammation as a trigger for depressive episodes. Their research explains how essential fatty acids can mitigate both chronic diseases and neurological conditions.

called lipoproteins. High density lipoproteins (HDLs) are commonly referred to as "good cholesterol" due to their ability to remove cholesterol deposits (plaques) from blood vessels. High levels of HDLs are associated with a decreased risk of cardiovascular disease. Low density lipoproteins (LDLs), or "bad cholesterol", are associated with an increased risk of cardiovascular disease. LDLs play a role in plaque formation. The American Heart Association (AHA, 2008) recommends a total serum cholesterol of less than 200 mg/dl, LDL levels of 100 mg/dl or less, and HDL levels of at least 50 mg/dl for a woman. The HDL/LDL balance is influenced by diet, exercise, and hormones. Endogenous estrogen favors the formation of HDLs and a reduction in the levels of LDLs. Research has documented the ability of a low-fat, high-fiber diet and exercise to lower serum cholesterol levels, lower LDL levels, and increase HDL levels (Corwin, 2008).

When polyunsaturated vegetable fats such as soybean, safflower, and sunflower oils are consumed, they lower cholesterol by enhancing its elimination from the body. However, these oils indiscriminately decrease HDLs as well as LDLs, and for this reason, the monosaturated oils such as canola, olive, or walnut, which reduce only the LDLs, may be preferable. In addition, omega-3 fatty acids, found in canola and olive oils and in large amounts in deep-sea fish, appear to be protective against heart disease as well as other conditions. In the body, trans fats behave like saturated fats, specifically raising the levels of unhealthy low-density lipoproteins (LDL) and lowering levels of the healthy high-density lipoproteins (HDL).

Proteins

The body contains large amounts of **protein**, which is essential to cell function and structure. Proteins are used for a wide variety of metabolic functions in the body. While proteins can be metabolized to provide energy, this function is secondary to their roles in normal growth and repair of the body's cells and tissues. The enzymes that catalyze metabolic reactions and many of the chemical messengers within the body are proteins.

Amino acids are the structural building blocks of proteins and contain carbon, hydrogen, oxygen, and nitrogen plus small quantities of other atoms such as sulfur. The 20 amino acids found in a woman's body are shown in Figure 16-7. Proteins are digested to amino acids, absorbed from the small intestine, and used by cells to construct new proteins. Protein synthesis, the process of assembling the amino acid in a specific order, can take place only when the necessary amino acids are present in an adequate supply. The lack of a single amino acid needed for a specific protein sequence can halt the formation of the protein chain. As long as there is enough nitrogen available (via protein food intake), cells are capable of manufacturing many of the amino acids normally present in animal proteins. Nine of the amino acids, however, cannot be synthesized in human cells. Those nine amino acids, called essential amino acids, must be obtained from the diet. They include isoleucine, leucine, lysine, methionine, phenylalanine, threonine, tryptophan, valine, and histidine.

Most foods contain some protein, but not all foods contain adequate amounts of all the amino acids. Animal proteins, such as meat, poultry, fish, eggs, and dairy products contain all the essential amino acids and are called complete proteins. Some nuts and a few grains, such as quinoa, are also complete proteins. Other foods are rich in protein but do not contain all of the essential amino acids. Most plant proteins are deficient in several of the essential amino acids, usually threonine, tryptophan, or lysine, and are referred to as incomplete proteins. Mixing incomplete proteins from different types of plant sources or with a complete protein can provide the full range of amino acids necessary for protein synthesis. For example, legumes, such as beans or peanuts, lack some essential amino acids while cereal grains lack others. Peanut butter on whole wheat bread, however, or beans and rice together provide the full range of amino acids. Another example is traditional Asian cooking which combines soybeans (a legume) with rice (a grain) and vegetables. Because the body has no mechanism for storing amino acids in the way that it accumulates fats or carbohydrates for future use, it is important to mix complementary protein foods in the same meal, if possible. In this way, all 20 amino acids necessary in the manufacture of protein will be present in the body cells at the same time. Once the quantities of amino acids needed for protein synthesis have been taken up by the cells and utilized, any additional amino acids are oxidized for energy. When proteins are used as an energy source, molecules called ketones are produced as a waste product. Ketones can alter blood pH, producing a condition called ketoacidosis which is seen in uncontrolled diabetes. Prolonged ketoacidosis damages the kidneys, alters enzyme functions, and can have deleterious effects on the nervous system.

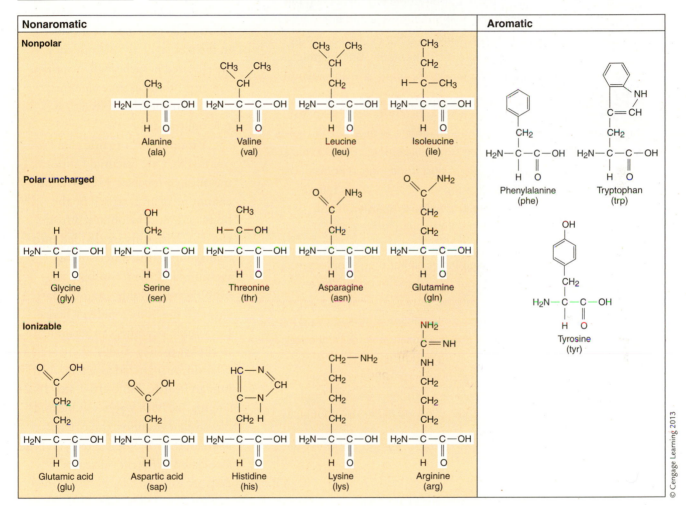

FIGURE 16-7: The general structure of an amino acid and the 20 amino acids found in the human body.

The body's need for protein increases during times of rapid cell growth, such as childhood, puberty, and injury. To ensure proper growth and development, there must to be an adequate supply of all the amino acids in the diet of growing children. For similar reasons, additional protein is also needed by a pregnant woman to support the placenta and fetus and by a lactating woman. Recovery from surgery increases the need for protein in the diet in order to repair and heal damaged tissues. For an athlete, a small extra amount of protein might be utilized during athletic training as the muscles get larger, but exercise or athletic performance does

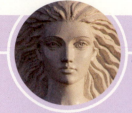

focus on

EXERCISE
Nutritional Requirements of Athletes

Talk with athletes intent on improving their performance, and the discussion frequently turns to the latest supplement or a special diet. Many athletes believe that dramatically increasing the amount of protein in their diet will build muscle and boost performance. Weight lifters and bodybuilders often eat large amounts of animal protein and take protein supplements. But do athletes really need exceptionally high levels of protein and special nutritional supplements?

Normally, a balanced diet with sufficient calories to match energy expenditures will provide an athlete with all the nutrients necessary. As always, there are some exceptions. Electrolytes are lost during heavy sweating. Water and fruits high in potassium like bananas can easily replace those. A French study found athletes may benefit from the protective properties of antioxidant vitamins like A, C, and E (Rousseau et al., 2004). The anti-inflammatory properties of many of the phytonutrients, found primarily in unprocessed foods rather than supplements, may also be of benefit to injured bones and muscles. The anti-inflammatory properties of omega-3 fatty acids may also benefit athletes, although again, adequate levels are obtained by eating a balanced diet (Simopoulos, 2007). Injured athletes may need additional protein to help in healing and tissue repair. For the average athlete, eating a low-fat, moderate protein diet based on whole grains, plant-based oils, and a variety of colorful fruits and vegetables will meet nutritional needs better than bottles of supplements.

not increase the requirement for protein (Figure 16-8). However, women whose diets do not contain adequate amounts of protein may need to increase the amount of this nutrient before beginning an exercise program. The recommended daily dietary allowance for women vary from 46 g to 109 g per day. The value is approximately 0.4 g protein per pound of body weight. A 125-lb woman should, therefore, eat about 50 g of protein per day. One ounce of lean meat yields an average of 7 g of protein. An ounce of cheddar cheese contains 7 g, and a cup of skim milk will provide 9 g. A half cup serving of dried beans contains 7 to 9 g of protein.

VITAMINS

Life cannot be sustained on pure protein, carbohydrate, fat, and water alone. Foods contain additional chemicals that are necessary for survival. These additional food substances—the vitamins and minerals—do not contribute energy, but they are nonetheless essential. The body stores only limited amounts of vitamins and minerals, so they must be included in the diet regularly. Because they are required in such small quantities, sometimes only in trace amounts, they are frequently referred to as micronutrients.

Vitamins are organic compounds that are essential for normal metabolic processes. Most vitamins cannot be manufactured by the body and must be obtained from the diet. Vitamins are divided into two groups—the water-soluble vitamins and the fat-soluble vitamins. Water-soluble vitamins pass through the body rapidly, whereas fat-soluble vitamins can accumulate in the fat tissues. Today, there are 14 vitamins recognized as essential to human health. Tables 16-1 and 16-2 summarize both water-soluble and fat-soluble vitamins, their richest sources, their biological role, and the associated deficiency diseases.

Vitamin needs are expressed by means of the Dietary Reference Intakes (DRIs). The DRIs are developed using tolerance limits, estimated average requirements and other factors (National Academy of Sciences, 2004) and replace the older recommended daily allowances (RDAs). The DRIs represent the quantity of any given nutrient that is needed daily to promote optimal health and to prevent chronic disease, based on the current research. As newer research becomes available, these recommendations are adjusted. The recommendations vary by age, sex, and individual considerations. For example, research indicates that women taking

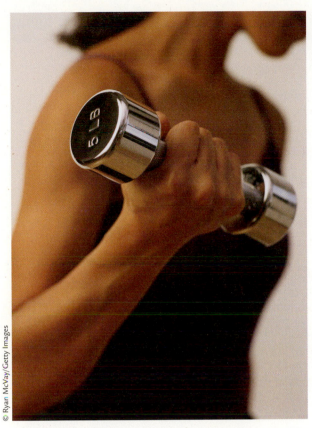

FIGURE 16-8: The body's need for protein increases during times of rapid cell development.

oral contraceptives often have lower than optimal levels of vitamins B_6 and B_{12} (Lussana et al., 2003). For this reason, they may need to increase their intake of these vitamins. Medications, either over the counter or medically prescribed, can cause vitamin depletion by interacting with the nutrients in foods. Some of the chemotherapeutic drugs used in the treatment of cancer, certain antibiotics, and various anticoagulants can interfere with vitamin absorption. Individuals who eat restricted diets—either by choice or circumstance—may not get adequate amounts of all the vitamins. For example, vitamin B_{12} is found only in animal-derived foods. Individuals who do not eat animal-derived foods may be deficient in B_{12}. Those who do not have access to fresh fruits and vegetables may find themselves short of vitamin C. Frequently, vitamins are recognized by the media for preventing specific diseases. For example, vitamin D has recently become very popular after studies linked increased levels of the vitamin with decreases in colorectal cancer (Soerjomataram et al., 2008) and pancreatic cancer

(Schwartz & Skinner, 2007). However, it is important to remember that no single nutrient is likely to be a silver bullet for preventing disease. The nutrients in foods often work together in ways that are not yet completely understood.

Most nutritionists maintain that taking vitamin supplements in the presence of an adequate diet is an unnecessary expense. There are no scientific data to indicate the necessity for supplementation when people are eating a healthy mixture of foods including a variety of fruits and vegetables. In fact, megadoses of some water-soluble vitamins can produce unpleasant symptoms and potential toxicity (Table 16-1). Fat-soluble vitamins are stored in the body and may build to toxic levels more easily than water-soluble vitamins. For example, vitamins A and D are stored in the body for long periods of time, are metabolized very slowly, and are excreted with great difficulty by way of the bile. Daily ingestion of more than 25,000 International Units (IUs) of vitamin A, 20 to 30 times the recommended dose, will cause toxicity, with neurological symptoms of irritability and headache, liver problems that can lead to cirrhosis, and dermatological problems such as brittle nails and dry, rough skin. Excessive vitamin A supplementation during pregnancy can also cause birth defects. It is less likely, however, to consume toxic levels by eating vitamin-rich foods. The levels present in food are minute and would require eating nearly impossible amounts of food to reach toxic levels.

In addition, supplements may not have the same effects as the whole foods that are rich sources of the vitamin in question. Epidemiological research that linked the antioxidant vitamins with disease protection was based on high fruit and vegetable intake in the populations studied and not on people taking vitamin supplements. Research has found that eating foods rich in carotenoids, which are precursors to vitamin A, appeared to lower the risk of developing lung cancer but taking vitamin A supplements did not (Holick et al., 2002). An extensive review of vitamin therapy by Huang et al. (2006) indicated that vitamins have use in cancer prevention in individuals not receiving adequate amounts through food, but provided no protection against cardiovascular disease. For women who are unable to consume adequate nutrition, an over-the-counter multivitamin

Table 16-1   Water-soluble Vitamins.

Name	DRI *	Functions	Rich Sources	Deficiency Symptoms	Potential Toxicity
Thiamine (B$_1$)	1.1 mg	component of coenzyme involved in energy release	whole grains, enriched cereals, legumes, pork	beriberi; impaired cardiovascular, nervous, and gastrointestinal systems	none
Niacin (nicotinic acid)	14 mg	component of coenzyme involved in energy release	lean meats, peanuts, yeast, cereal bran, and germ	pellagra; dermatitis; diarrhea; depression; death	none; may cause skin flushing, dizziness, and nausea
Riboflavin (B$_2$)	1.1 mg	component of coenzyme involved in energy release	milk, eggs, liver, oat bran, green leafy vegetables	dermatitis; light sensitivity; sores at corners of mouth	none
Pantothenic acid (B$_3$)	5 mg	component of coenzyme involved in energy release	liver, kidney, oat bran, egg yolk, wheat bran, fresh vegetables	fatigue; gastrointestinal distress; personality changes; numbness in hands and feet; muscle cramps	none
Pyridoxine (B$_6$)	1.3 mg	protein synthesis; central nervous system metabolism	yeast, oat bran, unprocessed wheat and corn, egg yolk, liver, kidney, lean meat	anemia	neurotoxicity and depression with megadoses
Cobalamin (B$_{12}$)	2.4 mcg	red blood cell formation; DNA synthesis; fatty acid synthesis; nerve function	beef, milk, eggs, oysters, shrimp, pork, chicken	anemia; nerve degeneration	none
Folic acid	400 mcg	red blood cell formation; neural tube formation	green leafy vegetables, whole grains, legumes, enriched cereals and breads	anemia; neural tube birth defects	none; possible neurotoxicity with megadoses
Biotin	30 mcg	coenzyme carrier of CO_2	milk, liver, kidney, egg yolk, yeast, intestinal bacteria	scaly skin	none
Ascorbic acid (C)	75 mg	collagen formation; capillary integrity; iron absorption; synthesis of corticosteroids	citrus fruits, tomatoes, green vegetables	scurvy; bleeding gums; bruising; swollen joints; slow wound healing	inconclusive

* Dietary Reference Intake recommended for adult females (National Academy of Sciences, 2004)

Table 16-2 Fat-soluble Vitamins.					
Name	DRI *	Functions	Rich Sources	Deficiency Symptoms	Potential Toxicity
retinol; retinal (A)	400 mcg	night vision; growth; cell membrane; reproduction	full-fat dairy products, liver, yellow and green vegetables; fruits	night blindness; skin lesions	neurological toxicity and birth defects at high doses
ergocalciferol (D$_2$) cholecalciferol (D$_3$)	5 mcg	bone formation; absorption of calcium and phosphorus	fatty fish, eggs, liver, fortified milk, sunlight	soft bones; rickets	highly toxic at high doses
alpha-tocopherol (E)	15 mg	antioxidant; prevention of cell degeneration	wheat germ, vegetable oils, beef liver, milk, eggs, leafy vegetables	none identified in humans	none
naphthoquinones (K)	90 mcg	Normal blood clotting; intestinal bacteria	lettuce, spinach, cruciferous vegetables	increased clotting time for blood	none

* Dietary Reference Intake recommended for adult females (National Academy of Sciences, 2004)

taken according to the label instructions would provide nutritional insurance, but is not necessary for individuals eating a well- balanced and varied diet (Figure 16-9).

MINERALS

Of the naturally occurring chemical elements in nature, more than 50 are found in human body tissues. Fewer than half of these **minerals** are known to be essential to human body function. Some, such as calcium, phosphorus, sodium, potassium, chlorine, magnesium, and sulfur, are required in fairly large daily doses for use as structural components and for metabolism.

Calcium is well known for its role in building strong bone and teeth. Women who have a diet insufficient in calcium or who suffer from malabsorption of calcium are prone to osteoporosis, particularly after menopause. Calcium is also essential in muscle contraction and blood clotting. A study of over 28,000 women found that low-fat dairy products and increased dietary calcium were associated with decreased rates of hypertension (Wang et al., 2008). Calcium, along with potassium, is involved in the transmission of nerve impulses. Other minerals are

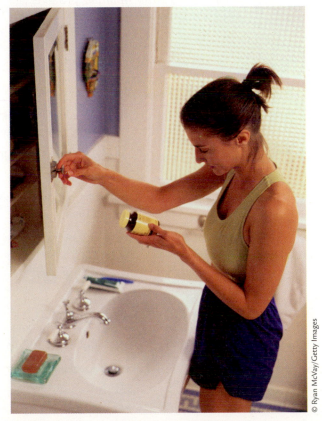

© Ryan McVay/Getty Images

FIGURE 16-9: For women eating a well-balanced, varied diet, multivitamins are not necessary; however, if a woman cannot get adequate nutrition, multivitamins used properly can provide nutritional insurance.

identified as trace elements because they are needed in daily amounts of a few milligrams (mg) or micrograms (mcg) daily. Iron, in the form of the heme molecule, is a major component of hemoglobin. Found on red blood cells, hemoglobin is responsible for carrying oxygen to the tissues. Insufficient intake of iron leads to iron-deficiency anemia, especially among menstruating women. Table 16-3 lists the minerals known to be necessary to human health, their dos-

age, sources, and functions. This list is not exhaustive. New research is continually identifying new functions for many minerals.

Some minerals, including tin, nickel, silicon, and vanadium, are found in minute quantities in the body. These are minerals that may be essential to human metabolic processes, but their functions are still being investigated, and no human requirements have been established for them.

Table 16-3	Essential Minerals.		
Name	**DRI ***	**Rich Sources**	**Functions**
Calcium	1000 mg	dairy; legumes; leafy vegetables; whole grains; nuts	tooth and bone structure; muscle contraction; blood coagulation; nerve transmission
Chlorine	2.3 g	salt; most foods	water balance; osmotic pressure; digestive HCl
Chromium	25 mcg	meat; corn oil	normal glucose metabolism
Cobalt	Unknown	animals proteins	part of vitamin B_{12}
Copper	900 mcg	liver; kidney; shellfish; nuts; legumes	enzyme component; hemoglobin formation
Fluorine	3 mg	fluoridated water; milk	resistance to tooth decay
Iodine	150 mcg	seafood; iodized salt	thyroid hormones
Iron	18 mg	organ meats; egg yolk; fish; beans; molasses; green vegetables	hemoglobin; cellular respiration
Magnesium	310 mg	vegetables; milk; meat; cocoa; nuts	enzyme activity; energy release; nerve and muscle function
Manganese	1.8 mg	bananas; whole grains; leafy vegetables	normal bone formation; reproductive and nervous system function
Molybdenum	1.8 mcg	beef kidney; legumes; some cereals	enzyme component
Phosphorus	1250 mg	dairy; meat; fish	normal tooth and bone structure; ATP; acid/base buffer
Potassium	4.7 g	most foods	muscle contraction, nerve function
Selenium	55 mcg	seafood; meat; grains	enzyme component
Sodium	1.5 g	most foods; table salt	osmotic pressure; muscle and nerve function
Sulfur	1.6 g	protein-rich foods	hormones; enzymes; protein formation
Zinc	8 mg	meat; eggs; seafood; milk; grains	enzymes; insulin production

* Dietary Reference Intake recommended for adult females (National Academy of Sciences, 2004)

Taking megadoses of mineral supplements in the belief that they can enhance energy or protect against disease is risky. For example, Broun et al. (1990) described cases of a life-threatening form of anemia and bone marrow depression caused by ingestion of excess zinc. The authors concluded that daily consumption of 100–150 mg of elemental zinc resulted in increased copper excretion, and a negative copper balance, which increased the likelihood of anemia. In addition, iron overdoses produce heart, brain, and liver damage as the body tries to store the excess iron in these tissues. This damage can lead to heart attack, stroke, and liver failure.

PHYTONUTRIENTS

In addition to vitamins and minerals, a third class of non-caloric nutrients has been identified. These bioactive compounds are most commonly called **phytonutrients**. Typically found in only trace amounts in plants, these compounds have diverse chemical structures. Some are plant pigments; others are structural components of plant cells. Phytonutrients have a variety of effects in humans, and can act as antioxidants, and anti-inflammatory agents. They also play a role in preventing diseases such as cancers and cardiovascular disease (Kris-Etherton et al., 2002).

Flavonoids are a group of phytonutrients that include hesperidin, rutin, flavonones, flavones, and flavonols. They are widely distributed in plant foods, found particularly in citrus fruits, berries, cabbages, brussels sprouts, onions, tea, vinegar, and red wine. There is evidence that some flavonoids have antibacterial and antiviral capabilities (Cushnie & Lamb, 2005). There has also been research to indicate that many of the flavones appear to have a tumor-inhibiting effect (Guo et al., 2010; Cárdenas et al., 2006). The substances also have a vitamin C-like activity, and large doses have been used therapeutically in patients with increased capillary fragility or permeability (Benavente-García & Castillo, 2008). While a flavonoid deficiency has been produced in animals, it has not yet been demonstrated for humans.

Phytoestrogens are plant molecules that bind to the same cell receptors as the hormone estrogen. They are most concentrated in soy, flax, whole grains, and nuts (Kris-Etherton et al., 2002). Phytoestrogens have been suggested as possible substitutes for hormone replacement therapy. Lignin, a common phytoestrogen, has been found to bind to both estrogen and progesterone receptors and to protect against the hormone-dependent breast cancers (Touillaud et al., 2007). Additional metabolic activities of phytoestrogens are topics of active research.

Lycopene is a phytonutrient most commonly found in tomatoes and watermelon. This antioxidant has demonstrated both anticancer and anti-inflammatory properties. It has been shown to reduce asthma attacks in children by reducing inflammation in the bronchioles (Sackensen et al., 2008). In combination with soy, lycopene has been shown to slow the growth of prostate cancers in both hormone-dependent and hormone-insensitive tumors (Vaishampayan et al., 2007). By inhibiting tumor growth, lycopene may have implications in the treatment and prevention of other hormone-sensitive cancers including breast and ovarian cancer. Resveratrol, a phytonutrient found in red wine, grapes, and nuts, may protect against cardiovascular disease. Research has shown it inhibits blood clot formation and has strong antioxidant properties (Kris-Etherton et al., 2002) which should help maintain blood vessel integrity and limit plaque formation. Other phenols appear to protect against type 2 diabetes by controlling blood sugar levels.

Many herbs and spices have strong antioxidant properties as well as other biological activities (Tapsell et al., 2006). Traditionally, seasonings have been strongly associated with specific cultures. Turmeric (Nandal et al., 2009) and hot peppers (Kang et al., 2007) have shown strong anti-inflammatory properties. Eating a diet high in a broad range of plant-based foods provides the best method of obtaining these beneficial chemicals. The seasonings associated with individual cultures may explain some of the epidemiological difference in disease rates, especially those diseases associated with chronic inflammation. This is by no means an exhaustive list of phytonutrients, and research continues to find both new compounds and new functions for those already identified.

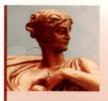

Cultural Considerations
HEALTH BENEFITS OF TWO TRADITIONAL DIETS

While obesity and its health complications plague the United States population in general, the problems are particularly severe in Native Americans and Hawaiians. Shifts in the diet from traditional foods to the "Americanized" diet are frequently blamed (Lombard et al., 2006). With the change in diet, many traditional and potentially protective foods have been replaced, often with less nutritious substitutes. However, the benefits of these traditional foods should not be underestimated. In a study of a traditional Native American diet, wild berries, including service berry (*Amelanchier* sp.) and high-bush cranberry (*Viburnum* sp.), show levels of phytochemicals capable of modifying lipid metabo-

lism, reducing blood sugar levels, and inhibiting inflammation, indicating the potential of the berries to fight type 2 diabetes (Burns Kraft et al., 2008). In recent years, programs that attempt to reintroduce traditional foods have had some success at battling health issues related to dietary shifts. The Uli'eo Koa Program reintroduced a traditional Hawaiian diet to program participants. The diet consisted of plant-based foods high in complex carbohydrates, limited amounts of protein, and less than 10 percent total fat. The program has been successful in reducing serum cholesterol and triglycerides, blood glucose levels, hypertension, and weight in program participants in Hawaii (Leslie, 2001).

SYNTHETIC FOODS

Concerns about calorie intake, the desire to avoid certain types of foods, and commercial interests have lead to the development of a variety of chemically derived substitutes for naturally occurring foods. Artificial sweeteners and synthetic fats have been available for several years. Synthetic, lab-cultured meat is currently being developed. In addition, the inclusions of genetically modified organisms have been added to the human diet. Many of these synthetic foods have raised safety concerns, but, because they are a relatively new development, the long-term implications of their inclusion in the diet are still unknown.

DIETARY GUIDES

Food availability, tradition, and personal preference all influence what people eat. The range of information about nutrition available can make determining what to eat a confusing endeavor. While there are many approaches that can be taken, one practical approach is the use of MyPlate, developed by the United States Department of Agriculture (Figure 16-10). MyPlate is tailored for sex, age, and activity level, a major change

Critical Thinking

How Do Popular Diets Stack up Nutritionally?

In the push to remain thin, many people will try anything. During the 1970s, the grapefruit diet was popular. Later, liquid protein diets were all the rage. While many of the popular diets will promote weight loss, their ability to meet the minimal requirements of vitamins and minerals remains questionable.

Research one popular diet and analyze its nutritional value—vitamins, minerals, phytonutrients, carbohydrates, proteins, and lipids. Could a person survive on that diet? What nutrients are available at adequate levels? What is it lacking?

from the basic four food groups used previously. The United States Department of Agriculture updates the dietary guidelines every 10 years, and the latest review was released in 2010.

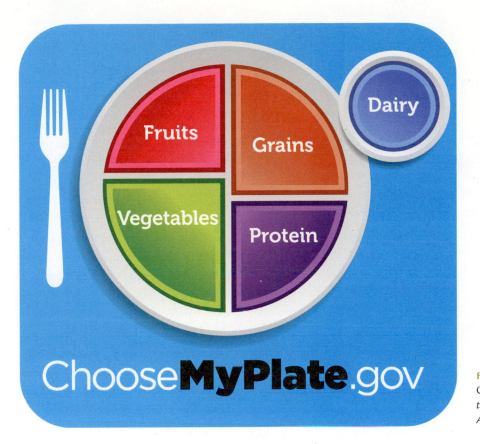

FIGURE 16-10: MyPlate Food Guidance System. *(Courtesy of the United States Department of Agriculture, www.choosemyplate.gov)*

MyPlate helps consumers by making food choice recommendations for each of five major categories. These categories are:

- Grains, half of which should be whole grains
- Vegetables
- Fruits
- Dairy
- Protein foods

The MyPlate guidelines stress a diet based on grains, fruits, vegetables, and lean proteins with minimal levels of sodium, added sugar, and saturated fats. For the average 20-year-old woman who gets 30–60 minutes of moderate exercise daily, MyPlate recommends a 2200 calorie diet with 7 ounces of grains, 3 cups of vegetables, 2 cups of fruit, 3 cups of milk, and 6 ounces split between the meat and nuts/seeds/legume groups. The average 40-year-old woman who gets less than thirty minutes of exercise daily is cut back to 1800 calories with 6 ounces of grains, 2 ½ cups of vegetables, 1 ½ cups of fruit, 3 cups of milk, and 5 ounces split between the meat and nuts/seeds/legume groups. Fats, oils, and sweets should be eaten sparingly because they provide food energy while contributing few nutrients. Coffee and tea and most herbs and spices contain few calories and can be used freely by most people. A variety of nutrition guides have been published in recent years, most with some pictorial format designed to be both familiar and easy to use. The majority of nutrition guides, no matter the country of origin, encourage a primarily plant-based diet with minimal consumption of sweets and fats.

Vegetarianism

Large numbers of people, for a wide variety of reasons, have eliminated or limit animal-based products from their diets. Using data gathered from a 2006 poll, it is estimated that there are 4.7 million adult vegetarians in the United States (Stahler, 2006). The label "vegetarian" covers a spectrum of diets. The lacto-ovo-vegetarian diet, one that includes milk, eggs, and other dairy products, provides a balance of essential amino acids and adequate vitamins and minerals. A vegan diet excludes animal products

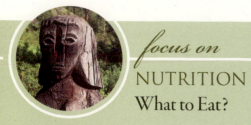

focus on

NUTRITION
What to Eat?

Walk into any bookstore and there are shelves lined with books about what to eat. Almost monthly, someone is promoting the newest fad. First, it is all carbohydrates, then no carbohydrates; unlimited meat then no meat. The diets range from reasonable and healthy to truly dangerous in their recommendations. But how to decide what is healthy?

A comparison of several different dietary guidelines from government health services, medical institutions, and current research finds several common threads. Recommendations include increasing the amount of plant-based foods (fruits, legumes, whole grains, and vegetables), replacing trans fats and animal fats with plant oils, and cutting back on added sugar and saturated fats. The United States Department of Agriculture's MyPlate includes adjustments for different age groups as well as ethnic variations. These variations are based on traditional diets combined with commonly available foods. The Native American diet includes wild rice, berries, corn, beans, squash, nopales, and game (canfit.org, 2008). The Mediterranean diet focuses on minimally processed seasonal foods, whole grains and legumes, minimal red meat, plenty of fish, and olive oil. The Asian diet is based on rice, soy products, vegetable oils, and large amounts of fresh fruits and vegetables (oldwayspt.org, 2008). A review of dietary guidelines from around the world found disagreement in serving sizes and the placement of some foods within the schemes, but overall most countries that have some form of nutritional guidelines for their citizens promote eating a broad variety of fresh produce and whole grains and minimizing fats, meats, and refined sugars (Painter et al., 2002).

in any form and relies on cereals, legumes, nuts, fruits, seeds, and vegetables. Plant-based foods are low-density foods, having relatively few calories per unit of volume. It is important to include protein-rich legumes in the diet and to combine them at the same meal with cereal grains to ensure that the essential amino acids are present. Since vitamin B_{12} is found only in foods of animal origin, a diet devoid of animal-based foods must be supplemented with vitamin B_{12}. Including almond or soy milk fortified with vitamin B_{12} or taking a supplement can prevent deficiency symptoms. Nuts and seeds play an important role in many vegetarian diets. These foods are a source of both protein and fat necessary for absorption of fat-soluble vitamins. The American Dietetic Association (ADA) and the Dietitians of Canada found that vegetarian diets are lower in cholesterol and saturated fat and higher in magnesium, potassium, folate, and antioxidant than diets high in meat, but are often low in iron. Epidemiological studies show those eating a balanced vegetarian diet have lower blood pressure, lower rates of death from heart disease, lower rates of type 2 diabetes, and lower rates of colon cancer (ADA, 2003; Meyer et al., 2006).

Fast Food versus Slow Food

In the 1950s, major changes took place in the diets of people in Europe and North America and has continued to spread across the globe. New categories of foods began to appear—"health foods," "junk foods," "fast foods," and engineered or synthetic foods. In the United States there has been a dramatic increase in the number of carryout, take away, and fast food restaurants which offer convenient and relatively inexpensive meals. Preparing meals from scratch takes time, time that a working woman may not feel she has, and convenience foods have become a major component of the diets of many people around the world. However, with few exceptions, the calories in fast food are primarily in the form of saturated and, until recently, trans fats. Fruits and vegetables rarely figure prominently in the menu of fast food restaurants, although recently there have been

Case Study

Why Am I So Tired?

Marie, a 19-year-old college student, showed up at the campus health service complaining of complete exhaustion. After falling asleep repeatedly in class despite full nights of sleep and several bouts of dizziness, her roommates convinced her that something was not right. A physical examination found her blood pressure was normal, but both her heart rate and respiratory rate were well above normal. A health history indicated no smoking, an occasional glass of wine with meals, no medications, and a vegetarian diet. She exercised regularly, walking the two miles to campus daily and playing volleyball three nights a week. However, in the last two weeks, just walking to and from campus had required frequent stops for muscle cramps and weakness. Her skin was exceedingly pale. Blood work indicated her hemoglobin levels were only 6.5g/100mL, a value well below normal, indicating she was severely anemic. Because her diet lacked red meat, a common source of iron, she was given a daily iron supplement and told to increase the iron-rich vegetables in her diet. After a week, she returned for further testing. Her hemoglobin levels had not increased, and her symptoms had not improved. The doctor suggested that she add red meat back into her diet, explaining that plant sources are a non-heme iron not well absorbed by some people. Animal sources contain heme iron which is sometimes better absorbed. Within two weeks, her energy returned, her color improved, her heart rate and breathing slowed, and her hemoglobin levels returned to normal.

1. Why does anemia produce the symptoms seen in the patient?

2. Which plant sources are iron-rich?

3. Are there plant-based foods which contain heme iron?

some shifts toward including them. The Slow Food Movement was launched in 1989, as a backlash against fast food and large agribusiness. The Slow Food Movement is now international and works to educate people about the pleasures and benefits of good food carefully prepared with locally produced foodstuffs. Promoting biodiversity and the protections of traditional and heirloom plants, members enjoy traditional foods in season. Many of the crops being protected are heirloom and local varieties of limited commercial value. These varieties ship poorly due to tender skins and short shelf life, ripen at their own pace, and are not uniform in shape, characteristics which make them undesirable to large mechanized agribusinesses and commercial food preparation companies. However, the genetic diversity, history, and rich range of flavors found in these varieties have endeared them to many people and have helped to fuel the interest in local cuisine made with seasonal, local produce.

The interest in local foods has lead to a recent increase in the number of farmers markets around the United States, and many grocery stores now carry locally grown produce (Figure 16-11). Many areas of the United States, Europe, and Japan have community-supported agriculture (CSA) farms to which an individual pays a fee in exchange for a share of the produce and other farm products. While most agribusinesses use pesticides, herbicides, and antibiotics in the production of food, CSA farms typically minimize or eliminate the use of these chemicals. The use of antibiotics as growth promoters and to prevent disease in farm animals has encouraged the development of antibiotic-resistance microbes, including some human pathogens. Many of the agricultural chemicals used in

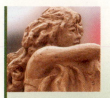

Economic Considerations
ENSURING ADEQUATE NUTRITION FOR POOR WOMEN

Let's face it, eating well can sometimes be expensive. However, there are things that women can do to ensure they get the nutrition that they need, without sacrificing their bank accounts. It is important to limit the purchasing of inexpensive, empty-calorie foods that do little to nourish the body. While the discount donuts may look appealing, they do not help the body to get the nutrients it needs to thrive. Eating healthy foods such as apples, bananas, carrots, dark leafy greens, potatoes, eggs, beans, yogurt, canned or frozen fruits, juices and vegetables, peanut butter, even whole grain bread, provides the vitamins, minerals, and fiber that are needed every day, without costing a fortune. While eating well does not have to cost a lot, the truth is that there is a price to be paid for *not* investing in good nutrition. Poor diets have been linked to many kinds of cancer, diabetes, heart disease, osteoporosis, and iron deficiency in women.

Still, there are millions of women in the United States who face serious economic challenges when trying to meet their nutritional needs. Poverty is not just about hunger, it is also about under-nutrition and inability to access the right kinds of foods. In the United States, 4.5 million Americans receive emergency food assistance in any given week, and single moms with children are more likely to face food insecurity (PBS, 2008). For these women, finding the right foods and ensuring that they get enough food can be a struggle. While food assistance programs such as the Supplemental Nutrition Assistance Program (formerly known as 'food stamps') and local food shelves can help to alleviate some of the burden, they have not been enough to ensure food security for all Americans. For women, who are often paid disproportionately lower wages than men and who often bear a greater responsibility for child care and ensuring that everyone in the family has enough to eat, rising food prices in recent years have also made it increasingly hard to make ends meet. For low-income families, food expenses are often cut so that the family can meet the costs of housing, medical care, transportation, and child care.

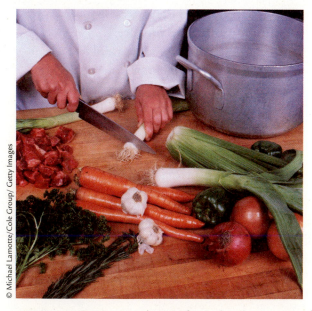

FIGURE 16-11: Concern over the use of agricultural chemicals has lead to a rise in interest in local foods and an increase in farmer's markets and grocery stores providing fresh, locally-grown foods.

large-scale production of foods leave residue on the surface of foods. A number of these chemicals have not been adequately studied to determine their long-term effects on the human body. Some, however, have been shown to act as endocrine disruptors, which mimic the natural hormones in the body, and neurotransmitters. The actions of these chemicals may have consequence on many body systems. A recent study found that two common agricultural chemicals, maneb and paraquat, increased the risk of developing Parkinson's disease (Costello et al., 2009).

CONCLUSION

A woman's body can carry out its biological functions best when it is supplied with the nutrients it needs. The current state of nutritional science has identified major nutrients, but the science continues to change as new discoveries are made. A woman can have a dramatic impact on her health by choosing a healthy diet. However, much is still unknown about the relationships between what a woman eats and chronic diseases such as cancer and diabetes. Consider genetic differences between individuals, and it becomes clear that there is no one nutritional pathway that can guarantee a longer life span, free from cancer, diabetes, or heart disease. However, consuming adequate nutrients from a wide variety of foods, choosing healthier fats rather than unhealthy ones, and increasing the number of plant-based foods are well-documented ways of pursuing a healthy lifestyle.

REVIEW QUESTIONS

1. What is an incomplete protein?

2. What foods should someone eat to increase the amount of omega-3 fatty acids in the diet?

3. What are the functions of calcium in the body?

4. Why do high levels of vitamin A pose a risk?

5. Based on MyPlate, the healthiest diets get the majority of their calories from which foods?

6. Which vitamin is now used to enrich breads, cereals, and pastas to help prevent neural tube defects?

CRITICAL THINKING QUESTIONS

1. Why must vegans and vegetarians take care to balance their protein intake? How is this done?

2. Why is having an abundance of food and calories not necessarily a guarantee of good nutrition?

3. Women have nutritional needs different from men. Identify three of these and explain why women need different levels of these nutrients than men.

WEBLINKS

California Adolescent Nutrition and Fitness Program (CANFIT)
   www.canfit.org
Oldways Preservation Trust
   www.oldwayspt.org
Slow Food International
   www.slowfood.com
US Department of Agriculture
   www.usda.gov

World Health Organization
   www.WHO.int
Centers for Disease Control
   www.cdc.gov
MyPlate
   www.choosemyplate.gov

REFERENCES

Adler, U. C., Marques, A. H., & Calil, H. M. (2008). Inflammatory aspects of depression. *Inflammation & Allergy - Drug Targets, 7*(1), 19–23.

American Dietetic Association. (2003, June). Position of the American Dietetic Association and Dieticians of Canada: Vegetarian diets.

Journal of the American Dietetic Association, 103(6), 748–765.

American Heart Association. (2008). Facts about women and cardiovascular diseases. Retrieved May 15, 2008 from http://www.americanheart.org/presenter.jhtml?identifier=2876.

Benavente-García, O., & Castillo, J. (2008). Update on uses and properties of citrus flavonoids: New findings in anticancer, cardiovascular, and anti-inflammatory activity. *Journal of Agricultural and Food Chemistry, 56*(15), 6185–6205.

Broun, E. R., Greist, A., Tricot, G., & Hoffman, R. (1990). Excessive zinc ingestion. A reversible cause of sideroblastic anemia and bone marrow depression. *Journal of the American Medical Association, 264*(11), 1441–1443.

Burns Kraft, T. F., Dey, M., Rogers, R. B., Ribnicky, D. M., Gipp, D. M., Cefalu, W.T., Raskin, I., & Lila, M. A. (2008). Phytochemical composition and metabolic performance-enhancing activity of dietary berries traditionally used by native North Americans. *Journal of Agricultural Food Chemistry, 56*(3), 654–660.

Cárdenas, M., Marder, M., Blank, V. C., & Roguin, L. P. (2006). Antitumor activity of some natural flavonoids and synthetic derivatives on various human and murine cancer cell lines. *Bioorganic & Medicinal Chemistry, 14*(9), 2966–2971.

Cochrane, W. A. (1965). Overnutrition in prenatal and neonatal life: A problem. *Canadian Medical Association Journal, 93*, 893–896.

Colin, A., Reggers, J., Castronovo, V., & Ansseau, M. (2003). Lipids, depression and suicide. *Encephale, 29*(1), 49–58.

Corwin, E. (2008). *Handbook of pathophysiology* (3rd ed.). Philadelphia, PA: Lippincott Williams, & Wilkins.

Costello, S., Cockburn, M., Bronstein, J., Zhang, X., & Ritz, B. (2009). Parkinson's disease and residential exposure to maneb and paraquat from agricultural applications in the central valley of California. *American Journal of Epidemiology, 169*(8), 919–926.

Cushnie, T. P., & Lamb, A. J. (2005). Antimicrobial activity of flavonoids. *International Journal of Antimicrobial Agents, 26*(5), 343–356.

Guo, W., Wei, X., Wu, S., Wang, L., Peng, H., Wang, J., & Fang, B. (2010). Antagonistic effect of flavonoids on NSC-741909-mediated antitumor activity via scavenging of reactive oxygen species. *European Journal of Pharmacology, 649*(1–3), 51–58.

Holick, C. N., Michaud, D. S., Stolzenberg-Solomon, R., Mayne, S. T., Pietinen, P., Taylor, P. R., Virtamo, J., & Albanes, D. (2002). Dietary carotenoids, serum beta-carotene, and retinol and risk of lung cancer in the alpha-tocopherol, beta-carotene cohort study. *American Journal of Epidemiology, 156*(6), 536–547.

Huang, H. Y., Caballero, B., Chang, S., Alberg, A., Semba, R., Schneyer, C., Wilson, R. F., Cheng, T. Y., Prokopowicz, G., Barnes, G. J., 2nd, Vassy, J., & Bass, E. B. (2006). Multivitamin/mineral supplements and prevention of chronic disease. *Evidence Report - Technology Assessment (Full Report)* (139), 1–117.

Kang, J. H., Kim, C. S., Han, I. S., Kawada, T., & Yu, R. (2007). Capsaicin, a spicy component of hot peppers, modulates adipokine gene expression and protein release from obese-mouse adipose tissues and isolated adipocytes, and suppresses the inflammatory responses of adipose tissue macrophages. *FEBS Letters, 581*(23), 4389–4396.

Kris-Etherton, P. M., Hecker, K. D., Bonanome, A., Coval, S. M., Binkoski, A. E., Hilpert, K. F., Griel, A. E., & Etherton, T. D. (2002). Bioactive compounds in foods: Their role in the prevention of cardiovascular disease and cancer. *American Journal of Medicine, 113*(Suppl. 9B), 71S–88S.

Leslie, J. H. (2001). Uli'eo Koa Program: Incorporating a traditional Hawaiian dietary component. *Pacific Health Dialog, 8*(2), 401–406.

Lombard, K. A., Forster-Cox, S., Smeal, D., & O'Neill, M. K. (2006, Oct-Dec). Diabetes on the Navajo nation: What role can gardening and agriculture extension play to reduce it? *Rural Remote Health, 6*(4), 640.

Lussana, F., Zighetti, M. L., Bucciarelli, P., Cugno, M., & Cattaneo, M. (2003). Blood levels of homocysteine, folate, vitamin B6 and B12 in women using oral contraceptives compared to non-users. *Thrombosis Research, 112*(1-2), 37–41.

Martin, C. M. (2008). Omega-3 fatty acids: Proven benefit or just a "fish story"? *Consultant Pharmacist, 23*(3), 210–221.

Mayo Clinic Health Letter. (2006). April 24(4), 7.

Meyer, T. E., Kovács, S. J., Ehsani, A. A., Klein, S., Holloszy, J. O., & Fontana, L. (2006). Long-term caloric restriction ameliorates the decline in diastolic function in humans. *Journal of the American College of Cardiology, 47*(2), 398–402.

Nandal, S., Dhir, A., Kuhad, A., Sharma, S., & Chopra, K. (2009). Curcumin potentiates the anti-inflammatory activity of cyclooxygenase inhibitors in the cotton pellet granuloma pouch model. *Methods & Findings in Experimental & Clinical Pharmacology, 31*(2), 89–93.

National Academy of Sciences. (2004). *Dietary reference intakes.* Washington, DC: National Academy Press.

O'Keefe, J. H., Gheewala, N. M., & O'Keefe, J. O. (2008). Dietary strategies for improving postprandial glucose, lipids, inflammation, and cardiovascular health. *Journal of the American College of Cardiology, 51,* 249–255.

Painter, J., Rah, J. H., & Lee, Y. K. (2002). Comparison of international food guide pictorial representations. *Journal of the American Dietetic Association, 102*(4), 483–489.

Moyers, B. (2008, April 11). Hunger in America (television series episode). In B. Moyers, *Bill Moyers journal.* Washington, DC: Public Broadcasting System.

Pollan, M. (2008). *In defense of food: An eater's manifesto.* New York, NY: Penguin Press.

Rattan, J., Levin, N., Graff, E., Weizer, N., & Gilat, T. (1981). A high-fiber diet does not cause mineral and nutrient deficiencies. *Journal of Clinical Gastroenterology, 3*(4), 389–393.

Reedy, J., & Krebs-Smith, S. M. (2008). A comparison of food-based recommendations and nutrient values of three food guides: USDA's MyPyramid, NHLBI's dietary approaches to stop hypertension eating plan, and Harvard's healthy eating pyramid. *Journal of the American Dietetic Association, 108*(3), 522–528.

Reisner, R. (2008, January 10). The diet industry: A big fat lie. Retrieved March 19, 2009 from http://www.businessweek.com/debateroom/archives/2008/03/the_diet_industry_a_big_fat_lie.html.

Rousseau, A. S., Hininger, I., Palazzetti, S., Faure, H., Roussel, A. M., & Margaritis, I. (2004). Antioxidant vitamin status in high exposure to oxidative stress in competitive athletes. *British Journal of Nutrition, 92*(3), 461–468.

Rousset, X., Vaisman, B., Amar, M., Sethi, A. A., & Remaley, A. T. (2009). Lecithin: Cholesterol acyltransferase–from biochemistry to role in cardiovascular disease. *Current Opinion in Endocrinology, Diabetes & Obesity, 16*(2), 163–171.

Sackesen, C., Ercan, H., Dizdar, E., Soyer, O., Gumus, P., Tosun, B. N., Büyüktuncer, Z., Karabulut, E., Besler, T., & Kalayci, O. (2008). A comprehensive evaluation of the enzymatic and nonenzymatic antioxidant systems in childhood asthma. *Journal of Allergy and Clinical Immunology, 122*(1), 78–85.

Sadiq Butt, M., Tahir-Nadeem, M., Khan, M. K., Shabir, R., & Butt, M. S. (2008). Oat: Unique among the cereals. *European Journal of Nutrition, 47*(2), 68–79.

Schwartz, G. G., & Skinner, H. G. (2007). Vitamin D status and cancer: New insights. *Current Opinion in Clinical Nutrition & Metabolic Care, 10*(1), 6–11.

Siegel, C., Barker, B., & Kunstadter, M. (1982). Conditioned oral scurvy due to megavitamin C withdrawal. *Journal of Periodontology, 53*(7), 453.

Simopoulos, A. P. (2007). Omega-3 fatty acids and athletics. *Current Sports Medicine Reports, 6*(4), 230–236.

Snow, J. T., & Harris, M. B. (1989). Disordered eating in southwestern Pueblo Indians and Hispanics. *Journal of Adolescence, 12*(30), 329–334.

Soerjomataram, I., Louwman, W. J., Lemmens, V. E., Coebergh, J. W., & de Vries, E. (2008). Are patients with skin cancer at lower risk of developing colorectal or breast cancer? *American Journal of Epidemiology, 167*(12), 1421–1429.

Stahler, C. (2006). How many adults are vegetarians? *Vegetarian Journal, 4.*

Tapsell, L. C., Hemphill, I., Cobiac, L., Patch, C. S., Sullivan, D. R., Fenech, M., Roodenrys, S., Keogh, J. B., Clifton, P. M., Williams, P. G., Fazio, V. A., & Inge, K. E. (2006). Health benefits of herbs and spices: The past, the present, the future. *Medical Journal of Australia, 185*(4 Suppl), S4–24.

Touillaud, M. S., Thiébaut, A. C., Fournier, A., Niravong, M., Boutron-Ruault, M. C., & Clavel-Chapelon, F. (2007). Dietary lignan intake and postmenopausal breast cancer risk by estrogen and progesterone receptor status. *Journal of the National Cancer Institute, 99*(6), 475–486.

United States Department of Agriculture and U. S. Department of Health and Human Services. (2010). *Dietary guidelines for Americans, 2010* (7th ed.). Washington, DC: U.S. Government Printing Office.

United States Federal Trade Commission. (2004, November). FTC - Weighing the evidence in diet ads. Retrieved March 31, 2009 from http://www.ftc.gov/bcp/edu/pubs/consumer/health/hea03.pdf.

Vaishampayan, U., Hussain, M., Banerjee, M., Seren, S., Sarkar, F. H., Fontana, J., Forman, J. D., Cher, M. L., Powell, I., Pontes, J. E., & Kucuk, O. (2007). Lycopene and soy isoflavones in the treatment of prostate cancer. *Nutrition and Cancer, 59*(1), 1–7.

Waladkhani, A. R., & Hellhammer, J. (2008). Dietary modification of brain function: Effects on neuroendocrine and psychological determinants of mental health- and stress-related disorders. *Advances in Clinical Chemistry, 45,* 99–138.

Wang, L., Manson, J. E., Buring, J. E., Lee, I. M., & Sesso, H. D. (2008). Dietary intake of dairy products, calcium, and vitamin D and the risk of hypertension in middle-aged and older women. *Hypertension, 51*(4), 1073–1079.

WHO Report. (2007). Cardiovascular disease. Retrieved February 10, 2009 from http://www.who.int/mediacentre/factsheets/fs317/en/index.html

Young, G. S., Conquer, J. A., & Thomas, R. (2005). Effect of randomized supplementation with high dose olive, flax or fish oil on serum phospholipid fatty acid levels in adults with attention deficit hyperactivity disorder. *Reproductive Nutrition Development, 45*(5), 549–558.

WOMEN AND STRESS

INTRODUCTION

Stress has always been a part of life. To deal with the stress, animals evolved coping mechanisms, physiological responses designed to protect the body from threats and then re-establish homeostasis. The human body makes use of the sympathetic and parasympathetic divisions of the nervous system to accomplish this. Under normal circumstances, activation of the sympathetic response helped an animal escape or defend itself—the classic "fight-or-flight" response. Once the threat passed, the parasympathetic response countered the changes and returned the body to a more relaxed state.

Threats in today's world have expanded beyond those of the past to include global issues such as climate change, pandemics, and economic hardships. Many women are part of the "sandwich generation", caught between caring for their children and aging parents while working to support themselves (Statistics Canada, 2004). In the United States, women make up 56.2 percent of the workforce, with 75 percent of women working full time, yet women, on average, earn less than men (United States Department of Labor, 2010). This places a greater financial stress on women, particularly female heads of households (Figure 17-1). Demands on a woman's

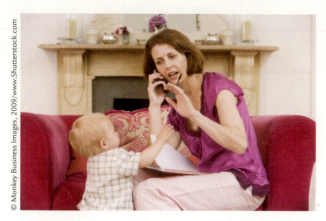

FIGURE 17-1: Women today experience significant stress as they are pulled by their many responsibilities both at home and in the work world.

time can, also, be a source of stress. Even when they work full time outside the home, women are still responsible for the majority of housework—17 hours per week for women versus 12 hours for men (Mixon, 2008).

Modern life is stressful, but the traditional outlets for stress—run or fight—are less viable today. Stress-related diseases can occur when there are no outlets for stress and the body cannot return to homeostatic levels. One significant aspect of stress-related disease is how an individual perceives and interprets the stressor. Each person responds to stress differently. Something that is devastatingly stressful for one person could be seen as unimportant to another or even pleasurable to a third. How the body copes with stress has a major impact on a person's health.

TYPES OF STRESS

Physical stressors include those things which have a direct effect on the body and alter its function through excessive demands on or damage to the body. Childbirth and extreme sports are common examples of physical stressors. Physical trauma, starvation, and prolonged illness are examples of physical stressors. Psychological stressors do not cause direct physical changes to the body, but, instead, influence thought processes or emotions. Concerns about finances, personal or professional relationships, and family issues should not be physically damaging in and of themselves, but they produce a stress response that is similar to that caused by a physical stressor. Not all

psychological stressors are associated with threatening or unpleasant situations. Weddings and births are considered joyous events, but they can also produce stress.

The duration of a stressful situation can influence the extent of its effects. **Acute stress** is a response to a single event, and its effects are short term. A fire alarm going off or a suspenseful movie can cause an acute stress response. The sympathetic nervous system activates, and the hormone **adrenalin**, or **epinephrine**, floods into the bloodstream, increasing the heart and respiratory rates. However, homeostatic mechanisms return the body to baseline levels within moments after the stressor is removed. **Chronic stress** takes place over an extended period of time, and the effects are longer lasting. A woman balancing the care of her young children with the care of her aging parents while working full-time may experience chronic stress. This situation can last for years. The pain caused by chronic disease or injury can also cause chronic stress. Post-traumatic stress disorder (PTSD) is a form of chronic stress response that results from an acute stress response that the body keeps reliving long after the initial traumatic event has passed.

THE FIGHT-OR-FLIGHT RESPONSE

Whatever the cause, the body's response to stress follows a predicable pattern. The nervous and endocrine systems coordinate a series of physiological actions aimed at minimizing the potential damage of stress on the body and re-establishing the homeostatic balance.

Actions of the Sympathetic Nervous System

Within moments of perceiving a stress, the sympathetic nervous system releases a surge of adrenalin that travels throughout the body. Under the influence of adrenalin, several changes occur that comprise what is called the fight-or-flight response. Adrenalin increases the heart rate and blood pressure. Blood vessels respond to adrenalin, increasing the blood flow to the heart, brain, and skeletal muscles while decreasing blood flow to the digestive system and skin. In the lungs, the bronchioles dilate and the respiratory rate increases. These changes increase gas exchange and allow more oxygen into the blood while increasing the removal of carbon dioxide. Adrenalin also decreases insulin secretion from the pancreas. This is coupled with an increase in secretion of the hormones glucagon and cortisol which increase blood sugar levels. The combination makes more energy available to fuel the skeletal muscles and nervous system.

Stimulation of the sympathetic nervous system also activates the **hypothalamic-pituitary-adrenal (HPA) axis** (Figure 17-2). This leads to the release of a collection of interconnected hormones, including the primary stress hormone **cortisol**, that support the nervous system's responses to stress (Charmandari et al., 2005).

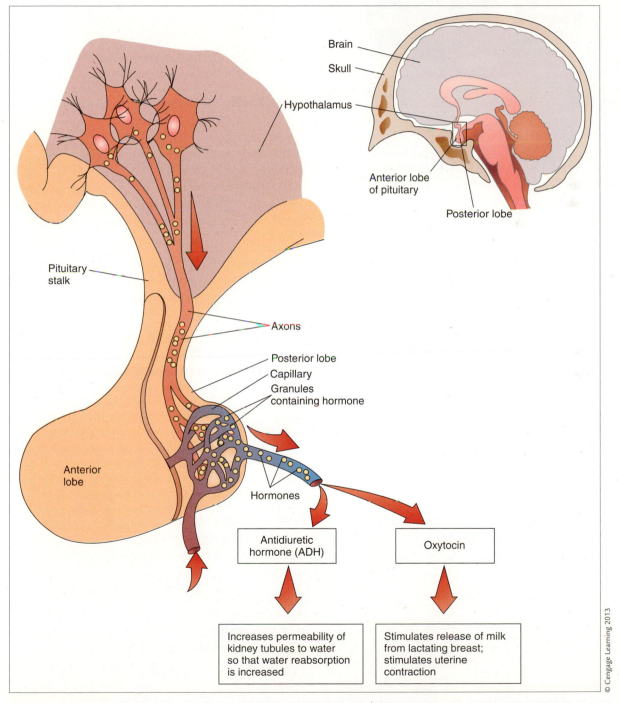

FIGURE 17-2: Secretions from the hypothalamus travel to the pituitary causing the release of other hormones, which have effects throughout the body.

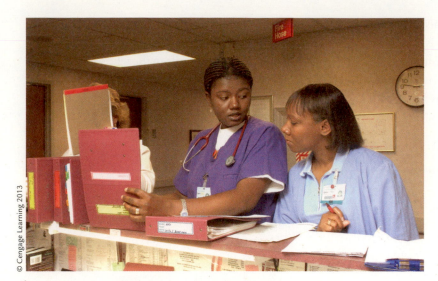

© Cengage Learning 2013

FIGURE 17-3: When women encounter stress, for example in a high-stress occupation, they are more likely to seek social interactions to help provide a calming effect.

THE ACTIONS OF THE PARASYMPATHETIC NERVOUS SYSTEM

The parasympathetic nervous system is responsible for re-establishing homeostasis after a stressful situation has passed. Stimulation of the parasympathetic system lowers the heart rate, lowers blood pressure, and reduces the respiratory rate. Hormones associated with the parasympathetic response include **endorphins** and oxytocin.

Research has suggested that, especially in women, endorphins are associated with increased socialization. When experiencing stress, women are more likely than men to seek out others, a behavior referred to as "tend and befriend" (Talyor, 2003). These social interactions produce a calming effect which helps to counter the negative effects of stress (Figure 17-3). Endorphins can also block pain and are responsible for producing the "runner's high" experienced by some athletes. They also decrease blood pressure and inhibit the stress response of the HPA axis (Drolet et al., 2001).

Another hormone which mitigates the effects of stress on the HPA axis is oxytocin. Oxytocin is released from the pituitary as a result of nervous

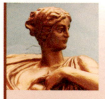

Cultural Considerations
LIVING TO BE 100

For many years, research has focused on how to lengthen the human lifespan. Robbins (2006) studied populations with unusually long, healthy lifespans and found that these populations shared a number of common characteristics including reduced stress levels, a plant-based diet, and physically and socially active lifestyles. Consider the Abkhasians of the Caucasus Mountains, where people typically live to be over 100 years old. Abkhasians usually live without the schedules and deadlines that are so common in other parts of the world. Their celebrations focus on enjoying the company of friends and family rather than gorging on fattening foods. In addition, they are lacto-vegetarians and base their diet on fermented milk and plant-based foods. Even the elderly continue to work the land, interacting with and helping out neighbors daily. Strong social support networks form the framework for nearly every activity, and domestic violence is almost unheard of. For the people of Abkhasia, good friends, healthy food, and taking the time to enjoy life appear to be major keys to a very long and healthy life.

system stimulation. Women typically produce higher levels of oxytocin than men do. This hormone is involved in both labor and nursing and is associated with nurturing behaviors. Higher levels of oxytocin trigger social bonding, and women under stressful conditions secrete more oxytocin and tend to seek friends for support. Men, on the other hand, secrete lower levels of oxytocin and exhibit less social behaviors and increased aggression when placed under stressful conditions (Taylor et al., 2006). Increased oxytocin levels also inhibit the activity of the **amygdala** (Baumgartner et al., 2008). The amygdala's role in processing emotional memories, specifically traumatic memories, would be decreased when oxytocin is present, dampening the effect of the stressor and helping the body to cope. The ability of oxytocin to alter memories may be responsible for the reduced memories of pain associated with giving birth.

THE CHRONIC STRESS RESPONSE

While endorphin secretion produces pleasurable sensations and lessens the effects of acute stress, chronic exposure to stressors can actually lower endorphin levels. As endorphin levels are depleted, the perception of physical pain may increase. This increased perception of pain is one of the common symptoms of chronic stress (Ribeiro et al., 2006). Stress has been identified as a contributing factor to conditions associated with chronic pain, including fibromyalgia (Bradley, 2009), headache, and shoulder and neck pain (Leistad et al., 2008).

Under chronic stress conditions, the sympathetic nervous system also triggers the release of **neuropeptide Y (NPY)**. NPY causes blood vessels to constrict and may contribute to the increase in chronic high blood pressure associated with long-term stress. In addition, NPY acts as a growth factor, leading to increased replication of the cells that line blood vessels. This causes narrowing of the vessels, which contributes to increased blood pressure. In studies of rats exposed to chronic stress, injured vessels underwent such extensive cell growth that some sealed closed (Li et al., 2005).

Endocrine Response to Stress

The hormones associated with the HPA axis form the primary endocrine response to stress. The pituitary gland releases adrenocorticotropic hormone (ACTH) and antidiuretic hormone (ADH). ACTH travels to the adrenal gland triggering the release of glucocorticosteroids, most notably cortisol. Cortisol primes the body to respond to stressors and affects nearly every system in the body. Under the influence of cortisol, peripheral tissues decrease their glucose uptake while the liver increases its conversion of fats into glucose, raising blood sugar levels and making glucose available to core organs such as the heart and brain, as well as providing the raw materials for cell division and repair. Cortisol also temporarily suppresses the immune system, decreasing inflammation, inhibiting production of white blood cells, and limiting the activity of both B-cells and T-cells, which decreases antibody production. Elevated levels of cortisol suppress the secretion of the reproductive hormone GnRH. This can reduce fertility due to decreased sperm and testosterone production in men and ovulatory inhibition and disrupted reproductive cycles in women.

While cortisol is the hormone most associated with stress, several other hormones are influenced by stress. Antidiuretic hormone (ADH) secretion increases under the influence of stress and causes the kidneys to retain more water. Animal studies have shown that estrogen exerts some control over ADH secretion (Ghuman et al., 2008) and is one potential factor in the differing response to stress both between the sexes and at different points in the reproductive cycle. Under stress conditions, aldosterone secretion increases. Aldosterone coordinates with ADH to control blood pressure. However, research shows that, under stress conditions, aldosterone impairs the normal reflex, interfering with the normal blood pressure response (Monahan, Leuenberger, & Ray, 2007). The loss of this control mechanism contributes to the high blood pressure characteristic of stress.

General Adaptation Syndrome

The body's response to stress can be divided into a three-stage process referred to as **general adaptation syndrome (GAS)** (Figure 17-4). The initial, or alarm, phase of the stress response is the fight-or-flight response, which initiates the sympathetic response in an attempt to protect the body from the perceived threat. This is followed by the resistance phase during

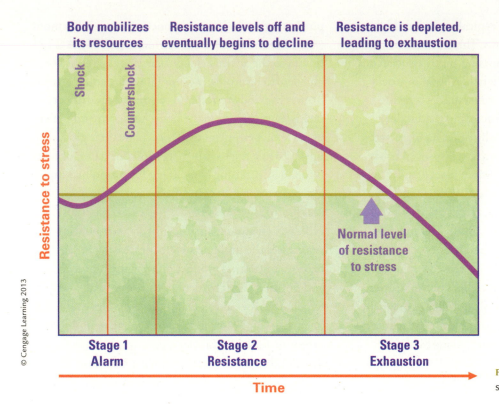

Body mobilizes its resources

Resistance levels off and eventually begins to decline

Resistance is depleted, leading to exhaustion

Resistance to stress

Shock

Countershock

Normal level of resistance to stress

Stage 1
Alarm

Stage 2
Resistance

Stage 3
Exhaustion

Time

© Cengage Learning 2013

FIGURE 17-4: General adaptation syndrome (GAS).

which the compensation mechanisms triggered during the alarm phase return to homeostasis. If, however, the stressful situation persists, the body may enter the exhaustion phase. During exhaustion, homeostasis cannot be reliably maintained, leaving the body vulnerable to stress-related illnesses.

STRESS-RELATED ILLNESS

Under normal circumstances, acute stress resolves itself quickly without serious consequences. However, chronic stress is associated with a variety of illnesses primarily related to the effects of elevated levels of circulating cortisol and a prolonged sympathetic response. The majority of these diseases fall into the following categories—neuropsychiatric diseases, cardiovascular disease, endocrine disruptions, digestive disturbances, immune system disorders, and musculoskeletal conditions.

Neuropsychiatric Diseases

The influence of stress on emotions and behavior is something nearly everyone has experienced at some time in their lives. The role of the nervous system in

the stress response makes it particularly vulnerable to stress-related disease. Under stressful conditions, the brain releases chemical messengers that cause localized inflammation. Unlike other organs of the body, outward swelling of the brain is limited by the skull. As inflammation increases, the spaces within the brain are compressed, decreasing blood flow to some areas of the brain at a time when the metabolic demands of the brain cells are increasing, potentially leading to the death of some cells. This inflammation and cell death are recognized as contributing factors in depression, schizophrenia, and post-traumatic stress disorder (García-Bueno et al., 2008). Other behavioral changes associated with chronic stress include increased aggression, an inability to concentrate, and alterations in memory, which are functions associated with the amygdala (Phelps & LeDoux, 2005).

Research indicates that men and women process stress, particularly emotional stress, differently (Kilpatrick et al., 2006), and these differences contribute to the difference in how stress manifests differently between the sexes. Depression, mood swings, and anxiety are more common in women who

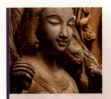

Social Considerations
PTSD AND NEUROLOGICAL CHANGES

Trauma, either physical or emotional, triggers a stress response. As homeostatic mechanisms repair the body, a person may recover from the trauma with no lasting effects. Some individuals, however, are unable to recover, reliving the trauma again and again in a condition described as post-traumatic stress disorder (PTSD). While much of the recent media coverage of PTSD is associated with returning veterans, combat is not the only cause of this disorder. In a study of homeless teens, more than a third were diagnosed with PTSD (Whitbeck et al., 2007). Natural disasters, childhood trauma, or sexual assault—anything which produces a severe emotional trauma—can trigger this condition. In response to new stressors,

individuals suffering from PTSD secrete higher levels of cortisol and norepinephrine. **Norepinephrine** has many roles as a hormone and a neurotransmitter and can alter brain chemistry in ways that lead to increased activity in the amygdala. In addition, individuals with PTSD appear to have a higher than normal sensitivity to cortisol, serotonin, and dopamine, resulting in changes in behavior and memory (Grossman et al., 2006). PTSD also appears to produce structural changes in the brain, most noticeably a decrease in the volume of the hippocampus, a region of the brain located adjacent to the amygdala (Bremner et al., 2008). The hippocampus is involved in memory processing.

---

experience chronic stress. Men, however, are more likely to respond using a self-rewarding behavior such as alcohol use or other cravings (Chaplin et al., 2008) or to respond aggressively to stress (Verona et al., 2007), striking out at those around them.

Cardiovascular Disease

Under stressful conditions, blood pressure and cardiac output both increase as a result of sympathetic stimulation. When stress becomes chronic, there is an increased risk of heart attack or stroke. Some individuals develop arrhythmias, or irregular heart beats. Blood vessels become less responsive to changes in blood pressure under the influence of HPA axis hormones. Elevated C-reactive protein levels in the blood indicate systemic inflammation and are associated with an increased risk for cardiovascular disease. Both LDL and C-reactive protein levels increase with chronic stress. Higher LDL levels are associated with the development of plaques within the vessel walls, which contribute to the risk of cardiovascular disease. Narrowed vessels may limit blood flow to the heart muscle and cause angina pectoralis, a cramp in the heart muscle due to inadequate blood flow.

Endocrine Disruptions

As described earlier, the stress response involves the HPA axis. The hypothalamus, pituitary, and adrenal glands release multiple hormones, some associated directly with the stress response, some not directly related, but still influenced by HPA axis hormones. Rosmond (2003) has linked stress-related disruptions of the normal HPA axis function with both the accumulation of fat in the abdomen and with type II diabetes. Leptin, a hormone secreted by fat cells, influences both eating and metabolism, interacting with NPY and cortisol (Kyrou & Tsigos, 2006). A low level of leptin or insensitivity to the hormone contributes to stress-induced obesity through uncontrolled eating and altered metabolism. Growth hormone levels initially increase after an acute stress event. Growth hormone triggers cell division that would help repair tissues damaged during an acute stress event. However, prolonged stress decreases growth hormone levels. This would slow healing, decrease metabolism, and inhibit cell division. In children exposed to chronic stress, this inhibition of growth hormone secretion leads to a condition called failure to thrive (Skuse et al., 1996). Other endocrine disruptions associated with stress include disruptions of the reproductive cycle, infertility, type II diabetes, and dysfunction of the HPA axis.

Digestive Conditions

Common stress-related conditions affecting the digestive system include inflammatory bowel disease, aggravation of ulcers and Crohn's disease, and peristaltic disruptions resulting in either diarrhea or constipation. Eating disorders, including obesity, bulimia, and anorexia, can occur when chronic stress alters the hormone balance of the HPA axis. Cortisol also encourages fat breakdown in the peripheral tissues and increases fat deposition in the trunk and abdomen. Increased cortisol works in concert with NPY and insulin (Adam & Epel, 2007). Stress eating appears to be influenced by alterations to endorphin, cortisol, leptin, insulin, and NPY levels. Research by Adam and Epel (2007) suggests that interactions between these hormones can lead to obesity by altering fat storage and glucose metabolism and by triggering overeating.

Immune System Disorders

Cortisol has both anti-inflammatory and immunosuppressive effects in the body. Suppression of the immune system conserves proteins that can then be used for clotting factors, enzymes, and energy—more immediate protein demands, which are needed during an acute stress response. However, long-term immunosuppression leaves a person vulnerable to disease. Chronic stress and the associated higher cortisol levels predispose individuals to infections. For example, students frequently become ill after the stress of final exams. In contrast, Nelson et al., (2008) found that reducing stress levels strengthened the immune system by increasing helper T white blood cell populations in women with cervical cancer.

Under conditions of chronic stress, additional cortisol receptors are activated throughout the body, which may actually increase rather than decrease inflammation and aggravate autoimmune conditions. Asthma, an excessive inflammatory response which narrows the bronchioles, is more common in women than in men. While a number of factors contribute to asthma, estrogen, progesterone, and stress appear to be major factors in determining the severity of the disease, most likely due to their influence on immune function (Melgert et al., 2007). Thyroid dysfunction, rheumatoid arthritis, and cancer are also linked to disruption of the immune system related to chronic stress.

Musculoskeletal Conditions

Muscle tension is a common response to stress. Tension headaches and muscle pain typically occur

---

Case Study

Sandwich Generation

A 48-year-old woman goes to her doctor with symptoms of insomnia, headache, and difficulty remembering things. She has been coming down with every cold her children bring home from school. The doctor finds her blood pressure is elevated and the she has gained weight since her last visit. The doctor asks about her home life. She comments that she has been experiencing more stress than usual lately. Her husband is an over-the-road truck driver and is frequently away from home for extended periods of time. One of her children is playing on a traveling soccer team and also plays with the band at school.

Her twins, age 12, are in dance lessons and a school play. Her elderly mother-in-law moved in with them about five months earlier after her husband of nearly 60 years passed away. With all the added responsibilities, she has had to cut back her hours at a very competitive ad agency and has even turned down a promotion. Her reduced hours at work have contributed to financial strain in the family.

1. What are the stressors in this woman's life?

2. What physiological causes lead to the symptoms?

How Much Stress Is Too Much?

The level of stress a person can experience before it does harm remains an important question. In a study of medical students, many working between 70-80 hours per week, nearly half suffered from extremely high levels of stress. In general, the more hours worked, the greater the level of stress experienced by the student. Higher levels of stress often corresponded with unhealthy coping strategies, including drug and alcohol abuse (Kasi et al., 2007). In addition, the study found that the students' stress level also put their patients at risk. Stressed residents were more likely to make errors and to compromise patient care (Pitt et al., 2004).

What can be done to reduce the impact of stress on medical students and others in high stress positions? Physiologically, why would individuals in chronic high stress situations be more prone to drug or alcohol abuse?

as a result of the sympathetic response. If the body tenses, preparing to fight or run, but there is no opportunity to release the tension, muscle readiness can become muscle pain. The pain associated with chronic stress can aggravate conditions such as **fibromyalgia,** a condition characterized by fatigue, sleep disruptions, and chronic pain The pain often radiates out from one of the tender points used for diagnosing the condition. Women have more tender points, more morning fatigue, and more pain in general with the condition than men (Yunus, 2001). The exact cause of the condition is unknown, but one study found individuals with fibromyalgia had abnormalities in the hippocampus and its response to estrogen (Emad et al., 2008) perhaps explaining why this condition affects women 10 times more often than men.

Human behavior in response to stressors is variable, so it is impossible to determine precisely how stress influences human illness. As new research explores the impact of stress on the body and the role other factors such as environment, genetics, and culture, play in the stress response, it is possible that additional stress-related illnesses will be identified.

COPING WITH STRESS

Each person copes with stress in their own manner—sometimes in beneficial ways and sometimes not. Some find that physical releases and exercise reduces stress. Others may choose less healthy coping mechanisms such as chain smoking, alcohol, or drugs. How a person manages stress by developing coping mechanisms plays an important role in mitigating the negative impacts of stress on the body (Dimsdale, 2008). In a study of hypertensive African-American women, therapeutic massage and breathing exercises helped to reduce blood pressure (Jefferson, 2010). Variation in the body's response may explain why stress-reduction methods employed by one individual are ineffective in another. There is no one "perfect" coping strategy when dealing with stress.

Physical Activity

Physical activity provides a healthy outlet for the fight-or-flight response (Figure 17-5). Research has demonstrated that regular exercise lessens the negative effects of stress on the body. With regular exercise, the body becomes less sensitive to stress

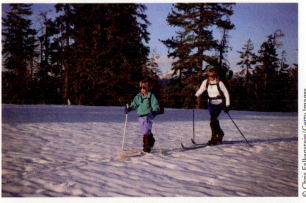

FIGURE 17-5: Regular physical activity can help the body better cope with stress.

© Chris Falkenstein/Getty Images

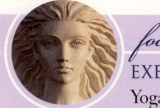

focus on

EXERCISE
Yoga and Stress Reduction

Many sports programs now include yoga as a component of their training. Styles of yoga range from the gentle, almost meditative Hatha to the perpetually moving, intense workout of Ashtanga, with many variations between. Each style has asanas, or poses, that focus on stretching, muscle control, and breathing, providing an excellent workout (Figure 17-6). Yoga has been shown to reduce stress in individuals who show stress-related conditions. In one study, as little as 10 days of training in yoga produced a significant reduction in anxiety (Gupta et al., 2006). In addition to the reduction in anxiety levels, measureable improvements in other stress-related conditions can result. For individuals with coronary artery disease, a six-week course of yoga training was found to lower heart rate, blood pressure, and body mass index. In addition, there was improvement in the ability of participants' arteries to respond to the circulatory challenges and reestablish homeostasis.

(Tsatsoulis & Fountoulakis, 2006). This, in turn, limits the metabolic aberrations associated with stress and reduces the chances of developing stress-related disease conditions. Exercise also increases the body's sensitivity to insulin, which has the effect of lowering blood sugar, and reducing the risk of type II diabetes. Cardiovascular fitness improves with regular exercise, increasing the oxygen delivery to the tissues and reducing the metabolic stresses on the body. Exercise also increases the level of endorphins, countering the fight-or-flight response.

Some people find team sports soothing. Others prefer more solitary activities such as weight training or swimming laps in the pool. Exercise need not take place in the gym. Dancing provides excellent exercise, increasing the heart rate, and working muscles. Getting outdoors for a hike or bike ride can also release stress. Many people find that gardening reduces stress and improves their mood. A recent study identified a soil microbe, *Mycobacterium vaccae*, that increases serotonin levels in the brain (University of Bristol, 2007). Serotonin is a neurotransmitter associated with mood, and increased levels improve mood, potentially helping with stress management. Gardeners working in soils with *M. vaccae* had higher levels of serotonin leading to an improved mood and feeling less stressed.

The Effects of Diet on Stress

Individuals in stressful situations often gravitate toward familiar foods such as chocolates, creamy pasta dishes, or cookies that are associated with pleasant memories. These high-sugar, high-fat, low-protein foods are termed "comfort foods", and they offer short-term benefits, but potential long-term ill effects for stress management. Eating comfort foods causes the brain to release endorphins (Gibson, 2006). High-carbohydrate, low-protein foods also increase serotonin release in the brain (Takeda et al., 2004). While eating comfort foods may have some short-term benefits, they come with a cost. Research has

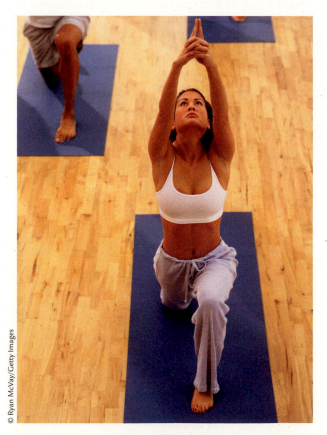

© Ryan McVay/Getty Images

FIGURE 17-6: Yoga can be an excellent work out and can reduce anxiety and stress levels.

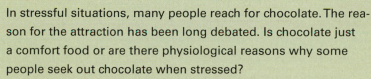

demonstrated that rats who ate high-sugar, high-fat, low-protein foods have increased glucocorticosteroid release levels which inhibit the activity of the HPA axis. This is associated with the development of belly fat in humans (Gibson, 2006).

Diet can affect the inflammatory response and influences how the body responses to stress. While some foods exacerbate the effects of chronic stress; others such as phytonutrients and omega-3 fatty acids have anti-inflammatory effects that can reduce the physiological effects of stress on the body. Waladkhani and Hellhammer (2008) suggest that diet modification be used as a coping mechanism to counteract the physiological effects of stress.

Relaxation

Any activity that engages the parasympathetic system can reduce the negative effects of stress on the body. Different people use a variety of methods for relaxing. Meditation, guided imagery, and controlled breathing work for some women. Others find escaping into a book soothing. Hobbies that engage a person's creativity can have a positive effect on heart rate and blood pressure. Many people find water soothing, whether they experience it by enjoying a soak in a bathtub, sitting by a river, or listening to a fountain (Figure 17-7). Many people find music relaxing whether performing it or listening to it.

CONCLUSION

Stress, whether emotional or physical, activates both the sympathetic nervous system and the HPA axis. While the body is designed to respond to an acute stress and then re-establish homeostasis, under the conditions of chronic stress, defensive mechanisms can overwhelm the body's coping mechanisms and trigger a series of stress-related illnesses. Finding ways to activate the parasympathetic response can mitigate these detrimental effects.

focus on
NUTRITION
Chocolate and Stress

In stressful situations, many people reach for chocolate. The reason for the attraction has been long debated. Is chocolate just a comfort food or are there physiological reasons why some people seek out chocolate when stressed?

Dark chocolate and cocoa are rich in phytonutrients such as polyphenols, sterols, and flavonoids. Typically, the darker the chocolate is, the richer it is in phytonutrients. Theobromine and methylxanthines found in dark chocolate have been shown to be psychoactive and improve mood (Smit et al., 2004). This may account for chocolate's "feel good" reputation, but the benefits go well beyond the emotional. Dark chocolate improves insulin sensitivity (Grassi et al., 2005) and helps to lower blood sugar levels in type II diabetics. One study of postmenopausal women, a group prone to cardiovascular disease, found that cocoa improved blood vessel function and lowered the levels of blood factors that promote clot formation (Wang-Polagruto et al., 2006). This can increase blood flow, lower blood pressure, and decrease the risk of heart attack and stroke. Consumption of dark chocolate with added plant sterols was found to decrease LDL levels by over five percent (Allen et al., 2008). A German study found that in individuals with slightly elevated blood pressure, small daily doses of dark chocolate lowered blood pressure and increased production of nitric oxides, a natural vasodilator (Taubert et al., 2007). Since hypertension and cardiovascular disease are common stress-related illnesses, including a small amount of dark chocolate as part of a healthy diet should benefit those experiencing stress.

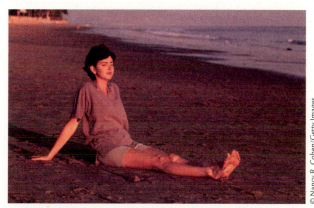

FIGURE 17-7: To reduce stress and relax, each individual should have an activity or hobby she finds soothing and enjoyable.

REVIEW QUESTIONS

1. What happens physiologically when the sympathetic nervous system is activated?

2. What are the components of the HPA axis?

3. What are some of the negative effects of stress on the body?

4. What are the major types of stressors?

CRITICAL THINKING QUESTIONS

1. Why are many stress-related illnesses difficult to treat?

2. Why won't the same coping mechanisms relieve stress for every individual?

WEBLINKS

Centers for Disease Control
www.cdc.gov (search stress management)

National Fibromyalgia Association
www.fmaware.org

REFERENCES

Adam, T. C., & Epel, E. S. (2007). Stress, eating and the reward system. *Physiology & Behavior, 91*(4), 449–458.

Allen, R. R., Carson, L., Kwik-Uribe, C., Evans, E. M., & Erdman, J. W., Jr. (2008). Daily consumption of a dark chocolate containing flavanols and added sterol esters affects cardiovascular risk factors in a normotensive population with elevated cholesterol. *Journal of Nutrition, 138*(4), 725–731.

Baumgartner, T., Heinrichs, M., Vonlanthen, A., Fischbacher, U., & Fehr, E. (2008). Oxytocin shapes the neural circuitry of trust and trust adaptation in humans. *Neuron, 58*(4), 639–650.

Bradley, L. A. (2009). Pathophysiology of fibromyalgia. *American Journal of Medicine, 122*(12 Suppl), S22–30.

Bremner, J. D., Elzinga, B., Schmahl, C., & Vermetten, E. (2008). Structural and functional plasticity of the human brain in posttraumatic stress disorder. *Progress in Brain Research, 167,* 171–186.

Chaplin, T. M., Hong, K., Bergquist, K., & Sinha, R. (2008). Gender differences in response to emotional stress: An assessment across subjective, behavioral, and physiological domains and relations to alcohol craving. *Alcoholism: Clinical & Experimental Research, 32*(7), 1242–1250.

Charmandari, E., Tsigos, C., & Chrousos, G. (2005). Endocrinology of the stress response. *Annual Review of Physiology, 67,* 259–284.

Dimsdale, J. E. (2008). Psychological stress and cardiovascular disease. *Journal of the American College of Cardiology, 51*(13), 1237–1246.

Drolet, G., Dumont, E. C., Gosselin, I., Kinkead, R., Laforest, S., & Trottier, J. F. (2001). Role of endogenous opioid system in the regulation of the stress response. *Progress in Neuro-Psychopharmacology & Biological Psychiatry, 25*(4), 729–741.

Emad, Y., Ragab, Y., Zeinhom, F., El-Khouly, G., Abou-Zeid, A., & Rasker, J. J. (2008). Hippocampus dysfunction may explain symptoms of fibromyalgia syndrome. A study with single-voxel magnetic resonance spectroscopy. *Journal of Rheumatology, 35*(7), 1371–1377.

García-Bueno, B., Caso, J. R., & Leza, J. C. (2008). Stress as a neuroinflammatory condition in brain: Damaging and protective mechanisms. *Neuroscience and Biobehavioral Reviews, 32*(6), 1132–1151.

Getting dirty may lift your mood. (2007, April 10). *ScienceDaily.* Retrieved April 29, 2009

from http://www.sciencedaily.com/
releases/2007/04/070402102001.htm.

Ghuman, S. P., Prabhakar, S., Smith, R. F., & Dobson, H. (2008). Noradrenergic control of arginine vasopressin release from the ewe hypothalamus in vitro: Sensitivity to oestradiol. *Reproduction in Domestic Animals, 43*(2), 137–143.

Gibson, E. L. (2006). Emotional influences on food choice: sensory, physiological and psychological pathways. *Physiology & Behavior, 89*(1), 53–61.

Grassi, D., Lippi, C., Necozione, S., Desideri, G., & Ferri, C. (2005). Short-term administration of dark chocolate is followed by a significant increase in insulin sensitivity and a decrease in blood pressure in healthy persons. *American Journal of Clinical Nutrition, 81*(3), 611–614.

Grossman, R., Yehuda, R., Golier, J., McEwen, B., Harvey, P., & Maria, N. S. (2006). Cognitive effects of intravenous hydrocortisone in subjects with PTSD and healthy control subjects. *Annals of the New York Academy of Science, 1071,* 410–421.

Gupta, N., Khera, S., Vempati, R. P., Sharma, R., & Bijlani, R. L. (2006). Effect of yoga based lifestyle intervention on state and trait anxiety. *Indian Journal of Physiology and Pharmacology, 50*(1), 41–47.

Jefferson, L. L. (2010). Exploring effects of therapeutic massage and patient teaching in the practice of diaphragmatic breathing on blood pressure, stress, and anxiety in hypertensive African-American women: An intervention study. *Journal of National Black Nurses Association, 21*(1), 17–24.

Kasi, P. M., Khawar, T., Khan, F. H., Kiani, J. G., Khan, U. Z., Khan, H. M., Khuwaja, U. B., & Rahim, M. (2007). Studying the association between postgraduate trainees' work hours, stress and the use of maladaptive coping strategies. *Journal of Ayub Medical College Abbottabad, 19*(3), 37–41.

Kelley-Hedgepeth, A., Lloyd-Jones, D. M., Colvin, A., Matthews, K. A., Johnston, J., Sowers, M. R., Sternfeld, B., Pasternak, R. C., & Chae, C. U., for the SWAN investigators. (2008). Ethnic differences in C-reactive protein concentrations. *Clinical Chemistry, 54*(6), 1027–1037.

Kilpatrick, L. A., Zald, D. H., Pardo, J. V., & Cahill, L. F. (2006). Sex-related differences in amygdala functional connectivity during resting conditions. *Neuroimage, 30*(2), 452–461.

Kyrou, I., & Tsigos, C. (2007). Stress mechanisms and metabolic complications. *Hormone and Metabolic Research, 39*(6), 430–438.

Leistad, R. B., Nilsen, K. B., Stovner, L. J., Westgaard, R. H., Rø, M., & Sand, T. (2008). Similarities in stress physiology among patients with chronic pain and headache disorders: Evidence for a common pathophysiological mechanism? *Journal of Headache and Pain, 9*(3), 65–75.

Li, L., Jönsson-Rylander, A. C., Abe, K., & Zukowska, Z. (2005). Chronic stress induces rapid occlusion of angioplasty-injured rat carotid artery by activating neuropeptide Y and its Y1 receptors. *Arteriosclerosis, Thrombosis, and Vascular Biology, 25*(10), 2075–2080.

Melgert, B. N., Ray, A., Hylkema, M. N., Timens, W., & Postma, D. S. (2007). Are there reasons why adult asthma is more common in females? *Current Allergy and Asthma Reports, 7*(2), 143–150.

Mixon, B. (2008). Chore wars: Men, women, and housework. Retrieved April 28, 2009 from http://www.nsf.gov/discoveries/disc_summ.jsp?cntn_id=111458.

Monahan, K. D., Leuenberger, U. A., & Ray, C. A. (2007). Aldosterone impairs baroreflex sensitivity in healthy adults. *American Journal of Physiology - Heart and Circulatory Physiology, 292*(1), H190–197.

Nelson, E. L., Wenzel, L. B., Osann, K., Dogan-Ates, A., Chantana, N., Reina-Patton, A., Laust, A. K., Nishimoto, K. P., Chicz-DeMet, A., du Pont, N., & Monk, B. J. (2008). Stress, immunity, and cervical cancer: Biobehavioral outcomes of a randomized clinical trial. *Clinical Cancer Research, 14*(7), 2111–2118.

Phelps, E. A., & LeDoux, J. E. (2005). Contributions of the amygdala to emotion processing: From animal models to human behavior. *Neuron, 48*(2), 175–187.

Pitt, E., Rosenthal, M. M., Gay, T. L., & Lewton, E. (2004). Mental health services for residents: More important than ever. *Academic Medicine, 79*(9), 840–844.

Ribeiro, S. C., Kennedy, S. E., Smith, Y. R., Stohler, C. S., & Zubieta, J. K. (2005). Interface of physical and emotional stress regulation through the endogenous opioid system and mu-opioid receptors. *Progress in Neuro-Psychopharmacology & Biological Psychiatry, 29*(8), 1264–1280.

Robbins, J. (2006). *Healthy at 100: The scientifically proven secrets of the world's healthiest and longest-lived peoples.* New York, NY: Random House.

Rosmond, R. (2003). Stress induced disturbances of the HPA axis: A pathway to Type 2 diabetes? *Medical Science Monitor, 9*(2), RA35–39.

Sivasankaran, S., Pollard-Quintner, S., Sachdeva, R., Pugeda, J., Hoq, S. M., & Zarich, S. W. (2006). The effect of a six-week program of yoga and meditation on brachial artery reactivity: Do psychosocial interventions affect vascular tone? *Clinical Cardiology, 29*(9), 393–398.

Skuse, D., Albanese, A., Stanhope, R., Gilmour, J., & Voss, L. (1996). A new stress-related syndrome of growth failure and hyperphagia in children, associated with reversibility of growth-hormone insufficiency. *Lancet, 348*(9024), 353–358.

Smit, H. J., Gaffan, E. A., & Rogers, P. J. (2004). Methylxanthines are the psychopharmacologically active constituents of chocolate. *Psychopharmacology (Berlin), 176*(3–4), 412–419.

Statistics Canada. The sandwich generation. (2004). Retrieved April 14, 2008 from http://www.statcan.ca/Daily/English/040928/d040928b.htm.

Takeda, E., Terao, J., Nakaya, Y., Miyamoto, K., Baba, Y., Chuman, H., Kaji, R., Ohmori, T., & Rokutan, K. (2004). Stress control and human nutrition. *Journal of Investigative Medicine, 51*(3–4), 139–145.

Taubert, D., Roesen, R., Lehmann, C., Jung, N., & Schömig, E. (2007). Effects of low habitual cocoa intake on blood pressure and bioactive nitric oxide: A randomized controlled trial. *Journal of the American Medical Association, 298*(1), 49–60.

Taylor, S. E., Gonzaga, G. C., Klein, L. C., Hu, P., Greendale, G. A., & Seeman, T. E. (2006). Relation of oxytocin to psychological stress responses and hypothalamic-pituitary-adrenocortical axis activity in older women. *Psychosomatic Medicine, 68*(2), 238–245.

Taylor, S. E., Klein, L. C., Gruenewald, T. L., Gurung, R. A. R., & Fernandes-Taylor, S. (2003). Affiliation, social support, and biobehavioral responses to stress. In J. Suls & K. Wallston (Eds.), *Social psychological foundations of health and illness.* Malden, MA: Blackwell.

Tsatsoulis, A., & Fountoulakis, S. (2006). The protective role of exercise on stress system dysregulation and comorbidities. *Annals of the New York Academy of Science, 1083,* 196–213.

U.S. Department of Labor, Bureau of Labor Statistics. (2009). Women in the labor force: A databook (2009 ed.). Retrieved January 20, 2011 from http://www.bls.gov/cps/wlf-databook2009.htm.

Verona, E., Reed, A., 2nd, Curtin, J. J., & Pole, M. (2007). Gender differences in emotional and overt/covert aggressive responses to stress. *Aggressive Behavior, 33*(3), 261–271.

Waladkhani, A. R., & Hellhammer, J. (2008). Dietary modification of brain function: Effects on neuroendocrine and psychological determinants of mental health- and stress-related disorders. *Advances in Clinical Chemistry, 45,* 99–138.

Wang-Polagruto, J. F., Villablanca, A. C., Polagruto, J. A., Lee, L., Holt, R. R., Schrader, H. R., Ensunsa, J. L., Steinberg, F. M., Schmitz, H. H., & Keen, C. L. (2006). Chronic consumption of flavanol-rich cocoa improves endothelial function and decreases vascular cell adhesion molecule in hypercholesterolemic postmenopausal women. *Journal of Cardiovascular Pharmacology, 47,* Suppl 2, S177–186.

Whitbeck, L. B., Hoyt, D. R., Johnson, K. D., & Chen, X. (2007). Victimization and posttraumatic stress disorder among runaway and homeless adolescents. *Violence and Victims, 22*(6), 721–734.

Yunus, M. B. (2001). The role of gender in fibromyalgia syndrome. *Current Rheumatology Reports, 3*(2), 128–134.

chapter 18

BIOLOGY OF APPEARANCE

Upon completion of this chapter, the reader will be able to:

- Describe the anatomy and physiology of the integument including skin, nails, and hair
- Discuss why people alter their appearance
- Describe the functions of cosmetic ingredients including potential benefits and risks

- Understand the potential risks associated with body alterations
- Define eating disorders and describe their effects on individuals

KEY TERMS

acne	cosmetic surgery	melanocytes	sebaceous glands
alopecia	dermis	melanoma	sudoriferous glands
anorexia	epidermis	reconstructive	
bulimia	hypodermis	surgery	

INTRODUCTION

Beauty is in the eye of the beholder, or so the saying goes. In many countries, popular culture focuses on youth, and the dominant message is that to be beautiful, one must look young. In regions of the Caucasus Mountains, where people typically live to 100 and age is revered, older women are considered the most beautiful. In that culture, telling a woman she looks young is considered an insult (Robbins, 2006). The concept of beauty has changed with both time and place. Currently, based on the images depicted in mass media, women who are thin are considered the ideal of beauty. Yet many Renaissance paintings or the Venus figures uncovered from archeological digs show women with very curvy, plump bodies. Cultures place a great deal of significance on appearance, pressuring individuals to look a certain way. Maintaining a specific image has been considered important enough that some corporations have run "appearance training" to ensure all employees presented the proper company image. Some people respond by becoming obsessed with changing themselves to fit the image pressed upon them (Figure 18-1). Others ignore the outside expectations and create their own idea of what they see as beautiful.

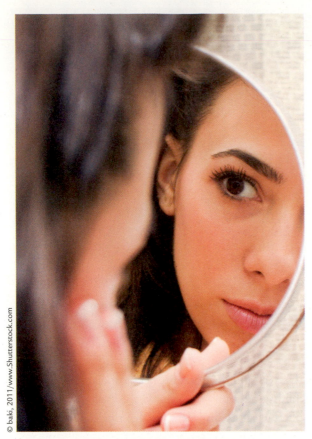

© baki, 2011/www.Shutterstock.com

FIGURE 18-1: Cultures around the world and throughout history have defined beauty in different ways, putting pressure on people to look a certain way.

INTEGUMENT

The integument, along with the bone structure and body fat distribution, contributes significantly to an individual's appearance. The skin, hair, and nails of the integument cover the body, and, unlike other organs, are completely visible. Along with its other functions of providing protection, and perhaps of greater importance to most people, the skin also defines the individual. It provides humans with an identity. Initial impressions are often determined based on how someone looks. Regardless of what this implies about human judgment, there are valid reasons for trying to change someone's appearance. According to Nancy Etcoff (1999), the skin provides information about social status and general health as well as reproductive fitness. Poor nutrition and disease produces physiological changes that show up in the skin. Understanding the structure of the integument and the effect cosmetics and body alterations have on it, can help women make informed decisions about how they want to appear.

The Skin

The skin functions as the only barrier between the outside environment and the body inside. In addition, the skin provides some protection against

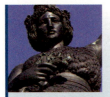

Historical Considerations
Body Politics

Beauty standards are not static, and, in fact, they change dramatically over time and from one culture to the next. In the United States, changing beauty standards have been linked to political and social changes. In the Roaring 20s, there were dramatic changes to both the social fabric of the nation and to the roles people played within it. People had money and the freedom to spend it. The sassy Flapper style became all the rage, with sleeveless dresses showing off more arm and leg than in previous periods. Women began to wear makeup in public, something which would have shocked the Victorians of only a few decades before. During the Great Depression, feminine modesty made a comeback and women's fashions became more reserved, mirroring the conservative mood of the country. During World War II, women first begin to wear pants in large numbers as they entered the paid workforce in greater numbers. The 1950s were embodied by the rise of Marilyn Monroe as the country's new female sex symbol, only to be followed in the 1960s by the stick-thin Twiggy as the new fashion ideal. In the 1970s, feminists publically took on 'beauty' as an oppressive tool of patriarchal culture, protesting beauty pageants and challenging conventional notions of beauty in popular media.

thermal, chemical, and physical injury. Relatively waterproof, the skin allows the body to exist in dry air without dehydrating as well as allowing a person to swim without becoming overhydrated. The skin is abundantly supplied with nerve endings and acts as a sensory organ, which constantly receives information from its surface for transmission to the brain.

Skin consists of three principal layers, each of which has its own subdivisions (Figure 18-2). Within the layers are the glands, nerves, and blood vessels. The layers do not occur in straight lines, but pocket and fold into each other based on the underlying topography of bone and muscle.

The exposed, outermost cellular layer of skin is the **epidermis**. The epidermis protects the body against the invasion of microorganisms, excessive fluid loss or gain, mechanical injury, and any other onslaught of an ever-changing environment. The skin is also host to a large population of normal flora that consume dead cells and repel potential invasions by pathogens. Cells reproduce rapidly in the deepest layer of the epidermis, called the basal layer or stratum basale. The new cells push toward

the skin surface into the stratum spinosum, or spiny cell layer, so called because the cells develop spiny projections, helping them attach to one another. As the cells move toward the skin's surface, they stop reproducing and start producing a tough protein called keratin. As they accumulate granules of keratin, they form a new layer called the granular layer, or stratum granulosum. Beyond the granular layer, the individual cell boundaries and nuclei begin to disappear, and the cells die. The cells appear glassy and closely packed, forming a clear layer called the stratum lucidum. Under mechanical stress, the stratum lucidum will thicken to form a callus. By the time the cells reach the top of the epidermis, they are flat, scaly, and lifeless, and they are retained in the stratum corneum. The lifeless cells of the stratum corneum are continually being sloughed off or removed by abrasion. As they are sloughed off, they are replaced from below by the rapidly dividing cells below. The flat, scale-like surface cells of the stratum corneum contain a soft form of keratin which has less sulfur content than does the hard keratin found in hair and nails. The rate of growth in epidermis is

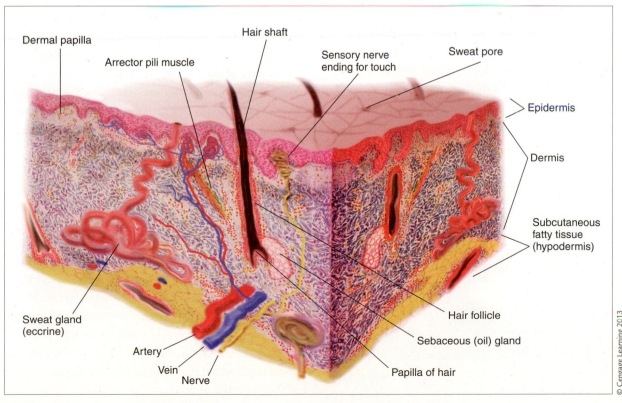

Dermal papilla

Arrector pili muscle

Hair shaft

Sensory nerve ending for touch

Sweat pore

Epidermis

Dermis

Subcutaneous fatty tissue (hypodermis)

Sweat gland (eccrine)

Artery

Vein

Nerve

Hair follicle

Sebaceous (oil) gland

Papilla of hair

© Cengage Learning 2013

FIGURE 18-2: The structure of the skin.

such that it completely replaces itself approximately every 15–30 days. The rate of replacement depends on the area of the body and on the individual's age and nutritional status. The epidermis also gives rise to specialized skin derivatives, such as the hair, glands, and nails. The surface of the skin is marked by numerous tiny ridges and furrows and the minute openings of the sweat glands and hair follicles. These openings are commonly referred to as pores.

Beneath the epidermis is the supporting layer called the **dermis**. Much thicker than the epidermis, the dermis contains the blood vessels that nourish the epidermis. The dermis and epidermis are held together by tiny elevations, or papillae, of dermis that project into corresponding depressions of the epidermis. Continued strong friction or heat can cause an accumulation of fluid and the separation of the epidermis from the dermis forming a blister. Hair follicles, tiny muscles, nerves, sudoriferous glands, and sebaceous glands originate in the dermis layer.

Below the dermal layer is the **hypodermis**, or superficial fascia, which anchors the skin to the underlying muscle. The subcutaneous layer is loosely constructed and contains adundant adipose tissue. In some areas of the body, this subcutaneous fat forms a continuous layer 2.5 cm thick or more. This adipose layer serves as a reserve energy supply, insulates the body, and cushions it from injury. Women store roughly half their total body fat in the hypodermis as subcutaneous fat. Hormones determine the locations for fat deposition. Estrogen encourages deposition of subcutaneous fat in the hips and breasts. The characteristic rounded body contours found in women result from this distribution and from their greater percentage of subcutaneous fat.

Skin Color

The activities of pigment-producing cells called **melanocytes** account for the wide range of skin colors found in human beings (Figure 18-3). Sandwiched between the dividing keratin-producing cells in the basal layer of the epidermis, the melanocytes synthesize a yellow, brown, or black pigment called melanin. Melanin is produced from the amino acid, tyrosine, with the aid of a copper-containing enzyme called tyrosinase. Gene mutations can prevent the conversion of tyrosine to melanin and are the cause of albinism, a condition that results in pale skin, white hair, and pale or pinkish eyes.

Melanin protects the skin from the harmful effects of ultraviolet rays from the sun. The pigment absorbs the damaging ultraviolet radiation that could, in excessive doses, cause sunburn and skin cancer. The more pigment produced, the darker the skin and the greater the protection from the ultraviolet radiation. Each person has the same number of melanocytes, one to two thousand per square millimeter of skin, no matter what the skin tone. Differences in skin color are determined genetically and result from greater melanin production by the melanocytes and a wider dispersal of the pigment throughout the epidermis.

In addition to melanin, other factors influence skin coloration. The fairer the skin, the more the skin color is modified by the presence of blood in the capillaries of the dermis and in the larger arteries and veins just under it. The translucent epidermis allows the blood vessels to show through, resulting in a pinkish skin tone. On the face and neck where the epidermis is thin and the blood vessels are close to the surface, dilation of the vessels during anger or embarrassment will cause the skin to blush. Fear or pain may cause a constriction of the blood vessels, and the skin blanches and turns pale as it takes on the color of the underlying connective tissue. Naturally rosy

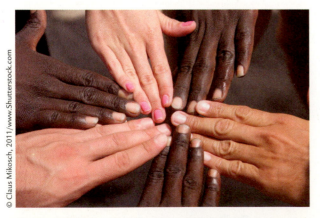

FIGURE 18-3: Melanocytes produce pigments that contribute to the different colors of skin.

cheeks or a ruddy skin tone indicates that blood-filled capillaries are close to the surface of the skin.

Accessory Skin Structures

Sudoriferous, or sweat **glands** are epidermal derivatives located in the dermis and are widely distributed over the entire body surface except on the nail beds of the fingers and toes, the margins of the lips, and on parts of the external genitalia. Sweat glands empty their secretion onto the surface of the skin through pores. Watery sweat, or perspiration, is a mixture of solids (mostly salts) in solution. It has a cooling effect on the body and also helps to eliminate wastes.

Sebaceous or oil **glands** are associated with hair follicles. The sebaceous gland drains its fatty secretion, sebum, into hair follicles and spreads over the skin surface. In some locations on the body, the glands develop independently of hair follicles and open by their own duct directly onto the skin. Sebum lubricates the skin and helps prevent dehydration and cracking. Sebaceous glands are largest and most numerous on the skin of the forehead, around the nose and mouth, and over the cheekbones, attaining a density of 800 glands per square centimeter compared with 100 glands per square centimeter in other locations. Their number and activity are under both hereditary and hormonal control. The production of sebum is greater in teenagers, the increase resulting primarily from the secretion of androgen but affected by estrogens and progesterone as well. There are vast individual differences in sebum production, and these differences cause the differentiation between dry, normal, and oily complexions.

The hair follicle openings on the surface of the skin are commonly called pores, although sweat gland openings are also pores. The diameters of the follicle openings are generally related to the size of the sebaceous glands they contain. People who have oily skin have larger glands and hence more conspicuous or enlarged pores. Any slight inflammation of the skin, such as a mild sunburn, can cause edema and make the pores less noticeable. Astringent facial toners cause slight inflammation which reduces the appearance of pores. Some cosmetics cover the pores, making them less obvious.

Hair follicles, with the exception of eyelashes, exit the surface of the skin at an angle. The sebaceous glands and a small bundle of smooth muscle fibers, the arrector pili, are associated with each hair follicle. The arrector pili muscles are controlled through the autonomic nervous system. When exposed to cold or when the fight-or-flight response is triggered, the arrector pili contract to pull on the follicles and make the hairs stand erect. At the same time, little dimples form where the pili attach to the dermis. This produces small bumps on the skin surface, commonly referred to as goose bumps.

Dry Skin, Oily Skin

The ideal in women's facial skin is a smooth, unblemished complexion in which the pores are not enlarged. It should not look dry, flaky, or chapped, nor should it appear greasy from too much oil on the surface. Many women have dry skin, not only on the face, but all over their bodies and consequently have either chronic or seasonal problems with itching and flaking skin. Other women have varying degrees of oiliness or possibly a combination of some areas that are dry and others that are oily. Oily skins are perceived as unsightly, but unless the condition precipitates a skin disorder, they are far less of a problem than dry skin.

Dry skin occurs when the water loss from the top layer of the epidermis occurs more rapidly than it can be replaced from the underlying tissues. The keratin in the epidermis must contain at least 10 percent water for the skin to be soft and supple. If the percentage of moisture falls below this level, the stratum cornium dries out, becomes brittle, and flakes off. The skin feels tight and dry, and in the extreme, the skin can crack and bleed. Water is constantly being supplied to the epidermis from dermis. The skin retains its hydration because there is a barrier layer in the epidermis to prevent rapid movement of water; without it, moisture would evaporate too quickly. Besides the barrier layer, two other factors promote water retention. Hydrophilic (water-loving) substances in the stratum cornium bind water. These water-soluble and water-attracting

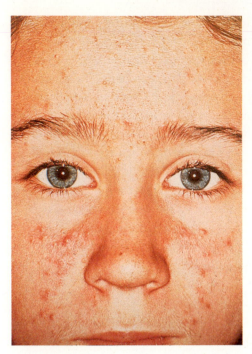

FIGURE 18-4: Acne. (From *Acne Vulgaris*, by G. Plewig and A. B. Klingman [Eds], 1975, Berlin/Heideberg, Germany; (*Springer-Verlag. Used with Permission*))

substances could be removed from the skin by washing or by perspiration, but they are protected from loss by a thin film of water-insoluble sebum. Sebum also coats the projecting edges of the dead keratinized cells, smooths them down, and reduces the surface area for evaporation. Creams, lotions, and moisturizers for dry skin attempt to duplicate and enhance the functions of sebum.

Any skin type can become dehydrated when water evaporation exceeds replacement. Environmental and hormonal factors play a role in inducing desiccation of the stratum cornium. Water loss is greater when the temperature is elevated and the humidity is low. In cold climates, the combination of cold, dry outside air and overheated, low-humidity indoor air can result in dry, cracked skin. Washing removes the oily sebum film from the skin. Ordinarily, this defatting of the skin surface is only temporary because the increased activity of the sebaceous glands soon renews the barrier effect of the sebum. The replacement is less rapid, however, in people who through heredity or age, normally produce less sebum. Once the skin has become dry, brittle, and cracked, it will take more than the application

of a lotion or cream to restore it. Hand lotions and creams are emulsions of water and oils. The water provides moisture to the skin, and the oils form a barrier to keep it there.

Acne

Acne is a disorder of the sebaceous glands, which are associated with the hair follicles of the skin. At least 75 percent of the population suffers from acne at one time or another, predominantly during the adolescent years (Figure 18-4). While the majority of acne cases occur during adolescence, the disorder sometimes appears or reappears during adulthood. Some men and women get acne in their late 30s, 40s, or 50s; some are troubled with acne all of their adult lives. Many women are troubled with premenstrual acne or by perimenopausal acne.

The sebaceous glands that are especially prone to acne lesions are most prevalent on the face and the upper trunk. Sebum production may occur too rapidly and accumulate in the sebaceous glands where it hardens, blocking the follicle. *Propionibacterium* and *Staphylococcus* bacteria can invade the glands, become trapped, and feed on the oils, producing irritation, pus, and inflammation. Sebum is normally synthesized by the sebaceous glands in response to circulating hormones, and the glands are especially sensitive to androgens. Suppression of androgens can limit acne outbreaks (Paradisi et al., 2010).

Another treatment option is to control the bacteria associated with acne (Kim et al., 2008). Mild scrubs and plant acids can be used to open blocked pores. Other successful treatments include oral antibiotics or the topical application of antibiotics, zinc compounds, or retinoids (Ochsendorf and Degitz, 2008). Phototherapy using lasers and blue light can also reduce some acne outbreaks (Smith et al., 2010). However, many of the treatments do pose potential risks. Oral antibiotics can disrupt the intestinal normal flora and interfere with digestion. Therapeutic levels of retinoids can be teratogenic and should be avoided by women who are pregnant or plan to become pregnant during treatment. The use of medications that suppress androgens can cause toxic effects in the liver (Paradisi et al., 2010) as well as having potential teratogenic properties.

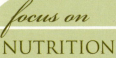

Wrinkles

Facial lines and wrinkles are a natural consequence of aging (Figure 18-5). They result from the normal deterioration of collagen and elastic fibers in the dermis. Much of the dermis is made of a loose interweaving network of collagen, elastic, and reticular protein fibers. The collagen and elastic fibers are responsible the skin's ability to stretch and contract to accommodate body movement. Generally, although there is great individual variation, skin loses this resiliency with age. The pace and characteristics of skin aging are influenced by heredity. Environment, however, also plays a role. Deterioration of collagen can be accelerated by UV light exposure. Smoking will also hasten the formation of facial wrinkles due to constriction of the capillaries that nourish the cells of the dermis.

The pull of the facial muscles to create facial expressions can influence the position of facial wrinkles. After years of facial expression, lines become accentuated and exaggerated, especially around the mouth and eyes. Over time, the natural degeneration of the elastic fibers accompanied by the decrease in hydration of the skin and the pull of gravity, results in the appearance of permanent wrinkles on the face.

There is no way to completely prevent the eventual appearance of wrinkles. Facial exercises merely tone the

focus on
NUTRITION
Food Choices for Younger-looking Skin

Cosmetics can be applied to the skin surface to mask imperfections, but can food choices influence the natural aging process and make skin look younger? In a clinical study of over 4000 North American women, ages 40–74, the answer appears to be yes. The study examined three factors to quantify skin aging appearance—skin atrophy, dryness, and wrinkles. Evaluation of these conditions was conducted by dermatologists, who found that women who ate a diet high in total fat and carbohydrates show more wrinkles and have greater skin atrophy. However, increasing vitamin C consumption was associated with decreased dryness and wrinkles. Increased intake of linoleic acid, found in nuts and fruits, decreased skin atrophy and dryness. The changes in skin condition occurred regardless of sun exposure, supplement use, physical activity level, race, or menopausal status (Cosgrove et al., 2007). So, sit down to a healthy low-fat, low carbohydrate meal with extra fruit and nuts to keep the skin looking young.

facial muscles underneath the skin and do not directly affect the skin above them. Facial massage can increase the blood flow to the skin which can support the production of collagen, but cannot erase existing wrinkles. Changes in nutrition can slow the aging of the skin. There are some cosmetics that can form a film that make tiny lines appear less apparent and others that plump and rehydrate the skin filling in the wrinkles.

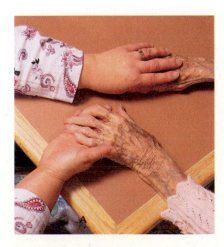
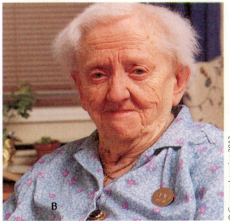

© Cengage Learning 2013

FIGURE 18-5: Wrinkles are a common sign of aging.

Botox, a purified form of the botulism toxin, can be injected to temporarily paralyze the muscles of the skin, which reduces the appearance of wrinkles. More than 5,000,000 people underwent botox treatments in 2008 (American Society of Plastic Surgeons, 2009). This treatment can be used successfully in place of more aggressive cosmetic surgeries (Levy, 2007). However, the procedure can produce an emotionless, mask-like appearance in some cases when the facial muscles cannot respond to nervous system stimulation. Botox injections also run the risk of infection, inflammation, and allergic reactions (Binder et al., 1998).

Other wrinkle treatments include dermabrasion and chemical peels that remove the outer layers of the epidermis. Radio waves or heat can be used to increase collagen formation in the dermis, and filler compounds composed of fatty acids and collagen can be injected directly into the wrinkles. However, injections can cause serious immune-related side effects, including fever, swelling, hardening of nodules of tissue near the injection site, arthritis, and dry eyes or mouth.

Soaps and Cleansers

The skin and hair are constantly exposed to dirt and dust. The sebaceous glands produce oils that coat the skin, and sweat glands deposit salts on the skin surface. As the normal flora consume dead skin cells and sebum, they produce metabolic by-products. Together, these factors can create an oily and sometimes aromatic coating on the skin and hair. Because water alone will not dissolve this film, soaps and cleansers are often used to remove it from the skin.

In their simplest forms, these cleansers have both hydrophilic (water attracting) and hydrophobic (water repelling) properties (Figure 18-6). The hydrophobic component of soaps dissolves the oils that are present, and the hydrophilic component allows them to be rinsed away with water. Cleansers remove the dirt, dead skin cells, oils, and bacteria.

The earliest versions of soap were based on a mixture of lye, which is a chemical derived from wood ashes, and animal fats. When the mixture undergoes a process called saponification, it becomes soap. A number of plants, such as yucca (*Yucca elata*) and soapwort (*Saponaria officinalis*), produce saponins and have traditionally been used as cleansers,

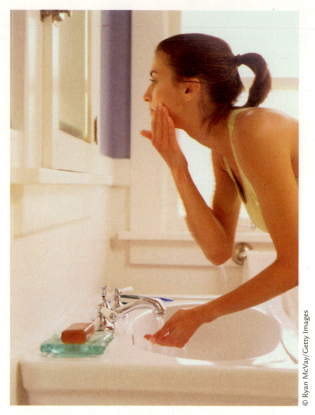

© Ryan McVay/Getty Images

FIGURE 18-6: Soaps and shampoos contain two properties, hydrophilic and hydrophobic, that allows them to cleanse skin and hair.

as well. Many modern cleansers are based on synthetically prepared surfactants which dissolve both water- and oil-based compounds. In addition, most commercial cleansers contain fragrances, coloring agents, and chemicals to adjust the pH. Plant extracts, fatty acids, and fillers also appear in many products.

Cosmetics for the Skin

Cosmetics are treatments that are applied to the skin to change appearance. They have been used for millennia to add decoration, provide protection, and convey information. Pots of cosmetics have been found in Egyptian tombs dating from 1400 B.C., and sticks of red pigments mixed with fats which are thought to have been used to decorate the skin have been found at archeological sites that are 40,000 years old (Etcoff, 1999). Examples of modern cosmetics include foundations, bronzers, eyeliners, eye shadows, mascara, and lipstick.

Reading the list of ingredients on most modern cosmetics is like opening a page in a chemistry book. While cosmetic formulas have changed over the centuries and vary from product to product, the basic components have remained the same. Pigments provide color and coverage. In the past, potentially toxic metals such as lead, mercury, and copper were used as pigments. Titanium, iron, zinc oxides, talc, kaolin clay, and coal tar-based colors are used as pigments today. Traditionally, rice, corn, and wheat flours have been used as face powders to lighten the skin. Current federal regulations in the United States prohibit the use of any organic pigments in eye make-up, but earlier recipes included flower petals, leaves, and fruits to impart color. Cochineal, an organic acid derived from the bodies of a small insect, is still used to produce brilliant red pigments for lip products. Carriers are necessary to spread the pigment over the skin, and the most common carriers are oils and waxes. These hold the pigments in place and also act as emollients to soften the skin and retain moisture. Glycerin, sugars, or propylene glycol are often added to draw moisture into the skin (humectants). Fragrances are often added to cosmetics to cover the rancid odor that can develop as the carrier oils age. Modern makeup usually contains antioxidants and preservatives to prevent this. Mica and ground fish scales can be used to add sparkle. Other additives include hydroxy acids and collagen to reduce wrinkles. Additional fillers alter the texture of the cosmetic and emulsifiers allow the water- and oil-soluble components to blend smoothly.

Some women are sensitive to the chemicals that are used in cosmetics. Contact dermatitis is an inflammation or rash that is caused by an allergic response, and it can result from exposure to cosmetic ingredients. In addition, the oils and waxes in cosmetics can block the pores and increase acne in some people. Historically, cosmetics contained a number of toxic compounds. For example, the white facial powder that was used throughout the seventeenth and eighteenth centuries contained lead, which was absorbed into the body, producing neurological damage. Today, a number of untested chemicals are still found in many cosmetics. Unlike drugs, food, color additives, and medical devices, cosmetics do not have to be pretested for safety before being sold. In addition, cosmetic companies are not required by law to report the results of their product safety tests to the FDA. There is no mandate that cosmetic companies inform the FDA of consumer complaints concerning adverse reactions to their products. In the United States, an estimated 8,000 chemical ingredients are used in formulating cosmetics, and for only the color additives is there any requirement for documenting safety and effectiveness. While the industry maintains that it can regulate itself, a Government Accounting Office study released in 1990 found that 884 chemicals used by the cosmetics industry are on a federal toxic substances list, and that companies rarely disclosed safety test results to the FDA or filed consumer injury reports under the voluntary provisions of the law.

Cosmetics are exempt from the regulations governing all other substances under the purview of the FDA because of the Food, Drug, and Cosmetic Act, which was passed by Congress in 1938. This law defines cosmetics as substances applied to the surface of the body for cleansing, beautifying, promoting attractiveness, or altering the appearance without affecting the body's structure or function. Under this definition, some cosmetic products which do alter body structure or function, such as deodorants or anti-dandruff shampoos, are legally considered drugs and have to undergo safety and efficacy tests before marketing. However, many cosmetics that are, by definition, excluded from regulation contain ingredients that can be absorbed by the skin, ingested, or inhaled and result in the same kind of health problems as those caused by the chemicals in drugs and food additives which are regulated by the FDA. The FDA does maintain a voluntary cosmetic review program which compiles information on the chemicals used in cosmetics, reports on safety issues related to cosmetics, and maintains a list of cosmetics and their components recalled for safety issues.

Cosmetics are prone to contamination by bacteria and fungi from the environment and by the skin's normal flora. Eye makeup, in particular, is prone to contamination, and use of infected cosmetics can lead to eye infections and even potential blindness. Because of the risk of infection, any cosmetic which develops an unusual color or odor should be discarded. Even without noticeable changes, cosmetics should be discarded after three to six months due to the probability of microbial contamination.

Skin Cancers

It is estimated that over 1,000,000 new cases of skin cancer were diagnosed in 2010 (NCI, 2010). The relationship between ultraviolet radiation exposure and skin cancer is well established. The most common forms of skin cancer are basal cell cancer (Figure 18-7), which rarely metastasizes, and squamous cell cancer (Figure 18-8), which occurs less frequently but is more likely to spread. Most basal and squamous cell cancers occur on the parts of the body that are most frequently exposed to the sun. Among fair-skinned individuals, more cases of the disease occur in areas of the world where there is greater sun exposure. Naturally dark-skinned individuals are not immune to skin cancer, however, their risk of skin cancer is less due to the natural protection of melanin.

A third type of skin cancer, **melanoma**, is produced by melanocytes which become cancerous and is highly dangerous but much less common.

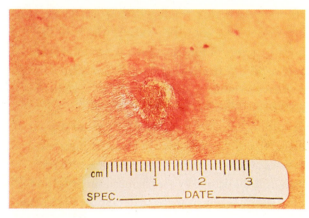

FIGURE 18-7: Basal cell carcinoma. *(Courtesy of Robert A. Silverman, MD, Clinical Associate Professor, Department of Pediatrics, Georgetown University)*

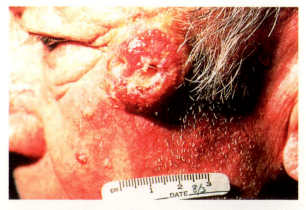

FIGURE 18-8: Squamous cell carcinoma. *(Courtesy of Robert A. Silverman, MD, Clinical Associate Professor, Department of Pediatrics, Georgetown University)*

This type of skin cancer is not as strongly correlated with overexposure to sunlight, but melanomas do occur more frequently in people with fair complexions and those with increased sun exposure. Two oncogenes (BRAF and NRSA) have been linked to the development of melanomas. Melanomas that result from a BRAF gene mutation are more heavily pigmented cells and characterized by sharper boarders and raised surfaces. BRAF melanomas are more likely to metastasize to internal organs. Melanomas resulting from mutated NRSA genes are difficult to identify because the cells have fewer distinguishing characteristics (Viros et al., 2008).

Skin cancers are most successfully treated at their earliest stages. The National Cancer Institute (2010) recommends examining the skin changes which may indicate cancerous cells. Moles which display asymmetry or have uneven borders are suspicious and should be investigated. In addition, moles that are multi-colored, larger than the size of a pencil eraser, or are raised above the skin surface should be examined by a healthcare provider.

Tanning and UV Protection

When skin receives a heavy exposure to sunlight, the melanin that is present oxidizes and darkens. This oxidation is followed by increased production of melanin by the melanocytes and a thickening of the epidermis to block more of the UV radiation. Over a period of several days, the skin becomes tanned or darker. Skin that is darker to begin with tans more readily. Well-tanned or naturally dark skin is protected to some extent against the harmful effects of sunlight, but even the darkest skin is not immune to overexposure and can become sunburned. Exposure to excessive UV rays—either from the sun or from tanning booths—is associated with skin aging, wrinkles, and skin cancers.

Many people dislike sun blocks because they minimize tanning and often have a thick and greasy consistency. Sunscreen preparations either block the rays of the sun or absorb them, mimicking the body's own defenses against UV rays (Figure 18-9). Zinc oxide ointments and other opaque substances, such as titanium dioxide or kaolin, are very effective sun blocks and reflect the damaging rays. The most effective solar radiation absorbing agents are those containing para-amino benzoic acid (PABA) or its

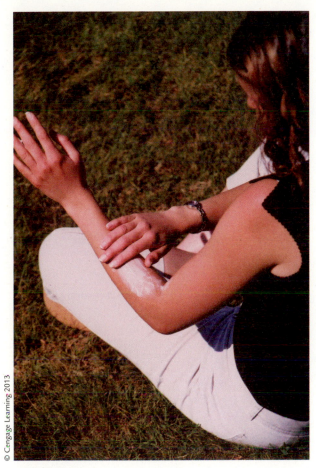

FIGURE 18-9: Sunscreens work by either reflecting the sun's rays or absorbing them.

derivatives. It is important to read the label before buying any suntan oil or lotion. A product that contains only vegetable fats, such as sesame seed oil, olive oil, or cocoa butter, may have some limited sunscreening properties but primarily just lubricates the skin. Baby oil has a mineral oil base and is ineffective as a sunscreen.

To help consumers determine which sunscreen to use, the Food and Drug Administration (FDA) has adopted a rating method called the "sun protection factor" or SPF of 2–45, which can be found on most brands of lotions. The numbers in the rating system refer to the amount of additional sun exposure that can be tolerated if the product is used. In theory, someone using a product rated SPF 8 could remain in the sun eight times longer without burning than when unprotected. As long as the sunscreen is reapplied often throughout the day, and especially after swimming, lower SPF products are usually sufficient. An SPF of 20 delivers protection to the fairest of skins for approximately 10 hours.

The kind of sunscreen preparation used may be important as well. Sunlight contains two kinds of solar rays, ultraviolet A (UVA) and ultraviolet B (UVB). A study by Hanson and Simon (1998) found that the appearance of prematurely aged skin—wrinkles, sagging, leathery looking—can be caused by ultraviolet A (UVA) radiation, a type not blocked by many of the preparations on the market that protect against UVB. Standard window glass blocks UVB rays, but allows UVA to pass (Hampton et al., 2004). Zinc oxide blocks UVA, and some sunscreens contain it, so it is important to read the label. The current FDA recommendations call for broad spectrum (both UVA and UVB) sunscreen application whenever someone goes outside. Sunscreens combined with insect repellents are not recommended, however (Hexsel et al., 2008). Clothing blocks some UV rays, and several companies market clothing designed to block 90 percent or more of the UV rays.

Hair

Humans may look hairless compared to other mammals, but have approximately the same number of hair follicles as gorillas, chimpanzees, and orangutans. However, in humans, most of the hair follicles give rise only to tiny colorless vellus hairs, or down. Hairs are present almost everywhere on the body except the palms of the hands, the soles of the feet, the nipples, and the skin around the nails and most body openings. Children have as many hairs as adults, but except for the scalp, eyebrows, and eyelashes, their hair is primarily vellus hair. With puberty and the increased production of sex hormones, the hair follicles enlarge and become more active. Heavier, darker, terminal hairs replace the vellus hairs in the pubic area and under the arms. In men, similar terminal hairs appear on the chest, face, shoulders, legs, and arms. Women have the same number of hairs on their bodies as men, even on their faces, but many of them are smaller and remain as vellus hair.

Hair follicles are formed before birth. The tubular hair follicle begins as a projection from the epidermis into the underlying dermis. This epidermal hair bud becomes bulb-shaped at its base and develops a concavity filled with connective tissue, blood vessels, and nerves called the dermal papilla. The epidermal cells that lie directly over the papilla are called the germinal matrix cells and are analogous to the basal

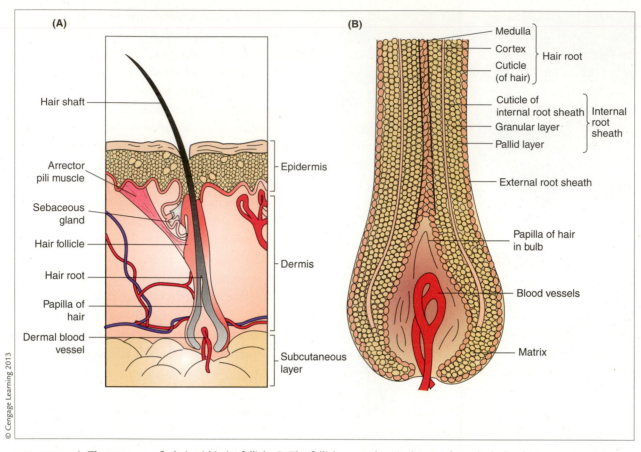

(A)

Hair shaft

Arrector pili muscle

Sebaceous gland

Hair follicle

Hair root

Papilla of hair

Dermal blood vessel

Epidermis

Dermis

Subcutaneous layer

© Cengage Learning 2013

(B)

Medulla
Cortex
Cuticle (of hair)
} Hair root

Cuticle of internal root sheath
Granular layer
Pallid layer
} Internal root sheath

External root sheath

Papilla of hair in bulb

Blood vessels

Matrix

FIGURE 18-10: A. The structure of a hair within its follicle. B. The follicle expands at its base to form the bulb which contains the dermal papilla.

cells of the epidermis. Nourished by the blood vessels in the dermal papillae, the matrix cells proliferate to form a hair shaft. As the hair shaft cells push toward the surface of the skin, they grow farther and farther from their source of nutrients. They become progressively keratinized, differentiating into an outer cuticle of dead cells, a middle keratinized cortex with variable amounts of pigment, and in some hairs, a central medulla. The hair shaft consists of the cuticle, the cortex, and the medulla and is almost completely composed of the protein, keratin. The root, enclosed within a tube-like follicle, expands at its base into the bulb, the only part of the hair with living cells (Figure 18-10). Hair contains trace amounts of DNA and hair samples, particularly those which retain traces of epithelium when they were pulled out, can be used for DNA analysis.

The cuticle and cortex are composed of hard keratin, similar to that found in the feathers and scales of birds and reptiles. Medullary keratin is softer and is similar to that found in the stratum

corneum of the epidermis. The medulla is often poorly developed and is not present in the vellus hairs. In addition, the medulla is missing from some of the hairs on the scalp, and is rarely found in blond hairs.

The cells that make up the cuticle are arranged like overlapping shingles on a roof. The cuticle is covered by a layer of sebum secreted by the sebaceous glands, and the cells move over each other, functioning as a flexible protective armor for the hair shaft. When the cuticle cells lie flat against the cortex, they reflect light evenly and the hair appears shiny. Disrupting the cuticle results in an uneven diffraction of light, and the hair will appear dull. Chemical exposure (chlorine or harsh shampoos, for example), UV exposure, and mechanical damage can disrupt the physical structure of hair. In addition, hair relaxers, color treatments, and other styling products may use strong alkaline chemicals to disrupt the cuticle in order to penetrate the cortex and change its configuration. Prolonged use of these products can result in scalp irritation or lusterless hair with decreased manageability and shine. Internal damage to the hair shafts caused by the chemical treatments can decrease their elastic properties and result in hair breakage or even loss.

Split ends result from the separation of the cell layers at the ends of the hair shaft. The longer the hair, the longer it has been exposed, and the more likely the cells are to separate (Figure 18-11). The cure for split ends is to cut them off.

Under some circumstances, hair falls out prematurely and does not regrow, a condition called **alopecia**. Alopecia can be caused by a variety of conditions including allergies , infections, or cancer (Richmand et al., 2008). In some cases, the immune system attacks the hair follicles, interrupting growth. In many cases, the specific cause is not identified. Braids and other hair styling techniques, if pulled too tightly, may cause traction alopecia. In these cases, the hair loss is due to excessive pressure on the hair follicles.

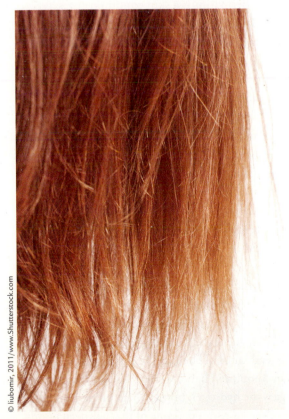

FIGURE 18-11: Longer hair is more likely to experience separation of the cell layers at the ends of the hair shaft forming split ends.

Hair Color

The pigments that give hair its color are produced by the activity of melanocytes in the germinal matrix. Pigment is deposited into the cortex of the hair shaft. The color of the hair depends on the size, number, and kind of pigment granules, or melanosomes in the cortex, and on the presence or absence of air bubbles in the cortex. The pigment melanin is the predominant color in black, brown, and ash blond hair. Golden blond, red, and auburn hair contain greater quantities of the yellow-brown pigment, phaeomelanin. White hair results from a lack of pigment and from air bubbles in the hair. Gray hair is caused by a progressive reduction in the activity of the melanocytes and the cessation of pigment production. The eventual loss of pigment in the hair is determined genetically and occurs in some people as young as 13. Initially, graying is more obvious in brunettes. Neither emotional stress nor traumatic events cause hair to go gray overnight. The process occurs gradually, following the growth pattern of the hairs. White hairs mixed in with partially pigmented and fully colored hairs results in the appearance of graying. Hairs that are actually gray in color are rare in humans.

Many people color their hair, either in an attempt to cover gray and look younger or simply for fun. A temporary color rinse contains a water-soluble color that coats the outside of the hair and does not actually dye it or change the hair structure. It can provide highlights, lessen the appearance of graying, or intensify and darken the natural shade, but the effect is removed by shampooing. A semi-permanent tint contains dyes that adhere strongly to the cuticle and provide a color coating that lasts through four to six shampoos. These products come in many shades, but cannot lighten the hair, only darken it.

Permanent dyes are coloring agents that provide a deeper and more lasting color effect. The chemicals penetrate the shaft and permanently change the color of the hair. As the hair grows, the new growth comes in the original color and can produce obvious "roots"—undyed hair close to the head. Permanent dyes are available in a variety of forms and some dyes use chemicals to remove the existing color from the hair and deposit the desired dye color into the cortex of the hair. This method can either lighten or darken the hair. These dyes can cause irritation, allergic reactions, or blindness if they accidentally get into the eyes. Beginning in the 1950s, reports began to surface linking permanent hair dyes to cancer. However, a meta-analysis by Kelsh et al., (2008) did not find a link between bladder cancer, one of the commonly claimed cancers, and hair dyes.

Metallic dyes have been used for centuries. These dyes use the salts of various metals such as lead, silver, and copper to add color to gray hair. These "color restorers," are said to make hair without pigment resume its natural pigmented shade. When a small amount of formula containing lead acetate, for example, is combed through the hair daily, the salt reacts with the sulfur of hair keratin to form lead sulfide, which coats the cuticle of the hair. Gradual color change from gray to yellow to brown to black is obtained with repeated applications. The result can be a flat-looking, unnatural color that is incompatible with other dyes or chemical processes and is very difficult to remove. In addition, lead is toxic so exposure can be harmful.

Vegetable dyes are a third class of permanent hair coloring agents. Henna has been used for centuries to color hair and, in its pure form, is an organic dye. A powder is made from the dried leaves and twigs of several varieties of a Middle Eastern bush, *Lawsonia alba, Lawsonia inermis*, or *Lawsonia spinosa*. It is mixed with mild acids and warm water to form a henna paste which is then applied to the hair. Pure henna produces a red-orange color on hair, creating copper highlights on dark hair and vibrant orange and salmon on light or gray hair. Henna alone is drying to the hair, so many people who use henna add oil to the paste for the added conditioning. Extracts from walnut shells produce a deep brown to black dye and have been used for centuries to darken the hair.

Shampoos and Hair Styling Products

Shampoos clean the hair by removing dirt, sebum, cosmetics, and dead scalp cells that have accumulated on the hair shafts. Since everyone's hair is different, qualities produced by using a particular shampoo may be more desirable to one person than to another. In addition, the condition of the water used to wash the hair can produce different results. Traditional beauty wisdom recommends washing hair in rainwater.

While the pH of rainwater varies depending on air quality, typical rainwater is acidic with a pH between 5 and 6. Under acidic conditions, the cuticle layer of the hair flattens, producing silky, shiny hair. Under alkaline conditions, the cuticle layers are more likely to be disrupted. True soaps are slightly alkaline, roughing up the cuticle, and can react with mineral deposits to coat the hair. The traditional method of dealing with this was to give the hair a final rinse in either rainwater or water acidified with lemon juice or vinegar. Most modern shampoos contain synthetic detergents or surfactants that emulsify oils and surround the oil and dirt so that they may be easily rinsed off.

Simple dandruff is the shedding of the top cornified layers of the scalp skin, and it is experienced by everyone to some degree. Dandruff usually appears several days to a week after shampooing. Any shampoo will control dandruff if the hair is washed frequently enough. Shampoos that are specifically formulated to treat dandruff may delay the return of dandruff symptoms for a longer period of time. Seborrheic dermatitis is a skin condition characterized by inflammation, severe itching, and flaking and can be treated with medicated shampoo. Some skin diseases such as psoriasis produce dandruff-like symptoms but will not respond to anti-dandruff shampoos.

The function of hair conditioners is to reduce the static electricity that causes the individual hairs to repel one another. Conditioners also help to restore a shiny appearance, improve the texture, and increase the manageability of processed hair. Most conditioners contain cationic surfactants for controlling the hair and increasing the tensile strength of the hair shaft. Conditioners often contain protein to coat the hair and add thickness for body, and a variety of oils to provide sheen and lubrication. Shampoos and conditioners which claim to "feed the hair" would need to be absorbed through the skin to the root of the hair. Only the root of the hair, buried deep within the follicle, contains living cells that divide and grow.

Several kinds of chemical bonds hold the keratin protein complex in hair together. The most common linkage is the hydrogen bond, which influences the shape of the hair strand. Some of the hydrogen bonds are easily broken by wetting the hair, and this forms the basis for setting hair while it is wet. If the wet hair is stretched, the bonds reform into a new and temporary curl position when the hair subsequently dries. Heat will also break hydrogen bonds so that they may be realigned. Electric rollers and curling irons can set in a curl, but the result is generally not as lasting as one formed through wetting and setting. Blow-drying works on the same principle. The hairstyle is directed into place by stretching the hair over a brush while drying it with hot air. But, because wet hair in the presence of heat is highly susceptible to mechanical damage, the brush or comb that stretches the hair during a blow-drying should be used slowly and gently. Hair sprays are aqueous solutions of shellac or the resin polyvinylpyrrolidone (PVP) which stiffen the hair to hold in shape. The curl formed by wetting and setting is only temporary, lasting a day or less. A permanent realignment of the protein chains to form a permanent wave, or perm, can be accomplished by breaking the disulfide bond. This sulfur to sulfur link is responsible for the strength, great stability, and cohesiveness of keratin. Water alone cannot disrupt the disulfide bonds. Consequently, strongly alkaline thioglycolate compounds are required to rupture the bond. Thioglycolates are the essential ingredients in permanent wave solutions.

Nails

The fingernails and toenails develop from differentiation of the epidermal cells. Each nail is a cornified plate of hard keratin that rests on a thickened surface of epidermis called the nail bed (Figure 18-12). The exposed portion of the nail covering the nail bed is pink because the blood in the capillaries of the dermis is visible through the translucent nail. The nail grows from a root which is hidden beneath the skin. The root is covered by a curved fold of skin, the cuticle, and a half-moon-shaped whitish area, the lunule, appears on the part of the nail body closest to the cuticle. The lunule may be completely hidden by the nail fold. If visible, the half-moon is largest on the thumbnail and becomes progressively less apparent in the other fingers. The white spots that occasionally appear on the nails are caused by air bubbles between the keratinized cells and are caused by an interruption of keratinization during growth of the nail, often due to injury. Nails grow an average of 0.5 mm per week and faster in the summer than in the winter.

Hangnails are the result of cracks or splits of the skin alongside the nails. They may stem from excessive skin dryness due to frequent washing of the hands, harsh cleansers, or dry environmental conditions. Hangnails may also be caused by picking at the skin surrounding the nail or other physical damage. Brittle, splitting nails can be caused by exposure to harsh environmental agents (detergents, solvents, nail polish remover), dehydration of the nails, or extreme cold. Nails absorb water and swell when immersed in water for long periods. As they dry out, they shrink and weaken; wearing protective gloves when working with water, cleansers, detergents, or any other chemicals can prevent damage to the nails. Nail polish can strengthen weak nails, but most modern nail polish contains several toxic chemicals including toluene and formaldehyde (both known carcinogens) and phthalates (an endocrine disruptor). Nail polish removers usually contain acetone or ethyl acetate, both of which dry the nails and surrounding cuticle.

ALTERING APPEARANCES

There are a number of reasons people change their appearance. For some, it is an attempt to look older; for others, a method of fighting aging. A change in social status can be indicated by a change in appearance. In some cultures, unmarried women wear their hair long and loose; once married, they put it up or cover it. Tattoos and scarification have been used for decoration or as part of coming of age rituals to indicate a woman is now considered to be an adult. Cosmetics can be used to cover skin damage, enhance specific features, protect the body, or to display a

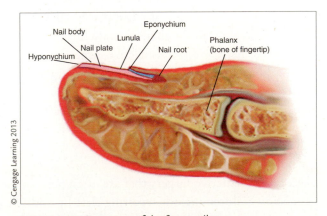

FIGURE 18-12: Structures of the fingernail.

message. Furthermore, changes can make someone blend in with a specific group or stand out from the crowd. Some modes of alteration, such as cosmetics and hair dyes are reversible, while others like cosmetic surgery or tattoos are more permanent.

Temporary Body Art

Decorating the body seems to be an inborn characteristic of humans. Children draw and paint on themselves almost as soon as they can grip a pen. Temporary body art can be applied and removed fairly easily because it does not go beyond the epidermis. The most familiar type of temporary body art is the makeup many women apply daily. Body painting and henna are other examples.

Permanent Body Art

Permanent body art—tattoos, scarification, and piercings—appears in many, many cultures and across time. These permanent means of decorating the skin fluctuate in popularity and cultural acceptability. The famous Otzi, the ice mummy discovered in the Alps, bore tattoos as do the ancient ice mummies from the Russian steppes. Native peoples around the Pacific Rim have used tattoos for centuries. Decorative scarification is practiced across many areas of Africa. Today, piercings and tattoos have also become common in the United States and Western Europe. Permanent body art has moved to the mainstream (Braverman, 2006).

While pierced ears have been common for centuries, piercing of other body parts is now becoming more popular. Piercings can be kept open with metal jewelry, wooden plugs, and any of a variety of other materials. Some piercings also include stretching to enlarge the hole. This form of body art is not without potential risks. According to Mayers and Chiffriller (2008), 19 percent of university students sampled experencedi complications from piercings, primarily infections. However, piercings associated with chipped teeth, tissue tears, allergies, and infections were reported in 45 percent of participants surveyed in a European study (Antoszewski et al., 2006).

Tattoos involve the introduction of pigments into the dermis layer of the skin using a needle. Designs range from tiny images to full body designs. Tattoos can indicate familial associations, identify tribal linkages, commemorate an event in the wearer's life, or they can simply be body art. Because the tattoo needle pierces the skin, there is a risk of infection, including the blood-borne pathogens HIV and hepatitis. Most professionals tattoo artists are well-versed in universal precautions and infection risks. Contracting an infection now rare among reputable artists. Neither Mayers and Chiffriller (2008) nor Laumann and Derick (2006) reported infections associated with tattoos in their research.

Aesthetic branding involves producing burns using heat, laser, or freezing to generate permanent scars. While traditional in many parts of the world, this form of body art is not widespread in the West. As with any burn, the risk of infection is high. In addition, branding is associated with a number of high risk behaviors in adolescents (Karamanoukian et al., 2006).

Surgeries that Alter Appearance

Plastic surgery is surgery that alters a person's appearance, and its history goes back to at least the eighth century B.C. There are two types of plastic surgery: cosmetic surgery and reconstructive surgery. **Cosmetic surgery** is elective, and it is performed to alter some aspect of a person's face or body to what is perceived as a more aesthetic appearance. Breast augmentation, eyelid lifts, liposuction, tummy tucks, and nose reshaping are the most common cosmetic surgeries (American Society of Plastic Surgeons, 2009). **Reconstructive surgery** is completed to restore parts of the body that may have been destroyed or injured by birth defect, accident, or disease. In some cases, reconstructive surgery corrects a problem that has developed due to aging, although in this case the line between cosmetic and reconstructive surgery can become blurred. In general, reconstructive surgery is performed to restore and improve function or to approximate an average or typical appearance. In the United States, most health insurance policies will cover reconstructive surgeries, but they will generally not cover cosmetic surgeries. Some examples of reconstructive surgery that are often performed on children include repairing cleft-lip and cleft palate, removing birthmarks, and correcting

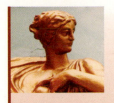

Cultural Considerations
THE HENNAED HAND

For over 5000 years, henna has been used to decorate the body. While most people are familiar with henna's use as a hair dye, the application of henna to the skin to create designs that last several weeks has been limited to Africa, the Middle East, and Asia until recently. Traditions link henna to important events. In India, brides are decorated before the wedding. In Morocco, henna was used as both a protective charm and for celebrations (Fabius, 1998). Each region developed its own designs, a practice that continues with modern henna artists. Today, henna artists can be found throughout the world.

The leaves of the henna plant, *Lawsonia inermis*, are ground to a fine, green powder and mixed with mild acids, usually tea and lime juice, to produce a paste. The recipe for henna paste varies from artist to artist. Applied to the skin and allowed to stay on the skin for several hours, the green paste dyes the layers of the epidermis (Figure 18-13). After 12–24 hours, the design is coated with a vegetable oil to soften the dried paste, and it is removed, revealing the stained skin (Figure 18-14). The final color varies from orange to rust to brown depending on the henna mixture and the thickness of the skin. The design stays until the epidermal layers wear off.

True henna does not damage the skin and actually has both astringent and antibacterial properties. A few people can have an allergic reaction to the henna itself or one of the other components in the paste, but this is rare. Black and other colored "hennas" have appeared on the market in recent years.

These are adulterated with sometimes toxic chemicals which can cause permanent damage to the skin. They are not true henna.

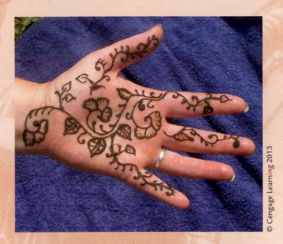

FIGURE 18-13: A design in henna paste.

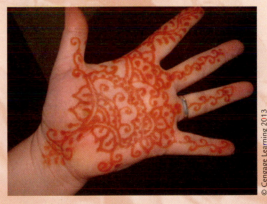

FIGURE 18-14: A henna design after the paste has been removed. The orange-brown color will remain for several weeks.

hand deformities. Some common hand deformities include syndactyly (webbed fingers) and extra or missing fingers. In some cases, large or unusually shaped ears can also be re-shaped. Reconstructive surgeries are sometimes required after tumor removal as part of treatment for cancer, such as breast reconstructive surgery after mastectomy.

Reconstructive surgery may also be necessary if a person suffers a severe burn or traumatic injuries such as a fracture of facial bones. Because most procedures involve incisions into the skin and the use of anesthesia, both cosmetic and reconstructive surgeries carry the same risks of infection or medication reaction that all surgeries do.

EVIDENCE BASED PRACTICE

Does Plastic Surgery Improve Body Image?

Elective cosmetic surgery is becoming more common among adolescents, but does surgery improve body image? Does it matter if the surgery is reconstructive (to repair a deformity) or elective (for aesthetic reasons)? In one 2002 study, Simis et al., examined these questions. Patients ranging in age from 12-22 received both preoperative and postoperative phone interviews and questionnaires asking about body satisfaction and attitudes, self rating of appearance, and other appearance-related issues. The results were then compared with a control group from the general population. The patient sample showed greater improvement in attitudes compared to the control sample. Those in the elective breast surgery group reported the greatest improvement, but surgery patients in both the elective and the reconstructive groups reported improved satisfaction with their appearance. This agrees with another German study which followed up a group of patients undergoing elective surgery. Eighty-four percent of those patients were highly satisfied with their surgery, 85 percent said they would undergo the same treatment again, and 94 percent would recommend their procedure (Papadopulos et al., 2007).

Mammoplasty: Breast Augmentation

From the pushed-up breasts of the 1940s pinup girls to the surgically enhanced and airbrushed stars of today, breasts are the objects of sexual attraction, at least in some cultures (Ectoff, 1999). In the United States, breast augmentation is the most commonly performed cosmetic surgery (Pelosi and Pelosi, 2010). However, the number of breast augmentation surgeries per year is dropping. In 2008, approximately 300,000 women underwent breast augmentation, a reduction of 12 percent from the year before (American Society of Plastic Surgeons, 2009).

Early surgeries to increase breast size used a woman's own adipose tissue that was transplanted to her breasts. While this method is still used, the results can be unpredictable because of the tendency for fat to be reabsorbed by the body. Another early method involved the injection of free silicone fluid into the breasts. This method proved unsatisfactory since a large quantity of silicon fluid dispersed away from the injection site causing infection and inflammation. Silicone liquid has been banned for breast augmentation in the United States since 1965. The most current methods involve either a flexible shell prefilled with silicone gel or an inflatable pouch that is filled with saline solution once in place. Saline inflatables feel softer than silicone gel implants and require a smaller incision for insertion. Their size can also be more easily adjusted. The implants can be inserted under the pectoral muscles or under the mammary glands, but above the muscles (Pelosi and Pelosi, 2010).

Breast augmentation is not without risks. Potential complications include capsular contracture, rippling, implant rupture, infection, or hematoma. Capsular contraction occurs when scar tissue forms, contracts, and hardens around the implant. Rippling most often occurs when wrinkles form in the implant or as a complication of contracture. This occurs most often in women who are underweight. In a 15 year longitudinal study, 14 percent of women with breast implants required additional surgery to correct complications (Codner et al., 2010). The United States Food and Drug Administration, in their 2004 Consumer Breast Implant Handbook, warns that women should expect to have additional surgeries to either remove or replace their implants. They also warn that many of the changes to the breasts following implantation can be cosmetically undesirable and also irreversible. Some of these changes include dimpling of the skin, wrinkling, and loss of breast tissue. For many women, these changes are unacceptable. In 2007, almost 27,000 women in the United States chose to have their implants removed (American Society of Plastic Surgeons, 2009).

Another concern associated with breast implants involves interference with the detection of breast cancer. Early detection of breast cancer, particularly of microcalcifications, can be more difficult when breast implants are present. However, in a study of over 4000 women, breast implants did not alter the rates of breast cancer detection, the stage at which the tumors were first identified, or the survival rates of the patients (Handel, 2007). Some implants now use a radiotransparent gel which does not interfere with mammograms but may require a slightly higher dose of radiation to obtain clear images (Garcia-Tutor et al., 2010). Finally, scar tissue surrounding the implants can either mask lumps or be mistaken for lumps in women performing BSE.

Leakage and rupture of breast implants can occur. During the 1990s, leaking silicone was linked with connective tissue disorders and autoimmune

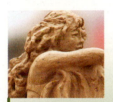

Economic Considerations
THE COST OF BEAUTY

The appearance of skin, hair, and nails contributes to sexual attractiveness. Enhancing their appeal has been part of every culture for thousands of years. Eons ago, some enterprising human being probably discovered that oils could be used to soften the skin and smooth the hair. Perhaps recognizing something powerful and splendid about the vivid colors of nature, primitive men and women mixed red clay or copper ore with water, daubed it on the face, and invented the first makeup. The face and body became the canvas for visible symbols, for dramatizing cultural ideas. Paint pots and implements to grind and apply eye shadow and liner have been unearthed in Egypt and dated to 10,000 years ago. Archeologists digging in Sumerian tombs have found 5000-year-old lip pigments. Throughout the ages, various substances have been applied to the skin to clean, perfume, or protect it. With the addition of colored pigments, these substances could even be used to cover flaws, camouflage the body, frighten enemies, or ward off evil spirits. As the use of makeup expanded, it began to be used by individuals to make a personal statement. There is nothing new about cosmetics; they have been in use for thousands of years.

What is new is the emergence of the cosmetics industry. Before the twentieth century, there was very little marketing of cosmetic products. Most preparations were created in the home from recipes that used household items or ingredients purchased from a pharmacist. In 1849, 39 manufacturers produced a total of $355 worth of cosmetics that cost only $164 to make (Corson, 1972). Today, the cosmetics industry has multibillion dollar annual sales depending on exactly which items are included in the thousands of formulations on the market. The dollar figure varies, according to whether sales of shampoos, deodorants, toothpaste, or mouthwash are contained in the totals. It is probably valid to include all such products in one mass group. All of them appeal to the buyer's desire to make themselves more appealing. With the largest advertising budget of any commercial enterprise in the United States, the cosmetics industry offers health, success, fulfillment, attractiveness, or a whole new lifestyle if only people will buy, buy, buy their products.

Currently, the primary focus of cosmetics advertising is directed toward women, who are the greatest consumers of the products. Even women who do not use cosmetics such as facial makeup or nail polish usually buy shampoos, hair conditioners, and toilet soaps. Even the most widely used cosmetic product, toothpaste, is sold as a beauty enhancer. The promotion of toothpaste may be based on sex appeal or plaque removal depending on whether the sales pitch is to enhance sexual attractiveness sex or to prevent cavities. And while skin-care products designed strictly for men are viewed by the industry as an additional opportunity for revenue, the major profit is derived from cosmetics purchased by women.

conditions. More recently, however, the National Cancer Institute reported that, in their opinion, there was no evidence that silicone breast implants were linked to lupus or rheumatoid arthritis, autoimmune conditions which attack connective tissues (Brinton et al., 2004). Another potential problem with silicone leakage is the transfer of platinum, which is used to give silicone gel its consistency, out of the implants and into women's tissues. Lykissa & Maharaj (2006) found that platinum does leak out of implants into women's tissues and can be found in their urine, hair, and breast milk. More importantly, they found the platinum in an oxidation form that can cause neurological damage.

Breast Reconstruction After Mastectomy

Until recently, the primary treatment for breast cancer was mastectomy, the complete removal of the breast. The loss of a breast is devastating to some women. For these women, postmastectomy breast reconstruction may be an option that can improve the quality of life after surgery. Both saline and silicone gel implants can be used for reconstruction, however, there is evidence that patients are more satisfied with the results of silicone implants (McCarthy et al., 2010). Postmastectomy breast reconstruction is subject to the same potential complications as breast augmentation. There is the possibility of rupture, capsular contracture, hematoma, and infection. In addition, the effects of other cancer treatment regimes may have an impact on patient satisfaction with the reconstruction. In a study of over 600 mastectomy patients, those who also underwent radiation therapy were less satisfied with the reconstruction results (McCarthy et al., 2010), implying that postmastectomy treatments should be taken into consideration when discussing reconstruction with a physician.

Reduction Mammoplasty

Macromastia, or disproportionately large breasts, can cause physical discomfort for a woman including neck and back pain, deep grooves in her shoulders from her bra straps, and difficulty in performing ordinary activities. She may also experience uncomfortable chafing, a skin rash and itching under her breasts. For women with macromastia, reduction mammoplasty is an option. In 2008, over 88,000 breast reductions were performed in the United States (American Society of Plastic Surgeons, 2009). During this procedure, some of the breast tissue is removed, the skin over the breast is proportionately adjusted, and the nipple and the areola are relocated to a new position. Alternately, liposuction can be used to remove fat from the breasts (Habbema and Alons, 2010). In most instances, there is no loss of sensation in the nipples, and women are still able to breastfeed after surgery. However, some surgeons recommend that the operation be delayed until childbearing and breast-feeding are no longer desired. Postoperative complications can include scarring, infection, and inflammation.

BODY IMAGE AND BODY SIZE

While cosmetics, body art, and surgery usually focus on a single aspect of the body's appearance, size impacts the whole body and is a major factor influencing appearance. Body size is often expressed in terms of the body mass index (BMI), which equals one's weight (kg) divided by height in meters squared (m^2). The USDA defines a BMI between 19 and 25 as healthy. Individuals with a BMI below 19 are defined as underweight, and individuals with a BMI over 25 are defined as overweight. Individuals with a BMI of 30 or greater are considered obese. BMI is not a perfect measure. It does not take into account factors such as the ratio of dense muscle to less dense fat tissue. Individuals, such as athletes, with very low body fat and high muscle mass often have a higher BMI than a less active person of similar size.

Mass media messages on movie and TV screens and on the pages of many magazines promote the message that, for women, thin is sexier, thin is beautiful, and that the best-looking body is a tall and slender body. Many women starve themselves in an attempt to achieve and maintain that ideal. Eating disorders are one complication of the fixation with being thin (Figure 18-15).

Despite the current fixation with being thin, the Centers for Disease Control reports that 72.5 million Americans are obese (CDC, 2010). A number of serious health problems are associated with obesity, including hypertension, coronary heart disease, thrombophlebitis, diabetes mellitus, respiratory and gastrointestinal (liver and gallbladder) disorders, pregnancy difficulties in women, and certain kinds of

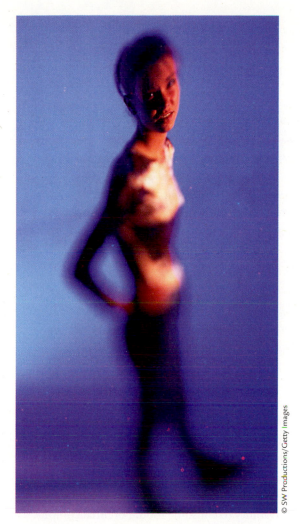

FIGURE 18-15: In an effort to conform to the ideal of beauty in early twenty-first century American culture, women who starve themselves to achieve extreme thinness run the risk of experiencing an eating disorder.

excess energy is stored as body fat. For many, weight gain or loss is just that simple. Too much food and a sedentary life, taking the elevator instead of climbing stairs, driving instead of walking, watching sports instead of participating in them, result in weight gain. Unfortunately, while overeating may be at the root of weight problems, the total picture of obesity is neither clear-cut nor simple. There is no one cause for obesity; excessive body fat is associated with a multitude of causes that include anatomical, neurological, behavioral, psychological, genetic, and social factors. The basis for obesity may be highly complex and different for different people. Current thinking places the major emphasis on several key areas—early over nutrition, inherited metabolic differences, lack of physical activity, and a combination of social factors that include home, family, education, economic status, and cultural influences.

Many obese people do not consume any more calories than the people of a healthy weight, and some actually eat less. That observation has led to the proposal that there may be some difference in metabolic efficiency. The role that brown adipose tissue might play has attracted recent attention. White adipose tissue, which is distributed throughout the body, is primarily a storage site for excess energy. Brown adipose tissue is responsible for producing body heat. In human babies, brown adipose tissue is found at the nape of the neck and in between the shoulder blades, but constitutes only about one percent of the total body weight.

cancer. Obese individuals are likely to experience an increased incidence of osteoarthritis in weight-bearing joints, have a greater number of accidents, and are at significantly greater risk when undergoing surgery. In addition to the risks to physical health, obese individuals are likely to experience greater emotional distress. They are often stigmatized as lacking willpower, and they may suffer not only social but also economic discrimination.

What Causes Obesity?

When someone takes in more calories than they are able to metabolize, the

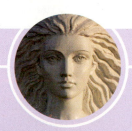

focus on
EXERCISE
Exercise Affects Girls' Self-Image

In a nine month school based study of formerly sedentary adolescent girls, Schneider et al. (2008) found that introducing supervised vigorous cardiovascular activity four times per week improved the girls', physical self-concept while improving their cardiovascular fitness. In addition to supervised physical activities, the girls received instruction promoting physical activity outside of the school one day per week. This is a potentially important finding since adolescence is a time when young women often struggle to maintain a positive self-image.

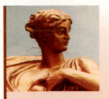

Cultural Considerations
WHERE BIGGER IS BEAUTIFUL

Beauty is in the eye of the beholder, and while the current media view of beauty generally promotes thin, athletic women, this is not the case everywhere. In Mauritania, a desert country on the western coast of Africa, the ideal woman is obese. Traditionally, being fat was seen as a sign of wealth and beauty, and men desired heavy women. In many areas of the world where food is scarce, the perfect beauty carries a good deal of extra weight (Harter, 2004). Women with extra body fat are more likely to have the reserves needed to carry a pregnancy to term. To obtain this ideal, young girls in Mauritania have historically been force-fed to gain weight. It is one of the few countries where girls receive more food than boys. While fewer girls are force-fed today, women are resorting to more modern methods including using steroids and other medications to stimulate the appetite and add weight (Harter, 2007).

Traditions are difficult to change despite the negative impact of obesity on health. The Mauritanian government has begun a campaign promoting a healthier weight as the ideal. Exposure to world media is also contributing to a glacial change in attitudes. Younger men, particularly in the urban areas, are rejecting fatness as a symbol of beauty.

In adults, there is evidence that this brown fat tissue has the potential to be activated to burn energy and facilitate weight loss (Saely et al., 2010).

Evidence for a genetic basis for obesity is supported by studies of identical twins. One study suggested that some people may have an inherited ability to turn excess food directly into fat tissue (Bouchard et al., 1990). Further genomic research has identified a number of genes linked to metabolic variation and heritable obesity (Jarick et al., 2010).

Several methods can be used to treat obesity. Calorie restriction, increased physical activity, and behavior therapy can be effective in reducing weight for many people. For others, medications that increase metabolism, alter the body's ability to absorb fat, and suppress appetite are effective. Unfortunately, serious side effects have been observed from some weight loss medication. For example, a commonly prescribed pair of weight loss drugs (fenfluramine and dexfenfluramine) was found to be associated with valvular heart disease, and the combination was removed from the market.

For the extremely obese adult who remains overweight despite maintaining a restricted diet, there are several surgical treatments that have been endorsed by the National Institutes of Health. Candidates for weight reduction surgery are individuals whose obesity is associated with potentially life-threatening health problems. Gastric bypass surgery and stomach banding (Figure 18-16) are used to diminish the capacity and the outlet of the stomach, thus restricting the ability to consume food. Potential complications of these treatments include postoperative wound infection, bleeding, ulcers, and long-term gastrointestinal complaints such as distressing diarrhea and excessive gas.

EATING DISORDERS

Based on National Institute of Mental Health research, eating disorders affect approximately six percent of women and less than one percent of men in the United States (Hudson et al., 2007). In most cases, eating disorders develop between puberty and the early 20s, but they can develop at any point in an individual's life. Two of the most common forms of eating disorders are anorexia and bulimia. A person with **anorexia** will starve themselves in an effort to avoid becoming what they perceive as overweight. An important component of this disease is a distorted body image, where the person with the disease sees themselves as heavier than they actually are. In some cases, the anorexic has

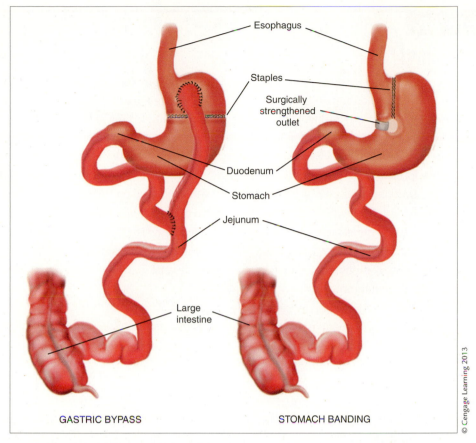

FIGURE 18-16: Gastric bypass and stomach banding.

Critical Thinking

Ban on Too-Thin Models.

As a step toward addressing the growing problems of eating disorders such as anorexia and bulimia, countries such as Spain, Italy, Brazil, and India have banned models that are too thin from being hired to display clothing during fashion shows in those countries. France considered such a ban, but instead implemented an education program to try to influence designers and to inform them about the health hazards of eating disorders. What is the best approach to reducing the number of women developing eating disorders?

unrealistic expectations of perfection for themselves that contribute to their distorted body image. The lack of calories and proper levels of nutrients have several negative impacts on the body. Short-term effects include amenorrhea, muscle weakness, skin and hair deterioration, slow healing, headache, and memory loss. In the long term, the lack of nutrition associated with this disease can lead to permanent impacts on brain and bone development and deterioration of other vital organs. In the case of

bulimia, a person may binge, eating hundreds of calories, only to purge in an effort to compensate for the additional calories consumed. Purging can take the form of vomiting, over-exercising, or the misuse of laxatives. Bulimics are often plagued by the deterioration of both tooth enamel and the lining of the esophagus caused by stomach acids and vomiting. Both anorexia and bulimia can lead to life-threatening electrolyte disorders which can lead to heart arrhythmias, coma, and death.

Case Study

A Sense of Control

Seventeen-year-old Tiffany is stressed and tired of doing what everyone else arranges for her to do. Her parents have enrolled her in a competitive, college prep high school. They plan for her to get into an Ivy League school. She has grown up with an appreciation of good food. Her mother is a caterer who practices new menus on the family before using them with clients. Tiffany has noticed she has put on some weight and this has her concerned. She is in dance line and works as a window model for a local clothing store. To her, the extra pounds are not acceptable. She needs to look good in dance line to get that on her college application, and she cannot afford to lose the modeling job because she needs the money to pay for school. She goes online and finds several websites with advice on quick weight loss. She has a big competition coming up in three weeks and wants to be thinner by then. She reduces her daily food intake to an apple, a salad, and glass of skim milk. She gets such positive feedback about her looks and such a sense of control about the weight loss that she continues the diet long after she reaches her initial goal. She becomes dissatisfied with her current weight and keeps lowering her weight loss goal. She knows what she's doing is unhealthy, but she can't stop. Finally she collapses at dance line practice and is rushed to the hospital. After an examination, the doctor explains to her parents that he suspects anorexia.

1. What are the short-term health risks of Tiffany's condition?

2. What are the long-term health risks of her condition?

3. What steps does Tiffany need to take to restore her health?

CONCLUSION

The integument protects the body from the environment and contributes significantly to an individual's appearance. Throughout history and across different cultures, the vision of perfect beauty has changed. To meet that ideal, people have modified their appearance through a variety of methods ranging from the temporary application of cosmetics to permanent alterations by surgery. While alterations of appearance has been practiced by women for centuries, striving to attain cultural ideals can result in destructive behaviors in the form of eating disorders.

REVIEW QUESTIONS

1. Describe the structure of the skin, including dermis, epidermis, and hypodermis.

2. What physiological effect does tanning have on the skin?

3. What is the role of the United States Food and Drug Administration in regulating the ingredients found in cosmetics?

4. Explain the two methods for dying hair.

5. Describe some of the potential complications of breast augmentation surgery.

6. What are some risks associated with being overweight?

7. What are some health risks of eating disorders?

CRITICAL THINKING QUESTIONS

1. Is a focus on appearance an inherent human trait, or is it a consequence of advertising and the cosmetics industry?

2. How might living in a "youth" culture influence people in ways that they might not be aware of?

WEBLINKS

FDA Handbook on Breast Implants
www.fda.gov/cdrh/breastimplants/ handbook2004/localcomplications.html
National Cancer Institute
www.cancer.org

National Association of Anorexia Nervosa and Associated Disorders
www.anad.org

REFERENCES

American Society of Plastic Surgeons. 2000/2007/2008 National plastic surgery statistics. Retrieved November 15, 2010 from http://www.plasticsurgery.org/Media/stats/2008-cosmetic-reconstructive-plastic-surgery-minimally-invasive-statistics.pdf.

Antoszewski, B., Sitek, A., Jedrzejczak, M., Kasielska, A., & Kruk-Jeromin, J. (2006). Are body piercing and tattooing safe fashions? *European Journal of Dermatology, 16*(5), 572–575.

Berg, N., & Lien, D. (2002). Measuring the effect of sexual orientation on income: Evidence of discrimination? *Contemporary Economic Policy, 20*(4), 394–414.

Binder, W. J., Blitzer, A., & Brin, M. F. (1998). Treatment of hyperfunctional lines of the face with botulism toxin A. *Dermatologic Surgery, 24*(11), 1198–1205.

Blandford, J. (2003). The nexus of sexual orientation and gender in the determination of earnings. *Industrial and Labor Relations Review, 56*(4), 622–642.

Bluhm, R., Branch, R., Johnston, P., & Stein, R. (1991). Aplastic anemia associated with canthaxanthin ingested for "tanning" purposes. *Journal of the American Medical Association, 264*(9), 1141–1142.

Bouchard, C., Tremblay, A., Després, J. P., Nadeau, A., Lupien, P. J., Thériault, G., Dussault, J.,

Moorjani, S., Pinault, S., & Fournier, G. (1990). The response to long-term overfeeding in identical twins. *New England Journal of Medicine, 322*(21), 1477–1482.

Braverman, P. K. (2006). Body art: Piercing, tattooing, and scarification. *Adolescent Medicine Clinics, 17*(3), 505–519, abstract ix.

Brinton, L. A., Buckley, L. M., Dvorkina, O., et al., (2004). Risk of connective tissue disorders among breast implant patients. *American Journal of Epidemiology, 160*(7), 619–627.

Centers for Disease Control. (2010). Vital signs: State-specific obesity prevalence among adults – 2009. *Morbidity and Mortality Weekly Report, 59*, 1–5.

Codner, M. A., Diego Mejia, J., Locke, M. B., Mahoney, A., Thiels, C., Nahai, F. R., Hester, T. R., & Nahai, F. (2010). A 15-year experience with primary breast augmentation. *Plastic & Reconstructive Surgery, 127*(3), 1300–1310.

Corson, R. (1972). *Fashions in makeup.* New York, NY: Universe Books.

Cosgrove, M. C., Franco, O. H., Granger, S. P., Murray, P. G., & Mayes, A. E. (2007). Dietary nutrient intakes and skin-aging appearance among middle-aged American women. *American Journal of Clinical Nutrition, 86*(4), 1225–1231.

Ectoff, N. (1999). *Survival of the prettiest: The science of beauty.* New York, NY: Anchor Books.

Fabius, C. (1998). *Mehndi: The art of henna body painting.* New York, NY: Three Rivers Press.

Garcia-Tutor, E., Alonso-Burgos, A., Marre, D., & Alfaro Adrian, C. (2010). Radiotransparency of polyvinylpyrrolidone-hydrogel and hydrogel breast implants: A quantitative analysis with mastectomy specimens. *Aesthetic Plastic Surgery, 35*(2), 203–201. doi:10.1007/s00266–010–9588–5.

Habbema, L., & Alons, J. J. (2010). Liposuction of the female breast: A histologic study of the aspirate. *Dermatologic Surgery, 36*(9), 1406–1410. doi:10.1111/j.1524–4725.2010.01649.x.

Hampton, P. J., Farr, P. M., Diffey, B. L., & Lloyd, J. J. (2004). Implication for photosensitive patients of ultraviolet A exposure in vehicles. *British Journal of Dermatology, 151*(4), 873–876.

Handel, N. (2007). The effect of silicone implants on the diagnosis, prognosis, and treatment of breast cancer. *Plastic and Reconstructive Surgery, 120*(7 Suppl 1), 81S–93S.

Hanson, K. M., & Simon, J. D. (1998). Epidermal trans-urocanic acid and the UVA-induced photoaging of the skin. *Proceedings of the National Academy of Sciences of the United States of America, 95*(18), 10576–10578.

Harter, P. (2004, January 26). Mauritania's 'wife-fattening' farm. Mauritania, Africa: British Broadcasting Company. Retrieved May 3, 2008 from http://news.bbc.co.uk/2/hi/africa/3429903.stm.

Harter, P. (2007, April 26). Mauritania's battle over beauty. In E. Rippon (producer), *Crossing continents.* Mauritania, Africa: British Broadcasting Company. Retrieved from http://news.bbc.co.uk/2/hi/programmes/crossing_continents/6567983.stm.

Hexsel, C. L., Bangert, S. D., Hebert, A. A., & Lim, H. W. (2008). Current sunscreen issues: 2007 Food and Drug Administration sunscreen labeling recommendations and combination sunscreen/insect repellent products. *Journal of the American Academy of Dermatology, 59*(2), 316–323.

Hudson, J. I., Hiripi, E., Pope, H. G., & Kessler, R. C. (2007). The prevalence and correlates of eating disorders in the National Comorbidity Survey replication. *Biological Psychiatry; 61,* 348–358.

Jarick, I., Vogel, C. I., Scherag, S., Schäfer, H., Hebebrand, J., Hinney, A., & Scherag, A. (2011). Novel common copy number variation for early onset extreme obesity on chromosome 11q11 identified by a genome-wide analysis. *Human Molecular Genetics, 20*(4), 820–842.

Karamanoukian, R., Ukatu, C., Lee, E., Hyman, J., Sundine, M., Kobayashi, M., & Evans, G. R. (2006). Aesthetic skin branding: A novel form of body art with adverse clinical sequela. *Journal of Burn Care & Research, 27*(1), 108–110.

Kelsh, M. A., Alexander, D. D., Kalmes, R. M., & Buffler, P. A. (2008). Personal use of hair dyes and risk of bladder cancer: A meta-analysis of epidemiologic data. *Cancer Causes & Control, 19*(6), 549–558.

Kim, S. S., Kim, J. Y., Lee, N. H., & Hyun, C. G. (2008). Antibacterial and anti-inflammatory effects of Jeju medicinal plants against acne-inducing bacteria. *Journal of General and Applied Microbiology, 54*(2), 101–106.

Laumann, A. E., & Derick, A. J. (2006). Tattoos and body piercings in the United States: A national data set. *Journal of the American Academy of Dermatology, 55*(3), 413–421.

Levy, P. M. (2007). The 'Nefertiti lift': A new technique for specific re-contouring of the jawline. *Journal of Cosmetic and Laser Therapy, 9*(4), 249–252.

Lykissa, E. D., & Maharaj, S. V. (2006). Total platinum concentration and platinum oxidation states in body fluids, tissue, and explants from women exposed to silicone and saline breast implants by Ic-ICPMS. *Analytical Chemistry, 78*(9), 2925–2933.

Mayers, L. B., & Chiffriller, S. H. (2008). Body art (body piercing and tattooing) among undergraduate university students: "Then and now." *Journal of Adolescent Health, 42*(2), 201–203.

McCarthy, C. M., Klassen, A. F., Cano, S. J., Scott, A., Vanlaeken, N., Lennox, P. A., Alderman, A. K., Mehrara, B. J., Disa, J. J., Cordeiro, P. G., & Pusic, A. L. (2010). Patient satisfaction with postmastectomy breast reconstruction: A comparison of saline and silicone implants. *Cancer, 116*(24), 5584–5591.

National Cancer Institute. (2010). Retrieved February 15, 2010 from www.cancer.gov

Ochsendorf, F. R., & Degitz, K. (2008). Drug therapy of acne. *Hautarzt, 59*(7), 579–589.

Papadopulos, N. A., Kovacs, L., Krammer, S., Herschbach, P., Henrich, G., & Biemer, E. (2007). Quality of life following aesthetic plastic surgery: A prospective study. *Journal of Plastic, Reconstructive & Aesthetic Surgery, 60*(8), 915–921.

Paradisi, R., Fabbri, R., Porcu, E., Battaglia, C., Seracchioli, R., & Venturoli, S. (2010). Retrospective, observational study on the effects and tolerability of flutamide in a large population of patients with acne and seborrhea over a 15-year period. *Gynecological Endocrinology.* Advance online publication. doi:10.3109/09513590.2010.526664.

Pelosi, M. A. 3rd, & Pelosi, M. A. 2nd. (2010). Breast augmentation. *Obstetrics & Gynecology Clinics of North America, 37*(4), 533–546.

Richmond, H. M., Lozano, A., Jones, D., & Duvic, M. (2008). Primary cutaneous follicle center lymphoma associated with alopecia areata. *Clinical Lymphoma & Myeloma, 8*(2), 121–124.

Robbins, J. (2006). *Healthy at 100: The scientifically proven secrets of the world's healthiest people.* New York, NY: Random House.

Saely, C. H., Geiger, K., & Drexel, H. (2010). Brown versus white adipose tissue: A mini-review. *Gerontology.* Advance online publication. doi:10.1159/000321319.

Schneider, M., Dunton, G. F., & Cooper, D. M. (2008). Physical activity and physical self-concept among sedentary adolescent females; An intervention study. *Psychology of Sport and Exercise, 9*(1), 1–14.

Simis, K. J., Hovius, S. E., de Beaufort, I. D., Verhulst, F. C., & Koot, H. M. (2002). After plastic surgery: Adolescent-reported appearance ratings and appearance-related burdens in patient and general population groups. *Plastic and Reconstructive Surgery, 109*(1), 9–17.

Smith, E. V., Grindlay, D. J., & Williams, H. C. (2011). What's new in acne? An analysis of systematic reviews published in 2009-2010. *Clinical and Experimental Dermatology, 36*(2), 119–123. doi:10.1111/j.1365–2230.2010.03921.x

Tiefer, L. (2008). New view campaign press release on female genital cosmetic surgery protest. Retrieved May 24, 2009 from http://www.newviewcampaign.org/userfiles/file/Final%20Press%20Release_11–08.pdf.

Tretinoin (Renova) approved for treatment of wrinkles. (1996, February). *Medical Sciences Bulletin, 18*(6), 2.

Viros, A., Fridlyand, J., Bauer, J., Lasithiotakis, K., Garbe, C., Pinkel, D., & Bastian, B. C. (2008). Improving melanoma classification by integrating genetic and morphologic features. *PLoS Medicine, 5*(6), e120.

APPENDIX A-WEB RESOURCES

American Congress of Obstetricians and Gynecologists www.acog.org
American Medical Association www.ama-assn.org
American Social Health Association www.ashastd.org
Center for Science in the Public Interest www.cspinet.org
Centers for Disease Control and Prevention www.cdc.gov
Gay and Lesbian Medical Association www.glma.org
National Cancer Institute www.cancer.gov
National Center for Health Statistics www.cdc.gov/nchs
National Institutes of Health www.nih.gov
National Women's Health Information Center www.womenshealth.gov
Planned Parenthood www.plannedparenthood.org
RESOLVE: The National Infertility Association www.resolve.org
U.S. Food and Drug Administration www.fda.gov
Women's Health Initiative www.nhlbi.nih.gov/whi/index.html
World Health Organization www.who.int

GLOSSARY

A

Abnormal uterine bleeding—A change in the frequency, duration, or amount of menstrual flow; may or may not indicate a medical problem.

Abortion—The termination of pregnancy before the fetus is able to live independently.

Acne—Localized skin inflammation associated with over activity of the oil glands at the base of hair follicles.

Acquired immunodeficiency syndrome (AIDS)—The last stage of the progressive human immunodeficiency virus (HIV) infection.

Activin—A peptide hormone that enhances secretion of follicle-stimulating hormone (FSH).

Acute stress—The response of the sympathetic nervous system to a single, abrupt event.

Adrenal gland—One of two glands located at the top of each kidney. Responsible for the production of cortisol, aldosterone, epinephrine, norepinephrine, and sex hormones.

Alopecia—The partial or complete loss of hair.

Amenorrhea—The absence of menstruation during a woman's reproductive years; a normal occurrence only during pregnancy.

American Medical Association (AMA)—National organization that promotes professionalism in medicine and sets standards for medical education, practice, and ethics.

Amino acid—Organic molecules composed of carbon, hydrogen, oxygen, and nitrogen that serve as the building blocks of proteins.

Amniocentesis—The withdrawal of a sample of amniotic fluid for the purpose of examination.

Amygdala—An almond-shaped mass of neurons associated with memory.

Anatomy—The study of the structure of the body.

Androgens—The male sex hormones.

Anorgasmia—The inability to experience orgasm.

Anovulation—The absence of ovulation.

Apgar score—A method for assessing a newborn's health status; a 10-point score rates color, reflex irritability, muscle tone, respiratory effort, and heart rate.

Aphrodisiac—A substance that arouses an individual to increased desire and the ability to engage in sexual activity.

Areola—Characteristic pigmented skin of the nipple that extends out onto the breast for approximately 1–2 cm.

Artificial insemination—A form of infertility treatment in which a partner's or donor's sperm is placed in a woman's reproductive tract prior to ovulation.

Assisted reproductive technology (ART)—A category of infertility treatment in which both eggs and sperm are collected, mixed, and placed into a woman's reproductive tract.

Assisted vaginal birth—A vaginal birth in which forceps or vacuum extraction are used to facilitate delivery of the baby.

ATP (adenosine triphosphate)—A high-energy molecule used for the storage of energy at a cellular level.

Axillary nodes—A cluster of small, bean-shaped nodes in the breasts; play an important role in immunity by filtering out harmful substances includes pectoral, lateral, and subscapular nodes.

AZT—A reverse transcriptase inhibitor; the first antiretroviral drug approved by the U.S. Food and Drug Administration.

B

Barr body—Sex chromatin mass seen within the nuclei of normal female somatic cells.

Barrier contraceptive—Any type of birth control that creates a physical barrier to prevent sperm and egg from meeting.

Bartholin's glands—In females, glands located in the cleft between the labia minora and the hymenal ring; responsible for secreting a clear, viscid, odorless alkaline mucus that improves the viability and motility of sperm along the female reproductive tract.

Basal body temperature (BBT)—Temperature taken upon awakening for the purpose of charting and determining the time of ovulation.

Basic research—Research conducted to expand knowledge rather than applied to a specific problem.

Blastocyst—An early stage of embryonic development consisting of a hollow ball of cells.

Braxton Hicks contractions—Uterine contractions that are irregular and painless; also known as *false labor.*

Breast self-exam (BSE)—A visual and manual examination performed by a woman on her own breasts.

C

Calorie—Also called *kilocalorie;* with a capital *C,* it is the amount of heat required to raise the temperature of a kilogram of water from 14.5 degrees Celsius to 15.5 degrees Celsius; the calorie (with a small *c*) is really 0.001 Calories, but it is used so often in association with food that it is usually understood to mean the kilocalorie.

Candida albicans—The fungus that causes candidiasis, thrush, and yeast infections.

Candidiasis—A name for vaginitis caused by genus *Candida,* primarily by the species *Candida albicans.*

Carbohydrate—Organic molecules composed of carbon, hydrogen, and oxygen, which act as the primary energy source for the cells.

Carcinogen—A substance or agent that is known to cause cancer.

Carcinoma—A new growth or malignant tumor that occurs in epithelial tissue.

Cardiovascular disease—Any disease of the heart or blood vessels, including heart attack, stroke, and atherosclerosis.

CD4 receptor—A cell surface receptor molecule; the target cells in the body attacked by HIV are those that have a CD4 receptor.

Central nervous system (CNS)—The brain and spinal cord.

Cervical cap—A thimble-shaped rubber cap used for birth control; covering only the cervix, it is used with spermicide.

Cervix—The narrow outer end of the uterus.

Cesarean section—An abdominal and uterine incision for the purpose of delivering a baby.

Chlamydia—A general term for three major groups of diseases caused by 15 recognized serotypes or strains of *Chlamydia trachomatis.*

Chlamydia trachomatis— A bacterial pathogen capable of infecting the mucus membranes of the eyes and reproductive tract.

Cholesterol—A lipid produced by the body and used in the synthesis of steroid hormones.

Chromosomes—Composed of protein and an exceedingly long and thin filamentous molecule called DNA; found in the nucleus of a cell.

Chronic stress—Repeated or long-term stimulation of the sympathetic nervous system.

Civil Rights Act—A U. S. law that bans discrimination based on race, religion, sex, color, or national origin.

Clinical breast exam—A visual and manual examination of the breasts performed by a healthcare professional.

Clinical investigation—Controlled research study designed to investigate the effectiveness of a specific treatment for a specific condition.

Clitoris—One of the structures of the female genitalia consisting of two crura, a shaft, and a glans; the homologue of the penis.

Coitus—Sexual intercourse between a man and a woman by insertion of the penis into the vagina.

Coitus interruptus—A method of contraception in which the male withdraws his penis completely from the vagina before orgasm and ejaculates well away from the vaginal orifice.

Colostrum—A thin, milky secretion expressed by the breast during pregnancy and for a few days after parturition; rich in antibodies and colostrum corpuscles.

Condom—A thin, flexible sheath closed on one end, manufactured from, and used for contraception and for the prevention of sexually transmitted disease.

Conjugated equine estrogens—A type of estrogen, administered clinically, derived from the urine of mares.

Contraction stress test (CST)—A diagnostic procedure performed to determine the fetal heart response under stress, that is, when contractions are induced by oxytocin.

Control group—A group of test subjects who are exposed to the same conditions as everyone else in the experiment, except that they are given a placebo instead of the medication being tested.

Cooper's ligaments—Supportive fibrous structures throughout the breast that partially sheathe the lobes shaping the breast.

Corpus luteum—Small, yellow endocrine structure that develops within a ruptured ovarian follicle and secretes progesterone and estrogen.

Corticosteroids—Hormonal steroids excreted by the cortex of the adrenal gland.

Cortisol—A naturally occurring steroid hormone, produced by the adrenal cortex and secreted in response to stress.

Cosmetic surgery—Any of a number of elective procedures performed to alter the body to make it more a esthetically pleasing.

Cystitis—Inflammation of the bladder.

D

Deoxyribonucleic acid (DNA)—The substance of heredity; a large molecule that carries the genetic information necessary for all cellular function including the building of proteins.

Depo-Provera—An injectable contraceptive manufactured by the Upjohn Company.

Dermis—The second layer of the skin; deep to the epidermis.

Diaphragm—A contraceptive device consisting of a soft rubber dome surrounded by a metal spring; used in conjunction with a spermicidal jelly or cream and inserted into the vagina to fit between the nooks of the anterior and posterior fornices creating a barrier that covers the cervix.

Diethylstilbestrol (DES)—A nonsteroid synthetic estrogen that has estrogenic properties, is effective when taken orally, and is less expensive than the real thing.

Double-blind study—An experiment in which neither the participants nor the researchers know which subjects in the study are receiving which treatment.

Ductal carcinoma in situ (DCIS)—A preinvasive malignancy likely to progress to cancer if no treatment takes place; with treatment, the outlook for a cure is about 98%.

Dysfunctional uterine bleeding (DUB)—A diagnosis of unpredictable, excessive, frequent, and/or prolonged bleeding from the uterus; arrived at after ruling out, through diagnostic tests and physical examination, all other possible causes.

Dysmenorrhea—Pelvic pain or cramps that occur during menstruation.

Dyspareunia—The experience of pain during sexual intercourse.

Dysplasia—Changes in the shape, size, or appearance of a cell.

E

Eclampsia—A seizure associated with pregnancy-induced hypertension.

Ectoderm—The innermost embryonic germ layer that develops into the digestive and respiratory systems and parts of the reproductive system.

Ectopic pregnancy—The implantation of an embryo outside the uterus; occurs most often in the fallopian tubes, where it is also known as a *tubal pregnancy*.

Ejaculation—The release of semen from the male reproductive tract.

Electrolytes—Essential chemicals in the blood such as sodium, potassium, and calcium ions.

Embryo—The developmental stage of a fertilized egg from implantation to eight weeks after fertilization.

Emergency contraceptive—A type of birth control that can be used up to five days after unprotected intercourse to prevent pregnancy.

Endocrine disruptors—A wide range of chemicals that can mimic the action of or interfere with hormone functions in the body.

Endocrine glands—Glands that secrete substances, including hormones, into the bloodstream.

Endocrine system—Hormones and the glands that secrete them. Consists of the pituitary gland, the thyroid gland, the parathyroid glands, the adrenal glands, the islets of Langerhans of the pancreas, the ovaries, and testes.

Endoderm—The outermost embryonic germ layer that develops into the nervous system, the skin, and some of the endocrine glands.

Endometrial cycle—The monthly shedding of tissue in response to the hormonal changes of the menstrual period.

Endometriosis—A condition in which functioning endometrial tissue is located outside of the uterine cavity.

Endometrium—The mucous membrane that lines the uterus.

Endorphin—A morphine-like neuropeptide produced by the body; blocks pain and reduces the effects of stress on the body.

Enzyme-linked immunosorbent assay (ELISA)—The most commonly used test to detect the presence of circulating antibodies to HIV virus proteins in blood serum.

Epidermis—Multilayered outer covering of the skin, consisting of four layers throughout the body, except for the palms of the hands and soles of the feet where there are five layers.

Epididymis—A 20-foot-long coiled tube that runs alongside the testis and serves as a storage site for sperm.

Epidural anesthesia—A popular anesthetic administered during labor and delivery; achieved by an injection into the epidural space between the dura mater of the spinal cord and the ligaments that connect the dura and the vertebrae.

Epinephrine—An adrenal cortex hormone produced in response to sympathetic nervous system stimulation.

Episiotomy—A small incision in the perineum, performed on a woman during childbirth to prevent the perineum from tearing.

Estradiol—A naturally occurring estrogen and the major hormone produced by the ovaries during the reproductive years.

Estriol—An estrogen that occurs naturally in the body.

Estrogen replacement therapy (ERT)—Administration of estrogen to menopausal and postmenopausal women.

Estrogen-receptor-alpha (ER-alpha)—One of the two estrogen receptors.

Estrogen-receptor-beta (ER-beta)—One of the two estrogen receptors.

Estrogens—A group of female sex hormones.

Estrone—An estrogen that occurs naturally in the body; primary form of estrogen found in postmenopausal women.

Exocrine gland—A gland that secretes substances outside the body.

F

Fallopian tube sperm profusion (FTSP)—A form of artificial insemination in which sperm are injected directly into the fallopian tubes prior to ovulation.

Fallopian tube—One of two tubes that extend from the cornu of the uterus to the ovaries and are supported by the broad ligaments; site at which eggs are fertilized.

Fatty acid—Organic molecules composed of carbon, hydrogen, and oxygen. Essential fatty acids cannot be produced by the body and must be ingested.

Female prostate—Surrounding the urethra and homologous to the male prostate, a collection of glands and ducts that manufacture secretions expelled by the urethra, and which contribute to the lubrication of the vulva.

Fetal alcohol syndrome (FAS)—Condition in which fetal development is impaired by maternal consumption of alcohol.

Fetus—The developmental stage of a fertilized egg from nine weeks after fertilization until birth.

Fibrocystic disease—A term for several benign (noncancerous) conditions of the breast characterized by lumpiness and cyclic pain.

Fibroid—A benign mass of muscle and connective tissue in the uterus; the most common gynecological tumor.

Fibromyalgia—A neuromuscular condition characterized by localized inflammation and joint and muscle pain.

Follicle—One of many spherical structures in the cortex of the ovary; consists of an oogonium or an oocyte and its surrounding epithelial cells.

Follicle-stimulating hormone (FSH)—Stimulates the growth and development of the primary follicles and results in hormone production in ovaries and sperm production in testes.

Follicular phase—The first of the three phases of the ovarian cycle.

G

Gamete intrafallopian transfer (GIFT)—A technique in which female germ cells required to begin formation of a human embryo are injected into a woman's fallopian tubes for fertilization.

Gastrulation—The formation of the three embryonic germ layers.

General adaptation syndrome—A series of physiological responses produced in response to chronic stress.

Genital warts/condylomata—A condition caused by the human papillomavirus (HPV); *condylomata* is Greek for warts.

Genome—The term for all the DNA in an organism.

Genotype—Genetic constitution.

Gestation period—The time that elapses between fertilization and birth, which encompasses the development of the embryo and fetus.

Gonadotropin-releasing hormone (GnRH)—Causes the release of both follicle-stimulating hormone (FSH) and luteinizing hormone (LH).

Graafian follicle—A mature ovarian follicle just prior to ovulation.

Granulosa cells—A layer of cells in the thera (outer layer) of an ovarian follicle; produces sex steroids.

Growth hormone (GH)—Controls the growth of all the cells of the body capable of growth, resulting in an increase in the numbers of cells and in enlargement of existing cells.

H

Health maintenance organization (HMO)—A type of health plan in which enrollees pay a fixed monthly premium for healthcare services and are required to receive all services from providers within a specific network.

Herpes virus—A group of viruses, some of which cause infections of the genital and perirectal skin characterized by repeated outbreaks of painful lesions.

High-order multiple pregnancy—A pregnancy in which three or more fetuses are developing at the same time.

Highly active antiretroviral therapy (HAART)—Therapy for HIV patients; includes three major classes of antiretroviral treatment.

Homeostasis—The maintenance of a stable internal environment, which allows the cells and tissues of the body to function optimally.

Hormone replacement therapy (HRT)—Therapy, typically administered to postmenopausal females, that includes some combination of estrogen and progestin.

Hormone—Endocrine secretions that influence the activities of cells, tissues, glands, and organs in the body.

HPA (hypothalamic-pituitary-adrenal) axis—An interconnected set of physiological responses linking the pituitary, hypothalamus, and adrenal glands in reaction to stress.

Human chorionic gonadotropin (HCG)—Hormone whose function is to preserve the corpus luteum and its progesterone production so that the endometrial lining of the uterus, and hence pregnancy, is maintained.

Human immunodeficiency virus (HIV)—The agent that causes acquired immunodeficiency syndrome (AIDS).

Human papillomavirus (HPV)—A virus that causes genital warts and is associated with some reproductive cancers.

Hymen—A membrane around the vaginal opening.

Hyperemesis gravidarum—An extreme form of morning sickness characterized by persistent vomiting.

Hyperplasia—An excessive proliferation of epithelial cells.

Hypothalamus—A region of the brain that controls the autonomic nervous system, regulates the release of pituitary hormones, and contributes to emotional responses.

Hysterectomy—Surgical removal of the uterus.

I

Iatrogenic disease—A health condition brought about by medical treatment, whether through negligence, medical error, or the adverse effects of a drug.

Impotence—The inability to achieve or maintain an erection.

In vitro fertilization—Fertilization outside of the body.

Infertility—The inability to conceive a child during the course of one year of regular sexual intercourse without contraception.

Inflammation—The human body's reaction as it fights infection or other foreign substances; typically characterized by swelling and fever.

Inhibin—A peptide hormone that suppresses FSH secretion from the pituitary gland.

Intercytoplasmic sperm injection—A technique in which a single sperm is injected into a single egg to fertilize it.

Intrauterine device (IUD)—Any of a group of devices inserted into the uterus to prevent pregnancy.

Introitus—An opening or entrance into a canal or cavity, such as the vagina.

K

Kaposi's sarcoma—A vascular malignancy characterized by lesions; the incidence of this condition has risen dramatically along with the incidence of AIDS.

Karyotype—Manner of viewing chromosomes in which the chromosomes are cut out of an enlarged photograph of chromosomes in metaphase, arranged in pairs, and systematically grouped.

Kilocalorie—See *Calorie.*

L

Labia majora—In females, the two longitudinal folds of skin that extend down from the mons pubis, narrowing to enclose the vulvar cleft and meeting posteriorly in the perineum; Latin for "major lips."

Labia minora—In females, the two inner folds of skin next to the labia majora enclosing the urethral opening and the vagina.

Lactation—In females, the production of milk in the mammary glands for the purpose of feeding a baby.

Lactiferous duct—Opening at the nipple through which milk and colostrum are excreted.

Lactobacillus—A genus of nonpathogenic bacteria that colonize the digestive and reproductive tracts.

Lamaze method—A method of childbirth preparation that emphasizes exercises to prepare muscles and joints for delivery, relaxation, and breathing techniques as an alternative to medication.

Laparoscopy—The examination of the pelvic cavity by an instrument inserted through a small incision in the abdominal wall.

Lipid—Organic molecules that are insoluble in water includes steroids, cholesterol, triglycerides, and phospholipids.

Lithotomy position—The position in which a woman lies for a gynecological exam, with feet in stirrups, buttocks hanging over the end of the table, and sheet draped like a tent over the knees and the upper part of her body.

Lobular carcinoma in situ (LCIS)—A condition caused by unusual cells growing in the lobules and ducts of the breast; although it may progress to cancer, it is generally not viewed as a true malignancy.

Luteal phase—In females, the third phase of the ovarian cycle during which the corpus luteum secretes estrogen, progesterone, and androgens.

Luteinizing hormone (LH)—A hormone responsible for ovulation, corpus luteum formation, and hormone production in the ovaries; the stimulus for hormone production from the interstitial cells of the testes.

M

Mammary gland—A specialized gland that produces milk for lactation.

Mammogram—Specialized X-ray used to detect abnormal tissues in the breasts.

Mastectomy—Surgical removal of the breast.

Melanocytes—Cells that produce pigmented substances that provide color to the hair, skin, and choroid of the eye.

Melanoma—A dangerous form of cancer of the melanocytes.

Menarche—In females, the onset of the menstrual period.

Menopause—The cessation of the menstrual periods; considered complete after menstrual periods have ceased for one year.

Menses—The shedding of the endometrial lining; menstruation.

Menstrual phase—Day 1 to day 4 of the endometrial cycle.

Menstrual synchronization—The phenomenon whereby women living in close proximity tend to menstruate at approximately the same time.

Menstruation—The periodic shedding and discharge of the uterine lining occurring at more or less regular intervals during the life of a woman from the age of puberty to menopause.

Mesoderm—The middle embryonic germ layer that develops into the skeletal, muscular, urinary, circulatory, and reproductive systems.

Midwife—One who assists women in childbirth.

Mineral—Inorganic chemical element.

Minipill—A small, low-dose progestin pill.

Miscarriage—Spontaneous loss of a pregnancy before the 20th week of gestation; also called a *spontaneous abortion*.

Mons pubis—In females, the cushion of fatty tissue and skin that lies over the pubic symphysis and, after puberty, is covered with pubic hair.

Morula—An early stage of embryonic development consisting of a solid ball of undifferentiated cells.

Mutagens—Anything capable of causing a gene change. Among the known mutagens are radiation, certain chemicals, and some viruses.

Myocardial infarction (MI)—A loss of blood supply to the heart resulting in tissue death; a heart attack.

Myotonia—Increased tension in both voluntary and involuntary muscles.

N

Nail—A cornified curved plate of hard keratin that rests on a thickened surface of epidermis called the nail bed.

National Institutes of Health (NIH)—Primary federal granting agency for research.

Negative feedback loop—A series of interconnected signals and reactions that coordinate with each other in a predicable pattern that results in conditions in the body being maintained around a "normal" set point.

Neisseria gonorrhoeae—The bacterial pathogen that causes gonorrhea.

Neural tube defect—A birth defect that occurs early in embryonic development when the neural tube fails to close.

Non-specific defenses—Immune defenses that target a wide range of potential infective agents.

Nonsteroidal anti-inflammatory drugs (NSAIDs)—Drugs used to control, stop, or regulate abnormal uterine bleeding.

Norepinephrine—An adrenal cortex hormone produced in response to sympathetic nervous system stimulation.

Normal flora—The collection of usually nonpathogenic microorganisms that colonize the human body.

O

OB/GYN—A physician who specializes in obstetrics and gynecology.

Observational study—A study in which the researchers observed the outcomes of groups they did not set up that gathered data on the prevention and treatment of a condition.

Oligoovulation—Irregular ovulation.

Oncogenes—Genes that have the ability to induce a cell to become malignant.

Oocyte maturation inhibitor—A peptide hormone in follicular fluid that suppresses final maturation of the dominant follicle until the time of ovulation.

Oral contraceptive—Commonly called "the Pill", this form of birth control suppresses ovulation by the combined actions of the hormones estrogen and progesterone or progesterone alone.

Orgasm—The physiological response to sexual stimulation representing the peak of the sexual cycle.

Orgasmic platform—The muscles that make up the outer third of the vaginal wall and those surrounding the turgid tissues of the vulva.

Osteoporosis—Disease characterized by reduced bone mass.

Ovarian cyst—A sac that develops in the ovary proper; consists of one or more chambers containing fluid.

Ovary—Small, almond shaped organ that, in pairs, comprise the female gonads; they create both gametes and hormones.

Oviduct—See *Fallopian tube*.

Ovulation—The periodic ripening and rupture of the mature graafian follicle and the discharge of the ovum from the cortex of the ovary.

Ovum—An egg; a female gamete.

Oxytocin—A hormone which stimulates uterine contractions and the milk let down reaction, also associated with emotional bonding.

P

Paraurethral gland—See *Female prostate*.

Parsympathetic nervous system (PNS)—A division of the nervous system that brings the body to a state of rest and relaxation.

Parturate—To give birth.

Parturition—The process of labor and delivery; childbirth.

Pathogen—A disease-causing organism.

Pathology—A condition produced by disease.

Pectoral nodes—A cluster of small, bean-shaped nodes in the breasts which play an important role in immunity by filtering out harmful substances. See *axillary nodes*.

Peer reviewed—Research which is reviewed by experts in the field before it is published.

Pelvic exam—A gynecological procedure in which a health professional palpates a woman's abdomen and inspects her internal genitalia. Cell smears of the cervix are usually taken for diagnostic analysis.

Pelvic floor—The muscles, ligaments, and membranes that hold organs in place in the pelvic cavity.

Pelvic inflammatory disease (PID)—Infection of the uterus, fallopian tubes, and adjacent pelvic structures that is not associated with surgery or pregnancy.

Penis—The organ that transfers semen from the body during coitus; also serves as the outlet for urine.

Perimenopause—The months or years leading up to menopause, which are usually accompanied by fluctuations and a gradual decline in reproductive hormone levels.

Peripheral nervous system (PNS)—All of the nerves in the body outside of the brain and spinal cord.

Physiology—The study of the function of the cells, tissues, and organs of the body.

Phytonutrient—A plant-based chemical that is biologically active in the body.

Pituitary gland—A small gland in the brain that secretes hormones that regulate many bodily processes.

Placebo—An inactive substance or treatment administered as if it were the prescribed active drug or test treatment.

Placenta previa—The result of implantation of the fertilized ovum in the lower part of the uterus instead of its more usual site higher up in the fundus; late in pregnancy or at the time of delivery, a part of the lower edge of the placenta may separate from its attachment to cause characteristically painless bleeding that is bright red in color.

Placenta—The special structure for fetal-maternal exchange; delivered from the uterus after the baby.

Placental abruption—(also called *abruption of the placenta*) Separation of the placenta from the uterine wall prior to the onset of labor.

***Pneumocystis carinii* pneumonia**—A type of pneumonia sometimes seen in AIDS patients that was previously seen only in cancer patients with profoundly suppressed immune systems.

Polycystic ovarian syndrome (PCOS)—An endocrine disorder characterized by a failure of ovulation, large numbers of follicular cysts, enlarged ovaries with thickened capsules, excessive androgen production, and amenorrhea.

Positive feedback loop—A series of interconnected signals and reactions that coordinate with each other in a predictable pattern that results in conditions in the body being moved away from the homeostatic set point.

Preeclampsia—A disorder in pregnant women that is a combination of symptoms, including hypertension, edema, and proteinuria (protein in the urine); can be categorized as mild or severe.

Preferred provider organizations (PPOs)—A type of health plan that contracts with selected doctors, clinics, and hospitals, which then constitute the plan's network.

Premature ejaculation—Inability to exert enough voluntary control to delay ejaculation resulting in the attainment of orgasm too rapidly.

Premenstrual dysphoric disorder (PMDD)—A more severe form of PMS that affects a small percentage of women.

Premenstrual syndrome (PMS)—Physical, psychological, or behavioral premenstrual changes that some women experience which can disrupt their usual activities.

Primary care physician—A physician who is the initial healthcare provider to examine a patient.

Progestational phase—Changes that occur in the superficial layer of the endometrium as a result of progesterone; typically corresponds with the luteal phase of the ovary. See also *Secretary phase*.

Progesterone—With estrogen, one of the sex hormones; in women, it is secreted primarily by the corpus luteum.

Progestins—A general term referring to chemical agents, both natural and synthetic, that produce changes in the uterine endometrium after it has previously been primed by estrogen.

Prognosis—The predictable outcome of a disease.

Prolapse—A protrusion of the uterus into the vagina.

Proliferative phase—The part of the endometrial cycle that occurs after day four and lasts until a day or two after ovulation.

Prostaglandins (PGs)—A closely related group of fatty acid derivatives with a variety of effects; belong to a group of compounds called *eicosanoids.*

Prostate—In males, a single gland that surrounds the urethra as it leaves the bladder; secretes a milky, alkaline fluid to neutralize the acidity of the vagina during intercourse and enhance sperm motility.

Protein—A polymer composed of amino acids.

Pseudoscience—The phenomenon of trying to make something sound scientific when it really has not been evaluated scientifically.

Puberty—Transition period between childhood and adulthood; during this period, the physical and psychological changes associated with reproductive ability take place.

R

Randomized clinical trial—Study in which participants are assigned to a treatment group randomly to avoid researcher bias.

Randomized sample—A method of assigning participants to a study in which all subjects have an equal probability of being selected for any of the treatments.

Receptors—Sites located on the cell membranes or in the cytoplasm of the target cells; their job is to transmit the message of the hormone's arrival to the area of the cell that is involved in the response.

Reconstructive surgery—Surgery to repair or reconstruct damaged body parts.

Reproductive neuroendocrinology—The study of the integration of the nervous system and the endocrine organs of reproduction.

Retroviruses—A viral class composed of a core of RNA surrounded by a protein coat, which is further surrounded by a protein envelope; they produce a unique enzyme called reverse transcriptase.

Rosacea—A form of adult acne associated with reddened skin across the cheeks, nose, and forehead.

S

Sample size—The number of subjects in a scientific study.

Sebaceous glands—Sebum-producing glands that are found almost everywhere in the dermis except for the palmar and plantar surfaces.

Secretory phase—The second half of the endometrial cycle, also called the *progestational phase;* the glands of the endometrium become dilated as they fill up with secretions of substances such as glycogen and fats, and the endometrium increases in thickness from the previous phase, forming a hospitable site for implantation of a fertilized ovum.

Selective estrogen receptor modulators (SERMs)—"Designer estrogens" that possess some, but not all, of the actions of estrogen and are used therapeutically in the treatment of complications of menopause and some breast cancers.

Semen—Consists of sperm suspended in a semigelatinous fluid that contains substances to nourish and protect the sperm and facilitate their movement.

Seminal vesicles—In males, glands located at the base of the bladder; produce a viscous, alkaline fluid rich in fructose to provide a direct source of energy for sperm.

Sepsis—The spread of an infection from its initial site to the bloodstream, initiating a systemic response that adversely affects blood flow to vital organs.

Seroconversion—The production of antibodies to HIV.

Skene's gland—See *Female prostate.*

Skin cancer—A form of uncontrolled growth of cells in the skin; most common forms are basal cell and squamous cell; a third type, melanoma, is highly dangerous but much less common.

Specific defenses—Mechanisms in the immune system that target specific microbes and other infective agents.

Speculum—An instrument used to examine body canals including the vagina.

Spermicide—A birth control method which kills sperm.

Staphylococcus aureus—The bacterial pathogen that causes toxic shock syndrome and MRSA infections.

Steroid hormones—Sex hormones and hormones of the adrenal cortex.

Steroid—General term applied to a group of substances derived from cholesterol; found in both plants and animals; includes some vitamins, drugs, and hormones.

Sunscreen preparations—Products designed either to reflect the rays of the sun or to absorb them, mimicking the body's own defenses against radiation.

Superovulation—Increased follicle production and ovulation, usually facilitated by fertility drugs.

Surrogate mother—A woman who donates the use of her uterus to gestate a baby for another individual, either altruistically or for compensation.

Sweat glands—Dermal glands that produce sweat.

Sympathetic nervous system (SNS)—A division of the nervous system that brings the body to a state of alertness and excitement that enables it to respond to emergencies.

T

Teratogen—A substance that can cross the placental barrier and impair an embryo's normal growth and development.

Testes—The male gonads that produce sperm and testosterone.

Testosterone—One of the sex hormones; produced by the testes in males; trace amounts are produced by the adrenal glands in women.

Theca externa—The outer fibrous layer of an ovarian follicle; produces sex steroids.

Thelarche—The onset of female breast development at puberty.

T-helper lymphocyte—A type of white blood cell that helps other white blood cells combat foreign antigens.

Thrombus—An abnormal blood clot that forms in an unbroken blood vessel.

Title IX—An amendment to the Civil Rights Act that prohibits educational discrimination based on gender by any agency that receives federal funding.

Toxic shock syndrome (TSS)—A disease caused by the toxin produced by *Staphylococcus aureus,* a bacterium commonly present on the skin and mucous membranes.

Treponema pallidum—The bacterial pathogen that causes syphilis.

Trichomonas vaginalis—A protozoan that infects the reproductive tract causing irritation and inflammation.

Trichomoniasis—A sexually transmitted infection caused by a parasite of the genus *Trichomonas*.

Tubal ligation—In females, a medical procedure in which the fallopian tubes are closed to prevent the possibility of future pregnancies.

U

Urethra—The muscular tube that transports urine from the bladder to the exterior of the body.

Uterus—In females, an inverted pear-shaped, hollow, muscular organ in which a fertilized egg resides as it develops into a fetus.

V

VACTERL syndrome—A combination of abnormalities that includes vertebral, anal, cardiac, tracheal, esophageal, renal, and limb defects.

Vagina—In females, a muscular tube connecting the uterus to the vulva.

Vaginitis—In females, a generic term for inflammation and infection in the vagina.

Varicocele—In males, a condition in which varicose veins in the testicles interfere with sperm production, reducing fertility.

Vas deferens—In males, the muscular tube that transports sperm from the epidididymis through the inguinal canal.

Vasectomy—Male sterilization; the removal of all or part of the vas deferens.

Vasocongestion—The engorgement of the vaginal blood vessels that results in vaginal lubrication as a consequence of sexual arousal.

Vestibule—In females, the area enclosed by the labia minora.

Vitamin—Organic molecules that play a role in the body's metabolic processes.

Vulva—In females, the visible external genitalia; sometimes called the *pudendum*.

Vulvodynia—A condition characterized by chronic burning or painful itching of the vulva with none of the perceptible physical findings present in the usual forms of vaginosis.

W

Wise woman—A woman who acts as an herbalist, midwife, or physician usually without formal medical training.

Women's Health Initiative—A large, federally funded study focusing on the prevention and treatment of major causes of death in middle-aged and older women.

Z

Zygote intrafallopian transfer (ZIFT)—A technique in which a woman's egg is fertilized outside the body, then implanted in one of her fallopian tubes.

Zygote—A fertilized egg.

INDEX

exogenous hormones and, 187
genetic factors and, 186
hormone replacement therapy and risk
of, 371
lifestyle factors to reduce risk of, 188–89
lycopene for reducing, 401
overview of, 185–86
risk factors for, 186–88
screening and diagnosis of, 189
staging, 189
treatments for, 189–93
types of, 186
worldwide patterns in, 160
Breast Cancer Detection Demonstration
Project, 371
Breast cancer treatments, 189–93
adjuvant, 190–93
surgical, 190
Breast changes
with age, 147
menstrual cycle and, 147
during pregnancy, 147, 255–56
Breast development, puberty and, 147
Breast-feeding, 148f. *See also* Lactation and
breast feeding
breast pumps, 153f
breast reduction, following, 444
nutrition during, 387
Breast implants
autoimmune disorders, linkage to, 444
breast cancer, association with, 443
lupus, linkage to, 444
rheumatoid arthritis, linkage to, 444
Breast milk
composition of, 148–49
environmental toxins found in, 154
Breasts, 143–65
anatomy of, 144–47
augmentation of, 440
cancer of, 443
disproportionately large, 444
introduction to, 143–44
lactation and breast feeding,
147–55, 149f
lifespan changes in, 147
non-cancerous conditions of, 155–57
of pregnant/nonpregnant woman, 256f
reconstruction of, 444
screening for conditions of, 157–65
Breast self exam (BSE), 158–60
guide for performing, 159f
overview of, 158
technique of, 158–60
Breech presentation, 265
cesarean section, for performing, 303
Broad spectrum sunscreen, 435
Brown, Lesley, 355
Bulimia, 377, 446–47
stress, caused by, 418

C

Cabbage soup diet, 389
Caffeine, 378
Calcitonin, 379–80
Calcium, 399–400

hypertension, decreased risk of, 399
osteoporosis, malabsorption of, 399
Calories, 388
recommended intake of, 403
reduction in, 446
Cancer. *See also* specific types of
antioxidants, decreased risk of, 388
inadequate nutrition and increased risk
of, 406
mortality caused by, 387
phytonutrients, role in preventing, 401
stress, caused by, 418
vitamins for prevention of, 397
Candida albicans, 119, 124f, 176, 349
Candidiasis, 124–25
Capacitation, 354
Capsular contraction, 442
Carbohydrates, 264
complex, 390–91
defined, 389
sources of, 390–91
Carbon dioxide, 389
Carcinoma, 174
Cardiovascular disease, 10
chocolate and decreasing risk of, 421
cholesterol and risk of, 393
female statistics for, 393
hormone replacement therapy and
protection with, 371
mortality caused by, 387–88
omega-3 fatty acids, reduced risk of, 393
phospholipids for reduced risk of, 392
phytonutrients, role in preventing, 401
resveratrol for preventing, 401
stress-related illness, caused by, 417
trans fats and increased risk of, 392
vitamins for prevention of, 397
Cardiovascular system, 33–38
blood and, 36–38
blood flow and, 34f, 35–36, 37f
blood flow to extremities and, 257–58
blood vessels and, 34f, 35
exercise benefits to, 420
generalized edema and, 259
heart and, 34f, 257f
overview of, 33
varicose veins and, 258–59
Carotenoids, 397
Carriers, 433
Cataracts, antioxidants for decreased risk of, 388
Catheter, 298f
Caudal block continuous, 297
Cavitations, 29
CD4 receptor, 137
Cell division by mitosis/meiosis, 227–28, 228f
Cells, 223–27, 224f
chromosomes and, 223–25
code reading of, 225
DNA structure and, 223, 225f
Human Genome Project and, 225–26
overview of, 223
pre-implantation genetic diagnosis and, 227
Cellular metabolism, 387
Cellular respiration, 389
Cellulose, 391

Centers for Disease Control (CDC), 120, 125,
129, 135, 259, 266, 272, 350, 357, 444
Central nervous system (CNS), 22, 287
Central placental abruption, 282f
Cephalic presentation, 265f, 266
Cerebral palsy and preterm labor and
delivery, 287
Cervical abnormalities, non-cancerous, 176,
178–79
cervical erosions as, 176, 178–79
cervical polyps as, 179
cervicitis (cervical inflamation) as, 176
Cervical cancer, 174–76, 174f
causes of, 176
economic considerations for, 177–78
invasive, 175
overview of, 174–75
prevention of, 175
symptoms of, 174
TNM categories of, 175
treatment of, 176
vaccines for, 175
Cervical cap, 327–28, 328f
defined, 327
disadvantages of, 327–28
Cervical erosions, 176, 178–79
Cervical intraepithelial neoplasia (CIN), 174
Cervical mucus, 59f
abstinence and, monitoring of, 323–24
female infertility, examination of, 349
Cervical polyps, 179
Cervicitis (cervical inflammation), 176
Cervix, 56, 58–59
dilation of, 268, 270
effacement of, 267f
parturition, changes prior to, 267
reproductive changes to, 254–55
Cesarean section (C-section), 302–5
breech presentation and performing, 303
defined, 302
dystocia resulting in, 303
emergency, 304
fetal distress resulting in, 303
following vaginal birth after cesarean, 303–4
incision locations for, 303f
infant mortality, decline of, 304
long-term risks of, 304
placental abruption with prior, risk factor
of, 282
risks of, 303
statistics for, 302–4
Chadwick's sign, 250, 255
Chemical peels, 432
Chemicals
male infertility and exposure to, 349
man-made, 347, 353
semen and exposure to, 349
Chemotherapeutic drugs, 397
Childbirth Connection, 294, 304
Childbirth fever, 5
Childbirth pain
Apgar score for, 270–71
cervical dilation and, 270
perineum stretching and, 270
postpartum care and, 271–72